Animal Handling and Physical Restraint

D0905547

Animal Handling and Physical Restraint

C. B. CHASTAIN, DVM, MS, ACVIM

Emeritus/Adjunct Professor
College of Veterinary Medicine
University of Missouri
Columbia, MO

Line drawings by **LYNN VELLIOS**

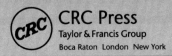

CRC Press
Taylor & Francis Group
Boca Raton London New York

CRC Press is an imprint of the
Taylor & Francis Group, an **informa** business

CRC Press
Taylor & Francis Group
6000 Broken Sound Parkway NW, Suite 300
Boca Raton, FL 33487-2742

First Issued In paperback 2010

© 2018 by Taylor & Francis Group, LLC
CRC Press is an imprint of Taylor & Francis Group, an Informa business

No claim to original U.S. Government works

ISBN: 978-1-4987-6193-2 (hbk)
ISBN: 978-0-367-02832-9 (pbk)

This book contains information obtained from authentic and highly regarded sources. While all reasonable efforts have been made to publish reliable data and information, neither the author[s] nor the publisher can accept any legal responsibility or liability for any errors or omissions that may be made. The publishers wish to make clear that any views or opinions expressed in this book by individual editors, authors or contributors are personal to them and do not necessarily reflect the views/opinions of the publishers. The information or guidance contained in this book is intended for use by medical, scientific or health-care professionals and is provided strictly as a supplement to the medical or other professional's own judgement, their knowledge of the patient's medical history, relevant manufacturer's instructions and the appropriate best practice guidelines. Because of the rapid advances in medical science, any information or advice on dosages, procedures or diagnoses should be independently verified. The reader is strongly urged to consult the relevant national drug formulary and the drug companies' and device or material manufacturers' printed instructions, and their websites, before administering or utilizing any of the drugs, devices or materials mentioned in this book. This book does not indicate whether a particular treatment is appropriate or suitable for a particular individual. Ultimately it is the sole responsibility of the medical professional to make his or her own professional judgements, so as to advise and treat patients appropriately. The authors and publishers have also attempted to trace the copyright holders of all material reproduced in this publication and apologize to copyright holders if permission to publish in this form has not been obtained. If any copyright material has not been acknowledged please write and let us know so we may rectify in any future reprint.

Except as permitted under U.S. Copyright Law, no part of this book may be reprinted, reproduced, transmitted, or utilized in any form by any electronic, mechanical, or other means, now known or hereafter invented, including photocopying, microfilming, and recording, or in any information storage or retrieval system, without written permission from the publishers.

For permission to photocopy or use material electronically from this work, please access www.copyright.com (http://www.copyright.com/) or contact the Copyright Clearance Center, Inc. (CCC), 222 Rosewood Drive, Danvers, MA 01923, 978-750-8400. CCC is a not-for-profit organization that provides licenses and registration for a variety of users. For organizations that have been granted a photocopy license by the CCC, a separate system of payment has been arranged.

Trademark Notice: Product or corporate names may be trademarks or registered trademarks, and are used only for identification and explanation without intent to infringe.

Visit the Taylor & Francis Web site at
http://www.taylorandfrancis.com

and the CRC Press Web site at
http://www.crcpress.com

CONTENTS

PART 2: HOUSEHOLD AND LABORATORY ANIMALS

PART 3: RANCH, FARM, AND STABLED ANIMALS

Proper handling and restraint are essential to the welfare of captive animals. Animals that are properly handled and restrained can be examined, groomed, and treated in ways that contribute to their optimum quantity and quality of life. However, as society moved from its rural origins toward an urban and suburban environment, many people who handle animals, or wish to, do not have the knowledge and experience to do so properly.

Veterinary medicine is both art and science. The most basic part of the art of veterinary medicine is the safe handling of animals. The needs of pre-veterinary and veterinary students to become knowledgeable in safe, humane animal handling was the impetus to write this book, but animal handlers of all types should know safe, humane, and effective handling methods.

Instruction in animal handling is time-consuming, expensive, and unglamourous. As a result, many animal science students receive inadequate training in proper animal handling and normal animal behavior. Much more time is often devoted to studies disengaged from animal handling and less expensive to teach, such as formulating rations and transgenics. Animal handling is also undervalued in many modern veterinary curricula. The teaching of handling and physical restraint typically receives lower priority than teaching specialty topics, such as neurosurgery. Proper animal handling should not be a realm of veterinary practice limited to technicians, and it should not be relegated to only a brief orientation to clinical rotations in colleges of veterinary medicine.

The goals of this book are to assist future veterinarians, veterinary technologists, technicians, and assistants, and others who deal with animals to be able to handle animals more safely and humanely. The additional benefits of becoming better animal handlers are gaining the confidence of animals and their owners and being able to instruct animal owners in proper handling methods. No handling or restraint of animals is without risk, but proper animal handling and restraint aids in reducing the chance of the handler or animal experiencing physical injury or mutual infectious diseases. Proper handling of farm and ranch animals raised for meat, milk, or fiber also aids the producer in gaining greater profits.

Animal handling and physical restraint can be taught without great difficulty, but to translate knowledge of the art into practical skills requires long practice of proper procedures. Early training, life-long practice, and an open mind to acquiring better techniques are the keys to successful animal handling. Practice yields improvement but not perfection. Each animal is an individual and each handling environment provides its own advantages and disadvantages.

Some aspects of animal handling and restraint, specifically chemical restraint and handling of wild and exotic animals, are not included here. Chemical restraint of animals with prescription drugs has been left to other books intended exclusively for licensed veterinarians. Private ownership of wild and exotic animals as pets is opposed by the Council on Public Health and Regulatory Veterinary Medicine, in part because the wholesale industry in wild and exotic animal sales has an animal mortality rate estimated at 70%.

It should be noted that a clear division does not exist between animal handling, animal behavior, and animal training. These three are separate but intertwined. Handling an animal safely, humanely, and efficiently requires practical knowledge of the species' normal behavior. And, each time a handler handles or restrains an animal he or she is training it how to accept the next time it is handled. Ideally, the response to the next time it is handled is better than the last.

C.B. Chastain

It would be fascinating to know when, with whom, and where did most of the animal handling and restraint techniques described here originate. Most are anonymous and their contributions may be hundreds or thousands of years old. However, I wish to personally thank the people who taught me many of the techniques described in this book.

Most animal handling mentors in my life have been veterinarians. Leonard E. Palmer, DVM generously let me observe him practice veterinary medicine and provided my first lessons in animal handling and restraint. Without his kind guidance and encouragement I would not have pursued a career in veterinary medicine. Other key veterinarian mentors were Ed Ebert, Toney Reynolds, Joe McGinity, Tom Eagle, Jim English, and Art Dobson. Bill Donaldson, head herdsman for the University of Missouri, was instrumental in teaching me low-stress handling of beef cattle. Horsemen who were the most influential in teaching me horse handling were Jerry Stone in Missouri and Bill and Fannie Robinson in Colorado. Herpetological handling guidance was provided by Karen Lucy and David Doyle. Proper handling of small mammals and birds was shared by laboratory animal specialist veterinarians Cynthia Besch-Williford and Scott Korte. The many preceding contributions to safer, more humane food animal handling by Temple Grandin are gratefully acknowledged.

Ultimately, the greatest instructors I have had are the animals that I have handled and restrained, who taught me more about safe, humane, and efficient animal handling each time I had the privilege of working with them.

Many thanks go to June Kelly and Hannah West for proofreading early drafts of this book.

The line drawings, done by Lynn Vellios, have permitted clean backgrounds and emphasis on key visual aspects of animal handling. In addition to providing her art, Lynn was highly diligent, responsive, and encouraging to reach the goals of this book.

Few productive efforts would have been possible in my life without the years of support from my wife, Joyce, and daughters Andrea and Danielle. I enthusiastically look forward to handling more animals with my grandchildren and best assistants: Rylee, Caroline, and Simon.

C.B. Chastain

CAUTION

Serious injury or death can result from handling and restraining animals. Safe and effective handling and restraint requires experience and continual practice. In addition to knowledge, conditioned reflexes must be developed and maintained by an animal handler. The purpose of this book is to provide an appreciation of best practices for animal handling and physical restraint. The methods described may not be suitable for everyone. Acquisition of the described skills should be under the supervision of an experienced animal handler whenever possible. Practice should be done on a regular basis with an open mind toward means of possible improvement. Knowledge gained from this book should enable the reader to differentiate a good mentor from those who are less qualified.

AAALAC	Assessment and Accreditation of Laboratory Animal Care International	FeLV	feline leukemia virus
		FIV	feline immunodeficiency virus
ACVB	American College of Veterinary Behaviorists	Hz	hertz
		IC	intracoelomic
ACUC	Animal Care and Use Committee	IM	intramuscular
ADA	Americans with Disabilities Act	IO	intraosseous
AG	anogenital	IP	intraperitoneal
AI	artificial insemination	IV	intravenous
AIDS	acquired immunodeficiency syndrome	NIH	National Institutes of Health
ANSI	American National Standards Institute	OIE	Office International des Epizooties/ World Organization for Animal Health
ASTM	American Society of Testing Materials		
AVBT	Academy of Veterinary Behavior Technicians	OLAW	Office of Laboratory Animal Welfare
		POTZ	preferred optimal temperature zone
AVMA	American Veterinary Medical Association	PPE	personal protection equipment
		REM	rapid eye movement
AWA	Animal Welfare Act	RV	recreational vehicle
BETA	British Equestrian Trade Association	SC	subcutaneous
CAFOs	concentrated animal feeding operations	SEI	Safety Equipment Institute
DAP	dog-appeasing pheromone	USDA	United States Department of Agriculture
DEET	N, N-diethyl-m-toluamide		
EMDD	electromuscular disruption device	UVA	ultraviolet A
FBI	Federal Bureau of Investigation	UVB	ultraviolet B

Part 1

PRINCIPLES OF SAFER HANDLING AND PHYSICAL RESTRAINT

1

SAFER ANIMAL HANDLING AND PHYSICAL RESTRAINT

Domestication is the process in which an animal species is habituated to survive in the persistent company of human beings. They are selectively bred for human-desired disposition, appearance, food or fiber production, or work ability. Prior to the domestication of the dog, animal–human interactions were hunter–prey. Animal handling and restraint began with the domestication of the dog (*Canis familiaris*), which is estimated to have occurred as early as 12,000 BC. The next animals to live dependently on the care of humans were goats (*Capra hircus*, circa 10,000 BC) and sheep (*Ovis aries*, circa 9,000 BC), followed by cattle (*Bos taurus* and *Bos indicus*) and swine (*Sus domesticus*, circa 8,000 BC). The cat (*Felis catus*) may have been domesticated by 7,500 BC, before the donkey (*Equus asinus*, circa 5,000 BC) and horse (*Equus caballus*, circa 3,500 BC). Chickens (*Gallus domesticus*), llamas (*Lama glama*), and alpacas (*Vicugna pacos*) were domesticated around 3,500 BC. The turkey (*Meleagris gallopavo*), guinea pig (*Cavia porcellus*), rabbit (*Oryctolagus cuniculus*), and hamster (*Mesocricetus auratus*) were domesticated about 100, 900, 1500, and 1930 AD, respectively.

Other animals such as reptiles, birds, and rodents are contained and handled by humans, but are not domesticated. They may be tamed individually (made tractable) and tolerant of being handled. Domesticated species can be made tolerant of the presence of humans much more easily. In general, domesticated animals are safer to handle than tamed, non-domesticated animals.

Physical restraint of animals is often necessary when training. If reasonable restraint is not tolerated, proper training has not been achieved. Chemical restraint by veterinary medical professionals is needed if the procedure to be done on an animal may cause moderate to severe pain without analgesia or anesthesia. The use of chemical restraint has to be weighed against the drug's potential adverse effects, including prolonged exposure to ambient temperatures, sunlight, risk of trauma inflicted by herd mates, and other factors. For many common handling procedures on animals that require restraint, physical restraint methods are easier, quicker, less expensive, and safer than chemical restraint, if physical restraint is properly carried out.

Effective, safer (none is entirely "safe") animal handling and restraint has therefore evolved over 14,000 years. The basic principle is well established: restrain as little as possible, but persist and do as much as it takes as long as it is safe and humane. Excessive, unnecessary restraint or initial failure will be magnified as greater resistance by the animal to handling in the future.

The reasons to handle or restrain individual animals include physical examination, prophylactic, medical, or surgical treatments, grooming, training, recreation, and companionship. Carnivores can be handled individually without others of their species present. Herd animals are handled as individuals with less stress if they are allowed to remain in a group or in close proximity to a group.

> The single action that veterinary medical personnel do for each and every patient is the application of handling techniques.

Many animals become bonded to a handler, thus establishing a level of bilateral trust. Older animals that have had several handlers, all of whom did not mistreat the animals, often transfer trust in their past handlers to a new handler. Because of these situations of trust, it is common to see handlers put themselves in harm's way with animals believed to be well behaved. For example, horse handlers may walk under the lead rope of a tied horse. Although this is extremely dangerous, the handler has become lulled into a false sense of safety. Giving into a false sense of security and not always exercising basic precautions is the major cause of handler injuries.

All animals that are not properly socialized to humans early in their life, or are subjected to circumstances in which they feel pain or feel they are endangered, can injure handlers in an attempt to escape or defend themselves. Animal handlers remain safer by not taking unnecessary chances with dogs that are said to "never bite," horses that "never kick," and similar scenarios.

ATTRITION OF PROPER HANDLING

Handlers should become familiar with animals in their care, including their normal habits of eating, drinking, sleeping, urinating, defecating, and exercising, so that problems can be identified early and corrected when possible.

Throughout the more than 14,000 years of domesticated animal handling, the benefits of good handling practices for the animal and for the handler were obvious, not only to the handlers but also the observing public. Starting with the Second Industrial Revolution that began in 1850 and accelerated by the advent of the automobile in the early 1900s, humans have become more detached from working directly with animals. A disconnect has developed between the decision makers, those who actually handle animals, and the general society. More than 95% of the U.S. population is three or more generations removed from farm or ranch living.

In addition to urbanization resulting in fewer young people being exposed to proper animal handling, there has been a de-emphasis on animal handling and containment in veterinary medical education. The *Journal of Veterinary Medical Education* dedicated an issue in 2007 to animal handling education in international veterinary colleges that were accredited by the American Veterinary Medical Association (AVMA). The conclusions expressed in this issue were that more animal handling teaching was needed in veterinary medical education. However, the idea of adding or expanding animal handling courses has had to complete with teaching an ever-expanding body of knowledge in specialized

fields that have strong advocates in academic veterinary specialists.

To aid in filling the void of training in animal handling of small animals, commercial postgraduate education has marketed Fear Free® (VetFolio, a joint partnership of the North American Veterinary Community and the American Animal Hospital Association) and Cat Friendly® (American Association of Feline Practitioners) training courses and certification for individuals and veterinary practices. Although some of the principles involve the use of synthetic pheromones and nutraceuticals, which may or may not be advantageous in decreasing stress, sensitization of veterinarians and veterinary technicians to the possible presence of discomfort and fear in their patients is beneficial in motivating change. Any renewed emphasis on improved animal handling is desirable. It is unfortunate, however, that veterinary practices that do not elect to participate in the copyrighted "Cat Friendly Practices" could be perceived as not being cat friendly, and the copyrighted name "Fear Free Practice" is hyperbole for stress reduction techniques. No veterinary practice is fear free to all patients.

Handling animals in seclusion, and thus without public visibility, by employees or agents of owners fosters an environment that allows the attrition of good animal handling. Several states in the U.S. have passed "ag gag" laws, which intentionally or unintentionally protect handlers of livestock from public scrutiny of inhumane handling of animals. Shielding of animal handling occurs with both livestock and companion animals (*Table 1.1*).

Streptomycin, discovered in the 1940s, was the first of many antibiotics that made possible the raising of food animals in greater confinement with lower risk of communicable disease. In the 1930s, chickens were the first to be raised in large-scale extreme confinement. Large feedlots for cattle became widespread in the 1960s. By 1990, most sows were kept in gestation crates.

The move from small farms to industrial-level raising of livestock has exacerbated the desensitization of on-site handlers to how animals are confined and handled. Ironically, the raising of animals in low physical and mental stress environments has repeatedly been shown to result in faster gains

Table 1.1 **Examples of contributors* to the attrition of good animal handling**
• Animal trainers who require appointments for owners to see training practices
• Veterinary hospital personnel who remove dogs and cats from the owners' observation in providing non-emergency handling, exams, and treatments
• Close confinement of livestock and poultry that prohibits public observation
• State laws that prohibit photographing animals in confinement

* These situations do not innately cause poor animal handling, but they permit and protect environments without transparency to the public that can harbor poor animal handling.

in productivity. However, since higher expenses in facilities and labor costs offset some of the gain in productivity, the pressure for extreme confinement persists. Fortunately, public knowledge of the disadvantages of raising animals in extreme confinement has grown. Responding to this, Burger King became the first U.S. corporation to announce it would begin switching to cage-free eggs and gestation-crate-free pork. Similar actions by Safeway, Kroger, Oscar Mayer, McDonalds, and other food companies have since followed the lead by Burger King. Smithfield Foods and Tyson Fresh Meats announced in 2014 proactive plans to improve hog housing and handling.

Evaluation of the quality of animal handling and restraint is not an exact science. The best, and only meaningful, source of evidence for good animal handling, restraint, and confinement is what the animal reveals by its behavior when the handling and restraint are repeated or persist. If the behavior is unnatural (stereotypic or exaggerated fear), poor handling or restraint methods have taken place. Stereotypic behaviors beyond random occurrence can be caused by excessive confinement and include pacing, weaving, chewing cages or stalls, and self-mutilation (feather picking, excessive grooming). Unnatural behavior caused by poor handling, restraint, or confinement is one of the primary means of assessing the need for improved management of animals, as well as the number of animals with excessive lameness, external injuries, and vocalizations.

Animal welfare is the state of the animal and how it is coping with the conditions in which it lives. When humans domesticated animals, they took on the responsibilities to provide shelter, food, and a painless death. Fulfilling these responsibilities has been erratic. In the 1700s, animals were believed to lack a soul and were therefore without feelings. The ability to work or produce food or fiber was used as the only indicator of sufficient welfare. The first law to protect animals from abuse did not exist until 1822; this was the Act to Prevent the Cruel and Improper Treatment of Cattle, which was passed in Britain. The American Society for the Prevention of Cruelty to Animals was later established in 1866, and in 1915 the Mayo Clinic became the first U.S. institution to have a veterinarian oversee the care of its research animals.

In the 1960s, responding to pressure for humane handling of production animals inspired by Ruth Harrison's book "Animal Machines," the British government commissioned the Brambell report on intensive animal production. In 1965, the Commission listed five freedoms that animals should be ensured (*Table 1.2*). The five freedoms are currently used to assess animal welfare by the World Organization for Animal Health, formally known as the Office International des Epizooties (OIE). In the U.S., provisions for the ability to exhibit normal behavior are not always provided for production animals (livestock and poultry). In some cases, farm animal welfare has been erroneously evaluated by producer groups solely on the basis of whether the animal grows or produces milk sufficient to meet the producer's expectations.

The AVMA has defined animal welfare as "when an animal is healthy, comfortable, well nourished, safe, able to express innate behavior, and not

Table 1.2 **Five basic needs (freedoms) of domesticated animals**
1 A suitable environment
2 A suitable diet
3 The ability to exhibit normal behavior
4 To be housed with, or apart from, other animals
5 Protection from pain, suffering, injury, and disease

suffering from unpleasant states such as pain, fear, and distress." In 2010, the AVMA amended the Veterinarian's Oath by adding the word *welfare*: "I solemnly swear to use my scientific knowledge and skills for the benefit of society through the protection of animal health and welfare." This oath is the basis for the handling, restraint, and confinement techniques that follow.

TYPES OF HANDLERS AND HANDLING

The need to handle animals varies and so do the approaches as based on need. Pet owners and stockmen have the luxury of time to develop a relationship and trust with their animals. These handlers are at some disadvantage in handling new animals, however, because they do not see the range of behaviors animals of the same species can exhibit, as do veterinarians and veterinary technicians. Pet owners and stockmen are more likely to drift toward the extremes of either ignoring potential dangers of handling animals or exaggerating the potential danger.

Veterinarians and veterinary technicians usually do not have much time for every patient to develop a deeper level of trust with the animal. However, veterinary professionals are more familiar with the range of animal behaviors and need for pre-handling plans, including judicious measures to protect the animals being handled and the handlers involved. Veterinarians have the option of using chemical restraint, when needed. Still, they should be able to advise animal owners on how they should handle their animals effectively and safely, for the sake of both the animal and the owner.

Advances in chemical restraint have changed veterinary medicine, in some ways for the better and in other ways not. Chemical restraint of animals, when used appropriately, can reduce physical and psychologic stress on animals, their owners, and veterinary personnel. However, chemical restraint, induction, and recovery can add expense, procedural time, and risks of adverse drug effects or injury, particularly during induction and recovery periods. Chemical restraint should be used only when the handling and physical restraint techniques are less safe for the animal or the handler, and not just for convenience or as a substitute for good handling or physical restraint methods. It could also interfere with a physical exam by altering vital signs (heart rate, respiratory rate, body temperature, etc.).

Animal handlers do not benefit anyone or any animal by using inappropriate or unnecessary restraint on an animal. This raises the questions: What is inappropriate and unnecessary? And what are the appropriate and needed alternatives?

THE MORE EFFECTIVE HANDLER: THE ART OF FIRM KINDNESS

Formal guidelines for handling animals do not exist, but there are official guidelines on the physical restraint of animals. Appropriate handling of an animal and physical restraint of an animal can overlap. Guidelines for physical restraint of animals are contained in the AVMA's position statement. The August 2012 revision of its Physical Restraint of Animals document states: "Humane and safe physical restraint is the use of manual or mechanical means to limit some or all of an animal's normal voluntary movement for the purposes of examination, collection of samples, drug administration, therapy, or manipulation. The method used should provide the least restraint required to allow the specific procedure(s) to be performed properly, and should protect both the animal and personnel from harm. Every effort should be made to ensure adequate and ongoing training in animal handling and behavior by all parties involved, so that distress and physical restraint are minimized. In some situations, chemical restraint may be the preferred method. Whenever possible, restraint should be planned, formulated, and communicated prior to its application" (*Table 1.3*).

Table 1.3 **Essentials of proper animal restraint**
• The least restraint required to allow the procedure(s) to be performed properly
• Protection of both the animal and personnel from harm
• To plan, formulate, and communicate restraint prior to its application
• The use of chemical restraint when physical restraint presents excessive risk of injury

Proper animal handling for husbandry, treatment, and safety should be quiet, methodical, and leave the animal easier to handle the next time. In addition to achieving the initial purpose for handling animals, each handling event should have three goals: (1) safety for the animal and the handler, (2) minimum stress for the animal and the handler during animal capture and restraint, and (3) a calm release of the animal at a time of the handler's choosing. Safety is paramount and, if necessary, supersedes minimizing stress or a desirable release. Handler safety is of higher priority than animal safety, but all possible effort should be made to ensure the safety of both.

An effective animal handler has a proper attitude, which includes allotting sufficient time; using his or her voice, touch, and body language appropriately; constantly guarding against the risk of human or animal injury; adapting to special circumstances; and having proper attire and grooming to reduce the risk of injury. A common question that an effective animal handler asks him- or herself is: Would going slower make things happen faster?

The traits of superior animal handlers have been found to be emotional stability and being assertive, serious, pragmatic, forthright, self-assured, sensitive, and conscientious. Better handlers are more reserved than outgoing, more suspicious than trusting, and more controlled than uncontrolled in their responses to animal actions. Lack of empathy is the hallmark of a poor animal handler. Handlers may be empathetic toward one species and effective with that species but dislike other species and be ineffective with them. Use of derogatory terms toward animals, such as "dumb," "stupid," and "mean," affect handler attitude and actions and should disqualify that person from handling the animals to whom the terms were directed.

Affection for the animals

A good animal handler has to like the type of animal that will be handled. Bob Loomis, member of the Hall of Fame of the National Reining Horse Association, said, "There are people who like horses and people who like what horses can do for them. I like horses." He wisely attributed his successes in horse breeding, training, and showing to his affection for horses. When a handler dislikes a type of animal to be handled, the handler should excuse himself or herself or the supervisor should remove the handler from the situation whenever possible.

In the early 1600s, Rene Descartes, a French mathematician and scientist, advocated a philosophy called Cartesianism. According to Cartesianism, animals have no soul, and thus they cannot reason, have no feelings, and simply react to stimuli like a robot. As such, animals were viewed as dumb creatures to be used like machines. Believers in Cartesianism denied the human–animal bond, but good animal handlers always have been able to see the value and benefits of treating animals in their care well. Animal behavior studies that began in the 1950s have provided evidence that animals are not biological machines and thrive better with empathetic care.

Since the time of Hippocrates, the first rule of medicine has been *primum non nocere* ("first do no harm"). Proper handling techniques should also not cause harm. Some may cause temporary discomfort for distraction reasons, such as horse twitches and hog snares, but none should cause physical harm. This includes the use of inappropriate enclosures. Enclosures that can cause mental harm, manifested in such stereotypic behaviors as self-mutilation and cannibalism, through intense confinement or the lack of minimal mental stimulation should not be used.

> Ultimately, it is dangerous to offer food rewards by hand to horses and livestock.

Positive reinforcement (clicker training, food rewards) can be appropriate for companion animals that are predators. Using food rewards, petting, scratching, grooming, and verbal praises are beneficial under the correct circumstances. However, larger prey animals can endanger people if they invade human personal space. With these animals, negative reinforcement is important. Food treats should be offered to horses and livestock in pans or buckets only. They should not be taught to associate hands or pockets as a source of food. Established respect of human personal space and trust of protection by a handler is far more likely to keep a frightened horse from running over the handler than when it is expecting a food reward or being petted when it is frightened.

Proper attitude

Extroverted behavior, such as direct stares, exaggerated facial expressions, frequent hand and arm movements, and loud or spiking speech patterns, may attract the attention of humans and engender a good first impression, but these mannerisms do not gain or maintain trust from animals. However, quiet demeanor does not mean being submissive. An effective animal handler is gentle and calm but assertive enough to remain socially dominant over the animal being handled. Animal handlers should move and act calmly, deliberately, and patiently. The best animal handlers are confident, empathetic introverts. The most effective veterinarians and other servants of the animal owning public are *ambiverts*, people who are able to have some extrovert tendencies around humans but be a confident, empathetic introvert around animals.

Being organized and having a plan before handling or restraining animals is important for success for each handling event and all future handling events with the animals. Determination is an essential quality of a good handler. A handler must be confident and determined that the plan to handle or restrain an animal will be successful. Allowing the animal to escape the first attempt at handling will make subsequent efforts at least twice as difficult. The release must be as quiet and calm as possible, and it must be under control of the handler, not the animal.

> Each handling, especially the restraint experience, is a lesson learned by the animal, and the release is most remembered.

Animals resent or fear forced restraint. Excessive restraint can cause increased aggression toward handlers. Regardless of the species being handled, the least restraint possible (without risking animal escape) should be attempted. If restraint is to be used, it should be as humane as possible while ensuring a reasonable level of safety to humans and animals.

Allocation of sufficient time: the power of patience

Sufficient time to observe the animal or animals to be handled is important in determining the best approach to handling and to allow the animal or animals to adapt to handler presence. Once a plan of handling is determined, sufficient time must be allocated to perform the handling with minimum stress to the handler and the animals. Plans and decisions made in haste or executed hastily are always temptations when a handler is pressed for time because of other responsibilities or is concerned about the expense of spending longer than the minimum feasible time. In the long run, trying to rush proper handling leads to increased risk of injuries or excessive procedure time because of animals being stressed and scared. Longer times need to be allocated, particularly for handling young or new animals. The luxury of adequate time is always subject to weather conditions.

An excellent example of the power of patience and working with animals is the Texas cattle drives that took place in the 20 years following the American Civil War, from 1866 to 1886. These so-called drives, which were actually herding, consisted of 10–15 men moving 2,000–3,000 wild cattle over 200–1,000 miles of open country without the cattle losing weight. This was made possible, in large part, by the patience shown when herding the cattle and doing so as a slow, quiet trek. Cattle handlers, called drovers, spent 10–12 hours riding horseback, herding the cattle primarily with quiet finesse, communicating by hand signals, and moving the herd 10–12 miles per day for 25–100 days to railheads in Kansas. Texas cattle drives to California took 5–6 months.

Use of voice, touch, and body language

Restraint begins with the handler's voice and body language. Animals like to hear a handler's voice, especially if it is soothing and has rhythmic tones, since soothing talk is not characteristic of a predator or a challenge for social dominance. Voice can be used to direct an animal's movement, gain its attention, or reprimand its misbehavior. An instructional voice has a lower pitch and is slightly louder than a soothing voice. A commanding or reprimanding voice is deeper and with conviction, but shouting, screaming, or high-pitched sounds should be avoided in all cases.

A handler's body language needs to be coordinated with the voice characteristics so that the animal will not become confused. Non-threatening body language includes keeping the arms down and close to the body with palms toward the thighs. Raising the arms is threatening, but can be used to drive animals in a desired direction. An erect posture is less threatening than slumped shoulders or a rounded back, which simulate a pouncing and threatening posture. A glancing gaze or indirect stare is less threatening that a direct stare. Staring directly at an animal's eyes in particular is threatening to prey animals and is a social dominance challenge to carnivores. Moderately rapid, rhythmically normal movements are less threatening than rapid, jerky, or slow and creeping actions.

Touch can readily convey handler confidence and intentions to an animal being handled. Excessively light touch or stroking does this poorly, causing signs of apprehension in most animals. A deliberate, moderately firm but gentle touch conveys more confidence and is less threatening than very light touch or stroking. Touching should be done with fingers together and applied with either the palm side or the back of the hand. Touching with the tips of the fingers while the fingers are spread or with the end of the thumb is less well tolerated and is likely to cause the animal to move its touched area away. Using spread finger tips or the end of the thumb can be a much more useful means of moving a horse in a desired direction than pushing with a flat hand. Very firm, pushy, or slapping-type touches may be perceived as a challenge to social position in the herd or pack or as a reprimand for misbehavior. However, it can be beneficial for handlers to desensitize horses to moderate slaps to prevent flight reactions if tack or clothing accidentally slaps them while mounting or riding or if the handler or rider needs to slap biting flies, especially horseflies.

The shoulders are not densely innervated by touch receptors, and this is not an area of the body to which fatal injuries can be inflicted. Because of this, animals tolerate touch on the shoulders better than touch around the more vulnerable areas such as the eyes, ears, throat, belly, or legs.

Animals use body language to a greater extent than any other means of communication. For example, dogs "play bow" to signal desire to play through body language. For them, a play face is one with an open mouth and erect ears, and they will bark while advancing and retreating with bouncing movements.

Animals can detect human body language that is imperceptible to humans.

Some animals are especially sensitive to human facial expressions and other body language. An Orlov Trotter horse in Germany, named Clever Hans, became famous through this ability in the early 1900s. He appeared able to perform arithmetic and other mental tasks, but it was later proven that he was doing so only by reading subtle human body language. In recognition of his ability, this type of observer effect is referred to as the Clever Hans effect. In the 1930s, a Llewellin setter in Missouri, Jim the Wonder Dog, was capable of similar feats. The Clever Hans effect may be what enables some animals to detect early signs of hypoglycemia in diabetics and impending seizures in epileptic humans.

Always on guard: safety first

Animals should always be handled with precautions for avoiding injury. The safest animals are safe 99% of the time, but handlers should always be prepared for the 1% chance that the usually safe animal will become dangerous because of pain, perceived territorial threats, illness, or a myriad of other situations different from those in the past.

Handlers must be constantly aware of the risks of injury to themselves, other people, and the animal being handled. A common error made by many who have worked around their own animals for years without injury is a false assumption that other species or animals of the same species will react to situations in the same way as their animals. But horses are not big dogs, and cats are not little dogs. Each species has its inherent species behavior, and within a species each individual has a unique temperament and behavior. Factors that affect an individual animal's reactions to handling are familial tendencies;

prior handling and training; trust, or the lack of it, in the handler; and stressful events preceding or during the handling. As a result, the assumption that all domestic species or animals within a species are the same can lead to serious injury.

Veterinary staff are at a relatively high risk of injury. Many animals they must treat have neither been socialized to humans nor previously handled. In addition, sick or injured animals may act atypically because of pain or fear. Sick or injured animals often hide their disease or injury until a handler disturbs them. Some owners do not appreciate the risk of handling sick or injured animals or animals being handled by new people with whom the animal has yet to established a bond of trust. Because of this, owners may interpret handler precaution as being afraid of the animal. The need for precautionary measures may have to be explained to owners.

Most injuries from animals are caused by the handler being overconfident or undercompetent. Animal handlers must always position themselves well and take other precautions to eliminate or minimize the chance of injury to all involved.

Distraction versus pain for restraint

Distractions are the basis for most humane and effective animal handling techniques and are not painful when correctly used. Pain is a message sent to the brain that body tissue is being injured. Distraction is applying a stimulus that supersedes competing stimuli. When a distraction technique is applied severely or incorrectly, it can inflict pain. For example, when a nose twitch, a pinching distraction technique most often used on the upper lip of horses, is applied correctly there is no tissue injured and therefore no pain. If used inappropriately, the twitch causes pain and there will be evidence of tissue damage, e.g. soreness persisting after the twitch is released, loss of function of the upper lip, or a change in the appearance of the tissue such as swelling, cuts, or bruising. Other indications of pain in animals can be a decrease in normal activities such as eating, grooming, or nesting. A hunched posture, tooth grinding, glazed stare, and elevated heart or respiratory rate may also suggest the presence of pain. Animals, particularly prey animals, may mask some signs of pain if in unfamiliar surroundings or

if otherwise feeling threatened. Observation from a hidden location or with surveillance cameras may be necessary to monitor for pain in these animals.

Some animals will react to distraction with fear, as if the distraction is painful. When this occurs, chemical restraint may be needed if there is a reasonable possibility that fear will be intensified and will hinder future efforts to handle the animal.

Respect for handlers

Animals should be respectful, not fearful, of human handlers. Respect is gained by animals knowing that pleasure (praise, food treats) or discomfort (not pain) will consistently occur with certain behaviors. Fear can result from the expectation of pain. If a fear is instinct-based, it can be moderated. If it is the result of having experienced pain, it is often permanent.

> Animals that are either fearful of handlers or have no respect of humans are the most dangerous to handle.

The social dominance (leadership) of a handler should be based on respect, not fear of injury. The dominant animal in a group establishes its social position by its control of movement and access to resources. Effective handlers do the same. For example, well-trained dogs are required to sit before receiving food and taught to wait before going through doors or up or down stairs. Food is provided only with permission of the handler. In the case of large animals such as horses, the use of food rewards can be impractical or dangerous owing to the risk of the animal invading the handler's personal space. Livestock wish to be left alone. Requiring them to respond to a stimulus and then removing that stimulus so that they are again undisturbed is a great reward. Rather than through food rewards, large animal's respect for human personal space is more safely established by simply staring at the animal or moving a hand away from the handler's body. The stimulus is immediately removed after a desired response from the animal. Additional positive reinforcement with food rewards may be desirable in some cases, but the large animal's access to the food should never be associated with being close to the handler, particularly hands or pockets.

Adaptation to special circumstances

Animal handling is not a set recipe that fits all situations. An effective animal handler must adapt techniques to the species, the surroundings, and the individual. Each animal handled should first be observed to assess its current attitude and physical condition.

Young, elderly, and pregnant animals need special handling. How immature animals are handled can ingrain their responses to handling for the rest of their life. Young animals may be more easily injured because of the risk of the growth plates in bones becoming damaged or through their uncoordinated attempts to resist handling. Elderly animals may have a lifetime accumulation of good or bad experiences from being handled and have a greater probability of failing organ function and arthritis. Pregnant animals may be more fearful from the instinct of knowing that their escape, if needed, will be more difficult.

Appropriate attire, grooming, and personal habits

Proper handler attire for the type of animal handling to be done is important for handlers and animals. Inappropriate attire can be dangerous (*Table 1.4* and **Figure 1.1**). Clothing should be reasonably clean and not torn. Attire for animal handling should be worn only when handling or restraining animals and then changed afterward to reduce the risk of transmitting disease to other animals and to humans. Fingernails should not extend beyond the end of the finger to reduce the risk of injury to other handlers or to animals being handled and because longer fingernails are more capable of

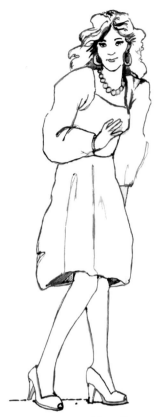

Fig. 1.1 Inappropriate animal handling attire.

entrapping disease agents. If ID badges are needed, they should either be attached to the clothing or worn using a safety breakaway lanyard around the neck. Handler cuts or abrasions should be treated and covered before handling animals. Smoking or consuming food or drink while working with animals or in animal handling areas should be strictly avoided owing to the danger of introducing infectious organisms to the handler's mouth.

Dogs, cats, and other small companion animals

A clinical or laboratory coat and water-impermeable shoes are appropriate for handling dogs, cats, and other small animals (**Figure 1.2**). Long-sleeved coats can aid in protecting handlers from cat scratches. However, when sick animals are to be handled, a short-sleeve length on shirts and coats may be preferable because of the risk of long sleeves becoming a fomite (an inanimate carrier of infection). Waterproof aprons should be worn when bathing animals. Safety glasses or goggles should be

Table 1.4 Inappropriate attire and grooming for animal handlers
• Loose clothes
• Loose long hair
• Dangling jewelry (earrings, bracelets, necklaces)
• Bulky rings
• Hoods or other head gear that obstruct peripheral vision
• Tight boots or boots with slick soles around large animals

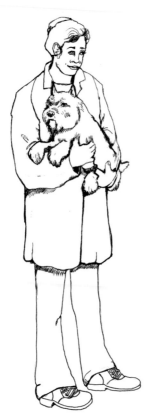

Fig. 1.2 Appropriate small animal handling attire.

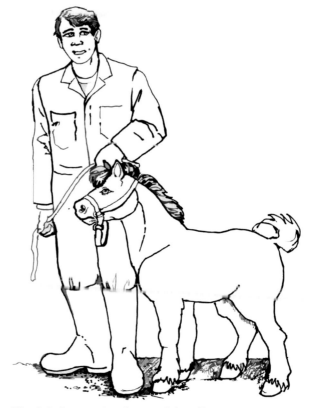

Fig. 1.3 Appropriate livestock handling attire.

worn if handling animals whose nails or beaks are being trimmed, especially when using a high-speed electric grinder (Dremel). Face masks or shields must be worn when handling birds with pointed beaks or assisting with teeth cleaning or other dental procedures. Latex rubber or nitrile gloves should be worn if hands have cuts or cracks and should always be worn when handling small mammals other than dogs and cats to protect from infectious diseases and allergens.

Livestock and poultry

Proper attire for handlers of livestock and poultry differs from the attire needed for small-animal handling (**Figure 1.3**). Hats for handlers of livestock or poultry help protect them from overexposure to sunlight and head injury. Ball caps are popular, but a simple brimmed hat will also help protect against sun on the ears and back of the neck. When working in tight quarters, brimmed hats give handlers an early warning of the possibility of hitting their heads on structure beams or handling equipment. They

also help keep spider webs in barns out of face and hair. Hoods or other head gear, or long hair styles that obstruct peripheral vision or might become snagged and entrap the head, should not be worn when working with livestock, particularly cattle, horses, or swine. Goggles should be used if working with horses or cattle in wet or muddy conditions. Temporarily not being able to see, particularly around horses, can be dangerous.

Coveralls or thick trousers in muted green or khaki color are appropriate for routine handling of livestock or poultry. A strong belt can be used as a temporary lead rope around an animal's neck or as a flag to direct animal movement. Leather leggings are advisable when handling ratites to protect legs from forward strikes. Boots should be loose fitting, water impermeable, and with non-skid soles. Metal toe caps may be advisable when working with cattle, small ruminants, or ratites.

Disposable rubber gloves and nose and mouth masks (N95 or N100) are needed in circumstances that could involve infectious diseases or dusty

Table 1.5 **Common courtesies when working on farms or ranches**
• If you open it, close it
• If it was open, leave it open
• If you unlock it, lock it
• If you move it, put it back
• If you make a mess, clean it up
• Do not climb on fences or gates without permission
• Do not leave an animal in a dirty stall; clean it as often as you find it dirty
• Unless certain of probable safety or animal welfare risks, do not tell owners how to handle their animals without being asked

environments, particularly in total-confinement poultry environments. Ear protection is often needed when working with swine and other situations likely to cause hearing damage. Dangling jewelry or long hair can catch on chains used for leads or cross ties.

If working on a farm or ranch, trust and respect from owners of animals are gained by adhering to common farm and ranch rules (*Table 1.5*).

CONDITIONS FOR HANDLING AND RESTRAINT

Outcomes of handling and restraint of animals can be affected by the health of the animal, time of day, lighting, ambient temperature, setting and facilities, personnel, and duration.

Pre-handling considerations

An unhealthy animal can have an altered temperament, requiring special handling techniques, or have an elevated risk of injury from being handled owing to an illness or previous injury. Before handling any animal, it and its surroundings should be visually inspected. The animal should be observed for signs of possible injury or disease, which could alter the means appropriate for handling the animal. Knowledge of the animal's normal posture, movements, and activities, including how and how often it lies down, is important. The animal's normal vocalizations should also be known. The area of containment (stall, pen, cage, run, etc.) should be examined

for urine and feces. Handlers should be familiar with the normal amount, consistency, odor, and color of feces for the type of animal to be handled, since these vary considerably from species to species. If food or water has been present, evidence of whether or not the animal has been eating or drinking should be noted. The containment area should be assessed for safety – for example, for protruding nails, especially those with hair on them, or other objects that could injure the animal, and whether blood is evident in the area of confinement.

The animal's attitude should be observed for signs of depression or aggressiveness. Its ambulation and other movements should be screened for lameness or other impairments. The respiration rate and depth should be monitored. Impaired respiration can make any handling method particularly dangerous to the animal.

Pre-restraint considerations

Restraint, if needed, must be applied effectively on the first attempt or the animal will learn to escape the restraint in the future. Pre-restraint planning should include considering the effects on the animals and what safety precautions will be appropriate.

Although a plan for restraint should be designed to be successful on the first attempt, a contingency plan should be formulated in case the initial plan turns out to be inappropriate or unexpected circumstances arise. A plan needs to include a check of equipment. If others will be assisting, everyone must be physically capable and trained to handle animals, and they must know the current plan thoroughly. When dealing with large or otherwise dangerous or potentially aggressive animals, an escape should be planned in advance. For some animals chemical restraint should be ready to be administered without delay if physical restraint fails.

Effects on animals

The effects of handling and restraint on animal safety should be considered. What will be the lesson that will be learned by the animal? Gordon Wright, circa 1930, a famous cavalry instructor in horsemanship, said, "Every time you ride, you're either teaching or unteaching your horse." The same principle applies to any handling of any type of animal. To yield the best lesson that might be learned by the animal, a handler should use the minimum restraint needed, maintain a calm environment, and carefully manage the final release so that the animal perceives it to be the handler's choice, not the animal's.

If adverse effects occur when handling or restraining an animal, the animal will associate with it any events, people, and objects that immediately preceded the handling and that occurred during the animal's handling. It may then respond with signs of stress or fear when subsequently exposed to similar handler clothing, locations (cage, pens, etc.), or sounds on re-exposure. Such displayed distress may seem inexplicable to a new handler.

Poor handling of dairy cattle can reduce milk production and increase the incidence of lameness. Bad handling experiences can cause reduced reproductive function and impaired growth and wool production in sheep. In sows, such experiences can result in smaller litters, decreased growth rate, and delayed age of first estrus.

Surroundings and conditions

The time of day or amount of light can affect animal handling. Nocturnal (night active) animals are more docile when handled in bright light. Diurnal (daytime active) animals are more docile when handled in subdued light.

Livestock and horses (prey animals) avoid shadows and darkened areas and will move willingly to well-lit areas, although not if the light is glaring and impairs their vision. The same intensity or moderately brighter light than in their present surroundings should be provided where diurnal animals are wanted to move.

Ambient temperature affects animal handling. Pigs and sheep are particularly susceptible to heat stress and should be handled early in the cooler part of the day. Fans and water spray on legs and lower abdomen should be applied when needed. Cool, brisk temperatures enliven horses, making handling more difficult. Hot weather makes them more tractable.

The setting for handling animals should be well prepared. For small animals, room doors and windows should be closed and all counter tops cleared. Before working cattle in chutes, a check of all chutes, alleyways, and stalls should be conducted. Stalls and stocks should be inspected for potential hazards to horses before their use. Areas for casting a large animal (lay an animal down) should be checked for hazards, especially where the animal could get its legs caught underneath a nearby structure.

Personnel

If an assistant is present to help a primary handler, it is the primary handler's responsibility to make sure that the assistant is knowledgeable in proper animal handling and is fully aware of the handling or restraint plan. An assistant should also be behaviorally mature and physically strong enough to carry out the needed assistance. Otherwise, if the assistant or the animal is injured, the primary handler can be liable for damages.

In the case of veterinarians or veterinary technicians being a primary handler, animal owners should not assist with the handling and restraint of their own animal. In less than ideal circumstances, when no one else is available to assist, an owner may insist on helping in a desire to ensure proper care of their animal or to prevent injury to it or the veterinarian. If assistance from an owner is the only means to provide reasonable safety for the animal or people present, the owner must not be allowed to assist without first being instructed in the proper technique, made aware of the risks involved, and have a stated willingness to defer to the veterinarian's directions during the procedure, preferably in writing.

Duration

The duration of animal handling or restraint should be as short as possible to complete the task. Longer durations cause unnecessary stress to the animal and exhausts their patience to tolerate the handling. Pre-handling preparation is absolutely essential to minimize the duration of handling and restraint.

RISKS OF INJURY

General risks

Few domestic animals are naturally aggressive toward humans. When fearful or stressed, most animals' first reaction is to attempt to flee. When fleeing is not an option, they will resort to their means of offense or defense, which may involve teeth or beaks that bite; hooves that kick, stomp, or strike; claws that puncture or scratch; heads that butt or crush; horns that gore – or some combination of these.

More than four million dog bites are estimated to occur annually in the U.S. About one-sixth of these require medical attention, and 10–20 deaths occur each year. Children, the elderly, and letter carriers, in that order, are at highest risk of dog bites. Five percent of all emergency room visits are caused by dog bites. Dogs that receive inadequate early socialization with humans or no continued gentle handling, as well as those that are tethered for long periods, are the most likely to bite. Bites from cats are common but less life-threatening than most dog bites. The risk of infection from cat bites is greater, and impairment of hand function is a significant risk.

Animals are responsible for approximately 1% of occupational fatalities in the U.S. One of six farm injuries are animal related, from bites, kicks, and crushing. Male and elderly handlers are demographically at highest risk. Cattle, especially bulls, are responsible for 40% of deaths, horses for 27%, dogs for 3%, and hogs for 1%.

Cattle cause deaths in humans by mauling, charging, goring, kicking, or knocking down. Most deaths are the result of attacks by bulls or cows with newborn calves. Beef cattle are handled less than dairy cattle and are more inherently dangerous than dairy breeds. However, dairy bulls are considered the most dangerous of all domesticated animals. Dairy handlers are most often injured during the milking process or treating mastitis, sustaining leg or facial injuries.

Most horse-related human deaths are associated with riding, such as falling off or being thrown off. Other people are killed by being crushed, trampled on, or kicked (particularly in the head) by horses. Brain and craniofacial injuries from animals are most often caused by horses. More than 100,000 people are admitted to emergency rooms in the U.S. from horse-related injuries each year. Approximately two-thirds of horse-related injuries are from riding,

and more than 12,000 injured people suffer head injuries.

Animal-related physical injuries to humans can be intentional by the animal, involving butting, goring, bites, and kicks from aggression or fear. In other cases, the injury may be unintentional, such as crushing from falls, stepping on feet, and scratching while struggling to get free.

Human-related physical injuries to animals can be intentional, from the inappropriate release of anger or from a sadistic impulse. Intentional mistreatment of dogs typically occurs with dogs being trained for fighting. Unintentional injuries to animals can occur to those that are handled or restrained inappropriately. Many unintentional injuries of animals involve horses and are caused by handlers without adequate training on the proper handling of horses.

Reactions of animals who are familiar with a particular handler are not the same as those of animals that have no prior experience with the handler. A perceived lack of handler confidence will elicit actions of social dominance or fear in animals. Equipment failure is an easily avoided but common cause of handler injury (*Table 1.6*).

Risks to veterinary personnel

Based on most of the reported epidemiological studies of animal-related injuries to veterinary personnel, more than half of all veterinarians will be seriously injured by animals some time in their careers. About one-fourth of the injuries will require surgery. The body location of about half of animal-related injuries are the hands. About one-fourth are to the arms and nearly the same to the head, with many fewer to the chest, followed by the abdomen and groin. The species inflicting injury are from, in

Table 1.6 **Causes of handler injury**
• Lack of animal handling competence
• Overconfidence or underconfidence
• Being rushed
• Becoming angered
• Error by an assistant
• Pain experienced by the animal
• Equipment failure

decreasing order of frequency, cattle, small animals, and horses. Injuries that are reported are primarily kicks and bites, followed by crushing injuries, butting, being run over, and other less common injuries.

Large-animal veterinarians are injured at 1.75 times the rate of injuries to companion-animal veterinarians, but veterinary technicians in companion-animal practice have more than six times more injuries than large-animal veterinary technicians (these figures include other job injuries in addition to those directly from animal handling). The most common large-animal-related injuries are from being kicked, followed by being crushed (both occur more often from cattle than horses). The percentage of injuries in large-animal practice are, from highest to lowest, dairy, cow-calf, and equine. The number of veterinarian or veterinary technician injuries from horses are fewer than the injuries to non-professional handlers and equestrians, a consequence of the latter's lesser training and the greater danger involved in riding.

In companion-animal practices, bites are the most common animal-related injury. Cat bites to veterinarians occur 50% more often than dog bites, and they are three times more common in veterinary technicians than dog bites. Scratches from cats are more common than bites but less frequently a reason for seeking medical attention.

When a sick large animal is being examined, an assistant should always be present to provide a diversion for the examiner. Mature bulls, stallions, rams, bucks, and boars are always unpredictable. Handlers should never lose sight of their presence and attitude. Cows, mares, and sows with newborns can also be unpredictable and dangerous. Whenever handling mature male or nursing female livestock, handlers should always have a planned emergency exit.

RISKS OF DISEASE TO HANDLERS AND OTHER ANIMALS

Zoonoses: transmission of disease from animals to humans

A zoonosis is any infectious disease of animals that can be transmitted to humans under natural conditions. Of the more than 1,400 known infectious diseases of humans, 60% are zoonotic. Most are associated with the gastrointestinal tract, and transmission is fecal–oral. More than 50 zoonotic diseases are known to be present in the U.S. Examples include rabies, salmonellosis, cryptosporidiosis, plague, sporotrichosis, psittacosis, and ringworm. Routes of transmission of zoonotic diseases are primarily contact, aerosol, and vector-borne. Every animal can carry some diseases that humans could acquire. However, handling apparently healthy domestic animals using basic sanitary practices, such as keeping hands away from eyes, nose, and mouth, keeping skin cuts covered, and washing hands after handling animals, carries very little risk of acquiring zoonotic disease. Stressful handling, including prolonged transportation or overcrowding of animals, can increase the risk of animals shedding disease organisms. The actual incidence of diseases transmitted from animals to humans is not clear, but the reported frequency is no doubt low compared with actual occurrence. Non-fatal zoonoses are underdiagnosed and underreported.

The risk of disease transmitted from animals is greater among people with immature or impaired immune systems. Children 5 years old or younger should have supervised exposure to animals because of their immature immune systems and their inclination to put unwashed hands in their mouths. Animal handlers who are more than 70 years old may have an increased risk of zoonoses from declining immune responses. Some conditions, diseases, or treatments in humans, regardless of their age, may lower their resistance to zoonoses. Among the systemic diseases are AIDS, congenital immunodeficiencies, diabetes mellitus, chronic renal failure, alcoholism, liver cirrhosis, malnutrition, and certain cancers. Pregnancy may also reduce the immune response. Treatments for cancer, organ or bone marrow transplants, and autoimmune diseases can depress immunity. Splenectomy and long-term hemodialysis are also treatments that can suppress immunity. Young children and immunosuppressed adults should especially avoid nursing calves, all reptiles, and baby chicks and ducklings.

High-risk animals for transmitting zoonoses are the young, females giving birth, and unvaccinated, stray, or feral animals. Others include those fed raw meat diets, kept in crowded conditions, and with internal or external parasites. All reptiles and wild or exotic species are high-risk sources of zoonotic diseases.

Keeping animals healthy can also reduce the risk of zoonosis and transmission to humans. Routine veterinary care, vaccinations, and parasite screenings should be maintained. High-quality food is advisable. Dog, cat, or ferret foods that contain any supplementary egg, poultry, or meat products should have been adequately cooked. Raw pet foods can be sources of zoonotic bacteria such as *Salmonella*. Pets should be prevented from drinking from toilet bowls or eating garbage, hunting wildlife, or eating other animals' feces. All pets should be kept away from areas where human food is prepared.

Hand washing is essential to controlling the transmission of disease (*Table 1.7*). All animal handling locations should have a means for handlers to wash hands. Animal handlers should keep their fingernails short and, if necessary, use moisturizers to keep the skin from cracking and creating portals of disease entry. Alcohol-based rubs are effective against most disease-producing agents if hands are not visibly soiled with organic material.

If a bite or a scratch, the wound should be thoroughly cleaned with warm soapy water, compression should be applied if bleeding persists, and a physician should be consulted. Special precautions are needed if working with animals with diarrhea or skin or mouth sores. Pregnant women should not handle cat litter or ewes that are lambing.

All animal handlers should be vaccinated against tetanus every 10 years, as recommended by the U.S. Centers for Disease Control and Prevention. Horse handlers are particularly at risk. Handlers of hogs or poultry should be vaccinated with the current human influenza virus vaccine. Veterinary personnel are also advised to receive pre-exposure vaccination against rabies and have serum titers checked every two years.

Some animal-related diseases are transmitted to humans indirectly via ectoparasite vectors, such as mosquitoes (encephalitis viruses), ticks (Rocky Mountain spotted fever and many others), and fleas (cat-scratch disease). The animal carrying the ectoparasite may or may not become ill. Control of ectoparasites on animals to be handled is important to the animals' and the handlers' health. Ectoparasites are controlled in dogs and cats with individually applied topical insecticides and acaricides. Livestock are protected using dusters, dust bags, back rubbers and oilers, pour-ons, impregnated ear tags, feed-through larvacides, or boluses of insect growth regulators. Premise control may include sprays, traps, and baits. Yards need to be mowed frequently enough to keep grass short. Pastures and pens should be either cleaned of manure or harrowed on a weekly basis. Manure piles and other compost should be turned weekly.

Rodents and birds can also be disease vectors. These are controlled by eliminating entry to animal dwellings and hiding places. Access to food sources should be eliminated by maintaining food storage in rodent-proof sealed containers and proper disposal of garbage.

The greatest zoonotic risks to companion animal veterinarians have been reported to be ringworm, rabies, and antibiotic-resistant bacterial infections. For food-animal and mixed-practice veterinarians, significant zoonoses are *Campylobacter*, ringworm, and rabies. Equine veterinarian zoonotic risks have been greatest for West Nile virus (acquired from mosquitoes).

Means of exposure to zoonoses are varied (*Table 1.8*). Direct transmission can be through contact of animal saliva, blood, urine, or feces with handler's eyes, nose, or mouth, which can occur from the splashing of body fluids or eating, smoking, or touching the face. Contamination of a skin cut, scratch, or crack with animal saliva, blood, urine, or feces is also a form of direct transmission. Indirect transmission can include inhalation of contaminated dust. Vector-borne indirect transmission can be the bite of a fly, mosquito, tick, or flea carrying a zoonotic organism.

Table 1.7 **Proper hand washing**
1 Clean fingernails and remove rings
2 Wet hands
3 Apply an olive-size amount of liquid soap to a palm
4 Scrub both hands while counting to 20 slowly
5 Rinse thoroughly and dry with paper towels

Table 1.8 **Means of exposure to zoonoses**
DIRECT
• Bite/scratch
• Pre-existing breaks in the skin
• Through intact skin or mucous membranes
• Ingestion (fecal–oral or other)
• Inhalation
INDIRECT
• Fomites – inanimate objects (brushes, food bowls, etc.)
• Vectors – organisms that transmit disease agents:
• Biological – agent transforms to infective stage in vector
• Mechanical – only transported by vector
VEHICLE
• Air
• Food
• Water

Table 1.9 **Recommendations for preventing zoonotic diseases**
• Thoroughly wash your hands after feeding or touching animals or moving their waste; do not dry hands on clothing
• Do not permit animals to eat from human plates or utensils
• Keep pets supervised to prevent hunting at will and do not feed raw meat
• Do not eat or drink in animal handling areas
• Wear appropriate clothing when handling animals
• Do not kiss animals
• Wash cuts thoroughly
• Wear gloves when gardening
• Keep animal environment reasonably clean and prevent children from playing where there is animal waste, for example, covers should be kept on children's sandboxes when not in use
• Clean cat litter daily and wash your hands immediately afterwards
• Keep animals from household areas where human food is prepared or handled
• Do not bathe pets in sinks or bathtubs used by humans
• De-worm animals on regular basis and provide reasonable control of fleas, ticks, and mosquitoes
• Avoid stray animals
• Do not keep wild animals as pets
• Vaccinate animals against zoonotic diseases and maintain tetanus vaccinations in all animal handlers and rabies vaccinations in high-risk animal handlers
• Use proper low-stress handling techniques and containment practices and facilities to reduce stress-induced shedding of zoonotic diseases
• Routinely train animal handlers on the prevention of zoonotic disease and animal handling safety measures

Personal protective equipment (PPE) should be considered in possible zoonotic risk situations. PPE can include protection of the eyes with properly fitted goggles or American National Standards Institute (ANSI)-approved face masks. Protection for the torso can be lab coats, coveralls, gowns, or aprons. Long sleeves protect against scratches and splashes. The scalp can be partially protected from exposure to cuts, splashes of infectious liquids, and ringworm by wearing a hat. Ears should be protected from excessive noise with ear muffs or molded ear plugs (cotton plugs are insufficient). Feet may be protected with closed-toe, slip-resistant, water-impermeable shoes or boots. Hands are typically protected with rubber or nitrile gloves.

Essential recommendations for the prevention of zoonotic disease are listed in *Table 1.9*. Precautions for veterinary personnel handling overtly sick animals are beyond the scope of this book. For these circumstances, consult the current *Compendium of Veterinary Standard Precautions for Zoonotic Disease Prevention in Veterinary Personnel*, published annually in the *Journal of the American Veterinary Medical Association*, and the Veterinary Standard Precautions at www.nasphv.org.

Transmission of disease among animals by their handlers

Handlers can easily carry diseases from one animal to another. Sanitation (reduction of possible disease agents) and disinfection (complete or nearly complete elimination of disease agents) methods are needed to reduce the chance of inanimate objects (clothing, handling equipment, confinement structures) from becoming inanimate transmitters of disease (fomites). The degree of sanitation needed varies with the risk of transmission.

The risk of transmission of disease is low if all animals appear healthy and belong to the same household, farm, or ranch. When animals drink from the same water source, eat from the same ground or containers, touch noses, and have other frequent physical contacts and appear healthy, the risk of handling procedures spreading disease is mild to non-existent. The risk is lowered further if animals of different age groups are segregated. Older animals are more likely to be disease carriers without signs and capable of transmitting disease to younger animals.

On the other hand, sick animals should always be segregated and handled separately after handling tools, boots, and clothing have been disinfected or changed. When handling animals from different sources (households, farms, ranches), disinfection of handling tools, boots, and clothing should take place between handling the different groups of animals.

In low-risk disease-transmission situations, simple washing of handling equipment and hands may be sufficient. Higher risk cases require as much disinfection of equipment as practically possible. Disinfection should be preceded by cleaning off all organic matter (feces, blood, saliva, dust, urine, and hair) before using the disinfectant. Disinfectants can be sanitizers that reduce the number of microorganisms, antiseptics that kill or stop the growth of a few specific microorganisms, or sterilants that kill all microorganisms. The manufacturer's directions for dilution and use of the disinfectant should be closely followed. More disinfectant is not necessarily better. A common, effective, and inexpensive disinfectant (sterilant) is household bleach diluted to 1:32 (1 cup bleach per 1 gal [3.8 L] of water). Bleach (sodium hypochlorite) must never be mixed with an acid or ammonia, which would release toxic gases.

To prevent the transmission of disease, handlers should always wash their hands after handling animals. Water-impermeable boots should be worn for walking on surfaces that are or may have been soiled with urine or feces, and the boots disinfected before moving to another animal holding area. Clothes worn during handling of animals that may have been ill should be washed near the handling areas with commercial equipment. Animal confinement areas should be properly cleaned before introducing new animals. New animals being introduced to an established group of animals should be held in quarantine until the effects of transport stress and the typical incubation period for infectious diseases has passed (usually 10 days).

Anthroponosis: transmission of disease from handlers to animals

In rare cases, diseased handlers can transmit their infection, such as tuberculosis, to animals. This is referred to as reverse zoonoses, or *anthroponosis*. Animal handlers who are ill should not handle animals because of the risk of reverse zoonosis, as well as the added risk of physical injury from impaired judgement and delayed reactions.

ETHICAL CONCERNS

Ethics are based in part on social mores and are therefore not static. Methods of animal handling, restraint, and discipline once considered acceptable might not be tolerated by society today. Acceptable techniques are changing.

The designation of what is proper handling, restraint, and discipline is often murky. There are no universally accepted guidelines. Agreement exists only for extremes. The reason is simple: there may be 100 ways to restrain an animal, but only 10 that are appropriate and humane and maybe just one that will work well for a particular handler on a particular animal under the circumstances at that moment. Because of this, state statutes on animal abuse usually prohibit forms of handling in vague extremes, such as overworking, overloading, and inflicting unnecessary cruelty. Certain actions have been proposed as inappropriate in veterinary practice for handling, restraining, and disciplining companion animals (*Table 1.10*).

Force is considered permissible if handlers are in full control of their emotions at the time and only the minimum amount of force needed is used to protect the safety of humans, the animal being handled, or other animals. Force must be used with consideration of the animal's nature and with empathy for the animal. An example of necessary force is using

Table 1.10 **Unacceptable handling, restraining, or disciplining animals**
• Use of force beyond that needed for self-defense or protection of others
• Use of force as punishment
• Punishment delivered in anger or to inflict pain
• Striking an animal on the head or other sensitive or injured body parts
• Choking an animal
• Shaking an animal violently
• Striking an animal with a rigid object, unless to avert a dangerous attack

a stout stick to strike a charging bull or boar on the nose in order to escape the attack.

Handlers who are supervisors of other animal handlers bear the responsibility to ensure that the other handlers are appropriately trained and supervised. Written guidelines, although they may only deal with extremes, should be provided along with a no-tolerance policy on cases of animal abuse. It should be read understood by all employees handling animals that immediate termination of employment will occur as a consequence of unequivocal animal abuse. There is a well-established link between willful abuse of animals and eventual domestic violence against humans.

LEGAL CONSIDERATIONS

Most states have laws that require animal handlers to exercise adequate control over an animal to prevent it from harming itself, other animals, people, or property. More serious charges may be filed against a handler who knowingly fails to exercise adequate control over an animal.

There is always a degree of risk in handling animals. A handler must assume the responsibility for the safety of the animal and that of the people who may become injured by the animal being handled. If all safety precautions are taken and cautions given to others, an injury to people or to the animal(s) may be attributed to inherent danger and involve an assumption of personal responsibility. For example, many states have passed horse activity

liability-waiver legislation with wording similar to: "Warning: Under State Law, an Equine Professional is not liable for an injury to or the death of a participant in equine activities resulting from the inherent risks of equine activities pursuant to the state statutes." Signs of this warning are required to be posted on the premises where horse handling occurs (**Figure 1.4**). Horse shows require participants to sign a statement something like: "I enter the above horse at my own risk, and release the horse association, show sponsors, show management and grounds from any claim or right to loss and/or damages which may occur to me and/or my horse and/or my property. I agree that in case of loss or injury involving either horse or exhibitor, I will make no claim whatsoever against this show or individuals connected with it." Liability waivers may help win a case for a defendant, but they do not prevent lawsuits and the cost of defense.

Waivers of responsibility also do not absolve handlers of liability in an injury or death that is due to their negligence or incompetence. Incompetence is simply not having the knowledge or ability to control an animal. Failing to properly contain or control an animal that causes injury to a human is negligence. Knowing that an animal is potentially dangerous and not taking extra efforts to protect others is also considered negligence.

Injury does not have to be direct. Injury received in an attempt to flee from an animal demonstrating threatening behavior could be attributed to owner or agent negligence. It is prudent to have adequate liability insurance that covers the activities of an animal handler. In some cases of animal handling that may involve people other than the primary handler, releases or hold-harmless agreements are advisable and legal counsel should be consulted. It is important to ascertain that any assistant animal handler is mature enough, strong enough, and trained sufficiently for each task to be performed. The assistant should also be adequately supervised during animal handling.

Some animals are considered inherently dangerous, such as lions, tigers, cougars, bears, monkeys, venomous snakes, and constricting snakes over 8 ft (2.5 m) in length. Inherently dangerous animals should be handled only by specially trained and

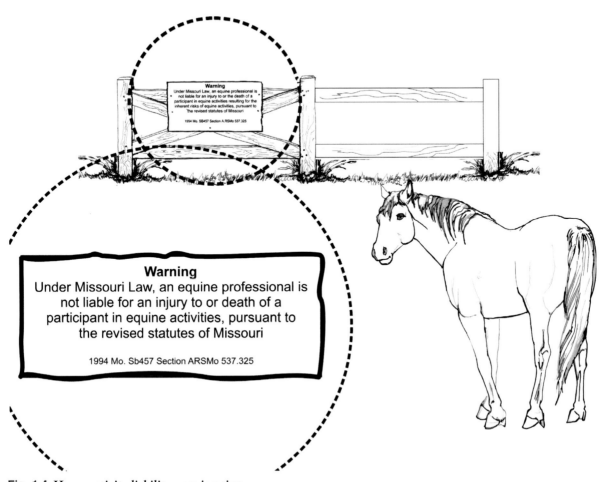

Warning
Under Missouri Law, an equine professional is
not liable for an injury to or death of a
participant in equine activities, pursuant to
the revised statutes of Missouri

1994 Mo. Sb457 Section ARSMo 537.325

Fig. 1.4 Horse activity liability warning sign.

experienced personnel. Animals considered rabies reservoirs (bats, skunks, coyotes, foxes, and raccoons) should not be handled except when absolutely necessary and only by professionals trained to handle wildlife. Currently five states in the U.S. (Alabama, Nevada, North Carolina, South Carolina, and Wisconsin) have laws prohibiting the keeping of dangerous wild animals as pets. Twenty-one states ban all dangerous exotic pets. Other states restrict only selected exotics.

If physical restraint results in unnecessary pain and suffering to an animal, a handler can be in violation of state animal cruelty and humane laws. In more than 30 states, at least one form of animal cruelty constitutes a felony. If the handler is a veterinary medical professional, there is risk of malpractice charges that could lead to disciplinary action under the state Veterinary Practice Act. Domestic animals have traditionally been viewed legally as property. Still, there are laws to protect the inhumane care of animals. This is not only to protect animal well-being; it also has benefits to human society. Willful abuse of animals is known to be associated with concurrent or eventual abuse of humans.

The most stringent restrictions on the handling of animals involve those used in federally funded research. The National Institutes of Health (NIH) Office of Laboratory Animal Welfare (OLAW) oversees all federally funded research institutions using laboratory animals.

Primarily as a result of articles in *Sports Illustrated* and *Life* magazines about the abuse of dogs in research, the Laboratory Animal Welfare Act (1966) was passed by Congress in 1966 regulating the use of dogs, cats, hamsters, guinea pigs, rabbits, and non-human primates used in research. It was designed to be enforced by the United States Department of Agriculture (USDA). In 1970, it was amended to the Animal Welfare Act (AWA) and broadened to include any warm-blooded animal used in research, exhibition, or wholesale animal trade. Horses, livestock, birds, mice, and rats not used in research were excluded in 1972. Reptiles were never covered by the AWA.

In 1985, the Improved Standards for Laboratory Animals Act, a part of the Food Security Act, and the Health Research Extension Act required the NIH to minimize the number of animals used in research and their pain and suffering. Institutions with federally funded research must have an Animal Care and Use Committee (ACUC) who monitor the care and use of research animals. ACUCs must be composed of at least one veterinarian, one non-scientist, and one person not affiliated with the institution. A veterinarian must be employed by the institution to oversee the care and use of the institution's research animals and be an advisor to the ACUC.

The Association for Assessment and Accreditation of Laboratory Animal Care International (AAALAC) requires a higher standard of care than the NIH, but membership is voluntary. AAALAC has standards that include provisions to provide social and other mental enrichments for animals. All social animals are expected to be housed in pairs or groups. Objects should be provided that create complexity in the animal's environment to create opportunities for decision making and other mental stimulation. Normal behaviors such as grooming, exploration, foraging, and burrowing are to be encouraged and monitored. Abnormal behaviors that include self-mutilation, stereotypic behaviors (pacing, bar biting), and aggression should be monitored and corrected, when possible.

The Federal Bureau of Investigation (FBI) reclassified crimes against animals in 2016 as a Group A offense and included cases in the FBI's National Incident-Based Reporting System. The motivation for the reclassification was the findings of studies that revealed a link between animal abuse and domestic violence, child abuse, and other violent crimes toward people.

EXTENDED BENEFITS OF ANIMAL HANDLING

Animal handling was needed to domesticate animals, and humans have reaped the benefits of dogs' protective tendencies and assistance in hunting, rodent control provided by cats, meat and fiber from livestock, and the work and transportation assistance of donkeys, horses, and oxen. There are even more benefits of living in close proximity to and handling animals.

To handle and restrain animal successfully, a handler must learn to control his or her emotions and reactions with animals and to more clearly interact with other people. Learning to handle animals correctly can train the handler to be more disciplined, fair, and clear in communicating with both animals and humans. Unnecessarily forceful commands, prolonged discipline, unclear or inconsistent instructions, and physical force will not be successful in handling animals and does not work in the long run when dealing with humans.

The personal benefits of handling animals have been long recognized. Antoine de Pluvinel, founder of the French School of Horsemanship, said in 1594: "In training horses, one trains oneself." More recently, the Hungarian dressage master Charles de Kunffy said: "The nobility of Europe was raised on horseback. The horse gives the rider courage, empathy, focus, self-discipline, and a sense of justice. The ruling classes became appropriate rulers by being on horseback." To varying degrees, such extended personal benefits are gained by handling all animals, not just horses, if the handler learns to enjoy and handle animals well.

Extended benefits can also apply to family members. Children raised in pet-owning families or on farms with livestock have fewer allergies and respiratory infections than children not exposed to animal dander and animal products containing dust.

ROLE OF CHEMICAL AND PHYSICAL RESTRAINT

Recent innovations in chemical restraint (sedation and anesthesia) have been highly beneficial to animals, owners, and veterinarians. The ease of chemical restraint has resulted in it being used unnecessarily at times. Chemical alteration of consciousness can alleviate some of the fear and resistance to restraint. However, the value of chemical restraint must always be weighed against the value of proper animal training and physical restraint. Chemical restraint is not void of risks, expense, and time required for supervision. It should never be used simply for the convenience of the handler. All sedatives and anesthetics have the potential to cause respiratory or cardiac arrest and physical injuries to animals or handlers during chemical administration, induction, or recovery. In addition, organ damage from overdosage, individual variations in response, or idiosyncratic reactions are possible. These are some of the reasons that most sedatives and all anesthetics are restricted for use by prescription or usage by a licensed veterinarian.

Chemical restraint should be the third and last option for handling and restraining animals. Proper animal training should be the first option. Careful application of humane physical restraint should be second. Furthermore, when chemical restraint must be used, it should be supplemented by sufficient humane physical restraint to optimize the animal's and handler's safety during administration, induction, and recovery from the drug's effects.

KEYS TO GOOD HANDLING OF ALL ANIMALS

Good handling of any type of domestic or tame non-domestic animal involves proper preparation (*Table 1.11*) and 10 basic keys (*Table 1.12*).

IDEALS AND REALITIES

Animal handlers should always be advocates of ideal animal handling conditions and scheduling. However, in the reality of day-to-day animal handling, animals often must be handled in less than ideal conditions and during less than ideal times because of medical or hazard emergencies or because owners are unwilling or incapable of providing ideal conditions. There are situations when delaying

Table 1.11 Proper preparation to become an animal handler

- Read about animal handling
- Observe normal animal behavior
- Gain guidance from a good handler
- Observe a good handler with animals
- Practice under a good handler's supervision

Table 1.12 Keys to good animal handling

- Frequently, but briefly and gently, handle young animals during their critical socialization period to reduce their natural fear of humans, while being mindful not to eliminate their inherent respect for humans
- Quietly handle healthy adults frequently for short periods to habituate the animals for handling without an association with fearful, painful events to follow
- Confine animals in environments as similar to their ancestor's natural habitat as reasonably possible; for example, crates as dens for dogs, pastures as steppes for horses, and deep substrate as desert sand for hamsters
- Provide environmental enrichments that will prevent or reduce boredom and stereotypic behaviors
- Confine animals with as much personal space as needed to prevent or minimize stereotypic behaviors
- Maintain social intraspecies support for animals by keeping prey, pack, and flock animals in groups with a size appropriate for the species
- Minimally handle elderly, neonatal, or sick animals to prevent their exhaustion or pain
- Handle animals with confidence, using smooth rhythmic movements along with a calm low-pitched voice
- Be able to recognize abnormal behavior for the species and the individual, including fear or signs of health problems
- Use correct timing and type of responses to favorable or unfavorable animal conduct to shape their future behavior to handling

handling is in the best interests of the animal, while other situations may mandate doing the best handling possible under less than ideal conditions in the timely best interests of the animal.

Unless a handler is comfortable with leaving animals in danger or being handled by less competent personnel, it is advisable for a handler to become familiar with, and skilled in, a variety of means of handling animals, some of which may not be needed in ideal conditions or at ideal times. For example, using a rope on a stick for capture, steel tube panels for traps, casting a cow with ropes, and using a detached tubular gate as an emergency glide are not needed in ideal conditions, but these might be the best, or only, methods to successfully handle animals in some handling conditions. To provide no assistance in handling animals whose welfare is in danger because conditions are less than ideal is a form of handler negligence. A good animal handler provides the best assistance for the animals in danger with the tools and techniques that are available at the time, as long as there is reasonable expectation of safety for the animals and the handlers.

SELECTED FURTHER READING

Austin HE, Hyams JH, Abbott KA (2007). Training in animal handling for veterinary students at Charles Sturt University, Australia. *Journal of Veterinary Medical Education* 34: 566–575.

Bender JB, Shulman SA (2004). Reports of zoonotic disease outbreaks associated with animal exhibits and availability of recommendations for preventing zoonotic disease transmission from animals to people in such settings. *Journal of the American Veterinary Medical Association* 224:1105–1109.

Busch HM, Cogbill TH, Landercasper J, et al. (1986). Blunt bovine and equine trauma. *Journal of Trauma* 26:559–560.

Cawdell-Smith AJ, Pym RAE, Verrall RG, et al. (2007). Animal handling as an integrated component of animal and veterinary science programs at the University of Queensland. *Journal of Veterinary Medical Education* 34:542–549.

Centers for Disease Control and Prevention (2011). Morbidity and Mortality Weekly Reports Compendium of Measures to Prevent Disease Associated with Animals in Public Settings 60(RR04):1–24.

Chapman HM, Taylor EG, Buddle JR, et al. (2007). Student training in large-animal handling at the School of Veterinary and Biomedical Sciences, Murdoch University, Australia. *Journal of Veterinary Medical Education* 34:576–582.

Cockram MS, Aitchison K, Collie DDS, et al. (2007). Animal-handling teaching at the Royal (Dick) School of Veterinary Studies, University of Edinburgh. *Journal of Veterinary Medical Education* 34:554–560.

Cogbill TH, Strutt PJ, Landercasper J, et al. (1989). Injuries from horses and cows. *Complications in Orthopedics* 120:112–114.

Epp T, Waldner C (2012). Occupational health hazards in veterinary medicine: zoonoses and other biological hazards. *Canadian Veterinary Journal* 53:144–150.

Epp T, Waldner C (2012). Occupational health hazards in veterinary medicine: Physical, psychological, and chemical hazards. *Canadian Veterinary Journal* 53:151–157.

Esch KJ, Petersen CA (2013). Transmission and epidemiology of zoonotic protozoal diseases of companion animals. *Clinical Microbiology Review* 26:58–85.

Farm and Ranch Safety and Health Association. *A health and safety guide for handling farm animals and poultry.* www.farscha.bc.ca (accessed 11/20/2015).

Frechette D (2008). Liability law: Reality check. *Equus* 374:45–49.

Hanlon A, Gath V, Mulligan F (2007). Practical animal-handling classes at University College Dublin. *Journal of Veterinary Medical Education* 34:561–565.

Hendricks KJ, Adekoya N (2001). Non-fatal animal related injuries to youth occurring on farms in the United States, 1998. *Injury Prevention* 7:307–311.

Kipperman BS (2015). The role of the veterinary profession in promoting animal welfare. *Journal of the American Veterinary Medical Association* 246:502–504.

Landercasper J, Cogbill T, Strutt P, et al. (1988). Trauma and the veterinarian. *Journal of Trauma* 28:1255–1259.

Langley, RL, Hunter JL (2001). Occupational fatalities due to animal-related events. *Wilderness and Environmental Med* 12:168–174.

Langley RL, Morrow WE (2010). Livestock handling – minimizing worker injuries. *Journal of Agromedicine* 15:226–35.

Lucas M, Day L, Shirangi A, et al. (2009). Significant injuries in Australian veterinarians and use of safety precautions. *Occupational Medicine* 59:327–333.

MacLeay JM (2007). Large-animal handling at the Colorado State University College of Veterinary Medicine. *Journal of Veterinary Medical Education* 34:550–553.

McGreevy P (2007). Firm but gentle: Learning to handle with care. *Journal of Veterinary Medical Education* 34:539–541.

McGreevy P, Hawke C, Celi P, et al. (2007). Learning and teaching animal handling at the University of Sydney's Faculty of Veterinary Science. *Journal of Veterinary Medical Education* 34:586–597.

McMillian M, Dunn JR, Keen JE, et al. (2007). Risk behaviors for disease transmission among petting zoo attendees. *Journal of the American Veterinary Medical Association* 231:1036–1038.

National Association of State Public Health Veterinarians Animal Contact Compendium Committee (2013). Compendium of measures to prevent disease associated with animals in public settings. *Journal of the American Veterinary Medical Association* 243:1270–1288.

National Association of State Public Health Veterinarians (2010). Compendium of veterinary standard precautions for zoonotic disease prevention in veterinary personnel. *Journal of the American Veterinary Medical Association* 237:1403–1422.

Patronek GJ, Lacroix CA (2001). Developing an ethic for the handling, restraint, and discipline of companion animals in veterinary practice. *Journal of the American Veterinary Medical Association* 218:514–517.

Poole AG, Shane SM, Kearney MT, et al. (1998). Survey of occupational hazards in companion animal practices. *Journal of the American Veterinary Medical Association* 212:1386–1388.

Poole AG, Shane SM, Kearney MT, et al. (1999). Survey of occupational hazards in large animal practices. *Journal of the American Veterinary Medical Association* 215:1433–1435.

Stafford KJ, Erceg VH (2007). Teaching animal handling to veterinary students at Massey University, New Zealand. *Journal of Veterinary Medical Education* 34:583–585.

Van Soest EM, Fritschi L (2004). Occupational health risks in veterinary nursing: an exploratory study. *Australian Veterinary Journal* 82:346–350.

White P, Chapman S (2007). Two students' reflections on their training in animal handling at the University of Sydney. *Journal of Veterinary Medical Education* 34:598–599.

Willems RA (2007). Animals in veterinary medical teaching: compliance and regulatory issues, the US perspective. *Journal of Veterinary Medical Education* 34:615–619.

CHAPTER 2

ANIMAL BEHAVIOR

Animals are not simply hairier versions of humans. Reacting to animals as if they are humans is called *anthropomorphism*, and anthropomorphism is not effective in establishing a safe and effective relationship with animals. Good animal handling is much more complicated. An important foundation for proper animal handling is learning the normal behavior for the species. Knowing the natural instincts of a species is essential to being able to handle, move, and contain them humanely with minimal stress and risk of injury to either the handler or the animals.

Most communication between animal species is silent, that is, it is "body language". The behavior and attitude of animals should be assessed by observing them at a distance before approaching for handling. Animals will begin assessing handlers by the handler's body language upon first noticing the handler and then modify their own behavior. For example, prey animals will often mask signs of illness or injury particularly in the presence of strangers. Not approaching them immediately will reduce some of the threat they might otherwise perceive. It is essential to not be perceived by animals as either their predator or being of lesser social rank to them.

The rank of all animals is primarily based on deference, not by actual fighting.

Most animals will telegraph, in advance, their intent to display open aggression. Their natural tendency is to avoid any possibility of injury or death. Therefore, barking or other vocalizations, lunging, pawing, fake charging, and other indications usually precede an attack on an apparent adversary. The human at which these behaviors are directed should know the meaning of these warnings and not ignore or minimize them. Avoidance of handling resistance in animals requires their early socialization with

Table 2.1 **Causes of irreparable handling resistance in animals**
• Failure to properly socialize animals in their juvenile period of life
• Infliction of pain at any age
• Exposure to extremely fearful situations at any age

humans and never causing them pain or extreme fear (*Table 2.1*).

PREDATOR AND PREY BEHAVIOR

All domestic animals evolved as either meat eaters (predators) or food for meat eaters (prey). Common small domestic animals, such as dogs and cats, are genetically predators. Common large domestic animals, such as horses, cattle, sheep, and goats, are genetically prey. Hogs and rats can be either, depending on the circumstances.

Predators

Predators have eyes that are positioned forward in their skulls, which permits greater overlapping of the field of vision from right and left eyes, and improves depth of vision. Predators stare directly at their prey and are able to track the movement and judge the speed of their prey.

Dogs are pack predators that run after their prey. They are instinctively more aggressive if in a group. They are more aggressive to humans with small stature, and to humans expressing fearful body language, especially when running away as a prey animal would do.

Cats are solitary stalking predators. High-pitched sounds and wiggly movements stimulate their predatory urges. They have explosive movements used to quickly pounce on their prey from a short distance away. If threatened and immediate escape is not possible, they will remain motionless at first. If the threat continues, they will attempt to warn the threat away by hissing and striking. Finally, there will be an explosive attempt to flee or to attack and then flee.

Prey

Prey animals have eyes that are located on the sides of their skulls. This reduces their depth of vision, but increases their range of vision and detection of motion, such that they are better able to monitor their peripheral environment to detect the presence of predators. They do not stare at predators, except to assess their intent and decide on a means of escape.

Cattle, sheep, goats, and horses are prey animals. Their primary defense tactic is to flee. They rarely attack, doing so only when fleeing is not an option. Prey animals seek protection in groups. Horses, cattle, and hogs should not be separated entirely from herd members, but they should be moved in small groups to avoid mob action by a large group. Sheep can be moved safely in larger groups.

Common situations that can elicit fear in prey animals are shiny objects, including sparkling reflections on water or shiny metal. High-pitched sounds are often made by prey captured by a predator, and therefore clanging, squeaky, or hissing noises, such as gates, squeeze chutes, dandling chains, exhaust fans, and air hoses, are frightening to prey animals. Rapid movements evoke fear, such as blowing plastic bags and fluttering banners or flags. Jerky movements by handlers can scare prey animals, as can fan blades that are turned off but blow with the wind. Anything that is unfamiliar in familiar surroundings can be frightening, including clothing, paper bags or cups, different flooring, different panels, puddles of water, and grates in an alleyway. Darkness and blinding glare is avoided by prey animals since either can impair their safety from predators.

Perception of handlers as predators or prey

A handler's body language may unintentionally mimic prey or predator behavior. Humans have predator eyes, directed forward. Because of this, staring at prey animals is perceived as a threat. Moving directly toward them is the pushing approach of a pack predator designed to encourage them to run before a kill. A human standing motionless is like that of a stalking predator, especially if the prey animals are being stared at. The least threatening actions are to have relaxed movements while approaching at an angle without looking directly at the animal. This is the demeanor of another grazing prey animal.

Dogs interpret a human running away from them as prey behavior. Staring directly at dogs or standing over them is considered a challenge for dominance. Playing with cats by wiggling a finger or toe can unintentionally invite a predator attack to a hand or foot.

ANIMAL HIERARCHY. SOCIAL DOMINANCE

Each animal is an individual, the sum of a unique combination of genes and past experiences. General assumptions about behavior might be made based on species, age, gender, and breed, but an individual animal may act and react in a unique fashion.

Nearly all domestic animals prefer to live in groups. Within animal groups there is a hierarchy, a social ladder. With birds this is referred to as the pecking order. Knowing the social rank of an individual animal mingling in a group can be helpful in determining the best means of handling or restraining a particular animal. When waiting for a group of gathered animals to settle, it is a good practice to assess the social interactions within a group.

Many animal behaviorists dislike the terms *dominance*, *dominate*, and *dominant* when applied to social rank among animals or to a handler of animals. To some, these terms imply forcing actions upon another individual, although the root word, from Latin, is *dominus*, which means "master". Being a master of animals denotes social rank but does not necessitate the use of force to acquire or maintain that status.

> Dominance in handling refers to social rank. Social dominance does not require fear or pain, but it does require leadership ability.

Being dominant requires the control of resources, such as access to food and movement of others. Dominant status is conveyed primarily by demeanor.

Force that inflicts pain is reserved for self-defense or defense of the species, such as conflicts during mating seasons. An effective animal handler must be dominant by his or her demeanor, not by applied force or micromanagement, to the animals being handled for the safety of all. On the other hand, a handler of large animals must be prepared and willing to exert force as a last resort for self-defense, as in the case of a charge, or threatened charge, by a large dog, bull, ram, buck, stallion, protective nursing mare or cow, or in similar situations.

Dominance within a group is generally related to height, weight, gender, age, or in the case of ruminants, the size of their horns. The oldest ewe is the most dominant sheep and the oldest doe goat is the herd leader. Dominant animals are identifiable by the deference given them by others, not by displays of aggression and force. Dominant animals are more calm and confident than others and will seek a position physically above others. For example, dominant horses prefer to be on rises in the land, dominant cats on ledges, and dominating dogs will attempt to stand over submissive dogs. Dominant individuals within a group of prey animals will seek the center of the group. Higher social rank is usually established by demeanor with direct stares, ritualized aggressive postures, vocalizing, and fake attacks without attempts to cause serious injury, such as boxing in young stallions and wrestling between young dogs.

The previous status of a group member, or that of an animal handler, can be altered within a group of animals if the demeanor of the group member or handler is different from usual. Acting ill, injured, or less confident, as with advanced age, can reduce the status of an individual within a group. Handlers who attempt to manage animal groups while ill, after being injured, or when acting uncharacteristically timid may be challenged by a group, particularly if the animal group is swine or poultry.

SOCIALIZATION WITH HUMANS

Handling animals gently, beginning early when their eyes have begun to open, is believed by some animal handlers to have a profound beneficial effect in handling these animals with less stress later in life. The process is often referred to as imprinting, although true imprinting is bonding with a mother and the acceptance of the proximity of members of the same species.

The length of the critical period for socializing animals to have less fear toward humans is related to the degree of species domestication. This period occurs later and longer in predators than in prey animals. Dogs, the longest domesticated species, have the longest period of critical socialization: up to 4 months of age. In contrast, wolves must be handled in the first 14 days of life to have lasting effects on their social behavior with humans. The period for domestic cats is up to 7 weeks of age.

There is a risk associated with prey animals becoming socialized with humans. If done improperly in a manner that startles or induces fear, the young animal may develop and retain a fear of being around humans. Exaggerated efforts to imprint large prey animals such as horses, cattle, and llamas may cause them to lose their respect for humans, and thereby make them increasingly dangerous as they mature.

More important than the imprinting of newborns is the routine handling and grooming of the mothers of young animals, particularly in the first 5 days of the young animal's life after its eyes have opened, so that it can see the mother responding to humans in a relaxed manner. The young foal, calf, or pig will be profoundly affected for life by how the mother responds to being handled by humans.

FLIGHT ZONE AND POINT OF BALANCE

Members of all species have invisible borders, *flight zones*, around them in the presence of possible danger. For example, the typical person without training in handling venomous snakes has an invisible surrounding border or zone such that if it is invaded by a poisonous snake the person will flee. The diameter of an animal's flight zone for humans varies by the animal species involved, its breed, the amount of prior exposure to humans, the quality of prior contact with humans, and the age of the animal when exposed to humans.

Flight zones are beneficial for handlers when moving groups of animals. The least stressful means of moving cattle forward is to calmly and quietly approach their flight zone behind their *point of balance*, also called the *drive line*, which is an imaginary line just behind the shoulder. The movement produced is like moving a positive pole of a magnet toward the positive pole of another. The approaching magnet at some point repels the other. On the other hand, if an animal is confined or physically restrained with a human in its flight zone, an effort to escape may occur, such as struggling, climbing or jumping fences, rearing, and kicking. Flight zones are larger for more dominant individuals. The zone is flexible and will shrink if the animal is very thirsty and must be in closer proximity to a human than usual to get to water.

Fight or flight arousal of prey animals is increased by hunger, sexual arousal, loud noises (barking, stock whips), sight of dogs, beating or electric prods, and unfamiliar objects or people. Familiarity with animals to be handled should be fostered in advance of need whenever possible. Handlers should walk among young livestock to habituate them to seeing and being near people. Range cattle in southern states often have a wider flight zone than northern range cattle, as northern cattle are fed hay in proximity to handlers during winter, thereby shrinking their flight zone. Along with being desensitized to humans, cattle, sheep, and goats should be desensitized to horses and dogs if either will be used in herding.

Invading a flight zone does not always result in flight of the animal. Some may be willing to fight and some may experience tonic immobility, i.e. they freeze with fear. *Freezing* is more common in prey animals. In those, freezing may be a dissociative state used to feign death and then attempt to escape, or be a resolution of impending death. One reason some dogs or cats are quieter after they are caged or kenneled without an owner present is that they are freezing from fear. Less severe dissociative behaviors that can be induced by fear are intense grooming in cats and repetitive yawning in dogs. Dogs and horses may exhibit an "adrenaline shake off" from a relief of fear.

SENSES AND BEHAVIOR

Olfactory (smell)

The sense of smell is more acute in all domestic animals than in humans. Animals monitor the odor of urine, feces, sweat, breath, and special skin organs,

such as anal glands in dogs, to identify others, assess their status in a reproductive cycle, and determine their social rank.

Animals are sometimes said to be able to smell fear in handlers who are unconfident. In the case of humans, animals "smelling" fear is probably detection of purposeless, unconfident, or hesitant body language. However, within the same species and same social group, animals can identify more submissive animals by smell. Because of this, handlers should always handle the most dominant animal in a group first, such as the largest boar in a herd of swine, or the smell of subordinate members on the handler may make the dominant member harder to handle. Cologne or other pungent cosmetic odors can also cause animals to resist handling and restraint.

Dogs

Dogs have the keenest sense of smell of any domestic animal. Some communications among dogs are by emitted pheromones from their body by secretions of saliva, urine, feces, and anal sacs.

> Dogs can detect odors that are 10,000–100,000 times fainter than what the human nose can detect.

Dogs can be trained to detect explosives, corpses, drugs, and other odoriferous objects by using their extraordinary ability to smell. The olfactory membrane of dogs is up to 150 sq cm, compared with cats (14 sq cm) and humans (4 sq cm). The olfactory area of the dog's brain is 14 times as large and 100 times more sensitive than that of humans. Humans have 6 million olfactory receptors in their nasal passages, while dogs have 300 million receptors. Dogs are capable of detecting airborne particles in 10 parts per billion to 500 parts per trillion.

Cats

Cats have scent glands under the chin, corners of the mouth, side of the forehead, and between their toes. They also emit odors by urine and feces. Urine spraying and odor from their front pads, which is left when scratching objects, are used to mark a cat's territory. The small cheek glands, near the corners of the mouth, are used to leave odors after rubbing on objects, including people, that they perceive as their territory. Facial pheromone has been synthesized and is used as a form of aromatherapy. Cats' olfactory epithelium is 14 times more developed than humans.

Reptiles and birds

Reptiles become excited at the smell of food. If the smell is on a handler's hands, the odor can entice a reptile to bite a hand.

The respiratory system of birds does not provide many of the protections of the respiratory system of mammals against airborne insults. Birds are particularly sensitive to odors and some can be lethal to birds. Canaries have been used to monitor for harmful gasses in mines.

Horses

Horse herd members defecate where they smell their dominant herd members defecate. These toilet areas are sacrificed from grazing, except when in desperation. They also use fecal smell to find their way home or to join other horses.

Cattle

Cattle have an excellent sense of smell, which they use to trace the trail of their calves and to find the right plants to eat. They can distinguish which is the most dominant animal and other members of the herd by their odors.

Vomeronasal organ

The vomeronasal organ, also called *Jacobson's organ*, is located in the roof of the mouth. It consists of two sacs that are connected to the nasal cavity by fine ducts. When domestic mammals smell sexual odors, many will lift their upper lip and open their mouth, a behavior called the *flehmen response*. The purpose of the flehmen response is to increase the opening of the ducts that carry the smell to the nasal cavity and the olfactory membrane. This enhances the detection of the odor.

Male horses do a flehmen response when smelling urine from mares in estrus. Cats "gape" (mouth open with tongue placed behind upper incisors) when smelling other cats' urine. Cattle will collect odors in moisture droplets on their muzzle, which are then licked off with the tongue and detected by

the vomeronasal organ. Snakes smell by using their forked tongue to collect particles in the air. The tongue then pulls the particles into the mouth where they are dipped into the vomeronasal pits in the roof of the mouth.

Aromatherapy for handling animals

Pheromones are chemicals used for communication by smell. Natural pheromones are well-established important communicators of individual identity and reproductive status in many, if not all, species. Synthetic pheromones and essential oils have been purported to be effective means of calming dogs and cats. Aromatherapy is a form of alternative therapy similar to nutraceuticals in that it is not required to prove efficacy to be marketed. Claims of efficacy are usually based on anecdotal statements or small studies without the sufficient controls and independent evaluations required of pharmaceuticals. Aromatherapy may be more of a means of non-threatening distraction than a mind-altering drug. Those that appear to affect cat behavior have a short duration of effects, less than 30 minutes.

Catnip

Nepetalactone is a volatile oil from the catnip plant (*Nepeta cataria*), a member of the mint family. It is an attractant for about three out of four cats. The playful activity it evokes in cats temporarily causes distraction from other non-threatening stimuli.

Feline synthetic facial pheromone

Facial glands in cats produce a pheromone involved in bunting, facial rubbing to mark possession. A synthetic facial pheromone of cats in an alcohol solution is a popular aromatherapy intended to calm cats.

Dog-appeasing pheromone

Dog-appeasing pheromone (DAP) is produced by the skin of the mammary gland of dogs after giving birth and during the nursing period. DAP is believed to aid in bonding pups to the mother. Synthetic DAP is an aromatherapy purported to calm adult dogs.

Lavender and chamomile oil

Oils from the plants lavender and chamomile are purported to have a calming effect on small animals.

Hearing

Sounds are an important communication method and stimuli that warn animals of potential danger. Animals are able to distinguish each member of their group's voices. Similarly, they know each of their handlers' voices. They are able to recognize and associate sounds that occur with feeding, distress, and breeding, among other things.

There are three aspects to hearing sounds: intensity, frequency, and directional ability. Intensity (amplitude) is measured on a logarithmic scale in units called decibels. Frequency is the number of vibrations per second, and measured in hertz (Hz).

Animals, particularly prey animals, are distressed by suspicious or loud noises. Small animals should be spoken to in a low-pitched, calm voice. Livestock should only be exposed to calm and relatively quiet sounds when being handled or moved. Handling facilities will require regular maintenance to reduce unnecessary noises.

Intensity

Soft, low-toned sounds are soothing to animals. High-pitched sounds are associated with distress signals and are stressful to prey animals. Conversely, predators (dog, cats) may become more aggressive if exposed to loud noises. Yelling with a high-pitched voice causes prey animals (horses, cattle) to panic and attempt to flee. Soothing background music can calm animals and is often used in kennels, milking parlors, and horse stables. Raucous music is not beneficial to animal handling. To reduce fear in livestock, it helps to attach rubber bumpers to metal gates and lubricate hinges, fans, and other moving equipment to control high-pitched noises during handling.

Yelling and waving arms should not be used to move animals, especially if they are in confinement. Cattle can be moved more efficiently and quietly by using canes, whips, or paddles as visual extensions of the handler's body without contacting the animal's body.

Birds have excellent hearing and pitch discrimination, which allows them to analyze sound. Their ears are funnel-shaped to concentrate sound waves, and are located behind and below their eyes, covered by soft feathers.

Frequency

The auditory range of humans is approximately 20–20,000 Hz, while dogs have a range to around 45,000 Hz, and cats can hear up to 75,000 Hz. Horses and livestock have upper ranges of 35,000–40,000 Hz. Rodents have a higher upper range of 75,000–80,000 Hz, similar to that of their chief predator, the domestic cat. Birds' range of hearing is similar to humans. Lizards react best to low frequency sounds below 5,000 Hz. Geckos are the most vocal lizards, using distress calls if threatened.

All domestic mammalian animals can hear higher frequency sounds than humans.

Snakes have internal ears that detect sounds only when a sound causes low-frequency vibrations. They feel the vibrations with their jaw from the surface that they are lying on. The vibrations are then transmitted to their internal ears. Snake charmers with a flute rely on the visual movement of the flute, not the sound of music, to mesmerize snakes.

Direction

The ability to hear can be enhanced by adjusting the external ear position toward the sound source. Ear position is an indication of expected behavior. Horses and cats turn their external ears in the direction of their current point of attention. A horse's ears moved toward a handler indicates that the handler has the horse's attention. Laid-back ears can be a sign of aggressiveness in horses, cats, and llamas. However, horses will lay their ears back when highly focused on any task, including working with great intensity, such as running hard or being intensely serious about wanting to eat grain. Laid-back ears in dogs and cats can be an indication of fear.

Erect external ears are best at detecting sound direction and amplifying sound to the ear drum. Dog breeds with erect ears are the most often used as sentry animals to guard property. Some breed standards expect ears to be trimmed so that they can be made erect to assist hearing. Although both have highly movable external ears, predators can locate the direction of sound more accurately than large prey animals.

Auditory communications

All domestic animals use sound as one means of communication, although not much is known about vocal communications among animals. The most that is known involves communication in dogs, cats, and horses.

Infantile sounds used in dogs and cats include meows (cats) and whimpering (dogs). Warning sounds are the growl or bark in dogs and hissing in cats. Eliciting or calling sounds in cats are meowing and howling. Withdrawal sounds of dogs are yelps, and in cats the sounds are screaming or chattering. Sounds of pleasure are moans and grunts in dogs. In cats, sounds associated with pleasure are purring and chirruping.

Horses neigh to acknowledge the location of other horses. Whinnies are louder and more questioning of location. A nicker is a welcoming sound. At feeding time a nicker means hurry up and do not forget about me. A snort is an alert to all around of a possible danger. A blow is a strong exhalation signaling a building of excitement. Squeals are intended to startle. Mares often squeal to tell another horse to back off. Grunts are an exclamation of extra effort. Screams mean extreme pain. A roar is a warning sign of an agitated stallion.

Cattle moo to convey their location. Grunts are used by new mothers as part of the bonding stage in the first days after giving birth. They use a louder call, a bellow, to locate their calf when separated, warn of possible danger, or express other reasons for distress. Snorting is a sign of agitation and may signal an attack from an angry nursing mother or from an irritated bull.

Camelids communicate vocally. Dams hum to their cria (babies). A clicking sound is made to warn of potential danger. A grumbling sound is made if irritated. They will scream if in extreme danger or pain.

Hogs grunt frequently. When excited, the grunts are short in duration. Long grunts are used when content or calling to establish location of other hogs. They squeal when disturbed and scream when hurt or frightened. Dominant hogs will bark at a subordinate to make them move, establishing or re-establishing their superior social rank.

Chickens have extensive vocal communications. Turkey hens bark when in an unfamiliar area to keep the flock together. A putting-sound alert is added if a threat may be near. Male turkeys (toms) make a gurgling gobble sound to advertise their presence to the hens, and if intending to attack, toms will make a purring sound.

Vision

Vision is the primary sense used for detecting danger for many species. Impaired vision can affect an animal's tractability. For example, diurnal birds are more easily handled in subdued lighting. Blindfolds can be effective means to improve the ability to handle horses, lizards, and ratites in some instances.

The sense of vision is adapted for a species' needs, particularly the needs of defense and communications. Visual ability encompasses field of view, depth perception (stereopsis, i.e. judgement of distances), acuity (focus), perception of motion, and color differentiation.

Field of View

The field of view in predators is narrower than in prey animals. Dogs have a horizontal field of view of approximately 240 degrees, slightly wider than in humans. Cats have a horizontal field of view similar to dogs but a wider vertical field of view due to their vertical pupils.

The eyes of grazing prey animals (horses, cattle, sheep, goats, rabbits) are located on the side of their head and protrude slightly in comparison to predator eyes. The side location and protrusion of their eyes allow grazing prey animals even greater horizontal peripheral vision. The horizontal vision of grazing animals is approximately 200 degrees or more with their heads raised and up to about 340 degrees with their head lowered in grazing position (**Figure 2.1**). The distance and peripheral vision of swine, a prey and predator, is poor.

Prey animals have both monocular and binocular vision. Prey animals' eyes work independently of each other (monocular vision), except when looking ahead with binocular vision in the attempt to perceive depth. The binocular range of horses is 60–70 degrees straight in front. Only monocular vision is used for monitoring threats when grazing.

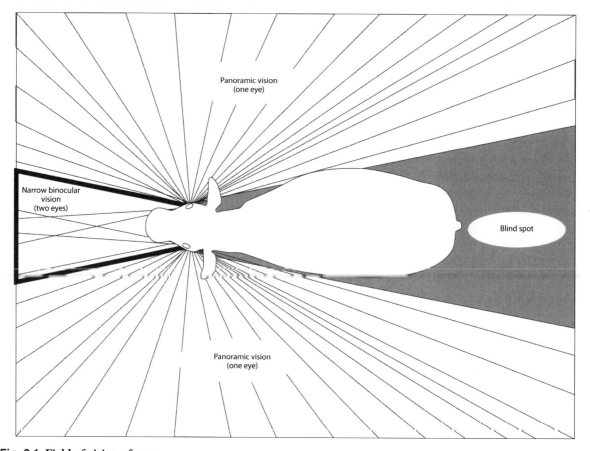

Fig. 2.1 Field of vision of a cow.

Pupil shape and light accommodation

The pupil of prey animals adapted to living on open grassland is often horizontally oval, which further enhances peripheral vision. However, vertical vision (being able to see above or below) is less in grazing prey animals than in humans and predators. Prey animals' range of vertical vision is only about 60 degrees. To properly place their feet on unfamiliar ground or to step into unfamiliar water, they have to lower their head. Horizontal pupils enable prey animals to see vertical lines better than horizontal lines, while cats, having vertical pupils, can see horizontal lines better. Containment fencing with more vertical lines is a more effective psychological barrier for grazing animals than the more common fences that have long sections of horizontal planks or rails.

Snakes, like cats, are low-profile hunters. Many snakes have vertical pupils, like cats, which may permit an enhanced ability to focus through thin vertical gaps in tall grass where they frequently hunt.

Taller predators, such as dogs, lions, and tigers, have circular pupils.

Dilation and constriction of the pupil is the primary means of accommodating to changes in lighting. Diurnal livestock species have pupils that accommodate slowly compared with humans. Bird pupils and pupils in nocturnal animals, such as cats, accommodate relatively rapidly.

Depth perception

Depth perception requires overlapping fields of vision from each eye. The central overlap that permits depth perception in dogs and cats is about one-half that of humans. Dogs and cats also have limited peripheral vision. Humans and predator animals have binocular vision. They always focus on objects with both eyes. Livestock have monocular vision and can focus on objects on both sides of their body at the same time. When looking forward, animals with monocular vision can view the same object with both eyes (binocular vision), which is needed for depth perception. Horses have an overlap of 65 degrees but 350 degrees of panoramic vision. Extreme panoramic vision has poor acuity but detects motion easily.

Horses and most other grazing prey animals have good distance vision, especially for moving objects, but their ability for depth vision and ability to focus on near objects is slow and poor, requiring them to face the object of interest. In prey animals, shadows appear as holes and water depth cannot be determined. Because of this, it is important to keep surfaces for them to walk on dry and lit by diffuse, shadow-eliminating lighting. Loading ramps that slant upward are easier for grazing prey animals to negotiate than steps. Consistent color, shading, and texture to prey animal handling floors are important to keep them from balking. A change in the color, shading, or texture of the surface of flooring will cause the animals to stop to reassess whether there is a change in the depth.

Grazing animals need to see potential predators while grazing. Because of this, their retinas have the best distance perception with light entering through the top of their eye. To facilitate good focus on where they step and the condition of areas to graze, light entering the lower portion of their eyes gives the best near-vision perception.

Grazing animals have a cone-shaped blind spot 4 ft [1.2 m] directly in front of their face. They also cannot see directly below their jaw. Objects that suddenly appear from a blind spot may startle them, particularly horses.

Acuity and perception of motion

Visual acuity is the ability to see details. Domestic mammals do not have the visual acuity of humans. Near vision is relatively poor. Normal humans have 20/20 acuity. Dogs are estimated to be 20/75 (normal humans can see clearly at 75 ft [23 m] with the clarity that dogs see at 20 ft [6 m]). Cats have 20/100 acuity, and horses have 20/33. Birds have exceedingly good visual acuity. The lens in birds is flexible, which aids their ability to rapidly focus on objects. Visual acuity of reptiles is poor. However, reptile vision depends on the species' lifestyle. For example, arboreal snakes have better vision than terrestrial snakes that burrow.

In most predators the area of greatest acuity is a circular area in the retina, called the *fovea* or *area centralis*. To visually evaluate the greatest detail, predators have to hold their head still and concentrate the image on the fovea. In contrast, grazing prey animals have a visual streak, an elongated band that runs across the retina. This permits grazing animals to better detect motion in their peripheral vision.

Color differentiation

The retina of the eye contains two types of light receptors: rods and cones. All mammals have more rods than cones and all other mammals have more than humans. For example, humans have nine rods per cone while horses have 20 rods per cone. Cones perceive objects best in bright light and can distinguish various colors. The area centralis or visual streak contains the highest concentration of cones and the lowest concentration of rods.

> **Most animals see better in low light than do humans but perceive fewer colors.**

Humans have three types of cones, which permits trichromatic color vision (tones of red, green, and yellow). Most domestic animals that are active during daylight have two types of retinal cones and dichromatic color vision (yellow and blue). They cannot distinguish colors in the range of 510–590 nm, which is the red wavelength. Dichromatic color vision in animals is similar to vision in humans with red-green color blindness. Animals with dichromatic vision appear to see blue and yellow best, and have trouble perceiving red and green. With dichromatic vision, red is dark and green is light gray. Dichromatic vision may aid in seeing sudden movements and objects in low light. Nocturnal mammals may be unable to distinguish colors.

Reptiles and tropical birds have four types of retinal cones and may perceive more colors, or colors in dim light, than humans can see. Birds can see ultraviolet, blue, green, and red. Bird vision peaks in the orange–red portion of the spectrum.

Night vision

Retinal rod cells are responsible for magnifying light impulses. Rods are able to detect low-intensity light and motion, and can differentiate shades of gray, but they provide poor resolution. Most domestic animals, especially nocturnal foragers (horses) or predators (cats), have many more rods than do humans. Species that are scotopic (having good vision in dim light) or nocturnal also have a *tapetum lucidum* (a reflective structure in the retina that increases the gathering of light). This results in superior night vision and more intense differences in grays, plus a better detection of motion. Horses and most other grazing animals are believed to see up to four times better at night, after accommodating to lighting, than can humans. The tapetum increases light detection at night up to seven times in cats.

Swine have forward-placed eyes, round pupils, and no tapetum lucidum. They are also dichromats. Swine are also nearsighted and cannot see well in dim light. Their depth perception is good for close objects, which aids their quest for food on forest floors.

Pupil shape affects the concentration of visual light. Diurnal species have round or horizontal pupils. The vertical pupil slit in cats provides some protection from bright light, but is able to quickly dilate in rapid darkness.

Tactile (touch)

Animals communicate with each other with a range of touching. Soothing or grooming touches reinforce the bonding within a group. Quick metered blows or bites are to reinforce early visual or vocal warnings of needed behavior change of another member of the group.

Excessively light touching by handlers may be perceived as fear by horses and cattle. Moderately firm stroking conveys a better impression of confident leadership of a good handler. Light to moderate slapping will first be perceived by horses as aggression, but they should be gradually desensitized to pats and gentle slaps for the safety of a handler, who might slap horseflies to protect himself or the horse, or unintentionally bump a horse.

Animals can feel vibrations of the ground through their feet, which is useful when herd members try to intimidate one another, initiate play activities, or signal the need to escape from danger. Snakes feel vibrations in the range of 150–450 Hz. Surface vibrations are transmitted via their jaw to their inner ear, enabling an auditory sensation.

Whiskers (*vibrissae*) are large, long, well-innervated hairs surrounded by a vascular sinus. Most species have vibrissae on the upper (maxillary) lips. Dogs also have supraorbital (above the eyes), genial (cheeks), and interramal (between the angles of the mandible) vibrissae. Cats also have carpal vibrissae. The function of vibrissae is to feel spatial limits, air movements, and movement of captured prey. Vibrissae on the muzzle of horses is trimmed for some show events. This can alter normal spatial sensations, causing some horses to temporarily quit eating or drinking.

Body heat

Some snakes (pit vipers, pythons, and some boa constrictors) have infrared receptors for tracking warm-blooded mammals. The receptors may be between the nostrils and eyes, as with pit vipers, or just below the nostrils, which is the case in pythons. This special organ can detect temperature changes of 0.002–0.003°C. The snake's brain is believed to form images from infrared rays in a way similar to visual images from the eyes.

RESISTANCE BEHAVIORS

Resistance to handling may be manifested as avoidance or aggression. Aggressive behavior can be caused by irritability or pain.

Maternal aggression

Animal mothers will protect young when they are not willing to protect themselves. This is most acute after birth to the time of peak milk production. In dogs, this is the first 3 weeks after birth. A cry from a young animal of any species may precipitate an attack on the handler from the animal's parents or other adults of the group. Before handling nursing pigs, sows should be separated from the pigs at a distance that none of the sows can hear the pigs squeal. Conversely, foals should be kept within sight of mares or both will become frantic. Female rabbits become fiercely protective of nesting boxes. Females must be taken to bucks for mating because they will attack bucks taken to their box.

Pain-related aggression

Pain-related aggression is a natural response to noxious stimuli. A major cause of people being bitten by dogs is that they trying to capture or move an injured dog that is in pain. Pain from saddle sores or arthritis are common causes for formerly mild-mannered horses to act resentful of handling or being ridden.

Anticipation of possible pain can induce fear-aggression. Frequent gentle handling of all parts of an animal's body, with no other purpose than training, can desensitize animals to anticipated pain aggression.

Predatory aggression

Predatory aggression can interfere with handling. Retreating from an aggressive dog, especially in the case of children running from them, can be perceived as fleeing prey and aggravate aggression. This is the same reason for the many dog bites suffered by joggers and bicyclists.

Predatory aggression in cats is characterized by a low posture, crawling, and freezing in place. Playing with cats by inviting them to pounce on wiggling fingers or toes can stimulate predatory aggression.

Territorial and possession aggression

Dogs or cats may establish their cage, run, yard, or family car as personal territory and become aggressive if they anticipate being separated from their territory. Even in veterinary hospitals, after they are maintained in a cage for a short period they can become protective of their cage. Some dog breeds are more prone to territorial aggression, such as Rottweilers and German shepherds, which have been selectively bred for the trait of territorial aggression.

Territorial and possession aggression are common causes of dog bites.

Protection of food while eating is a common possession aggression among dogs. Dogs should be trained to control that tendency while they are in their critical socialization period prior to 16 weeks of age. Horses assert dominance within their herd over individual feeding territory. Hay piles have to be separated into piles equal to or exceeding the number of horses to prevent or minimize possession aggression. Hogs become more aggressive at feeding time, especially when feeding times are unpredictable.

Hamsters are aggressive in protecting their territory. Males have scent glands on their back near the hips that are used for territorial marking. Adult golden hamsters need to be housed separately to prevent fighting. The less common Russian hamster can be housed in small groups if raised in the same small group as when young.

Fear-induced aggression

Fear-induced aggression in dogs or cats is very common in veterinary hospitals. Fear-based body language in dogs is a fixed stare, rigid neck, head lowered, ears laid back, lips pulled back, and tail between the legs. Cats crouch with their ears back, wrap their tail close to their body, raise the hair on their back, and hiss combined with a low rumbling, throaty sound. When the fear-inducing stimulus (a person) backs off, the aggression is rewarded and the animal will intensify its aggression the next time it feels threatened.

Inter-male aggression

Inter-male aggression can endanger handlers. Bulls, boars, rams, bucks, and stallions are particularly dangerous during mating season. Female animals in estrus will intensify male agitation and aggression. Male mice, rabbits, or bearded dragon should not be housed with other males of their species because of the risk of inter-male aggression. Feral tomcats may kill young kittens from another male when taking over a new clowder (group of cats).

Dominance aggression

A major factor of establishing dominance in a group is body size. For example, dogs attempting to dominate another will raise the hair on their back and elevate their stance in front to appear larger. Larger size means more food has been needed and successfully attained in a competitive environment. Larger individuals are more dominant than small individuals of the same breed, and larger breeds are more dominant to smaller breeds.

Male sex hormones are also major influences on displays of dominance. Castration prior to puberty does not eliminate the possibility of dominance aggression, but it significantly reduces it. Post-pubertal castration effects are less impressive since adult male behavior may become ingrained on the nervous system before the removal of male hormone stimuli. Bulls display dominance aggression by pawing the ground, shaking their head, and displaying the silhouette of their side. A bull that are ready to attack will stand with his side displayed to demonstrate how big he is to his opponent. A bull that charges a person in an open pasture should be culled and not sold at auction, which would put others at risk.

Orphaned male grazing animals should be castrated early or placed in a social group with their own species by 6 weeks of age. Stallions or bulls are more easily handled if they are raised with other horses or cattle, including older males of their species. Older or larger males teach the challengers that they cannot easily bully others. Dominant males learn as they gain their social position that unnecessary fighting risks serious injury. If raising young males together, sufficient room is necessary to allow subdominant males to escape a losing fight.

A dog that is aggressive in an attempt to establish dominance over a human is dangerous, and must be handled initially with higher levels of restraint by experienced handlers. Dominance aggression is more common in some dog breeds than others. For example, it is relatively common in spaniels. Signs of dominance aggression in dogs appear in early adulthood (1–3 years of age) and are manifested when guarding food or toys, being overprotective of some family members, or growling and snapping when told "no!"

Many owners will not risk a young stallion or bull possibly getting hurt during socialization with older, larger animals and will raise them in isolation from their own species. However, once the stallion or bull raised with his own kind reaches adult size, his social behavior is nearly completely set for life if it has been reinforced with continued good handling and opportunities to socialize with others of his own species.

When stallions must be kept in stalls, the stall should be as large as possible and as visually open as possible with good ventilation. At a minimum, they should be turned out daily in stallion-appropriate (at least 7 ft [2.1 m] tall) pens where they can see other horses and be provided forms of environmental enrichment.

Punishment or domination techniques, such as holding a dog on his back and staring at him (alpha-rolls), often make a fear-aggressive animal more aggressive. Dogs and horses tend to seek human attention. Ignoring their attempts to get their handler's attention is the first step in establishing handler dominance, followed by offering attention on the handler's terms and praise only if obedient to the handler's commands. Performing simple commands, such as "sit" or "down" for dogs and yielding a horse's hindquarters or backing it, place them in submissive positions and reinforce a handler's status as being their leader, which, in turn, increases his safety in handling them.

Well-adjusted dominant animals only become aggressive if they have to protect themselves or their group. Within a species, animals do not risk serious injury or death to establish dominance, with the exception of mature males during breeding seasons.

The social status among cattle is affected by age, weight, size of horns, sex, and breed. As with other species, adult males are more dominant than cows. Larger breeds of dairy cattle are dominant to smaller breeds, but breed dominance in beef cattle is not as closely linked to body size.

The size of a hog is directly related to its degree of exerting dominance within a group.

SPECIES DIFFERENCES IN AGGRESSION AND AVOIDANCE

Dogs

The dominance posture in dogs is head up, tail up, front end held high, rear end possibly slightly crouched, teeth maybe bared, and a fixed stare (**Figure 2.2**). The submissive posture is front end lowered, eyes not making direct contact with the handler's eyes, tail between the legs; submissive urination or defecation may occur, and the dog may roll on its back to expose its abdomen (**Figure 2.3**).

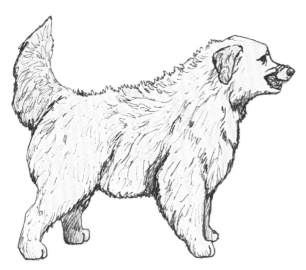

Fig. 2.2 Aggressive posture in a dog.

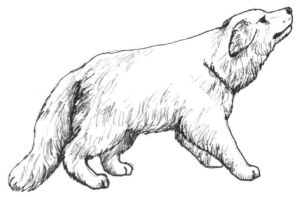

Fig. 2.3 Submissive posture in a dog.

Some dogs are aggressive in the presence of their owner; others, especially dogs strongly bonded to one person, may be more aggressive away from their owner.

Cats

Cats have an uncanny speed over short distances that allows them to stalk prey and then run and pounce for a rapid kill before the prey can escape. A common sign of irritability or anxiousness is flicking the end of the tail. Most cats will attempt to escape rather than fight with a handler. They are escape artists, so all exits from a handling room must be closed before handling cats. They can be highly aggressive if they feel endangered and trapped.

Small mammals

Most aggression and efforts to dominate are within a small mammal's own species and are related to breeding behaviors.

Companion birds

Companion birds seek high perches to establish dominance. Handlers should not permit companion birds to sit on their head or shoulders since this encourages dominance behavior toward the handler.

Reptiles

All reptiles regularly shed their skin by a process called *ecdysis*. Snakes typically shed their skin in its entirety at one shedding, which can impair their sight and make them less tolerant of handling. Shedding begins as a roughing of the skin while the belly turns a pink color. The skin around and over the eyes, called the spectacle scales, become opaque or blue colored. The shedding skin breaks at the mouth, and the skin is usually shed as one piece. Rough surfaces need to be provided in their containment enclosure to facilitate shedding. Young snakes shed every 2–3 months. Adult snakes shed just a couple times per year.

Lizards indigenous to arid lands are more docile than iguanas, which come from tropical forests, but bearded lizards, which are from deserts, will puff out their throat like a spiny beard if threatened.

Horses

Horses kept in stalls and those maintained without direct interaction with other horses are most likely to be aggressive. Stallions and horses that are handled in small confinements, or with training techniques that restrict natural movement, are more likely to be aggressive. Mares with foals can be very protective even if they are docile in other situations. Snappily swishing the tail from side to side can be a sign of frustration and irritation.

Cattle

Dairy bulls are the most dangerous of all domestic animals. They are unpredictable and extremely strong. They will inflict injury by crushing, goring, pinning to the ground, or smashing the victim. Dairy bulls are typically hand (bottle)-raised and so lose their flight zone and thus their natural respect for humans. Beef bulls, although also dangerous, are more predictable and respectful of human space. Being raised with other bulls and cows, beef bulls concentrate more on establishing their dominance over cattle, not people.

Dairy cows are usually handled frequently and become docile if handled well. Beef cows vary depending on frequency and quality of handling. Nursing cows are more likely to be aggressive, whether beef or dairy breeds.

Small ruminants

Sheep defend themselves by tightly flocking together and moving as a unit. Rams may attempt to butt handlers and can be dangerous particularly during breeding season. Dominance in goats depends on their age, gender, body size, and whether they have horns; and if they do, the larger the size of horns, the greater a goat's social status.

Swine

If not socialized properly or deprived of social interactions, boars can be very aggressive. Nursing sows are always aggressive if they hear pigs squeal. Young pigs should be penned in small groups since they like to huddle, climb, and shove each other. Introducing one new pig or hog into an established group will often initiate life-threatening aggression by the dominant members of the group; a group of new pigs or hogs can be more safely introduced to another group than an individual.

Poultry

Chicken pullets and turkey poults, in extreme confinement, have their beaks trimmed because of territorial aggression and the risk of feather picking and cannibalism. Turkeys and some chicken hens can become aggressive toward handlers who are timid in their body language when handling a flock.

TRAINING METHODS FOR HANDLING ANIMALS

Training animals to be handled should be the major part of preparing young animals to become socialized with humans. The most effective means of

Table 2.2 **The foundation for success at handling and training animals**
• Selection of a young animal that is an offspring of parents that have been willingly receptive to their own training
• A mother that has been properly socialized to humans and is quietly handled in the offspring's presence (observational training of offspring)
• Gentle repeated handling of the young animal during its critical socialization period

training depend on the species and what is to be learned. Success at training is dependent on animal genetics, observational learning from its mother, and the quality of handling an animal receives prior to puberty (*Table 2.2*).

Either *positive reinforcement* (adding a reward such as food treats) or *negative reinforcement* (removal of a noxious stimulus) are used to instill trained behaviors. The timing of either reinforcement is critical, and should occur within 3 seconds of the behavior to be reinforced with a treat or discouraged with a reprimand. Late negative reinforcement becomes simply punishment, and this can lead to the animal becoming aggressively defensive or developing an attitude of helplessness that inhibits further learning.

Small predatory companion animals (dogs and cats) can be trained effectively with positive reinforcement. Their natural behavior is to investigate (hunt) sources of food and be rewarded by food when the hunt is successful. Misbehavior within their social group is corrected by immediate warning (a growl or hiss) followed, if needed, by a sharp, brief vocal or physical reprimand by a more socially dominant member of the group. The reprimands must not be injurious, and proper timing is essential. Most effective handlers emulate this with food treats for desired behavior and sharp, brief reprimands, vocal or physical, such as a tug on a training collar when needed, for inattention or misbehavior. Treats for positive reinforcement of dogs should be the size of a pea or grape and be able to be eaten quickly. It should be a treat that the dog does not get at any other time. Food treats should be gradually supplanted with tactile and voice rewards, particularly if a dog is to become a working dog, guardian, or support companion. Negative reinforcement for dogs should not be so harsh as to lead to avoidance behaviors, such as avoiding collars or being unwilling to engage the handler visually. Aversive behaviors are commonly associated with shock-collar training.

Large prey animals (horses, cattle) can also be effectively trained to do tricks with positive reinforcement (food treats). However, this method can teach them to be a nuisance and dangerous since it can eliminate the animal's respect for human personal space that is needed for safer handling of large species. Food rewards are impractical for training horses for work or performance since carrying and providing treats is not possible when the work or performance is in progress.

Herd animals are also rewarded by being left alone by more dominant member of the herd. Work and performance horses are trained by providing a stimulus to elicit an action. The reward is an opportunity to rest. Behaviorists term this *negative reinforcement*, which carries an erroneous connotation that punishment is involved. Trainers refer to this instead as *pressure and release*, a more accurate descriptive phrase than negative reinforcement. For horses, the most desirable reward, and one that is safe for a human to easily provide within 3 seconds, is an opportunity for the horse to rest undisturbed.

It should be remembered that excessive handling can be harmful by exhausting young animals physically and mentally and may break down respect for the handler and his or her personal space. Advanced training of maturing or mature domestic animals involves *shaping*, breaking a task to be learned into small pieces, which are gradually refined. The refined small pieces of trained activity are then performed in sequence, a process referred to as *chaining*.

Aversive training methods should be avoided, but sometimes what is aversive is conditional. For example, spurs are used to train horses for lateral movement, and choke or prong collars are used in dogs to regain a distracted dog's attention. Spurs, choke collars, and prong collars can be aversive, but not if they are used with the correct timing and with the minimum effort to elicit an intended response.

Counterconditioning is rewarding a no response. Counterconditioning is useful in training animals to become used to something that might cause a fearful reaction. Counterconditioning is beneficial in training dogs and cats to accept veterinary hospitals, veterinary examinations, nail trims, blood collection, injections, and transport crates. Rewards are typically highly desired food treats, such as chicken or turkey baby food, peanut butter, braunschweiger sausage, or squeeze cheese.

Habituation and *desensitization* are similar training methods. Habituation means providing a steady stimulus that causes an undesired response until no response occurs. Desensitization is using a repeated stimulus with increasing intensity until no response occurs. Habituation and desensitization are often used to eliminate a flight reaction to a fearful stimulus in prey animals, particularly horses. Another technique called *flooding* is used to habituate or desensitize an animal by rapidly presenting several stimuli until mental exhaustion and no response occurs. Flooding is used in colt-starting contests to demonstrate rapid results for entertainment purposes, but flooding is a poor training technique with short-lived results.

HEALTH AND BEHAVIOR

Illness or injury can markedly alter the animal's tolerance to handling. Handlers should always observe the animal's overall appearance (body condition, hair coat condition), locomotion, interactivity with other animals, consciousness of the environment, evidence of food and water consumption, presence of fecal matter, feces that are characteristic of the animal's species, and appearance and quantity of voided urine.

It is natural for predator animals to become defensively aggressive if ill or in pain. Common maladies are injury, arthritis, skin sores, and febrile infections.

Conversely, prey animals tend to attempt to hide their illnesses. Some will fake eating and minimize lameness. They will become more social so they do not stick out from the herd. True behavior of sick or injured animals, particularly prey animals, often requires containment in familiar surroundings and monitoring behavior unobserved with hidden video cameras.

STEREOTYPIC BEHAVIOR AND ENVIRONMENTAL ENRICHMENT

The determination of psychological stress in animals is qualitative. This tempts some people to anthropomorphize by assuming that certain situations are mentally stressful to animals, which may or may not be the case. Efforts at quantitative measures have traditionally relied on the measure of cortisol levels and heart rates, both measures of parameters that change within minutes and are affected by multiple stimuli. Meta-analyses of salivary cortisol studies in animals have shown that cortisol as a single parameter and without the contexts of duration of possible stress, gender, and other effectors of cortisol concentrations is unreliable as an indicator of stress or welfare.

Visible reactions of animals to situations that induce apprehension, fear, trust, respect, and pain are very similar to observable human reactions. Recognition of these similarities is not anthropomorphism. It is pragmatism. Experienced animal handlers can recognize these primitive basic feelings in animals just as well as any human can recognize the visible signs of fear, pain, and other basic reactions in another human.

Failure to appropriately thrive and repetitive alternations in normal behavior are reliable indicators of stress in animals. *Stereotypic behavior* is dysfunctional behavior, usually induced by stress and influenced by genetics. The stressors are often excessive confinement, barren, boring environments, and isolation from their own species. Stereotypic behaviors are characterized by repetitive actions that have no obvious purpose. Common types are usually forms of pacing or oral behaviors (*Table 2.3*).

Table 2.3 **Examples of stereotypic behaviors**
• Circling and pacing in mice
• Feather pulling in caged birds
• Cribbing and weaving in horses
• Tongue rolling in cattle
• Bar biting in sows (female hogs); belly nosing and tail and ear biting in young pigs
• Wool eating in sheep

Stereotypic behaviors are most common in stabled horses without turnouts, caged birds without cage enrichments or time out of their cage, crate-confined hogs and pen-confined hogs without environmental enrichments, and chickens confined to battery cages.

Observed stereotypic behaviors may relate to the current environment or a past environment. Once the behavior has been established, it may become permanent through alterations in primitive brain locations. These behaviors are not seen in wild animals or those with relative freedom and adequate stimuli for mental exercises.

> The percentage of confined animals that show stereotypic behaviors can be an indication of the degree of stress from excessive confinement.

A lack of stereotypic behavior is not necessarily evidence of good current or past handling or good confinement. However, animals raised in a barren environment during their socialization period are more prone to stereotypic behaviors.

NUTRACEUTICALS AND BEHAVIOR

Nutraceuticals are over-the-counter food substances administered orally with the intention of improving health or having medicinal benefits. They are not considered pharmaceuticals and are therefore not regulated in the same as drugs. Often, the efficacy of a nutraceutical in achieving the purported effect has not been proven. Some nutraceuticals are claimed to have beneficial effects on animal behavior.

L-tryptophan

Tryptophan is a large amino acid that is a precursor to serotonin. Tryptophan dietary supplements are administered with the expectation that serotonin levels in the brain will increase, improving mood and behavior. However, the clinical benefits in humans are insignificant, and behavior improvement in treated dogs has not been scientifically validated.

Melatonin

Melatonin is a hormone produced by the pineal gland in the brain and also by plants. Oral melatonin administration is purported to successfully treat insomnia in people and modulate fear in dogs, but proof of efficacy is currently insufficient.

Alpha-casozepine

Alpha-casozepine is a trypsin hydrolysate of the mammalian milk protein casein. It has been associated with a decrease in signs of anxiety in dogs and cats, but the evidence is weak and more studies on clinical efficacy are needed.

L-theanine

Theanine is an amino acid found in tea leaves. Reduction of anxiety in dogs and cats has been attributed to the oral administration of theanine, but more studies are needed to confirm these claims. Health claims in humans were not substantiated by the European Food Safety Authority. The European Union now prohibits L-theanine health claims for humans.

ANIMAL BEHAVIOR SPECIALISTS

Knowing basic animal behavior is essential for anyone to become a good animal handler. Animal behaviorists and animal handlers are not synonymous, however. To be a good animal handler also requires an ability to interpret animal actions and the reflexes to respond in a timely metered fashion, appropriate to the situation, including the humane use of physical restraints. Some excellent animal handlers may only be able to describe normal animal behavior in colloquial language while some excellent animal behaviorists may be less than average animal handlers.

An animal behaviorist is trained in the investigation of how and why animals behave as they do. A certified animal behaviorist who is a veterinarian is the best source of information on how to diagnose abnormal behavior and what corrective measures to prescribe.

There are no state or federal regulations for becoming an animal behaviorist or trainer. However, for veterinarians two governing bodies exist with requirements for formal education and evidence of acquired knowledge and skills: the American College of Veterinary Behaviorists (ACVB) and the Animal Behavior Society. There are also the Society of Veterinary Behavior Technicians and the Academy of Veterinary Behavior Technicians (AVBT), which certify veterinary technician specialists in animal behavior. For help with behavioral problems in animals, contact the ACVB at www.dacvb.org or AVBT at www.avbt.net. Also helpful are the AMVA at www.avma.org and the Animal Behavior Society at www.animalbehavior.org.

SELECTED FURTHER READING

Cobb ML, Iskandarani K, Chinchilli VM, et al. (2016). A systematic review and meta-analysis of salivary cortisol measurement in domestic canines. *Domestic Animal Endocrinology* 57:31–42.

Frank D, Beauchamp G, Palestrini (2010). Systematic review of the use of pheromones for treatment of undesirable behavior in cats and dogs. *Journal of the American Veterinary Medical Association* 236:1308–1316.

Gilger BC (2010). *Equine Ophthalmology*, 2nd edition. Elsevier, New York.

Grandin T (2005). *Animals in Translation: Using the Mysteries of Autism to Decode Animal Behavior*. Scribner, New York.

Hammerle M, Horst C, Levine E, et al. (2015). AAHA canine and feline behavior management guidelines. *Journal of the American Animal Hospital Association* 51:205–221.

Hannah HW (1999). Malpractice implications of animal restraint. *Journal of the American Veterinary Medical Association* 214:41.

Herron HE, Shreyer T (2014). The pet-friendly veterinary practice: a guide for practitioners. *Veterinary Clinics of North America. Small Animal Practice* 44:451–481.

Hewson C (2014). Evidence-based approaches to reducing in-patient stress – Part 1: Why animals' sensory capacities make hospitalization stressful to them. *Veterinary Nursing Journal* 29:130–132.

Hewson C (2014). Evidence-based approaches to reducing in-patient stress – Part 2: Synthetic pheromone preparations. *Veterinary Nursing Journal* 29:204–206.

Hewson C (2014). Evidence-based approaches to reducing in-patient stress – Part 3: How to reduce in-patient stress. *Veterinary Nursing Journal* 29:234–236.

Houpt KA (2010). *Domestic Animal Behavior for Veterinarians and Animal Scientists*, 5th edition. Blackwell Publishing, Ames.

Kim YM, Lee JK, Abd el-aty AM, et al. (2010). Efficacy of dog-appeasing pheromone (DAP) for ameliorating separation-related behavioral signs in hospitalized dogs. *Canadian Veterinary Journal* 1:380–384.

Kipperman BS (2015). The role of the veterinary profession in promoting animal welfare. *Journal of the American Veterinary Medical Association* 246:502–504.

Kronen PW, Ludders JW, Erb HN, et al. (2006). A synthetic fraction of feline facial pheromones calm but does not reduce struggling in cats before venous catheterization. *Veterinary Anaesthesia and Analgesia* 33:258–265.

Ladewig J (2007). Clever Hans is still whinnying with us. *Behavioural Processes* 76:20–21.

Mills DS, Ramos D, Estelles MG, et al. (2006). A triple blind placebo-controlled investigation into the assessment of the effect of dog appeasing pheromone (DAP) on anxiety related behavior of problem dogs in the veterinary clinic. *Applied Animal Behavior Science* 98:114–126.

Murphy J, Arkins S (2007). Equine learning behavior. *Behavioural Processes* 76:1–13.

Murphy J, Hall C, Arkins S (2009). What horses and humans see: a comparative review. *International Journal of Zoology* Article ID 721798, 14 pages.

Patronek GJ, Lacroix CA (2001). Developing an ethic for the handling, restraint, and discipline of companion animals in veterinary practice. *Journal of the American Veterinary Medical Association* 218:514–517.

Phillips C (2002). *Cattle Behavior and Welfare*, 2nd edition. Blackwell, Malden.

Price EO (2008). *Principles and Applications of Domestic Animal Behavior*. CAB International, Cambridge.

Rushen J, Taylor AA, de Passille AM (1999). Domestic animals' fear of humans and its effect on their welfare. *Applied Animal Behaviour Science* 65:285–303.

Siracusa C, Manteca X, Cuenca R, et al. (2010). Effect of a synthetic appeasing pheromone on behavioral, neuroendocrine, immune and acute-phase perioperative stress responses in dogs. *Journal of the American Veterinary Medical Association* 237:673–681.

Timney B, Macuda T (2001). Vision and hearing in horses. *Journal of the American Veterinary Medical Association* 218:1567–1574.

Wells DL (2006). Aromatherapy for travel-induced excitement in dogs. *Journal of the American Veterinary Medical Association* 6:964–967.

Part 2

HOUSEHOLD AND LABORATORY ANIMALS

CHAPTER 3

CONTAINMENTS FOR HOUSEHOLD, YARD, AND LABORATORY ANIMALS

All domestic animals have basic containment needs that should be provided by handlers: adequate and accessible food and water; room to stand and raise their head, stretch, turn around, move forward, lie down, roll, and groom themselves without restriction; regular exercise; and social contact with humans and others of their own species. If the confinement is long term, an area of seclusion (hide box) and means of continually stimulating mental activity, such as environmental enrichments, should be provided. Aspects to consider for small animal containment are listed in *Table 3.1*.

Containment and handling of animals used for federally funded research in the U.S. requires oversight by an Institutional Animal Care and Use Committee that ensures compliance with the Public Health Service Policy and the Animal Welfare Regulations. The welfare of research animals is also guided by the National Research Council's Guide for the Care and Use of Laboratory Animals. The U.S. Department of Agriculture's Animal and Plant Inspection Service inspects animal facilities to evaluate them for compliance with the Animal Welfare Act.

CONFINEMENT AND BEHAVIOR

Confinement of animals should not result in physical injury or mental disability. Excessive confinement that does not permit normal physical movements, stimulation of the mind, interaction with other living beings, or establishment of a zone of personal space can lead to stereotypic behaviors, abnormal aggression, cannibalism, or self-mutilation. Areas of confinement of animals should thus be large enough to permit natural movement, provide mental stimulation and frequent interaction with other animals or humans, and have a private space for retreat and refuge.

Confined animals should be monitored for stereotypic behaviors, abnormal aggression, self-mutilation, and cannibalism. Additional room in the confinement area should be created at best before or at least by the time these abnormal behaviors exceed 2% of the animals maintained as a group.

Environmental enrichments are enclosures or activities that stimulate natural social interactions, provide exercise, and encourage decision-making activities for the species. These can include companionship or social interactions with other animals and humans, investigating hiding and exploration structures, playing with appropriate toys, having variable feeding routines, and playing with food mazes or puzzles. Small animals in the wild spend up to 60% of their waking hours searching for food. Besides the nutrition gained, hunting for food provides important mental challenges. Finding hidden food and extracting it from a food toy simulates natural food hunting. Companion dogs receive much mental stimulation from time with a handler going on long

Table 3.1 **Considerations for containment of small animals**
• Light exposure
• Temperature
• Exercise space and mental stimulation that encourage natural behavioral patterns
• Companionship
• Bedding
• Rest and sleeping area
• Suitability of containment materials for the species
• Species-normal behavior
• Escape prevention
• Location for enclosure

walks, jogging, chasing a ball or Frisbee, and other play activities.

Environmental enrichments are routinely provided to animals in zoos and research institutions. Privately owned small animals are too often not provided with appropriate containments and environmental enrichments.

CONTAINMENT ETHICS AND LIABILITY

Good animal handling begins with the safe and secure containment of the animal. Safety of the animal and of the handler depends on appropriate, well-maintained enclosures. Failure to provide or maintain adequate enclosures can result in injury to the animal while it is contained or attempting to escape, or it can result in successful escape with subsequent injury or loss of the animal or injury to humans, or both.

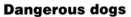

> Poor staff training on animal handling and inadequate facilities to avoid patient escape are among the ten most common legal problems of veterinarians.

Dangerous dogs

Locks on cages and runs are needed when containing dangerous dogs. Easily read warning signs should be attached to the cages. Runs should have contiguous roofing with the walls to prevent dogs from climbing corners and going over a wall. Secondary barriers, such as a series of closed doors, to rooms with cages and runs should be present. Whenever a dangerous dog is taken out of a locked cage or run, a short chain leash and a closed-end wire muzzle should be used.

Rural settings

It is common for people who live in rural settings to think that is appropriate to let their dogs constantly run free, but this is a risk to the health and welfare of the dogs and to people or other animals they may interact with outside the dog's property or range of voice command from its owner. When dogs are not on a leash or under voice control, they should be kenneled or inside a fence because of liability risks relating to the danger they might be to other people,

animals, or property, and for their own safety against larger, more aggressive, or stronger roaming dogs or predator wildlife.

Escape of reptiles

Many exotic reptiles can damage the ecosystem if they escape containment. Concern for this possibly led to legislation against wild-type red-eared slider turtles as pets in Florida. In addition to causing an imbalance in the ecosystem by preying on indigenous wildlife, some escaped reptiles can pose a hazard to humans or domestic animals. Conversely, the escape of pet reptiles into a hostile environment with predators or into an adverse climate can lead to the premature death of the escaped reptile. The escape or release of exotic animals into a foreign environment is called *biopollution*. Thousands of Burmese pythons have been released or have escaped into the Florida everglades and pose a serious problem to the ecological balance of southern Florida.

Recovering escaped small animals

Animal shelters and veterinary clinics should be contacted when small animals escape outdoors and their whereabouts are unknown. The owner should also be notified.

Escaped animals that are located should not be chased. Dogs or cats, if well socialized, may come to a familiar handler. The handler should slowly approach the animal. At a non-threatening distance the handler lowers his body and calmly calls the animal. Offering food treats, if available, can be helpful. If the animal approaches, the handler should attempt to pet the animal for 20–30 seconds before putting a leash on it or picking it up. The handler should not lunge at the animal or attempt to snatch it with his hands.

Another approach that can be effective for all small animals, including small mammals, birds, and reptiles, is to put the escaped animal's cage, with its door open and treats inside it, in a garage or shed and leave the people door open, but not the overhead sliding garage door for vehicles. Optionally or additionally, a preferred animal associate (buddy animal) can be placed in a nearby closed cage in the garage or shed. This can allow trapping of the escaped animal in the garage or shed by closing the door at the opportune time and then capturing the animal directly or in its cage.

DOG CONTAINMENT

Dog containment may be indoors or outdoors. Outdoor housing must provide protection from extremes of temperature (above 85°F [29.4°C]), air movements, moisture, light, and other climate elements.

Cages

Containment of a dog should be in a quiet area, and the front should not provide vision of animals in other cages. The size should be appropriate for the dog being contained. If the cage or crate is too large, the dog may feel that soiling an end or corner is permissible. If the containment size is too small, it may restrict the dog's ability to relax, and if it urinates or defecates, its hair coat could be soiled.

The U.S. Animal Welfare Act of 1966 states that dog cages for short-term confinement must provide a dog the ability to sit, stand up, turn around freely, and lie fully recumbent in a natural position. Flooring should be at least partial solid flooring. Dogs should never be restricted to bare wire bottom containment. This causes pressure sores that become smeared with excrement and leads to serious infections of the feet and bony points on the legs. Each dog should have at least the square of the sum of the dog's length from its nose to the base of the tail (without following body contours), plus 6 in (15 cm). This measurement provides the square inches required. The minimum square footage can be determined by taking the product of this measurement and dividing it by 144. For minimal height, at least 6 in (15 cm) of room above the dog's head is required when it is in a normal standing position. More than standard minimal room is needed for nursing dams with puppies. A minimal exercise area of at least twice the area for the cage is also required. Ventilation should be adequate to avoid drafts, noxious or harmful odors, excessive humidity, and temperature extremes.

Transport cages for temporary enclosure during travel, or crates for short-term restricted activity, can be smaller. Only enough room to stand, turn around, and lie down with legs stretched out is sufficient, since being crated should only occupy the inactive time of the dog's day (sleeping, naps, feeding, resting) and should never exceed 6–8 hours at a time (less for puppies).

Fixed cages are generally in banks two or three cages high. Banks of dog cages should not be positioned to face each other. Upper cages require extra vigilance to prevent a small animal from jumping in or out. Bending over to remove dogs from lower cages may intimidate dogs and result in defensive attacks from fearful dogs or be perceived as a challenge to an aggressive dominant dog. However, most dogs will be eager to get out and can be caught inside the cage at the door with a slip leash by opening the cage door just wide enough for a hand holding the slip leash to enter and apply the leash.

Dogs need environmental enrichment for mental stimulation, as do all confined animals. For example, providing food-filled toys or other enrichment activities improves the behavior of shelter dogs and increases the chances of being adopted. Social interaction is also important, and full body contact with compatible, healthy dogs should be permitted daily.

If dogs and cats are caged in the same facility, they should be in separate rooms.

Crates

Portable cages include rigid clamshell transport crates that can act as dens for training and help retain body heat (**Figure 3.1**). Wire transport cages

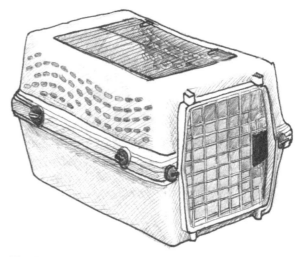

Fig. 3.1 Clamshell crate with front and top doors.

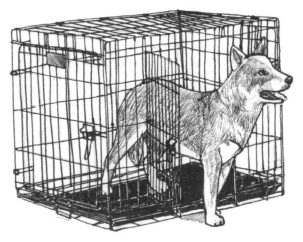

Fig. 3.2 Wire crate.

allow visual contact with handlers or other dogs (**Figure 3.2**). Wire cages are built to collapse flat for storage when not in use. Wire cages are also easier to see into to monitor for soiling. In addition, they allow air circulation, which reduces the risk of overheating. A solid-bottomed tray should always be used with wire-bottomed crates. Collars with tags should be removed from dogs in wire crates because of the risk of strangulation from being caught on a wire. Soft-sided bags are convenient transport cages for cats and small dogs. However, they provide less protection from injury and can be excessively confining.

Crates can be used as a source of refuge from various stresses for dogs. Placing a towel or blanket over wire crates can provide some dogs with a sense of security when in the crate. Crate training puppies can reduce the risks of several behavioral problems, such as house soiling, destructive chewing, digging, unnecessary barking, howling, and separation anxiety. Crate training aids in establishing the proper bond between dogs and owners since the owner is better able to control the dog's activities. The crate door should not be closed the first time the dog enters. The dog should enter voluntarily and be able to leave on its own for a couple of days before enclosing it for extended times. Soft bedding should be provided in the crate and treats offered when the dog enters the crate. Nothing adverse (no reprimands) should occur when the dog is in the crate. The dog should never be told to "come" and then shoved into the crate. Although most dogs seek out time in their

crate for rest and security, inappropriate training or excessive use of crates can lead to separation anxiety and stereotypic behaviors.

Crates should be matched to the size of the dog. A crate should be large enough for the dog to easily stand up, turn around, and lie on its side with its legs outstretched, but small enough to discourage the dog from soiling the crate. Growing dogs may need to have several crates of various sizes. Matching the dog's size with a crate provides the option to carry a small dog in its crate. Although crates have top handles for carrying them when empty, the handler should use both hands in carrying a crate with a dog in it to stabilize the crate's floor. The crate to be carried with a dog in it should be covered with a towel to avoid overstimulating the dog by making it fearful or excited.

Runs

Healthy dogs should be given the opportunity to exercise in a normal manner. For example, each day a dog should be allowed to achieve a running stride. Kennel runs should have a solid wall or at least 4 ft (1.2 m) of vertical visual isolation from other runs and to keep male dogs in adjacent runs from urinating from one run into another. The remainder of the run walls should be 3/8-in stainless steel rods to promote adequate air circulation. Urine should not be able to flow in any direction other than toward the run's floor drain. The door can be hinged or sliding. Hinged doors should open outward only to prevent accidental wedging of a struggling dog attempting to escape. Outdoor runs should have a contiguous, escape-proof roof (**Figure 3.3**). If not on concrete, wire mesh should be buried around the inside of the perimeter to prevent a dog from escaping by digging out.

Dog houses

Dog houses should be moisture and wind proof and provide shelter from intense sunlight, rain, snow, sleet, and hail. If properly constructed and sized for the dog, it can provide passive warmth. To fit the dog, the house should be just large enough for the dog to stand on all four feet comfortably, turn around, and lie on its side. If it is larger, it may not sufficiently entrap the dog's body heat in winter. The door should be relatively small, only slightly higher

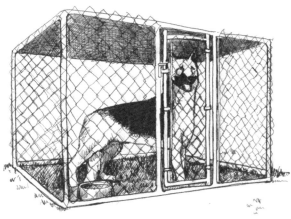

Fig. 3.3 Outdoor kennel with covered top for shade and prevention of escape.

than the top of the dog's shoulders. There should be a flexible water-resistant door flap, a self-closing door, or an interior partial partition that creates a small hallway entrance that prevents wind from blowing directly into the house. For further wind protection, the house should be located on the east or southeast side of a larger structure (house, garage, barn, shed) with the door to the dog house facing east or southeast, away from prevailing winds.

The floor of the dog house should be a solid floor raised at least 2 in (5 cm) from the ground for insulation. The roof should be hinged to permit easy cleaning. Soft insulating bedding (old shredded clothes, blankets, commercial dog beds, or hay) that cannot be dragged out of the dog house should be provided in winter months. Bedding should be replaced or cleaned on a regular basis. Straw is poor bedding for dogs, as it is typically dusty and will prick and irritate the skin.

Only dogs that have a dense hair coat for colder weather and have had time to gradually adapt to declining temperatures should be kept outdoors with a dog house.

Fences
Wire mesh
Wire fences are typical yard containments of dogs. A galvanized 2 × 2 or 2 × 4 in (5 × 5 or 5 × 10 cm) woven wire mesh yard and kennel fence 3–5 ft (1–1.5 m) tall is economical and safe fencing for dogs. It is flat surfaced, reducing the chance of dogs climbing out at the corners. Chain link is more common, but it is easier for dogs to climb over, especially at fence corners.

Invisible fencing
An invisible fence is an enclosure surrounded by buried perimeter wire that functions by delivering an electric shock to deter a dog from leaving the area. The system consists of a combination of a perimeter wire buried up to 8 in (20 cm) deep, a radio signal generator, and a special collar containing a battery-driven radio receiver. When a dog wearing such a shock collar approaches the perimeter, the collar will issue a warning beep. If this is not a sufficient deterrent, the dog will receive a shock. Ten minutes of training per day for 2 weeks is recommended to familiarize dogs to the system. Temporary flags marking the perimeter may aid in initial training. The dog must be shocked at least once to learn the consequences of ignoring the warning or perimeter flags.

Potential drawbacks to invisible fencing are system failure due to weak or dead collar batteries or a broken perimeter wire. No barrier exists to discourage animals without a special collar from entering the yard, which leaves the contained dog vulnerable to injury or death by roaming dogs. The charge may be insufficient for dogs with thick hair coats without the neck being groomed, and excessive shock can occur if a dog's hair coat gets wet. In addition, if the shock is perceived as painful, avoidance, submissive, or aggression problems could result.

Some dogs wearing a receiver collar will bound through an invisible fence line with high excitement but then refuse to return for fear of being shocked. Some dogs resist going past a perimeter fence even if the fence electricity is off or when they are not wearing a receiver collar. People or other animals may unknowingly venture into the confinement and be bitten.

An indoor version of invisible fence is available to limit a dog's range of movements inside a house. These electroshock devices are wireless and use either a base unit with a range that is permitted before a shock occurs to the dog wearing the receiver collar, or use a moveable transmitters that establish boundaries that if passed cause a shock to the dog.

Tethering

Tethering dogs for long periods on a chain, rope, or cable is contrary to the proper socialization of dogs. In 1996, the USDA issued a statement that tethering is inhumane. The majority of U.S. states have anti-tethering laws. Being tethered separates dogs physically and psychologically from members of dog, human, or any other surrogate family members. Tethered dogs become overly protective of their small territory and defensive, knowing they cannot escape. Tethers can become wrapped around or over objects or tangled, possibly causing strangulation or leg injuries, or preventing the dog from escaping an attack by another dog, malicious humans, or stinging insects. Tethers can also prevent access to food or water or escape from being forcibly bred. Tethered dogs usually wear down the vegetation, leaving only dirt or mud to lie on. In addition, owners who tether dogs are less likely to clean the area of feces. Many tethered dogs hang themselves to death attempting to jump or climb over objects or falling off elevated surfaces.

A study by the U.S. Centers for Disease Control and Prevention reported that tethered dogs are three times more likely to bite than dogs that are not tethered. Children under 12 years old are five times more likely to be bitten by a tethered dog. Tethering on a dog trolley, a tether attached by a slip ring to a horizontal line similar to a clothes line, permits the tether to slide along the horizontal line. This may increase the dog's territory but it does not eliminate the problems associated with tethering.

Putting dogs into and removing them from cages and runs

Entering an enclosure

Doors and gates on cages and runs should always open to the outside. When putting a dog into a cage, the dog should be placed in the cage while holding onto its collar and closing the cage door onto the handler's dog-restraining arm. The door is closed against the arm as the dog is released and the handler's arm is then slipped out of the cage.

When putting a dog into a run, the dog should be led in and then turned around. Trying to stand outside the run and force the dog in should be avoided. The run gate should be opened only wide enough to allow the handler's body enough room to exit sideways while blocking the dog from escaping with a handler's leg, if necessary. The handler's hands should not be used to attempt to block escape.

Exiting an enclosure

A slip leash should be applied to the dog while it is still in the cage or run, even if it is small and will be carried. Applying the leash can be done by opening the cage or run door just wide enough to insert an arm with the leash and slip it over the dog's head. If capturing a dog in a run, the handler can carefully enter the run and apply the slip leash if an assistant holds the run door closed after the handler enters and opens it when needed.

CAT CONTAINMENT

Cats are semi-*arboreal* (tree-living) predators. When maintained in an enclosure, cats will use raised structures more often than the floor. Those that spend the most time on the floor are higher-ranking, more dominant cats. Having an elevated area to rest and retreat is important for a feeling of security in cats, especially lower-ranking cats. Long-term enclosures should provide height with climbing frames, raised walkways, and platforms at various heights. Slanting boards, steps, and poles can help smaller or younger cats to move around the enclosure. The floor should be smooth and easy to clean but also provide enough traction to prevent slipping. Mesh flooring should never be used for cats because of resulting injury to their paws. Single- or multiple-cat enclosures with sufficient height for handlers to walk into are preferable. The enclosure should have no sharp points, edges, or protrusions.

Cages and catteries

Cats are social animals when active, but they like to rest alone. They can be housed in single cages or in group enclosures (catteries) if properly introduced to others in the group and if there is sufficient space, easy access to food and litter boxes, resting areas, and individual hiding spaces at various levels.

The introduction of a new cat to a group, called a *clowder*, should be done slowly by placing it in a nearby cage with a hiding box. Cats from either cage should not be able to reach into each other's cage. Exchange of bedding material or cage "toys" will aid adaptation. After about 2 weeks, if the cats seem adjusted to each other, the new cat can be released into the group. Under proper conditions, up to 20–25 cats can be housed together.

When single long-term cat enclosures are used, the minimum floor space should be 5 sq ft per (0.5 sq m) cat with a height of at least 3 ft (1 m). Cages for short-term hospitalization in veterinary hospitals can be smaller. Larger, multi-leveled cages are preferable (**Figure 3.4**).

Cats should have hiding boxes in their cages with non-skid tops to reduce stress and visibility when desired. Cardboard boxes with doors cut in one end can be used as disposable hiding boxes and perches for cats. A hiding area can be created by a towel attached

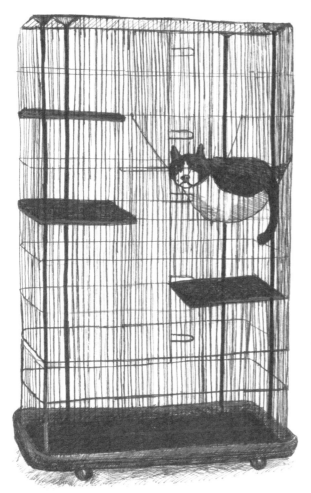

Fig. 3.4 Multi-level cage for cats.

to half of a cage door. Some commercial cages have built-in hiding boxes and litter boxes attached to the larger main compartment of the cage. Resting areas should have soft padding. Cats that sleep on soft surfaces have longer periods of deep sleep.

Scratching and kneading surfaces should be provided for cats to exercise their instinctual desire to mark their territory with their paws and sharpen their claws. Suitable surfaces may include scratch posts, carpet, and wood. Pheromones from cats' paws can be rubbed from a previously used scratching post to a new post to encourage its use.

Conventional litter boxes are smaller than that preferred by cats. Litter boxes are ideally 1 ft (0.3 m) in length, and cats should be able to get at least 3 ft (1 m) away from a litter pan to rest and eat. In group enclosures there should be at least 1 litter box per two cats. Litter boxes should be cleaned each time they are soiled or at least once per day. However, when sanitation permits, only spot cleaning a cat cage allows the personal odors to persist and provide stress release. Baskets or boxes provided in addition to litter pans will reduce or eliminate the desire for the cat to rest in litter pans. Cats allowed to roam in multi-leveled homes should have at least one litter box on each level of the house.

Enrichment toys should be provided for mental stimulation. Placing cages next to windows, screened-in porches or window boxes, or having glass backs on cages that permit cats to view activity in another room or outdoors, are good environmental enrichments. Favorite enclosure "toys" for cats can be small mobile objects with a complex surface texture such as a tennis ball. Puzzle toys in which pieces of dry food can be hidden for the cat to extract can provide good mental stimulation. Paper sacks and cardboard boxes are favorite toys of cats. Excessive confinement, or confinement devoid of environmental enrichment for cats, does not lead to the stereotypic behaviors in cats common to other species, such as cannibalism, pacing, or self-mutilation. Instead, cats respond to stressful environments primarily by not eating, grooming, or playing.

Crates

When acclimating cats to a transport crate, they should have constant access to the crate. The crate should be secured on an elevated surface, such as a table. A soft towel should be provided inside the crate to lie on. The cat should receive toys or food treats whenever entering it to prepare the cat for crate travel. A toy dangling from the top of the crate may be tried as an added incentive to spend more time in the crate. Commercial water-resistant cardboard boxes are available that permit perching, hiding, and transport.

Crates for cats should have a front and top door. Cats are more tolerant of being placed into and taken out of a top-opening crate than a front-opening crate. If a top door is not available, a clamshell crate that has an easily opened top half will suffice. Alternatively, a clamshell crate can be placed on its end with the front door on top. Then, introduce the cat into the crate from the top and gently right the crate.

Fences and tunnels

The AVMA recommends that companion cats should be kept indoors. Staying indoors is associated with a longer life span, decreased predation of songbirds, and decreased relinquishment of ownership. For some owners, allowing their companion cat time outdoors provides the cat with high-quality environmental enrichment. Cat fences and tunnels are a couple of ways that outdoor excursions can be relatively safe for the cat.

Cat fencing is polypropylene netting attached to stanchions angled inward to the containment yard. The netting should be attached to the fence above a typical jump height of cats, which is about 4 ft (1.2 m) (**Figure 3.5**).

Flexible, portable exercise tunnels with closable ends are commercially available for cats. The tunnels can be collapsed for storage when not in use. Tunnels provide an alternative to special fencing as a means of permitting outdoor exercise and mental enrichment while keeping a cat in confinement (**Figure 3.6**).

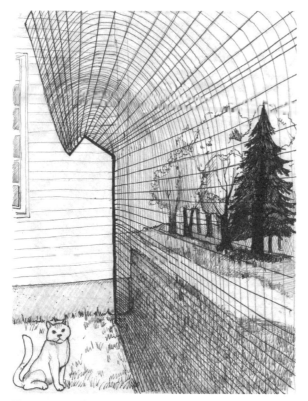

Fig. 3.5 Outdoor fence for cats.

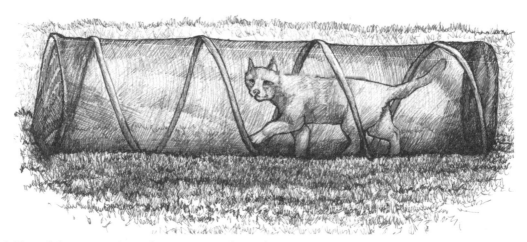

Fig. 3.6 Tunnel for cat exercise and environmental enrichment.

SMALL MAMMAL CONTAINMENT

Small mammals housed alone are more anxious about being handled than those kept in groups. Most small mammals should be contained in groups, but there are important exceptions. To prevent fighting, neither sexually mature male rabbits nor adult male mice should be housed together. Adult hamsters prefer to live a solitary life, especially adult females. For these reasons, as well as for managing reproduction within groups, is important to be able to correctly determine the sex of small mammals. Anogenital (AG) distance is generally used for sexing small mammals, except for guinea pigs and young rabbits. Females have shorter AG distance than do males. Pressure on either side of the prepuce in male guinea pigs or young buck (male) rabbits will cause the penis to extrude.

The safest approach to minimizing aggression within a group of small mammals is to group members of the same sex and same litter after puberty to control breeding and fighting. Spacious enclosures and small hide boxes that can be defended will minimize aggression among males. Introduction of new rodents to an established colony should take days to weeks, beginning with mixing used substrate material from both cages and sharing the mixture in each cage to allow adaptation to smells that will be in the new mixed group.

All small mammal containments should be free of sharp projections, easily cleaned, and well ventilated but free of drafts. Wood enclosures absorb urine and will foul the air with ammonia. Most small mammals will also gnaw through wood enclosures. Wire mesh lids are recommended for adequate ventilation. Drinking water should be constantly available and provided in a way that prevents the water from being spilled or contaminated. Shade from direct sunlight should always be present in the enclosure.

Substrates (bedding) should be kiln-dried pine, aspen, paper products, or good-quality grass hay. Cedar or fresh pine shavings should not be used owing to their irritant volatile oils, and cat litter should be avoided because of dust or possible ingestion with digestive tract compaction. Cloth materials such as towels should not be used for bedding:

strings could be ingested and cut the lining of the digestive tract or become caught around a leg or neck.

Small mammal pets should have exploration and exercise time outside their primary enclosure. However, no other animals that could be a predator (dogs, cats, rats, birds, ferrets) should be allowed within sight, hearing, or smell of the small mammals. Time outside of primary enclosures should be directly supervised.

Most small mammals, including rodents and rabbits, burrow and rest during the day to avoid heat and to thermoregulate. When in captivity, they can be at risk of heat stress, and the temperature of their containment should be carefully regulated.

Rabbits and many rodents produce and ingest *cecotropes* (also called *night feces*), which are important for their nutrition. Cecotropes are smaller, softer, and moister than regular feces. Rabbit cecotrope pellets stick together with a greenish mucus. Cecotropes have a high concentration of vitamin K and B vitamins, plus twice the protein and half the fiber of regular feces. Wire-bottomed cages could cause wastage of cecotropes, although, if they can, rabbits eat cecotropes directly from the anus.

Rodents

Wood or plastic cages can easily be gnawed through by rodents. Flooring should be solid to prevent foot and leg injuries from wire flooring. Plastic coating will be chewed off and should not be used on wire cages. Substrate should be 1 in (2.5 cm) deep. Cedar shavings should not be used, as wet cedar shavings release fumes that are toxic to the respiratory tract. Other unsafe wood substrates include cherry, citrus wood, pine that has not been dried, oleander, plum, and redwood. Aspen shavings, chopped straw, or stripped paper are safe. Sand can be used for gerbils. Mice, hamsters, and gerbils need mesh-wire lids to provide adequate ventilation. Substrates should not be dusty, especially if used in solid wall enclosures such as aquariums.

Cages for all rodents should be made of wire, sheet stainless steel, non-galvanized aluminum, or glass with solid gnaw-proof material.

Gerbils and hamsters can be satisfactorily housed in large aquariums so that at least 3 in (7.5 cm) of substrate can be provided to meet their burrowing desires while containing the substrate within the enclosure.

Hiding and sleeping areas should be provided. Small prey animals hide in small dark areas to escape being eaten in the wild and become stressed if they do not have a hiding area. Enrichments for mental and physical stimulation should be added, such as clay flowerpots, empty coconut shells, or tunnels of PVC pipe. Enrichments can include ladders and ropes for climbing as well as exercise wheels. Exercise wheels should not have any rough edges. Exercise balls should not be used if there is access to stairs or other ledges for the ball to roll off. Blocks of untreated wood should be provided for gnawing. All rodents and lagomorphs (rabbits) will gnaw wood. Their teeth continually grow, and gnawing is an instinctive means of wearing off the teeth to keep up with new growth. Containment contents should be routinely rearranged on a regular basis to maintain interest and mental simulation, except for hamsters, which prefer stability in the location of their possessions. Boredom and stereotypic behaviors will result from an inability to gnaw on objects and sort through mental challenges.

Mice should have substrate replaced every 2–3 days and their enclosures washed weekly. Gerbil and hamster cages can be cleaned less often, but at least weekly.

Rats and mice

Plastic or glass enclosures are recommended for mice and rats. Wire mesh sides allow drafts, and metal condenses moisture, which supports bacterial growth. Wire mesh lids should not have mesh openings of larger than 0.155 sq in (1 sq cm). The size of the enclosure and mesh lid should be large enough to provide adequate ventilation. An adult mouse should have 15 sq in (97 sq cm) of floor space and cage height of 5 in (12.5 cm), while an adult rat should have 40 sq in (258 sq cm) and a height of 7 in (17.5 cm).

The minimum space requirement for 2 or 3 mice is 18 × 18 in (45 × 45 cm) and 10 in (25 cm) high. Mice should have 1 in (2.5 cm) deep substrate, but rats do not require as much. Mice are excellent climbers and need a wire mesh lid on the top of their confinement.

Rats should have at least 12 × 24 in (30 × 60 cm) by 12 in (30 cm) height for each rat. Wire-bottomed perches for rats should not have mesh openings greater than ½ × ½ in (13 mm) to prevent a rat's foot from getting caught in the wire. Solid floors are preferred.

Vertical exercises with climbing structures such as ropes, ramps, and branches are desirable, especially for rats. PVC pipes and blocks of wood with drilled holes can provide tunnels to explore and hiding areas. Exercise wheels for rats should be at least 12 in (30 cm) in diameter. Chewing toys can include untreated wood blocks, cardboard tubes and boxes, and rawhide chews for dogs. Rats and mice like to create their own nesting material by shredding toilet paper, paper towels, straw, or other easily shredded materials.

Rats should be kept away from birds and dogs, cats, and other small mammals since they may be prey of some animals and predator of others. Male rats can be housed together, but adult male mice will often attack each other.

Enclosures should provide a temperature of 65–75°F (18.3–23.9°C) and humidity of 40–70%. Temperatures above 85°F (29.4°C) can lead to heat stroke. Humidity of less than 30% for rats can cause dehydration and necrosis of the tail, called *ringtail*.

Guinea pigs

Guinea pig containment is simple since they do not climb or jump. The cage should have at least 1 × 2 ft (0.3 × 0.6 m) of floor space per adult and wire-mesh sides that are at least 10 in (25 cm) high. Long-term enclosures should have 2 × 4 ft (0.6 × 1.2 m) of space for each guinea pig to provide sufficient exercise space. Ventilation and regular enclosure cleaning are important to reduce the risk of respiratory problems from urine-produced ammonia. Sides of the enclosure may be glass, plastic, metal, or wire mesh. Wood should not be used since it can absorb waste products and pathogens. Although guinea pigs do not climb well or jump, a top lid should be provided to protect guinea pigs from other animals and should be wire mesh to provide needed ventilation. An exercise area should be 1 ft (0.3 m) long. Environmental enrichments should include multi-levels with gentle sloping solid-bottomed ramps, PVC pipe tunnels, and chewables (wood blocks, rawhide chews).

To protect their small feet from injury, the floor, ramps, ledges, and exercise wheels should have a smooth, solid bottom. A sturdy plastic tub is sufficient if there is adequate ventilation. Guinea pigs will clog sipper bottles with food and contaminate water bowls with feces. Heavy, tip-resistant water bowls should be cleaned daily. Food bowls should be small enough to prevent the guinea pig from climbing in it. Guinea pigs of either sex can be kept in the same containment, but adult males will fight with newly introduced males.

For supervised outdoor excursions, guinea pigs can be contained in collapsible, portable fencing or small plastic pools made for children. Shade and hiding boxes should be provided.

Guinea pigs should be maintained at an environmental temperature of 65–75°F (18.3–23.9°C) and a humidity level below 50%. Heat stroke is a risk at temperatures above 85°F (29.4°C).

Chinchillas

Chinchillas are athletic and need multi-level ramps, perches, and platforms for jumping and the largest cage practical for their containment area. Metal cages should be used. Wood or plastic cages will be gnawed through. The minimum size for cages should be 24 × 24 in (60 × 60 cm) floor area and 24 in (60 cm) high for each chinchilla. Chinchillas are not very social and are usually housed alone in a cage. Pairs may be compatible, but much larger cages are necessary to reduce the tendency for aggression.

Mesh openings for wire sides should be no larger than 1 × 2 in (25 × 50 mm) Solid-bottomed cages are best. If wire-bottomed cages used, the mesh should be no larger than 0.5 × 0.5 in (12 × 12 mm) to prevent their feet from getting caught. Broken tibias from inappropriate wire flooring are common. Exercise wheels should have solid bottoms without rungs or cross bars. The diameter of the wheel should be at least 15 in (38 cm). When wire-bottomed cages are used, a portion of the floor should be a solid-bottomed area for rest from the wire. Chinchillas should also have access to some of their feces since they are coprophagic and will eat their feces at night.

Unprinted newspaper, kiln-dried pine, or aspen shavings are safe forms of substrate. Hiding places can be provided by PVC piping that is large in diameter compared with the size of chinchillas.

Chinchilla locomotion is primarily hopping. Hollow exercise balls may be dangerous since they force chinchillas to run, which can dangerously exhaust them.

Chinchillas clean their fur with dust. A shallow pan with 2–9 in (5–23 cm) of appropriate commercial dust (9 parts silver sand to 1 part Fuller's earth) should be offered for 5–10 minutes at least 2–3 times per week. The dust pan should not be left in the enclosure for longer periods to keep the sand clean from feces and food. Alternatively, a separate aquarium or similar enclosure may be used exclusively for a 5–10-minute dust bath every 24–72 hours.

Chinchillas are native to high altitudes and cold weather. They will have heat stress at temperatures above 80°F (26.7°C) and should be kept in well-ventilated enclosures at 35–80°F (1.7–26.7°C) with low humidity (less than 40%) and protection from direct sunlight. They need 12 hours of darkness at night with undisturbed rest during the day.

Gerbils

Gerbils are gregarious and can be housed together, regardless of gender. They are good jumpers, and the enclosure walls should be tall enough to prevent them from jumping out, with a lid for additional assurance of preventing escape. Gerbils are very active and need space to prevent behavioral problems associated with overcrowding. Therefore, enclosures should provide at least 12 × 24 in (30 × 60 cm) for a pair of gerbils with walls at least 12 in (30 cm) high.

The container floor should be solid and smooth. Gerbils like to frequently stand on their hind feet, which could lead to injuries of their small feet or delicate tail by the wire mesh flooring. Likewise, only solid-floored exercise wheels should be used for gerbils. Wheels that have spokes that might catch their tail should not be used. Glass aquariums or plastic tubs with wire mesh lids for ventilation are adequate containment structures. Five gal (US) (19 L) of space are needed for each gerbil. Gerbils are indigenous to desert, so a pan of sand should be provided for gerbils to bathe in for personal hygiene and mental stimulation.

The best temperature range is 60–90°F (15.5–32.2°C), and relative humidity should be near 30%. Aspen shavings, sand, or paper products are adequate substrates. Container enrichments should include PVC tubing for hiding and exercise, as well as ladders, cardboard boxes, toilet paper or paper towel tubes, ramps, and rocks.

Hamsters

Adult, sexually mature golden (Syrian) hamsters should be housed alone, except for breeding. Chinese or Russian hamsters are smaller, less solitary, and can be housed in groups of litter mates. Stainless steel cages are best with deep bedding for burrowing (aspen shavings or paper products). Enclosure walls should be at least 6 in (15 cm) above the level of the substrate. Solid-bottomed cages are more secure and permit a hamster's needed coprophagic behavior. A single hamster should have a cage of at least 12 × 16 in (30 × 40 cm) and 12 in (30 cm) high.

Cages should be well ventilated. Wire cages are preferable. Female hamsters come into estrus every 4 days accompanied by a strong odor.

Recommended cage enrichments include an exercise wheel of fine mesh or solid running surface, and ramps, ladders, and tubes for climbing and hiding. Exercise wheels should be at least 5½ in (14 cm) in diameter. A hamster exercise ball may be beneficial, but there can be risk of injuries from rolling down stairs or exhaustion.

When reassembling the enclosure after cleaning, hide boxes, chew blocks, and other items should be replaced in their original locations. Hamsters are finicky about the arrangement of their enclosure.

The temperature should be maintained between 64 and 79°F (17.8 and 26.1°C). At temperatures below 50°F (10°C), hamsters will *hibernate* (go into a prolonged dormant state), and above 80°F (26.7°C) hamsters will *estivate* (a sleep-like state similar to hibernation).

Degus

Degus (day-goos) are gregarious, territorial ground dwellers. They prefer to live in small groups of 5–10 animals of the same sex. Males should be introduced to each other prior to puberty or they are likely to fight.

Their housing needs are greater than other small mammals since groups need to be housed together and provided with areas for digging, storage of food, nesting, scent marking of each other, sand baths, and low-level climbing. They are larger than other rodents commonly kept as pets and can eat thick wood, plastic, and small gauge wire easily. Because they can climb and jump, they need very large cages. Minimum cage size for one pair of adults is 2 × 4 ft (0.6 × 1.2 m) and 2 ft (0.6 m) high. The minimum length of a cage for a group of degus is 5 ft (1.5 m) and a height of 4 ft (1.2 m). No wood or plastic should be used for the frame. Non-galvanized aluminum or steel should be used as framing for either glass or acrylic sides. Cages and exercise wheels should have a solid bottom to reduce the risk of foot damage and infection. The preferred temperature is 65–75°F (18.3–23.9°C).

A thick substrate (4 in [10 cm]) should be provided as chopped straw, hay, shredded paper, or aspen shavings, since degus like to burrow. Heavy food bowls and sipper bottles should be used to reduce territorial hoarding. Enrichment items can include tree branches, hollow logs, wood blocks, cardboard tubes, and large rodent all-wire exercise wheels. Sand or dust baths are needed twice per week for about 30 minutes.

Sugar gliders

Sugar gliders are very gregarious arboreal marsupials that may be tamed but are not domesticated. If housed alone, sugar gliders will develop stereotypic behaviors that can lead to self-mutilation, pacing, or cannibalism. At least four sugar gliders should be housed together. However, new sugar gliders must be gradually introduced over days to an established group.

Enclosures should be large enough, vertically and horizontally, to permit gliding with a variety of branches to glide between, and bright lighting should be avoided, which can damage their vision. Horizontal cage bars will facilitate climbing. An individual space of at least 24 × 24 × 36 in (60 × 60 × 90 cm) should be provided for each sugar glider. If sugar gliders are overcrowded, stereotypic behaviors of pacing, cannibalism, and self-mutilation may occur. Exercise outside of an enclosure must be closely supervised since they can reach and hide in areas that other pets cannot. Large, tall aviaries with wire mesh sides that have openings of less than ½ in (13 mm) are best for groups of gliders. Wire-bottomed cages may be used to allow droppings to pass through, but the mesh openings should be 1 × ½ in (25 × 13 mm) or smaller. Latches on cages must be secure. Sugar gliders are dextrous and can often open simple latches.

Materials must be used for housing that resist damage from sugar gliders' lower incisors, called gouging teeth, which point forward. Wood-frame enclosures are not sufficient containment. Tree branches should be added for climbing and moving exercises, but some fruit tree branches, such as cherry wood, may be poisonous. Ropes, ladders, and exercise wheels are other favorite diversions. Sleeping pouches or nest boxes lined with cloth, bark, or leaves should be provided at the top of the gliding enclosure for rest and warmth. Water and feeding bowls should also be fixed in an elevated location because gliders urinate and defecate indiscriminately and will unintentionally contaminate their water and food with waste products. Bowls should be too small for sugar gliders to climb in and soil.

Temperature should be maintained between 60 and 90°F (15.5 and 32.2°C). The preferred range is 75–85°F (23.9–29.4°C). Light exposure should be approximately 12 hours per day.

Hedgehogs

Hedgehogs prefer a solitary existence and are usually housed individually in at least 20-gal (76 L) aquariums or other smooth-walled, solid-floored enclosures with a thick substrate of aspen shavings, hay, or shredded paper to allow digging. They are good climbers and have little fear of heights but are susceptible to injuries from falls. Hedgehogs are nocturnal and need a hiding box to rest during the day with large floor space for exercise at night. Their hide box should be large enough for them to easily turn around in. They prefer to use one part of a cage to eliminate. Water and feed bowls should be attached to the cage wall or be too heavy to be pushed around and turned over. A litter pan of dust-free litter may be used to facilitate daily cleaning. The entire enclosure should be cleaned each week.

Hedgehogs like to use exercise wheels during their nocturnal activity. The floor of the wheel should be solid to avoid toe and leg injuries. Small enclosures can cause hedgehogs to develop stereotypic behaviors (excessive pacing and weaving). The enclosure's ambient temperature should be temperate to warm (70–85°F [21.1–29.4°C]). Cooler temperatures can cause hibernation, and hotter temperatures may induce estivation. Humidity should be maintained at 40–70%. A shallow pan of water for wading can also aid in maintaining desired humidity.

Rabbits

Rabbits are social and should be housed in groups of two or more, but bucks should not be housed together because of the risk of fighting. Adult males will try to castrate each other.

Allowing pet rabbits to run free in a house can be expensive and dangerous. Rabbits will eat carpet, gnaw on furniture, destroy houseplants, and bite electric cords. They can be harassed, injured, or killed by predatory pets (dogs, cats, ferrets). Just the smell of predators nearby can be stressful to rabbits. They should be confined to a rabbit-proof play enclosure, under immediate supervision, or kept in their hutch (rabbit cage).

Rabbits should be housed in wire cages to provide adequate ventilation, but they also need protection from drafts, sunlight, and dampness. The minimum size of the cage needed depends on the breed of rabbit. Medium-sized rabbits require a minimum of 24 × 30 in (60 × 75 cm) per rabbit with 18 in (45 cm) of height. Giant breeds should have a minimum floor space of 30 × 36 in (75 × 90 cm) per rabbit, and small-sized breeds should have a minimum of 18 × 24 in (45 × 60 cm) per rabbit.

Optimal size cages should be tall enough to permit rabbits to stand on their hindquarters to inspect their surroundings, and provide an opportunity to climb on elevated platforms. The length of the cage should be four times that of an adult rabbit with a total area of at least 8 sq ft (0.75 sq m). Improperly constructed or excessively confining containment can lead to stereotypic behaviors such as self-mutilation from over-grooming and repetitive cage biting and pawing at cage corners.

Wire cages can be partially self-cleaning and provide good ventilation, handler visibility, and parasite control. Cages with wood frames in direct contact with rabbits will be gnawed and soaked with urine and feces, making them incapable of being adequately cleaned. The floor should be ½ × 1 in (13 × 25 mm) mesh and at least 16 gauge. The sides and roof can be 1 × 2 in (25 × 50 mm) mesh and at least 12 gauge. Unlike front opening doors, top-hinged doors will remain closed even if accidentally left unlatched. In addition, open top-hinged hutch doors are not an obstruction to a handler's movement around the outside of the cage.

Outdoor hutches should be surrounded by a tall mesh or solid fence to prevent access by predators, especially roaming dogs. To keep walls free of urine, fur, and feces, aisles 3 ft (1 m) wide should be created between hutches and wooden walls of a shelter. Hanging hutches from the ceiling of enclosures facilitates removing manure and eliminates the rotting of wood or rusting of metal hutch legs. Some solid-bottomed area should be provided in an otherwise wire-bottomed cage to allow the rabbit to rest its feet from the pressure of wire, which does not distribute the pressure of the rabbit's body weight in a normal manner and can cause chronic foot problems. Cages should be waterproof and draft-free. Two sides of the hutches should have visual barriers, such as scrubs or buildings, for partial relief from predator surveillance for the rabbits and to block the wind.

Household pet rabbits can be offered outdoor exercise for environmental enrichment, if an outdoor enclosure is escape-proof and predator-proof, and a rabbit's time outdoor is closely supervised. Portable pens for dogs can be used on concrete surfaces to temporarily contain rabbits for exercise. If the pen is placed on a grassy area, the rabbit must be more closely monitored to keep it from burrowing under the fence.

Rabbits evolved to survive in the safety of burrows. All hutches should contain a hide box or other burrow-like shelter to relieve stress. Loose straw or hay can also be burrowed into as well as eaten. Alternatively, paper products, such as towels and newspaper, can be used as substrate. Hide boxes or shelters within an enclosure should be strong enough to support a rabbit if it decides to perch on top of it. A feeding and exercise area and a separate resting area should be provided.

Enclosure enrichments can include cardboard boxes, vegetable treats, untreated wood, paper bags, blankets, cat tunnels, and large-breed dog toys that cannot be gnawed into pieces. Since interest in specific enrichment objects will gradually wane, different enrichments should be regularly rotated in and out of the enclosure.

Nest boxes are needed for pregnant does (female rabbits) and does with litters. Nest boxes should be made of ½ × 1 in wire mesh (13 × 25 mm), 18 in (45 cm) long, 10 in (25 cm) wide, and 10 in (25 cm) tall for average-sized breeds. The top should be open to aid with ventilation and control of moisture in the nest. In cold weather, cardboard liners can be used outside the box to provide additional insulation.

The cage or box should be spot cleaned daily and all litter removed weekly. Pens should have a non-slip surface. Pine and cedar as substrate should be avoided, as their aromatic oils can irritate skin and respiratory tracts. Clay or corncob litter, which can lead to digestive impaction, should not be used. Pen walls should be at least 4 ft (1.2 m) tall to prevent rabbits from jumping out.

Exposure to environmental temperatures of lower than 40°F (4.4°C) and higher than 85°F (29.4°C) should be avoided. Colder temperatures are tolerated better than hotter temperatures since rabbits do not sweat. They dissipate heat primarily, but inefficiently, from their ears, and pant only when in desperation. Good ventilation is needed to control odors and assist cooling during warm weather, but not to the extent of creating drafts that could cause stress.

Pet rabbits should be trained to tolerate a travel crate and short car rides prior to the need to transport them for veterinary care.

Ferrets

Ferrets are nearsighted ground dwellers that live in burrows. Their enclosure should be a solid-bottomed wire cage with 0.5 × 1 in (13 × 25 mm) mesh and a hiding box. A cage for two adult ferrets should be at least 3 × 3 ft (1 × 1 m) and 2 ft (0.6 m) high. Ferrets should be kept in wire or sheet metal cages with adequate play time outside the cage, at least 1 hour twice per day of supervised activity out of the cage. Aquariums should not be used, because of inadequate ventilation. Solid-sided cages prevent ferrets from seeing their surroundings, which is stressful to them because they cannot satisfy their curiosity of what is going on around them. Wood construction should be avoided because of ferrets' chewing and wood absorption of urine. Multi-level cages with ramps and ledges pose a risk of falling injuries. Ferrets will learn to use a litter pan, but it must be cleaned daily.

Substrates that produce dust should be avoided. Water should be provided in heavy, wide-bottomed, tip-resistant bowls made of dense materials. Soft plastic bowls that can be gnawed and ingested should not be used. Sipper bottles should not be used because they do not permit ferrets to fulfill their natural desire to wash.

Ferrets are very energetic and quickly bored. Cage accessories for hiding, burrowing, and exploring should be provided. Towels and blankets can be used for hiding and burrowing, but ferret nails may catch in looped fabrics so these should be avoided. Ferrets toys need to be gnaw-proof and too large to be swallowed and cause choking. Flexible clothes dryer vent tubing or rigid PVC tubes can be used as simulated burrows for exploration and exercise. Cages should be placed in areas of early morning and early evening human traffic to provide mental stimulation.

The best temperature for ferrets is 59–64°F (15–17.8°C) with 40–65% relative humidity.

CAGED COMPANION BIRD CONTAINMENT

Companion birds are contained in cages or aviaries, or both. Cages are the most practical for pet birds. Since most birds need the social support of a flock, it is generally inadvisable to cage a bird alone, particularly budgerigars, canaries, and lovebirds.

Cages
Birds need cages for safety from predators or playful injuries when unattended and for psychological

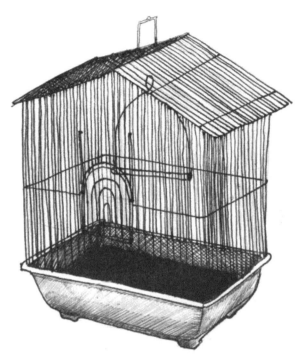

Fig. 3.7 Rectangular bird cage (preferable to circular cages).

security to relieve stress. Cages with angular corners are more conducive to grasping the birds than are circular cages (**Figure 3.7**). Square or rectangular cages are also easier to line with paper for cleaning.

Location
The respiratory system of birds does not protect from inhaled hazards as well as the mammalian respiratory system does. Cages should never be placed near open windows or doors or other areas with drafts or near fumes, such as paint, smoke, hair sprays, insecticides, scented candles, plug-in fresheners, ammonia-based glass cleaners, and stain-guard chemicals. They should not be located in or near kitchens with fumes from burned foods or from non-stick cooking pans coated with the fluoropolymer polytetrafluoroethylene (Teflon®). Silverstone® and Tefzel® are also coated with fluoropolymers. Vaporization of dangerous fluoropolymers begins at 464°F (240°C).

The cage should be located in a bright area, but not in direct sunlight. The location should be without drafts and away from kitchens and placed at chest level. If the cage is placed near the floor, birds will be stressed with concern about their vulnerability to predators. Placing cages above human eye level will decrease stress in timid birds. Locating a cage near an open window risks drafts, direct sunlight, stress from being on constant alert for predators, and transmission of disease from wild birds.

Birds that are well socialized to humans should be caged in family traffic areas during the day. The cage should be located against a wall, or the cage should contain a hiding area to reduce stress for rest periods. A separate cage for rest may be needed in a quiet, dark area for larger birds that are used to handling. Frequent interaction with people should be supplemented with toys and multiple perches for entertainment. Placing the cage near a closed window and out of direct sunlight can allow birds to watch outside activities and provide valuable mental stimulation. Boredom is a common cause for many behavioral problems in birds. Providing opportunities to simulate foraging for food and guarding against predators and to create nests avert stereotypic behaviors.

Most companion birds are from the tropics, where 10–12 hours of daylight occurs year round. Exposure to direct sunlight or a UVB light source 18 in (45 cm) above the cage should be provided for these companion pets at a near consistent 10–12 hours per day. For sleeping, some birds prefer for the cage to be covered. Others do not. Cage covering is optional.

Size
Minimum cage size in width, depth, and height for large birds should be 1½ times the wing span for each bird. Smaller birds need additional room to fly in the cage. All cages should be wider than tall. When perched, the tail should not contact the floor, walls, or any other object in the cage. Mynah birds require the largest cages (6 × 3 × 3 ft [2 × 1 × 1 m] minimum for one bird).

Construction materials
Bird cages should be constructed of non-rusting metal (stainless steel, anodized aluminum, or chrome plating) and inspected for sharp or pointed projections that might cut or stab an inquisitive bird's tongue. Cages should not be painted with lead-based paint or galvanized. Zinc used for galvanizing is

toxic to birds and the most common metal poisoning in caged birds. Better cages are made from stainless steel or wrought iron. Powder-coating can keep the metal from rusting.

> Birds can get metal poisoning from cages constructed of inexpensive materials.

Bars
The space between cage bars should be narrow enough to prevent entrapping a bird's head. Small birds (parakeets, finches, canaries) should have bars spacing no greater than ½ in (1.3 cm). Medium-sized birds (cockatiels, conures, lories) should have bar spacing of no more than ¾ in (1.9 cm). Large birds (African grey parrots, macaws, cockatoos) may have bar spacing of up to 1-¼ in (3.2 cm). Vertical bars cause less damage to tail feathers than horizontal bars. Wire grids above a sliding solid bottom prevent paper from shredding and the bird from eating wasted, spoiled food. Wire cages can be too stressful for nervous birds. Box-type cages are preferable for timid birds. Other birds enjoy viewing activity and receiving attention. Door latches should be substantial. Simple door latches on barred cages can be opened by many birds.

Perches
A cage should have at least two perches: one narrow perch for birds to grasp with their feet, and one that they can stand flat-footed on. Most perches should be wooden, preferably manzanita wood, which is dense without any harmful chemicals in it. Willow or fruit tree branches can also be used. Yew, oak, or rhododendron branches should not be used. All branches should be washed carefully to remove possible diseases from wild bird fecal contamination. Additional perches should vary in size to exercise the full range of the grasp of the feet and prevent tendon contracture, but all perches should be appropriate for the size of the contained birds' feet. Recommended perch diameters for small, medium, and large birds are ⅜–¾ in (9.5–19 mm), ⅝–1-¼ in (16–32 mm), and 1–2 in (25–50 mm), respectively. Sandpaper should not be used on perches in an attempt to wear down toenails. Perches should not be positioned over food

or water bowls. A sleeping perch should be located in the back of the cage. The location perches of different styles and diameters should be changed occasionally.

Concrete perches can be beneficial in maintaining needed abrasion to the toenails and beak for larger birds (200–1,000 g body weight), eliminating the need for nail and beak trimming. Concrete perches should be placed where the bird spends less time, such as in front of a feeding container. They should not be used where the bird spends more time at play, rest, or preening to avoid the possibility of excessive foot abrasion.

Substrate and cleaning

Paper should be used as substrate. Organic bedding, such as ground corncobs, can promote bacterial or fungal growth. Wood shavings and sawdust can cause respiratory problems and digestive tract impactions.

Food and water containers and floor paper should be cleaned daily. Perches should be cleaned whenever soiled. The entire cage should be cleaned once per week.

Enrichment

Inanimate toys are important to provide mental stimulation and prevent stereotypic behaviors caused by boredom, such as aggressive conduct, pacing along a perch, swinging the head from side to side or bobbing it up and down, feather picking, and screaming. Ropes, paper towel rolls, and plain cardboard boxes are simple toys that birds enjoy. Many bird toys are commercially available, including ladders, chains with bells, and blocks of wood on string. Another diversion is cuttlebones, the exoskeleton of saltwater cuttlefish. Cuttlebones are a source of calcium and iodine for small birds and an abrasive that can help keep the beak from overgrowing. Birds also enjoy tearing up paperback books and searching for treats hidden in toys that create a puzzle to solve.

Large psittacines, such as African grey parrots and macaws, are highly intelligent birds that are often kept alone in relatively small cages. Extra effort is needed to ensure these birds have room to exercise, interaction with their owners, and inanimate forms of environmental enrichment for mental stimulation. Otherwise, stereotypic behaviors, particularly feather picking, often occur.

Small passerines, such as canaries and finches, should be provided with a nest or hiding boxes attached to the top of the cage. Nest boxes should be easy to remove and clean.

Aviaries

Food and water containers and soiled perches in aviaries should be cleaned daily. Substrate should be raked clean once per week and all perches washed. All substrates should be replaced at least twice per year. Substrates for aviaries with concrete floors are usually a gravel or stone chip.

Indoor

Aviaries should have an enclosure within, or connected to, the flight area. Along with being large enough to accommodate the species size and number of birds, an aviary should be large enough to facilitate cleaning. The shape is commonly rectangular or square.

When more than one indoor aviary chamber is present, there should be enough space between adjoining aviaries to prevent birds in different chambers from pecking their neighbors. At least two perches should be provided. Perches should be placed at different heights and made of branches with bark, cotton ropes, and dowels with varied diameters. A portion of the aviary floor should be sandpaper to allow scratching and wear of toenails.

Tree limbs are useful and easily replaced when soiled. However, care must be taken in their selection. Some trees are poisonous. Willow or fruit tree branches are safest. The limbs should be thoroughly washed to prevent exposure to wild bird feces. Perches should be attached securely and positioned away from food and water containers. Bathing bowls or regular sprays of mist should be provided to encourage proper preening. Bathing water should be checked to monitor for bird mites.

Outdoor

Most aviaries have an indoor compartment and an external cage. In addition to having the same needs of indoor aviaries, an outdoor aviary should be sheltered from wind, noise, and stressful nearby activities by constructing the outdoor cage so that it is sheltered from the prevailing winds. Other visual barriers should be created between the cage and the public and other possible stresses to the birds. An aviary should not be located beneath overhanging trees because of the risk of exposure to feces from wild birds. Wire and wood frame is acceptable for most species, but parrots may chew wood and so should be contained in heavy (10–14 ga) mesh-and-metal-framed aviaries. At least one-third of the top of the aviary should be clear plastic for shelter from the weather and wild birds. The floor should be concrete to prevent entry of burrowing rodents and predators.

To prevent escapes, the ideal entry to an aviary is a chamber with an outside door and a door into the aviary. The second best entry is a door that opens inward. Water is best provided with tube drinkers to prevent contamination. Cuttlebones, mineral blocks, and bathing dishes with about 1 in (25 mm) of water should be provided. Supplementary heating and lighting may be necessary for some species.

REPTILE CONTAINMENT

Reptile health is highly dependent on their containment. They are high maintenance animals because of the complexities of maintaining an environment appropriate for the species. Enclosures must match the humidity, temperature, exposure to light, color of surroundings, walking surface, climbing options, hiding places, access to water, and, at times, social interactions of the species' native region.

Cramped containment, improper heating, difficult shedding, and territorial issues with others in the enclosure are just some of the ways in which containment can affect the attitude of reptiles and their handling safety.

General considerations

Vivariums are enclosures designed to mimic a natural environment. A terrarium is an enclosure for terrestrial (land) animals (**Figure 3.8**). Terrariums may be desert-like and some may be forest-like, including trees for arboreal reptiles to climb. An aquarium is for a water environment. Some reptiles are semi-aquatic and require a combination environment in their enclosure. Enclosures for reptiles should always closely match their natural environment.

Terrestrial species need horizontally elongated enclosures. Arboreal species require tall enclosures. Burrowing species need extra deep substrate. All reptiles should have a place to hide in their enclosure to reduce stress. In general, the space required per

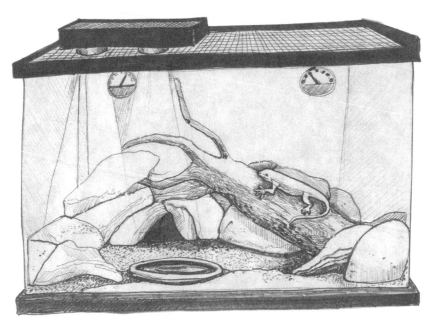

Fig. 3.8 Terrarium for reptiles.

reptile is at least 1½ sq ft (0.14 sq m) per 1 ft (0.3 m) of reptile. More active reptiles need additional space. Larger reptiles will usually bully smaller reptiles and opportunistic feeders can cannibalize others, so group housing should be restricted to reptiles of approximately the same size.

All reptiles require secure containment since they are all escape artists, especially snakes. Lids made of wire mesh or plexiglass with holes should be used to prevent escape but permit ventilation.

Wood cages should not be used because of the inability to be properly sanitized. All reptiles need appropriate space and hiding areas. Cage furniture that blends with the reptiles' coloring should be provided to reduce stress. Mirrors should not be present in enclosures as males will be stressed over an apparent invasion of their territory by a rival male and may injure themselves fighting their reflection. Males should also not be in view of other males in nearby enclosures. Therefore, transparent wall enclosures are undesirable.

Reptiles also all require an area to bask in warmth and a hiding location to relieve stress. Adaptation to new environments of about 1 week should be permitted prior to handling. Cages may be warmed with basking lamps or heating pads placed underneath the cage. Heat rocks often cause thermal injuries and should not be used. Because of the use of water and high humidity in many vivariums, all electric circuits should be wired with ground fault interrupters to disconnect the electricity in situations that could cause electrical shock to the animals or handlers.

Hide boxes, which may be fashioned from stacked rocks and a piece of slate or branches, are useful to relieve stress and reduce the risk of becoming aggressive or overly defensive.

Arboreal lizards and snakes need enclosures with vertical space and structures to climb and rest on. Branches from hardwood trees may be used, but prior treatment by baking, boiling, or soaking with diluted bleach solution is necessary to prevent introducing pathogens from wild reptiles or birds to the enclosure.

Substrate

Oils in cedar or pine shavings and walnut shells are potentially toxic to reptiles and should not be used as substrate. Safer substrates are artificial turf, orchid bark, alfalfa pellets, newspaper, peat moss, or sand. Corn cobs and mulch are hard to keep clean, mold easily, and may cause impactions if eaten. Neither soil nor sawdust should be used because of their ability to retain too much moisture, which can sustain disease-producing organisms and increases the risk of introducing parasites to the enclosure. Rocks or gravel should be large enough so as not to be eaten.

Reptiles, especially snakes, should be fed in a feeding enclosure separate from their primary enclosure. Only newspaper should be used on the floor of the feeding enclosure to prevent accidental substrate impaction.

Humidity

Optimum humidity for the species is needed for normal shedding, breathing, ability to eat properly, and elimination of waste products. Too low a humidity for the species involved can contribute to abnormal shedding of skin scales. Failure for lizards to normally shed skin on their legs, toes, or tail can lead to the partially shed attached skin drying and creating a constriction that cuts off blood supply to the affected extremity. Conversely, abnormally high humidity can promote skin infections.

Humidity needs vary widely depending on the species of reptile and the habitat in which the species evolved. Humidity should be maintained at 50–70% relative humidity for species from temperate climates, 30–50% for desert species, and 70–90% for tropical species. Low airflow is needed in the enclosure to maintain humidity.

A higher humidity environment can be more easily maintained in enclosures that have glass or acrylic sides. It can be enhanced with misting, drippers, foggers, waterfalls, pools or shallow bowls of water, and damp towels draped over the wire top of an enclosure. Plants can be attractive additions to enclosures but are difficult to clean and might be eaten by the inhabitants. Hide boxes with peat moss that is regularly misted is another means of enhancing humidity. Rocks with rough but not sharp edges to rub against may aid in the shedding process.

Warmth

Reptiles are ectotherms, which means that optimum external heat for the species is needed for normal activity, digestion, and immune functions. This is referred to as the *POTZ*: preferred optimal temperature zone. If reptiles get too hot, heat stress can develop. If they get too cold, indigestion or respiratory disease can result.

The warm environment they require can facilitate the growth of many disease agents. Good ventilation is essential to control odors and disease microbes. Frequent cleaning is also important.

The temperature needed throughout the day by reptiles fluctuates within their POTZ. The POTZ for species from temperate climates is 78–86°F (25.5–30°C). Semi-aquatic turtles prefer slightly lower temperatures. Tropical species should be maintained at 82–92°F (27.8–33.3°C), and desert species should be in 84–96°F (28.9–35.5°C).

Heat is provided in a basking area of the enclosure to allow self-adjustment by the reptile situating itself closer or farther from the source of heat. The difference between basking areas and resting areas should be about 15°F (8°C). Heat lamps should be 50–75 watts and positioned so that there is no chance of the reptile directly contacting them. Basking surfaces for most species should be 90–100°F (32.2–37.8°C). Basking lights should be at least 18 in (0.5 m) from the substrate. Ultraviolet lamps provide heat to objects in the enclosure without raising the air temperature. Supplemental heat can be provided with under-tank heaters that cover no more than one-third of the enclosure's floor. Overhead heat sources should be used for diurnal species and under-tank heaters for nocturnal species. Extra care is warranted for under-tank heaters, which can be hazardous for burrowing reptiles.

Lighting

The amount and type of lighting are important for indoor enclosures for reptiles. Lights should be timed to be on for 14 hours during summer months and 10 hours during winter months for tropical and subtropical species. Temperate region species need 16 hours of light in summer and 8 hours in winter.

Full spectrum light is needed as visible rays; UVA (long wave) light to control photoperiods, and UVB (290–310 nm) light for vitamin D formation in diurnal lizards and chelonians. UVB light can improve reptile activity and aid in maintaining healthy skin. Mercury halide or fluorescent lights can provide heat and UVB light. UVB light does not penetrate glass; therefore, lighting must be placed on the same side of glass enclosures as the reptile, in a way that prevents contact with the reptile, which could cause burns. UVA and UVB lights on timers are safer and more reliable than relying on natural sunlight for enclosures. Sunlight through windows does not provide sufficient UVB light and may lead to an unacceptably high enclosure temperature.

Water

Heavy objects in an enclosure, such as water bowls, should be wide based with a smooth bottom to prevent them from tipping over onto a reptile. Ceramic bowls are heavy and can be used for drinking and bathing water. Aquatic or semi-aquatic species should have two-thirds of the enclosure as water, with the remaining area for basking. Lizards and tortoises often defecate in water bowls. Water should be changed daily.

Small lizards such as chameleons drink water that accumulates from condensation on leaves. Misting the environment or providing a drip system is needed to encourage water consumption in these species.

Cleaning

Reptile cages should be cleaned daily to remove uneaten food, waste, shed skin, and food and water dishes. Once per week the cage, substrate, and enclosure objects should be disinfected.

Rocks should be boiled for 30 minutes. Sand and branches need to be heated to 200–250°F for 30 minutes.

Rubber gloves and eye protection should be worn while cleaning the cage and its contents with mild soap and water. After cleaning, disinfection should be performed with 1 cup of household bleach per 1 gal (3.8 L) of water. After disinfection, the enclosure and its contents should be allowed to dissipate volatile gases and dry out for 5–10 minutes in a well-ventilated area and then be rinsed thoroughly with water.

Turtles and tortoises (chelonians)

The most common turtles kept in captivity are red-eared sliders, painted turtles, and box turtles. Red-eared sliders and painted turtles are primarily freshwater turtles, while box turtles are primarily woodland dwellers and terrestrial. All tortoises are terrestrial. Turtles can usually be housed together, the exception being some territorial males.

Enclosures for chelonians may be glass aquariums or plastic boxes made for general storage. Opaque sides will reduce stress to the turtle and aid particularly in the first week's adjustment period to a new containment. Handling should be avoided when possible during the first week in a new containment. Tortoises need to be kept in pens. Pens should have buried wire mesh to prevent digging out and to provide additional protection from dogs.

A terrestrial turtle should have an enclosure at least six times as long and six times as wide as the turtle's shell. Aquatic turtles should have enclosure space at least five times as long and three times as wide as its shell. The height of the enclosure should be sufficient to prevent the turtle from climbing out. Water for terrestrial turtles should be provided in a shallow bowl no deeper than the height of the edge of the upper shell (carapace).

A swimming area should be provided at one end of the enclosure and a basking area at the other end. The pool water should be maintained at 70–75°F (21.1–23.9°C) with the use of a submersible aquarium heater. The water should be changed daily. Aquatic turtles prefer to defecate in the water so used water must be discarded carefully because of possible disease agents, such as *Salmonella*, being in the water. Sinks used for food preparation or personal hygiene should not be used for disposing of the used pool water.

A hiding spot for turtles can be provided with a hollow log, artificial vegetation, and other underwater objects. Terrestrial turtles should have deep substrate for burrowing, hide boxes, or heat-treated bark. Small rocks and sand may be used a substrate for digging. Absorbent substrate might harbor intestinal bacteria from the pool water.

Containment of aquatic chelonians is the most labor intensive of all reptile enclosures. Water needs to be as deep as the width of the turtle's shell, and the bottom should be at least four times the width of the shell. A dry basking area is also needed. The water temperature must be maintained within the range tolerated by the species, usually 75–85°F (23.9–29.4°C). Water filters and separate feeding enclosures are helpful but do not eliminate the need for frequent cleaning of the aquarium and replacement of the water.

Snakes

Appropriate enclosures for snakes vary widely because, depending on the species, snakes may be burrowing, arboreal, or semi-aquatic. Snakes that need higher humidity should be kept in glass or plexiglass tanks with adequate hiding areas to relieve the stress of any threatening activities that might be going on outside the transparent walls. Enclosures should have tight-fitting lids and be free of sharp protrusions. King snakes must be housed alone since they will eat other snakes.

The minimal size of the enclosure should be at least the length of the snake. Adult snakes should be in the size of a 30 gal (114 L) aquarium at least, with a secure lid to prevent escape. Rough rocks or branches should be provided to aid in shedding.

Substrates are play sand for burrowing snakes, and newspaper, brown packing paper, indoor/outdoor carpeting, or aspen shavings for surface-dwelling snakes, including semi-aquatic snakes. All snakes should have access to a large and heavy bowl of water to permit them to soak their entire body to aid in shedding. Arboreal snakes need branches or platforms sturdy enough to easily support their body weight to climb on. Hide boxes should be placed at each side of the enclosure so the snake will not limit its movement owing to possible stress of being in the open.

Snakes should be fed in a separate container from their main enclosure. They may strike at anything that is within reach if excited about being fed. The lid of the feeding box can serve as a shield while presenting the food, e.g. a thawed frozen mouse, in the feeding enclosure. Any uneaten food after 12 hours should be removed. Feeding enclosures should not contain substrate, in order to avoid accidental ingestion and resulting impaction.

Snakes only have one fully functional lung, the right lung. The left lung is vestigial or absent. Their containment must be kept clean to reduce the risk of lung infections. They cannot cough to clear their lungs of exudate.

Lizards

The most popular lizards kept in captivity are the bearded dragon (*Pogona*), leopard gecko (*Eublepharis macularius*), uromastyx (uros, or spinytailed lizards), blue-tongued skink (*Tiliqua*), and green iguana (*Iguana iguana*). All but the iguana and gecko are terrestrial lizards from arid or semi-arid environments. The iguana and gecko are arboreal from tropical forests. Many male lizards (geckos, water dragons, bearded dragons) are territorially aggressive and must be housed alone or with females.

Smaller lizards require at least 20 50 gal (76–190 L) enclosures depending on species age, size, and number of individuals. Small lizards should have at least a 12 × 12-in (30 × 30 cm) and 16-in (40 cm) high enclosure, or width and length at least four times the length of a smaller lizard. Small terrestrial species can be maintained in glass aquariums or plastic bins with screened or ventilated tops.

Large lizards, such as iguanas, need an enclosure at least 6.7 × 5 ft (2 × 1.5 m) and 5ft (1.5 m) high or at least as tall as the lizard, including its tail; a depth of two-thirds the lizard's length; and a width of twice the length of the lizard. The minimum size enclosure for a young iguana is a 50-gallon (190 L) aquarium. Enclosure requirements will increase with the growth of the lizard. Enclosures for all lizards need tight lids to prevent escape. Glass tanks are acceptable for small lizards, but larger lizards need hand-built structures.

Arboreal species (iguanas, anoles, chameleons, and some geckos) require branches and perches to climb on. Arboreal lizards need good air circulation and should not be enclosed in solid wall enclosures. Mesh-sided enclosures should rather be used.

Arid and semi-arid climate lizards should be provided with full spectrum UV light (UVA and UVB). The resting end of the enclosure should be about 80°F during the day and the basking area should be 90–100°F (32.2–37.8°C), or higher for uromastyx. Light sources should be mounted outside the cage and 18–24 in (45–60 cm) above a basking surface. Adding peat moss to the hide box and spraying it with water daily can add moisture that aids with shedding. If more than one lizard is in the same enclosure, each needs its own hide box.

Water bowls should provide lizards with a means to climb out of the bowl if they go or fall in. Some arboreal species need water from leaves, which requires misting the leaves daily.

SELECTED FURTHER READING

Allen CJ (2008). Letter of the law: 10 of the most common legal troubles for veterinarians. *DVM Newsmagazine* **Jan**:50–51.

Ballard B, Cheek R (2017). *Exotic Animal Medicine for the Veterinary Technician*, 3rd edition. Wiley-Blackwell, Ames/Oxford.

Bays TB, Lightfoot T, Mayer J (2006). *Exotic Pet Behavior*. Elsevier Saunders, St. Louis.

Bennett B (2001). *Storey's Guide to Raising Rabbits*. Storey Publishing, North Adams.

Campbell KL, Campbell JR (2009). *Companion Animals*, 2nd edition. Pearson, Upper Saddle River.

Heath S, Wilson C (2014). Canine and feline enrichment in the home and kennel. A guide for practitioners. *Veterinary Clinics of North America: Small Animal Practice* 44:427–449.

Warren DM (2002). *Small Animal Care and Management*, 4th edition. Cengage Delmar Learning, Albany.

The dog's partnership with humans has existed for at least 14,000 years. Dogs have been domesticated longer than any other species. Dogs have served as camp sentries, game hunting scouts, a source of thermal warmth, guardian of humans and livestock, scavengers, beasts of burden, trackers, and, in a few cultures, a source of food.

Domestic dogs are a subspecies of the Eurasian gray wolf (*Canis lupus*) and were thought to have evolved from the wolf in the Middle East about 100,000 years ago, but more recent evidence indicates they originally came from south of the Yangtze River in Asia. Its Latin name is *Canis lupus familiaris*, "the familiar wolf."

Dogs are not naturally indigenous to the western hemisphere, but were brought to the Americas by people from eastern Siberia across the Bering Strait land bridge to what is now Alaska about 14,000 years ago. Dogs are in more households as pets in the U.S. than any other animal.

The DNA of the domestic dog is nearly 99% identical to that of the gray wolf, but through selective breeding by humans, it has more diverse body shapes, sizes, and dispositions than any other species. The dog has an unusually large number of chromosomes (78 compared with 46 for humans and 38 for cats) and a short gestation period (63 days) which have allowed relatively rapid selective breeding for specific traits. Despite the diversity among dog breeds, 99.8% of the DNA is identical among all breeds.

The Kennel Club was formed in England in 1873 and was the first that formally recognized breeds of dogs. The American Kennel Club was formed 11 years later. Most breeds of dogs recognized since 1900 have been selectively bred just on their appearance, not their service.

The proper names for male dogs are *dogs*. Females are *bitches*, and young dogs are *puppies*.

NATURAL BEHAVIOR OF DOGS

The great majority of domestic dogs are highly social. If feral, they seek to form packs of two to five dogs and hunt in groups as do wolves. If a choice exists, they prefer to group with dogs of their same breed and same family. Although domestic dogs evolved from the gray wolf, dogs have been selectively bred and amplified into what humans have thought were beneficial qualities and have lost what were considered undesirable behaviors of wolves.

Close extrapolation of wolf behavioral studies to dogs may be without merit now that some studies have been done on captive wolves. Captive wolves socialize as packs, whereas wild wolves center their relationships around their family. Wolf behavior is based on family structures. Social rank and behavior are determined early in life and are not reflective of the interactions of adult dogs with strange, unrelated adult dogs or other species. For example, wolves will play fight as littermate pups to determine social rank. Strange adult dogs may fight to the death of an opponent to establish social rank.

All higher animals, including dogs, have a social strata of dominance and submission. Dominance hierarchy in dogs is a complex ranking system that serves to maintain order, reduce conflicts, and promote cooperation within a family unit (pack). An effective socially dominant relationship to dogs must be based on respect gained from controlling resources (food, treats) and movement (being on a leash, in or out of a cage or kennel), and not fear.

Dogs are protective of their territory, which radiates from a home. If feral dogs do not find human structures to serve as a home, they will dig to make a den. The den provides a place of security and protection from the weather and a hiding place for surplus food. Territorial aggression can supersede other factors and cause small dogs to be aggressive toward large dogs in protection of what the small dog considers its property. Their behavior when they are in their own perceived territory is markedly different from when they are in a strange territory. They are embolden and more aggressive in their own territory, have others (a "pack") with them, and have a known escape route.

Leadership in a pack is not based on fighting, which may lead to serious injury, except as a last resort. Leaders control resources and the movement of others, including breaking up squabbles among pack members.

Dogs watch and respond to their master's face and body language as much as, or more, than their master's voice. Some dogs are so sensitive to human body language that they can appear to read minds.

Body language

Communication among dogs involves body language, olfaction (feces, urine, anal glands and other glands), and vocalization.

Dogs have highly expressive body language. The body language of dogs that communicates dominance is a direct stare with ears forward and tail up. Midline hair over the shoulders and neck is raised, and the lips pulled up and back. A dog's manner of approaching another dog or a human presumed to be less dominant is direct. A submissive approach is to approach the other animal's side. To establish social dominance over another dog, a dog will jockey for a position above another dog by putting its head or front legs on the neck or shoulder of a lower-ranking dog. Because of this, a handler lowering a hand onto a dog's head is perceived as attempting to dominate the dog. It may also circle and sniff with growls if the other dog moves. Territorial marking, such as urinating on objects or where other dogs have urinated, is a dominance sign.

> Dogs trying to communicate assertiveness or dominance aggressiveness make themselves as large as possible by piloerection (elevating the hair on their back and rump), standing with stiff, elevated shoulders, lowering their pelvis with hind legs extended backward, and holding their tail high.

An aggressive dog will stare at its opponent with lowered upper eyelids. Its lips will be drawn back and the mouth is held open. Ears are pointed forward and the tail may slowly wag. Unlike dogs with fear aggression, dominance-aggressive dogs will not hesitate to bite at a handler's face. Dominance aggressiveness is characterized by calculated actions, while fear aggression is reactionary.

Submissive dogs demonstrate a lack of direct eye contact with their ears back and their tail held low. A submissive dog may freeze in place, or roll on its side and raise a hind leg to expose its belly. Muzzle or face licking another dog is a submissive gesture. Some may lick the air as if face licking. Profound submission may lead to a submissive pose along with urination. If a dog approaches in a submissive manner, its body is curved toward the other animal or a person and the tail wags.

Fearfulness is conveyed by repeated lip licking or yawning. Attempts to hide will occur, when possible. If hiding is not possible, cowering in a corner is common, with the head held at shoulder level, or lower. A fearful dog with its head down may glance upward with its eyes at whatever it considers a threat. The ears are held back and flat as possible next to the head. The dog may shiver or shake and lean away from the threat and snarl with its teeth exposed. The neck is held rigid and the tail is tucked down and between its legs. Freezing in place is common just before the dog attempts to bite at the threat.

Olfactory communication is important among dogs. Non-fearful dogs approach new dogs and will immediately attempt to sniff the other dog's anogenital region.

Dogs intending play will begin their interaction with another dog by assuming a *play bow* posture, rocking back on their hind legs while lowering their front end by stretching forward with their front legs. The dog's ears are placed forward and the tail is wagged rapidly. This posture is usually accompanied by a series of sharp barks.

Vocal communication

Growling and snarling are intended to intimidate opponents. Barking is a sign of territory possessiveness or simply attention getting. Whining is a request for care-giving or affection. Whining may be accompanied by raising one front paw or pawing the animal or person of attention.

Natural behavior by breed

The natural behavior of dogs has been modified genetically by selective breeding. These traits can be intensified or suppressed by training, but the trait will remain and can be manifested again under new circumstances such as a new home, owner, or handler, among many possibilities. Although breed behavior varies by family lines, the behaviors intentionally or unintentionally concentrated in breeds can be categorized by usage deemed desirable by past and present breeders.

Personal guard dogs, such as the boxer, St. Bernard, and mastiff, tend to be even tempered and have a strong bond to family. Livestock guard dogs (e.g. Great Pyrenees, Komondor, Kuvasz) are solitary, bond less with handlers, and have low reactivity. Herding dogs (collie and shepherd breeds) bond strongly to individual handlers, have a high desire to chase and herd things that move, and a low level of fear. Terriers and pinschers are highly alert, aggressive, and develop possessive bonding with individual handlers. Sighthounds (e.g. borzoi, greyhound saluki, whippet) are aloof and quiet, have low reactivity, and bond less strongly with handlers. Scent hounds (e.g. bloodhound, coonhound, basset hound, beagle) have low reactivity and low aggression with stoic dispositions. Sled dogs (e.g. malamutes, spitz, Norwegian elkhound, Siberian husky) are usually not aggressive but can be, bond weakly with owners, and have moderate reactivity.

SAFETY FIRST

Handler safety

All dogs need to be exposed early in life to what their world will be like as an adult. Breeds of dogs that were selectively bred to guard property or livestock or to herd livestock were selected for an extra degree of assertiveness. It is the owner's responsibility to socialize and control dogs, particularly those with aggressive tendencies.

Socialization: the key to handling ability

Dogs, and other domestic species, go through an early socialization period, during which social experiences have a greater effect on the development of their temperament and behavior than if the experiences occur in later life. In dogs, this period ranges between the end of the neonatal period, at 2½–3 weeks (the age when eyes and ears have first opened), to sometime between 12 and 14 weeks. However, others suggest that the effective period may be significantly shorter, while still others say that social maturity does not occur until 36 months. However, dogs that have little, or bad, experience with humans before 14 weeks of age rarely bond or respond to humans well for the rest of their lives.

Many social and behavioral deficits observed in adult dogs may be caused by removing puppies too early from the dam and littermates. Puppies need to learn social ranking between 3 and 8 weeks of age through play fighting, and how to interact with humans and other species from 5–12 weeks.

Preparation of puppies for socialization

The American Veterinary Society of Animal Behavior recommends beginning socialization at 7–8 weeks of age and 7 days after first vaccinations and deworming treatment. Vaccinated puppies attending socialization classes are at no greater risk of canine parvovirus infection than vaccinated puppies that do not attend those classes. However, classes should be held on surfaces that are easily cleaned and disinfected, and puppy exposure to dog parks, pet stores, or other areas that are highly trafficked by ill dogs or dogs of unknown vaccination status, or not sanitized regularly, should be avoided.

If adopted from a shelter, puppies should be kept in their new home for 2 weeks before socializing with other dogs to reduce the risk of them exposing other dogs to shelter-acquired diseases. Puppies should not socialize with other dogs that are sneezing, coughing, vomiting, or have diarrhea in order to reduce the risk of transmission of disease to the puppy.

Socialization should minimally include other people, children, other dogs, cats, vacuum cleaners, moving cars, bicycles, veterinary hospitals, and grooming parlors. A popular Rule of 7 is often applied (*Table 4.1*).

Table 4.1 **Rule of 7s. By 7 weeks of age, pups should have:**
• Been on 7 types of surfaces
• Played with 7 different objects
• Been in 7 locations
• Met with 7 new and different people (young, old, disabled, different races, etc.)
• Been exposed to 7 challenges (similar to an obstacle course)
• Eaten from 7 different types of containers
• Eaten in 7 different locations

Puppy classes

Well-organized puppy classes can be very helpful in socializing a weaned puppy. Ideally, puppies should be grouped by similar size. To limit distractions a group should be no more than six puppies, and each puppy should have only one or two people handling it.

Puppies should never be exposed to an experience that is perceived as harmful, painful, or excessively frightening. If the puppy becomes apprehensive, its handler should give it a command and then a reward, but not pet or cuddle the puppy immediately after it acts apprehensive or it will interpret fearful actions as yielding rewards.

Supervised play time should be scheduled each day. The play and training sessions should be short, about 15 minutes, and only 1% improvement expected each training session. When allowed play with freedom, a puppy's distracted attention can be regained as needed by having it wear a drag line leash at least 4 ft (1.2 m) long. Handlers should avoid sitting on the floor or ground when playing with a pup owing to the overstimulation of the puppy that generally results. Punitive methods, including scruff shakes, alpha rollovers, pinning to the floor, thumping the nose, swatting with rolls of paper, or shock collars should never be used for training puppies.

Socialization with humans must present the handler as a consistent, gentle leader. Interactions with humans should be gentle, not rough, and not submissive to any attempts by the puppy to dominate. Effective socialization must be one-on-one with each puppy, not as a litter. Direct attention from a handler should be only when the dog is obeying a command. When attention is shown to the dog, the dog should respond with its attention.

Positive reinforcements are initially small bits of food treats that are combined with petting and other praises. Training treats for basic training should be dry for ease of handling and to prevent spoilage. Treats should also be small enough to be consumed in a couple of seconds. Food treats are gradually phased out as the dog matures and responds to other forms of praise.

Petting should be reserved as only a reward for good behavior. Withdrawal of handler attention should be the penalty for poor behavior. Fearful behavior should not be rewarded with extra attention to try to comfort it, and apprehension should not be reprimanded. Rather, the handler should have the puppy obey a familiar basic command such as "sit" and then reward it for sitting. A familiar situation, direct attention from a handler, and reward for appropriate behavior will provide distraction from its apprehension and promote a feeling of security for the puppy.

It is important for a handler to establish a superior social rank to the puppy's during its socialization. This requires controlling the puppy's resources (food) and movements. One of the steps in acquiring higher social status is to make the puppy sit before feeding, then holding the bowl while it eats. The food bowl is withdrawn if the puppy demonstrates food aggression. Attempts to bite the hand are reprimanded by a sharp "ouch" or other word to startle the puppy and convey to it that biting is unacceptable. After the socialization period (16 weeks), controlling food aggression is a slower, more guarded procedure. Puppies' behavior should be controlled in certain situations, as in being taught to sit when approached by strange people or when a stranger comes to the door. Handlers should expect a puppy to learn to wait for permission to go through doors or up and down stairs when on a leash. The handler should remain still, avoiding any attention to the puppy until its attention is directed only to the handler. The puppy should not move before the handler moves and it is given permission to move.

A dog shows disrespect for a handler by putting its mouth around a hand or arm. If a puppy mouths a handler's arms, hands, or fingers, the handler should make a high-pitched sound and ignore the pup for about a minute before returning to more interactions with it. Puppies should not leave littermates and their mother until 8 weeks of age so they can better learn bite inhibition from each other.

Puppies should experience a wide variety of people, animals, and situations in non-threatening ways during their prime socialization period. Objects that make a loud noise should be introduced at a distance and gradually introduced to the puppy. The puppy should be exposed at a distance to a running vacuum cleaner and other noise makers in his new home and exposed to them again at a later time closer to the noise. This should then be repeated. The puppy should be taken to shopping centers, parks, veterinary clinics, and other sites where there are many people and much activity. It should be taken for short but frequent rides in a car. Stops for the puppy to get out and relax should be planned. Handlers should countercondition the puppy to being brushed, bathed, inspected, and having nails clipped and teeth and ears cleaned. This is accomplished by gentle, frequent, short-term handling sessions with small food treats whenever the puppy does not react adversely to the distracting stimuli.

Instruction of children
Handlers must always supervise interactions of puppies with other people, particularly children. Interactions need to be calm, gentle, brief, and controlled. Small children, in particular, should be closely supervised to insure against unpleasant or threatening experiences for the puppy. Children must be taught in advance to move slowly and be quiet around puppies. Although small children should learn to handle puppies in their lap gently while sitting and supervised by an adult, they should never pick up or carry puppies. Bites and scratches occur to children from struggling puppies, and bone-breaking falls occur to puppies when dropped. Children should also be advised not to bother puppies when the puppies are eating or resting in their crates.

Exposure to other animals
Exposure to other dogs during the socialization period should only be to good canine role models. Much is learned by puppies from observing how other dogs relate to humans and other animals.

The first socializing with other animals should be to other dogs that are introduced to a puppy's environment. The introduced dogs should at first be of similar size, friendly, healthy, and vaccinated dogs and other puppies. Larger and smaller dogs should be introduced later. Cats that are not afraid of dogs should be introduced to the puppy.

The second stage of socialization is to take the puppy outside of its own environment to the homes of other friendly, well-behaved pets. A puppy should be socialized to any type of animal that it may come in contact with during the rest of its life, which, in some cases, could include birds, horses, cattle, sheep, swine, and others.

Commercially bred (high-volume) puppies
There is no uniform definition of commercial dog breeders. One that is accepted in most states is breeding 20 or more dogs within a year. Another criterion that is often accepted to separate hobby breeders from commercial breeders is breeding more than three breeds of dogs. The AMVA defines a high-volume dog breeder as any person who whelps more than six litters a year or transfers ownership of more than 50 dogs per year.

Commercially bred puppies are generally at high risk of inadequate socialization. Many states do not mandate socialization for commercially bred puppies, and those that do have vague requirements. Interstate shipment of puppies falls under Federal Regulations on the Humane Handling, Care, and Treatment of Dogs and Cats (Code of Federal Regulations, Title 9, Chapter 1), which covers animals that are on display, being shipped interstate, or used in research. However, socialization is not a requirement for interstate shipment, and interstate shipment is permissible as early as 7 weeks of age. Retail pet stores are also not required to socialize puppies.

> Commercially bred (high-volume breeders') puppies are less socialized and more aggressive toward humans than puppies from hobby breeders.

Dogs obtained from pet stores are rarely socialized properly. They have significantly more aggressiveness toward humans, including family members and other animals, as well as separation-related issues and inappropriate urination and defecation problems.

Potential for injury

Overall incidence

Each year dogs kill about 20 people in the U.S., seriously injure at least 800,000 with bite wounds serious enough to require hospital attention, and are estimated to inflict a total 4.5 million bites. Still, the risks are low, considering that about 70 million dogs are kept as pets in the U.S. and that nearly all bites could be avoided with responsible care and handling.

Dog bites account for more than one-third of all homeowner liability claims. The average bite claim settlement is for more than $29,000. The most dangerous dogs are larger dogs, not because they necessarily bite more often, but because their bites inflict more damage. The ability to inflict a killing bite is instinctive. What is killed is not considered food by a dog unless taught by older dogs or by starvation.

Fatal dog bites occur most often to 1- to 4-year-old children (**Figure 4.1**). Based on a U.S. Centers for Disease Control and Prevention report, 90% involve a sexually intact male dog and 90% of 2-year-old children were unsupervised by an adult. The dog acts alone in 68% of cases, and in 25% of killings the dog is chained. Three-fourths of biting dogs

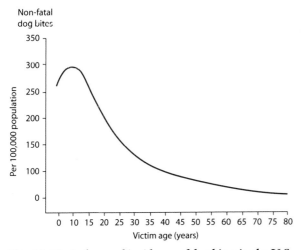

Fig. 4.1 Typical annual incidence of dog bites in the U.S.

are owned by family or friends of the person bitten. Most dogs involved in a killing are in the 50–100 lb (22.5–45 kg) body weight range.

Non-fatal wounds are usually to the arms, hands, or face of children less than 5 years of age or adults more than 65 years of age. In addition to the puncture wounds, a large dog can generate enough pressure to cause significant crushing injuries. Tearing injuries may also occur when, after making the bite and holding on, the dog shakes its head and sometimes its whole body, or the victim tries to withdraw quickly. Two-thirds of bite wounds to children occur to the head and neck. In addition to serious physical injury, dog bites can cause post-traumatic stress disorder in child victims.

Dogs involved in serious bites to humans are primarily male. Male dogs are 6.2 times more likely to bite people, and intact males are 2.6 times more likely to bite than neutered male dogs. However, once a dog develops the courage and ability to successfully bite a human, neutering has little effect in preventing future attempts to bite.

Breeds and bites

Breeds of dogs that have been selectively bred for aggressive behavior do not have the same temHorament as breeds that were not bred for that trait. However, members of aggressive breeds can have the trait of aggressiveness encouraged or discouraged by their socialization as a puppy and handling as an adult. A dog's handling, socialization, and training have more to do with the risk of bite or lethal ability than the breed. However, without proper handling, some breeds are more inherently dangerous owing to their size, gender, and breeding. For example, the Labrador retriever has been bred to willingly jump into water and most can be trained to retrieve ducks. A Yorkshire terrier will not willingly jump into water and cannot be trained to retrieve ducks. Breeds selectively bred to protect people or property or to move or fight other animals are more likely to develop the courage to bite a human. Pit bull-type dogs were bred from bulldogs and terriers to fight bears and bulls (bear-baiting and bull-baiting). Later, they were bred to fight each other in pits.

In a study of dogs causing fatal attacks on humans during the 1980s and 1990s in the U.S., dogs with a pit bull appearance were responsible for the majority of the attacks. A breed named pit bull is not recognized by the AKC (though it is by the United Kennel Club and the American Dog Breeders Association), but up to 20 breeds have some characteristics of what is popularly referred to as a pit bull. Pit bulls are derived from American Staffordshire terriers, American pit bull terriers, and/or Staffordshire bull terriers. Registered American Staffordshire terriers, American pit bull terriers, and Staffordshire bull terriers are usually properly socialized to other dogs and to humans and trained to be good canine citizens.

The pit bull-type dogs responsible for human fatalities are typically mixed-breed, poorly or unsocialized, tethered, intact males, and taunted or trained to become more aggressive. Any dog that is not properly socialized can become dangerous. Although pit bull-like dogs are the breed type responsible for the most fatalities, they are believed to constitute only 6% of the dog population in the U.S. Rottweilers were responsible for the second greatest number of fatalities and German shepherd dogs were third in a 20-year-long study of fatalities caused by dogs in the U.S.

It has been argued that pit bulls were bred for their temperament and have no standard appearance. Because of this, it has been claimed that many bite reports have misidentified other dogs as pit bulls owing to their unfortunate reputation. Misidentification of any breed is a common occurrence by the uninformed, but there are relatively distinct physical characteristics of pit bulls with which most people knowledgeable of common dog breeds are aware.

Pit bull terriers are dogs that have identifiable features of Staffordshire bull terriers, American Staffordshire terriers, or American pit bull terriers, including mixed breeds if they display predominant features of any of these three breeds. Features of pit bull terrier-type dogs include a height of 18–24 in (46–61 cm) at the shoulder and weight between 30 and 60 lb (13.5 and 27 kg). Their bodies are muscular with a wide chest. They have a large wedge-shaped head that is in proportion with the rest of the body. Slight wrinkles are present on the forehead. The hair coat is short and without an undercoat. They may come in any color except merle, and they may be solid-colored or have patches of color. Their eyes may also be any color but blue. The ears are either cropped or, when left natural, are rose-shaped or semi-pricked. The short tail is tapered. Since the body type is distinctive, breed-specific legislation is legally enforceable.

Many pit bulls are often used for illegal activities by irresponsible owners who do not socialize them to other dogs or to humans and taunt them to become aggressive. As a result, pit bulls are believed to be the most abused dog breed in the U.S. Pit bulls are the dog breed of choice for dog fighters, drug dealers, and people who want to project an image of intimidation. Dogs that inflict serious bites are often acquired and trained by thoughtless or sinister people to be a weapon or to give the appearance of a weapon. Aggressive pit bulls are exceedingly dangerous because of their tendency to not signal before a bite, to bite and hold, and to fail to be deterred by weapons or being kicked. They are more prone to attack the victim's face or the abdomen of a victim. Pit bulls are banned from being imported into the UK, France, Australia, and the Netherlands.

The U.S. Centers for Disease Control and Prevention has reported the dog breeds most often involved in fatal human attacks (*Table 4.2*). An association of liability lawyers lists pit bulls, Rottweilers, chow chows, and Akitas as the most dangerous dogs. In March 2009, the U.S. Army and Marine Corps prohibited pit bulls, Rottweilers, Doberman pinschers, chow chows, and wolf hybrids in U.S. military housing units because of the risk of severe bites. The dog breeds ineligible for insurance coverage for bites by some companies include pit bulls, Rottweilers, German shepherd dogs, chow chows, mastiffs, Akitas, and Doberman pinschers. For more information, visit:http://dogbitelaw.com/

Table 4.2 **Dogs most involved in fatal human attacks in the U.S., in descending order**	
• Pit bulls	• Doberman pinschers
• Rottweilers	• Chow chows
• German shepherd dogs	• Great Danes
• Huskies	• Akitas
• Alaskan malamutes	

Attempts to control bites by controlling breeds

Banning dog breeds associated with most dog bites is not the only answer, but it can play an important role in reducing dog bites. Veterinary, law, and animal control associations do not recommend attempts to legislate the prohibition of only one risk factor for dog bites, such as bans on breeds.

The American Veterinary Medical Association and the American Bar Association do not support breed bans, but they are concerned about public safety involving dangerous dogs. Although a single factor approach is inadvisable, only some breeds are big and strong enough to inflict serious injuries or become a lethal hazard. These breeds were genetically selected for their size, strength, fearlessness, and aggressiveness to serve as personal and property guardians. Their inbred tendencies may not be manifested unless the dog is not socialized or trained to express and refine their aggressiveness. A dog that can bite once and inflict great damage or death is far more significant threat to public safety than a little dog that bites frequently and hurts no one.

The choice should not be to ban all members of the breed or to give all pit bulls the benefit of the doubt. People should be allowed to own big, strong, and potentially aggressive dog breeds if they can prove that their dog has been properly socialized and is adequately controlled. They should also be required to have liability insurance that covers the possibility that their dog might bite and injure someone.

> The objective in controlling dog bites should be to ban the IRRESPONSIBLE ownership of dogs capable of inflicting serious injuries and fatal human attacks.

Requiring evidence of a pedigree and a certificate of American Kennel Club Canine Good Citizen training, getting the dog neutered, and having three or fewer dogs in the same household would significantly reduce the risk of serious or fatal dog bites. If a high-risk breed dog is pedigreed, the risk is usually not high. Fighting dogs and drug dealer dogs are usually mixed breeds. A certificate of professional training from a qualified trainer usually indicates the dog is not at high risk for biting. Dogs in households with three or fewer dogs are less likely to be a risk for aggressive biting. If a dog has been neutered, it suggests the owner is a responsible owner and that the dog is more likely socialized.

Whenever there is doubt that a dog is safe to be around, having the dog wear a harness with a chain lead and a basket muzzle, when among the public, is an alternative to a complete ban simply based on breed. Rather than bans based on breed, bans may be beneficial if they are on selected pit pulls, Rottweilers, and other strong personal or property protection dogs that are (1) not purebred, (2) have not been certified as having puppy classes before 4 months of age, and (3) are not always on a leash if not in another dog-proof enclosure.

Steps to avoid dog bites

Preventing bites includes selecting a dog appropriate for a family's living situation and family members, socializing the dog to other humans and animals in the first 4 months of its life, and training the dog to simple commands. The dog should also be kept on a leash in public, and owners need to avoid aggressive games like wrestling or tug-of-war with the dog. If the dog is male, it should be neutered early in life. A safe and secure containment (well-maintained fence, kennel, crates) should be maintained. Tethering dogs should be strictly avoided. Each dog should receive play time and short periods of training each day. Isolated dogs become irritable, unsocial dogs. Actions that provoke dog attacks should be avoided (*Table 4.3*).

Teaching children to avoid dog bites

Supervised contact between dogs and children is beneficial to both. However, a baby or small child

Table 4.3 **Actions that can provoke dog attacks**
• Tethering
• Teasing or taunting
• Invading a dog's territory
• Wrestling games with dogs
• Loud, sudden noises (firecrackers, gun fire)
• Competing for food (bothering a dog that is eating)
• Presence of a female dog in heat
• Demonstrating fear

(less than 6 years old) should never be left unsupervised with a dog, particularly larger ones (more than 50 lb [22.5 kg]). Children need to be told, and shown by example, how to properly handle dogs. No one should tease dogs by pretending to hit or kick them or to take their food, toys, or treats. A dog's ears or tail should not be pulled, and dogs should not be sat on, climbed on, or ridden. Children should never approach a strange dog or run from or past a dog. They should watch for and avoid unleashed dogs. If approached, a child should freeze ("be like a tree") but not stare directly at the dog. They should count slowly to five and then slowly move away backward or sideways. They should never turn their back on the dog. Dogs that are nursing, eating, in their crate, or sleeping should not be disturbed. A dog should not be petted without permission from its owner. Children should never reach over a fence or into a car or truck to pet a dog. If knocked down by a dog, the child should "be like a rock," that is, roll into a ball, cover their face and neck with their hands and arms, stay still, and not scream.

Adult handler response to dog attack

Defense in dog attacks can either be reactive or proactive, but preparation for both is advisable. Basic defense includes not screaming, avoiding eye contact, remaining motionless, and backing away slowly when the dog moves away or hesitates.

Preparation for an attack by a large dog begins by knowing not to run away from the dog unless you are absolutely positive there is time and a definitive way of escape. If an attack appears unavoidable, an obstruction (bag, backpack, umbrella, coat, bicycle, car, etc.) should be sought that is between the victim and the dog. The dog should be ordered to "BACK OFF" with a low stern voice and occasional yells for help. Wrapping an arm with a coat can help in fending off an attack. If the dog attacks an arm, it should be kicked hard and repeatedly until it releases. A nearby stout stick or similar object should be sought that can be used to keep the dog at bay while backing toward safety. If there is no escape evident and no nearby object to use as a weapon, a stationary object should be grabbed to prevent the dog from knocking or pulling a victim to the ground. If knocked to the ground, a victim should curl up in fetal position, with fists pressed into the neck, elbows held firmly against chest, and legs curled up and held tightly together. This position will protect the carotid, brachial, and femoral arteries as well as the abdomen.

Proactive defenses begin with never trying to handle an aggressive large dog without another capable handler present. It is also important to be mindful of both the dog's body language and the handler's. Handler body language suggesting fear of the dog can provoke an attack. Other proactive defenses can be non-lethal dog defense weapons. The policy of the AVMA is that electro-muscular disruption devices (EMDDs), also called stun guns or tasers, should not be used on any animal for routine capture or restraint. Animal control or law enforcement officers may use EMDDs with non-lethal force to respond to aggressive dogs. Sprays that use capsaicin, citronella, and similar irritants require close proximity and accurate aim. They may also infuriate an excited dog rather than deter it. Air horns can be effective deterrents at a greater distance and do not require aim. Using an air horn can also deter multiple dogs simultaneously and alert other people to either help or to avoid the aggressive dog.

Air horns are effective deterrents to dog attack.

Another proactive defense against dog bites is to encourage the elimination of bite-provoking stimuli. Actions or circumstances that can provoke a dog to bite include being tethered on a rope or chain, teasing, taunting, play wrestling, trying to protect food or puppies, presence of a female in heat, and loud noises such as firecrackers or gunfire. Dangerous dog legislation should also prohibit tethering, which has been shown to cause dogs to become more aggressive.

Dog safety

More dogs are subjected to pain and suffering by poor care by humans than there are humans who are seriously bitten by dogs. Lack of socialization and improper containment are the primary safety hazards to dogs. Many problems that lead to relinquishing dogs to shelters stem from poor socialization while a puppy.

Improper containment such as tethering or allowing dogs to ride loose in the cargo area of pick-up trucks puts dogs at several risks. A lack of containment can lead to dogs being hit by cars, running in packs, and other harmful sequelae.

Introducing a dog to an unknown dog can be hazardous. Distractions should be minimized. The introduction should be on neutral ground with both dogs on a short leash, preferably with just one handler per dog. Time for the dogs to assess each other by sight and smell at a distance from each other is important. Based on the body language of each, the distance can be gradually reduced until they can do anogenital smelling. Signs of over-stimulation or aggression should signal handlers to separate the dogs. Alert signs for separation include growling, teeth baring, prolonged direct stares, stiff-legged gait, and attempts to stand on top of the other dog.

Key zoonoses

(*Note:* Apparently ill animals should be handled by veterinary professionals or under their supervision. Precautionary measures against zoonoses from ill animals are more involved than those required when handling apparently healthy animals and vary widely. The discussion here is directed primarily at handling apparently healthy animals.)

Apparently healthy domestic dogs pose little risk of transmitting disease to healthy adult handlers who practice conventional personal hygiene. The risks of physical injury are greater than the risks of acquiring an infectious disease.

The most suitable pets for young children are dogs and cats because the risks of injury and infection are better known and more easily controlled than for other animals.

Directly transmitted zoonotic diseases from dogs can result in signs of disease systemically or primarily in the respiratory, digestive, or integumentary system of humans. In some cases healthy appearing dogs can transmit zoonotic diseases (*Table 4.4*).

Direct transmission
Systemic disease
Many zoonoses from dogs can cause generalized (systemic) illness. Nearly all are described as flu-like symptoms. None are common in adult handlers of healthy appearing dogs.

There can be serious damage in humans, primarily the liver or eyes of children, who acquire dog roundworm (visceral or ocular larvae migrans) by carrying the infective larvae in the soil to their mouth. Fecal material must be ingested to develop larvae migrans infections. Development of the larvae for at least 2 weeks after being passed in the feces is required for transmission. Fresh feces is not a risk for larvae migrans. Young children should be kept from playgrounds and beaches where dogs are allowed to defecate.

Echinococcosis (*Echinococcus granulosus* and *E. multilocularis*) are tapeworms of dogs that have contact with sheep or wildlife. They are acquired by ingesting fecal contaminated materials. The eggs are sticky, and exposure can occur by petting an infected dog's hair coat. Echinococcosis typically causes cysts in the liver or lungs in humans. It occurs wherever dogs are allowed to eat raw sheep parts (*E. granulosus*) or rodents (*E. multilocularis*) but is rare in the U.S.

Capnocytophaga canimorsus, a potentially fatal bacteria in the oral cavity of dogs, is a risk for humans with impaired immune systems, such as from chemotherapy, cancer, AIDS, or splenectomy.

Brucellosis is a systemic disease of humans that can be transmitted by dogs ill with the disease, particularly after a dog experiences an abortion.

Listeriosis can cause generalized disease in immunosuppressed humans that includes an atypical pneumonia.

Urogenital secretions from dogs may transmit canine brucellosis (*Brucella canis*), Q fever, or leptospirosis. Dogs with brucellosis generally have clinical signs of disease although they may be subtle. Coxiellosis (Q fever) is a bacterial disease that is transmitted by inhalation of dust contaminated by the body secretions of animals (urine, milk, feces, etc.) infected with *Coxiella burnettii*. Dogs from farms with livestock may transmit Q fever in placental fluids, although the risk from cats is better established. Dogs with leptospirosis can have subclinical infection, especially if previously vaccinated against leptospirosis or are in a recovery phase while transmitting the infective organism in the urine. Leptospirosis causes systemic disease and tends to

Table 4.4 **Diseases transmitted from healthy appearing dogs to healthy adult humans**

DISEASE	AGENT	MEANS OF TRANSMISSION	SIGNS AND SYMPTOMS IN HUMANS	FREQUENCY IN ANIMALS	RISK GROUP*
Bites	–	Direct injury	Bite wounds to face, arms, and legs	All dogs are capable of inflicting bite wounds	3
Visceral larvae migrans	*Toxocara canis*	Direct, fecal-oral	Enlarged liver, coughing	Very common in puppies	2
Ocular larvae migrans	*Toxocara canis*	Direct, fecal-oral	Defects in eye(s), blindness	Very common in puppies	2
Cutaneous larvae migrans	*Ancylostoma caninum, A. braziliense, Uncinaria stenocephala*	Direct, oral, transdermal	Linear, red, itchy eruptions on the skin	Common in puppies	2
Echinococcosis	*Echinococcus granulosus, E. multilocularis*	Direct, fecal-oral	Cough and shortness of breath, or abdominal pain and jaundice	Possible in dogs allowed to eat sheep or rodents	4
Leptospirosis	*Leptospira* spp.	Direct, oral, mucous membranes, broken skin	Flu-like signs and symptoms	Common if dogs are near wildlife	3
Campylobacteriosis	*Campylobacter* spp.	Direct, fecal-oral	Diarrhea	Common in puppies	3

* Risk groups (National Institutes of Health and World Health Organization criteria. Centers for Disease Control and Prevention, *Biosafety in Microbiological and Biomedical Laboratories*, 5th edition, 2009):
 1 Agent not associated with disease in healthy adult humans.
 2 Agent rarely causes serious disease and prevention or therapy possible.
 3 Agent can cause serious or lethal disease and prevention or therapy possible.
 4 Agent can cause serious or lethal disease and prevention or therapy are not usually available.

localize in the kidneys. In humans, symptoms vary, ranging from flu-like to meningitis, hepatitis, and renal failure.

Rabies is a fatal viral infection that is transmitted by bites or saliva contaminated wounds.

Respiratory disease

Dog respiratory or oral secretions can be a source of infection with *Bordetella bronchiseptica, Capnocytophaga canimorsus, Pasteurella multocida,* plague (*Yersinia pestis*), and tularemia (*Francisella tularensis*) in immuno-suppressed humans. Young children should not be permitted to kiss dogs and expose themselves to dog respiratory or oral secretions. It should be noted that strep throat, caused by Group A *Streptococcus*, does not originate in dogs.

Digestive tract disease

Ingesting material contaminated with feces is needed in order to acquire some of the bacterial diseases that cause diarrhea, such as campylobacteriosis or salmonellosis, from dogs. Of these, campylobacteriosis (previously known as vibriosis) is the most common, although the source (*Campylobacter upsaliensis*) is generally from puppies with diarrhea. However, campylobacteriosis can be transmitted to humans from healthy appearing dogs. Salmonellosis (*Salmonella enteritidis*) is uncommon in dogs, but the incidence has increased with the popularity of feeding raw meat or bones to dogs. Handlers become at risk from infected feces or handling raw meat or bones and accidentally ingesting the bacteria.

Both cryptosporidiosis and giardiasis have been listed as potential zoonoses from infected dogs, but the risk of transmission has been poorly characterized.

Zoonoses that are passed in the feces in the infective form and could be acquired from exposure to the rectum during handling a dog are salmonellosis, campylobacteriosis, cryptosporidiosis (*C. parvum*), yersiniosis (*Yersinia enterocolitica*), and perhaps giardiasis. Among these, salmonellosis and campylobacteriosis are the greatest risks, although the risks are still small if no clinical signs (diarrhea) are present and hands are washed after handling dogs.

Skin disease

The zoophilic skin fungus *Microsporum canis* is a common cause for ringworm, particularly tinea capitis, in young children. It is often carried on hair coats without clinical signs, especially in cats, and transferred to the scalp of children by contamination of their hands and fingernails. Young children should have their hands washed and fingernails cleaned after handling dogs and particularly cats to reduce the risk of acquiring ringworm. Ringworm is the most common reported zoonosis other than bites and scratches in small animal veterinarians. Dog handlers may develop transient infections by contact, often by infected hair being caught under a sleeve or collar and rubbed against the skin or caught under the fingernails and scratched into the scalp.

Mange mites (*Sarcoptes scabiei, Cheyletiella yasguri*) can be transmitted transiently to handlers, but transmission by animals without clinical signs of skin disease is highly unlikely.

Staphylococcal infection (*Staphylococcus pseudintermedius*) is a common cause of bacterial disease of dogs, but the species of bacteria is usually not the type that is found in people (*S. aureus*).

Exposing bare skin to feces-contaminated soil can result in hookworm larvae (*Ancylostoma braziliense* and less commonly *A. caninum* or *Uncinaria stenocephala*) penetrating the skin and causing inflamed, itchy tracts in the skin (cutaneous larvae migrans, "creeping eruption," "plumber's itch"). Larvae migrans diseases are not acquired from fresh feces. Larvae do not become infective until 1–3 weeks after elimination in the feces.

Vector-borne

Some zoonotic diseases are not acquired directly from dogs, but dogs may have a role in delivering the disease to humans. Ehrlichiosis (*Ehrlichia chaffeensis, E. ewingii*, and *Anaplasma phagocytophilum*) and Rocky Mountain spotted fever (*Rickettsia rickettsii*) are white blood cell diseases or blood platelet diseases

transmitted from ticks, which dogs could carry into a human's environment.

Tularemia (*Francisella tularensis*) is a bacterial infection of wild rabbits and rodents that can be transmitted by infected animal body secretions or biting insects and arachnids, especially deer flies and ticks.

Lyme disease (*Borrelia burgdorferi*) is another tick-transmitted disease that causes infectious arthritis and other symptoms in humans. Dogs might carry infected ticks to humans.

Plague can be transmitted directly by respiratory secretions or other body fluids, but the usual means of transmission is via rodent flea bites. Plague in the U.S. is most often associated with exposure to wild rodents or their burrows (and fleas) or the dogs or cats that become infected by eating wild rodents that carry plague.

Leishmaniasis is a protozoan disease that requires sandflies for transmission and causes skin sores that do not heal and can affect internal organs. Infected dogs can be reservoirs from which sandflies can acquire the organism.

The most common tapeworm in dogs (*Dipylidium caninum*) can be acquired by humans, if they swallow the intermediate host, a flea, or less commonly a louse.

Sanitary practices
Zoonosis prevention

Persons handling dogs should wear appropriate dress to protect against skin contamination with hair and skin scales or saliva, urine, and other body secretions. Handlers should not allow dogs to lick their face, wounds, or scratches. Fleas, ticks, deer flies, and other biting flies, should be controlled. Vaccinations in dogs should be kept current against rabies and leptospirosis. Dogs should be dewormed on a routine conventional schedule. Dog handlers should be vaccinated against tetanus at least every 10 years.

Basic sanitary practices should be adhered to, such as keeping hands away from eyes, nose, and mouth when handling dogs and washing hands after handling them. Feces should be removed from yards and properly disposed of at least weekly. Dogs should not be allowed around rabbit or rodent burrows or given the chance to kill or eat dead wild rabbits or rodents. Handlers should wash their hands each time they handle pet foods and treats. Dog food bowls and food scoops should be washed after each use. The Federal Drug Administration and Centers for Disease Control and Prevention discourage the feeding of raw meat or bones to dogs owing to the risks of transmitting the bacteria that cause salmonellosis, listeriosis, and colibacillosis. Dogs should be prevented from eating out of cat litter boxes.

Children should not handle dogs that have fleas or ticks. Dogs should be routinely examined and treated for external parasites. Avoiding ticks requires avoiding tall grass, brush, and bushes during warm weather and keeping grass maintained short in dog pens and yards. Wearing light-colored clothing facilitates seeing and removing ticks. Long sleeves and long pants that are tucked into socks, plus tall boots and a hat reduce the possible tick attachment sites. Ticks are picked up by brushing against vegetation that the tick has crawled out onto in order to *quest*; that is, to wait to grab onto a victim. To deter or kill ticks, skin and clothing can be treated with N, N-diethyl-m-toluamide (DEET) or just clothing can be treated with permethrin. Daily inspection of the skin, particularly under the long hair of children, and prompt removal of attached ticks will minimize or eliminate the risk of transmission of zoonotic diseases. Most tick diseases take 24–48 hours of attachment for disease transmission to occur.

Preventing spread of disease among dogs

When handling more than one dog from different households or kennels, proper sanitation is required to prevent the spread of disease from carriers without clinical signs to dogs immunologically naive to the disease. Dogs from different origins should not be confined in the same cage or run. A separation of at least 3 ft (1 m) is desirable to reduce the risk of the spread of airborne disease agents. Handlers should wash their hands before and after handling animals and clean and disinfect table tops and cages used in handling. Runs should be sanitized with chlorine (3 cups of bleach per 1 gal [3.8 L] of water) before being used by a dog that has not previously mingled with other dogs that have used the run. Restraint equipment such as blankets, muzzles, capture poles, grooming equipment, collars, harness,

and slip leashes should be disposable or cleaned and disinfected. Leather gloves should be kept as clean as possible and used infrequently.

Special precautions are needed if sick dogs are handled, and sick dogs should be isolated from apparently normal dogs. New household dogs should be quarantined for at least 2 weeks to reduce the risk of transmitting a disease to others dogs in the house.

APPROACHING AND CATCHING

Companion and working dogs

Whenever possible, handlers should allow a dog the opportunity to approach and be caught rather than the handler approaching a dog to catch it. If the owner is present, the handler should first speak with the owner and initially ignore the dog. This allows the dog to assess the handler's voice, body language, and acceptance by its owner.

The dog's attitude should be observed to determine if it appears friendly and calm (typical of most companion dogs); friendly and fearful; fearful and reclusive or aggressive; or dominance aggressive. The handler should avoid a fixed stare or staring at the dog's eyes. A normal, quiet managed tone with reassurance should be used. The dog should be called by its name, if known, when speaking to it. A quiet, cheerful tone should be used, and an overly excited, party-time voice should be avoided.

Dogs should not be approached or attempted to be caught in a small confined space. In a relatively open area, the dog should be approached only up to the edge of the dog's personal space zone (usually about 3 ft [1 m]). The handler then should stand sideways or crouch with his or her side to the dog and give it a chance to more easily approach submissively. If the dog is large and potentially aggressive, the handler should be positioned to be able to stand immediately and move, if needed.

Greeting an unfamiliar dog should NOT involve a direct confrontation, leaning over the dog, patting on top of the dog's head, thrusting a hand with outstretched fingers in front of it, high squeaky voices, or direct stares.

Food treats may be held out at the level of the dog's head or tossed near the dog to entice it to approach. The treat should be small and easily consumed in a couple of seconds. Dry dog food treats that are easily stored in a pocket and will not spoil are best. However, some handlers prefer to use pieces of boiled hot dog, dried shrimp, or canned cheese spread. Constant praise should not be used for the dog's approach. Praise should be metered and appropriate to each stage of the behavior to be effective.

After being approached by a dog, the handler should offer the back of his hand with fingers curled for the dog to sniff. The hand should be offered at the level of the dog's head, or lower. A possibly fearful or otherwise aggressive dog should never be approached by offering a hand with extended fingers to smell. If the dog's body is relaxed and the dog sniffs or licks the hand, it can then be stroked on the jaw or side of the face. Stroking should not be initially directed toward the top of the dog's head or shoulders, and the dog should not be leaned over. The rest of the dog's body should be gently stroked from the neck toward the hips before attempting to move or lift it.

Once the dog tolerates being petted, a slip leash should be placed over its head and around its neck. When possible, the leash loop should go around the neck and one front leg on small dogs. Large dogs can be led and small dogs are usually picked up. If present, the owner should first be asked whether the dog is known to be painful anywhere before it is picked up. The slip leash is gently pulled forward and upward for head restraint while the other hand reaches under the dog and supports its body. The hand with the leash can then be moved to the dog's neck to aid in support and loose control of the head.

If there is more than one dog, the dominant dog should be addressed first and control of it established before proceeding to other dogs. Most companion dogs know the command to sit. If the dog is fearful or overtly aggressive, it should be given the command to "sit." Not complying to this command could be an indicator of its continued apprehension or aggression and the need for greater physical restraint methods or for chemical restraint. Large, potentially dangerous dogs should never be handled by one handler alone.

Some dogs, particularly retrievers, herding dogs, and guard dogs, are more aggressive or defensive when the owner is nearby. Other dogs, such as terriers, may be more difficult to handle when the owner is gone. If a dog has a history of biting or is obviously aggressive, the owner, or any other non-professional handler, should not assist in the dog's capture or restraint.

The capture of an escaped dog should not involve chasing it. Once located, the dog should be approached slowly to the closest distance that does not appear to threaten the dog. The handler should kneel, speak calmly, and offer small food treats until it approaches and permits petting. Having a friendly dog on a leash accompany the handler can be an added lure when attempting to capture an escaped dog.

Service dogs

Service dogs, as defined by the Americans with Disabilities Act (ADA), are dogs that have been trained to assist people with disabilities. A properly selected and trained service dog can be of great help to people with a loss of sight, hearing, or mobility. They can also aid some people with seizures, autism, and other disabilities, but a true service dog is a working animal, not a companion pet whose presence is only for owner comfort or convenience. Unfortunately, in the U.S. no certification of training of service dogs is required by the ADA. Some certifications offered to people wishing to claim a dog (or other animal) as a service animal do not verify any professional training having been done on the dog or skills acquired from training. The training may range from a well-established program, such as that of Seeing Eye Inc., to an individual (owner) claiming training without any verification of the training.

Psychologists who certify animals as "emotional support animals" do so without recognition of the ADA. Mental health professionals also could face legal ramifications for such actions because of the lack of scientific guidelines and the risk of the animal causing disease or injury to others. Possible cases of true emotional-support animals should be certified by forensic psychologists who are capable of providing a legal defense service, if needed.

When approaching a service dog in a harness or on a leash, it is working and should not be distracted. It should not be talked to, except by the owner, or petted, except by the owner. The owner should not be distracted. Discussion with the owner must wait until he or she appears free to talk. The dog should not be offered treats or snacks by anyone other than the owner.

Service dogs are not required by the ADA to wear a vest or ID tags. The ADA permits only two questions to be asked of an owner of a possible service dog: (1) Is the dog required because of a disability? and (2) What assistance has the dog been trained to do? Questions may not be asked of the person's type of disability or for the dog to demonstrate its ability to assist. Documentation of a person's disability or the training of the dog has received cannot be requested

Assistance animals are a broader definition and do not necessarily fall under the ADA, although in the U.S., service dogs may be referred to as assistance dogs. Most other countries maintain a clear distinction between the designations of a service dog and an assistance dog. Also, owner training of service dogs is not permitted in some other countries. Since there is no federal oversight on certification of service animals, abuse of the special allowances given to service animals is currently common in the U.S.

HANDLING FOR ROUTINE CARE AND MANAGEMENT

Basic equipment

When handling a dog other than the handler's personal pet, a slip leash is the most useful equipment. All dogs (and cats) in a veterinary clinic or boarding kennel should have a slip leash on when taken outside a cage or kennel. All dogs taken outside a building without a secondary barrier (a fence) to prevent escape should have a chest harness with an attached leash.

Leashes

Slip leashes

A slip leash is a rope, cord, or flat woven strap with a metal ring honda or honda knot used for routine handling of dogs. Flat-strap slip leashes should not be used owing to their inability to maintain an open loop when being placed over the dog's head and neck. A slip leash serves as a sliding collar and lead rope in one piece. It can be tightened when needed to gain the dog's attention and released to reward proper responses. It also provides greater security against escape than a fixed collar and snap leash.

Handlers traditionally stand or walk with the dog on the handler's left side. For the slip leash to loosen when desired properly, the honda end of the leash should go clockwise around the dog's neck. This will orient the honda end of the leash pointing upward on the side of the dog's neck. This allows the neck loop to loosen when tension is released on the leash.

The handler should not stand in front and extend his hands toward the dog to place a slip leash. This posture is intimidating to dogs. When dealing with fractious dogs, a string should be tied to the leash's honda. The slip leash can then be loosened by pulling on the string and removed without placing a hand near the dog's head.

Slip leashes should not be used on dogs with breathing problems. If an alternative does not exist, the loop should be placed around the neck with one front leg through it to prevent pressure on the trachea. Dogs should never be tied and left unattended with a slip leash because either escape or strangulation may result.

Slip leashes should not be wrapped around the muzzle and held in place by the ends to form a temporary muzzle. The neck loop could be too tight when the loops around the muzzle are made. Moreover, a one-handed muzzle is more effective and better tolerated.

Snap leashes and retractable leashes

Snap leashes should be attached only to a choke collar, head collar, or chest harness. Attachment to a fixed buckle collar is not secure restraint for preventing an escape since many dogs will back away while pulling on the collar and shaking their head.

Training leashes are 4–6 ft (1.2–1.8 m) long. A retractable leash is a snap band or cord leash that is 10–26 ft (3–8 m) long and can be spring wound similar to the action of a retractable measuring tape.

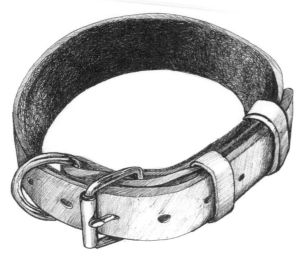

Fig. 4.2 Flat collar with buckle closure.

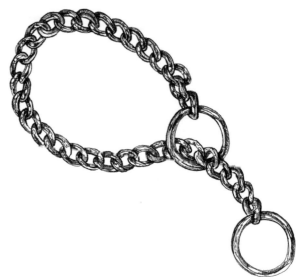

Fig. 4.4 Choke chain collar.

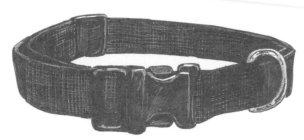

Fig. 4.3 Flat collar with snap closure.

Retractable leashes offer minimal control of dogs and should be used in open spaces only.

Collars

Flat and rolled (fixed buckle) collars

Flat fabric or flat or rolled leather collars with a buckle (**Figure 4.2**) or plastic snap closure (**Figure 4.3**) are used for identification purposes and routine restraint of puppies or sensitive small dogs. Collars should allow two fingers to be easily slipped underneath; if not, the collar is too tight.

For reliable restraint, leashes should not be attached to flat or rolled collars. Even if the collar is properly fitted, the dog may be able to back up, shake its head, and escape.

Choke (attention) chain collars

Choke chain collars are similar to slip leashes (**Figure 4.4**). The term "choke" is a misnomer since the goal is not to choke the dog. A choke chain

tightens quickly around the neck and releases quickly when tension is released on an attached leash. A more accurate name would have been "attention chain." Pulls should be to the side and not upwards, which can cause excessive compression around the neck. If the handler is to be on the right side of the dog's body, the collar's loop should go clockwise around the dog's neck. If applied counter clockwise, the loop will not fully release when tension is removed on the attached leash (**Figure 4.5**).

Dogs must continually walk on the same, traditionally left, side of the handler. The chain will not be oriented correctly when on the other side of the handler. Choke collars should be used for training purposes only and only when the dog is on a hand-held leash. Otherwise there is risk of strangulation if tied or if the collar becomes caught on an object.

Choke collars, as with any restraint equipment, can be misused and cause aversive behaviors. Unlike shock collars, choke collars are training tools that can deliver getting-attention-to-the-handler signals appropriate to situations that may quickly vary. They are not intended to cause injury or pain. Used with proper discretion and timing, a choke collar can be a safe, useful communication tool between handlers and dogs and does not cause aversive behaviors.

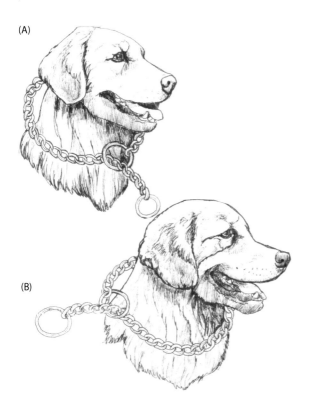

(A)

(B)

Fig. 4.5 Proper (A) and improper (B) placement of a choke chain.

Martingale and prong collars

Martingale collars are flat collars with rings at both ends and a chain that goes through each ring (**Figure 4.6**). The chain also has rings at each end. The size of the flat collar can be adjusted so that the extent of squeeze on the neck, when the leash is pulled, can be modified. Unlike choke collars, martingale collars cannot be put on backwards and will work the same if the dog changes from one side of the handler to the other. Since they are flat collars and the pressure delivered to the dog's neck from tension on the leash is less than a choke collar, martingale collars can be more easily ignored than choke collars by inattentive dogs.

Thick-haired dogs may have sufficient hair padding on their neck to ignore the pressure of a basic martingale collar. Blunted prongs can produce better responsiveness without causing injury (**Figure 4.7**).

Martingale collars are also called limited-slip collars because they are less likely to slip off if the dog

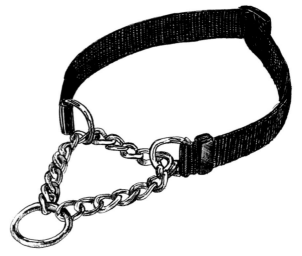

Fig. 4.6 Martingale collar.

pulls back on the collar and leash. For this reason, they are often used on sight hounds, such as Afghans, which have narrow heads.

Chest harnesses

Chest harnesses cannot strangle dogs and will not slip off if the dog pulls backward on a leash. All dogs without advanced leash or voice-command training taken outside a building or security enclosure, and all dogs being transported by car, should have a harness with attached leash on to prevent

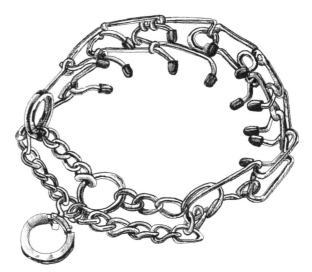

Fig. 4.7 Prong martingale collar.

escape or strangulation if they escape. Vicious dogs may be more easily handled and tractable if they are wearing both a harness and a leash that cannot be chewed in two (chain or heavy wire). Upon return of the dog to a cage, the harness is removed first and the leash is removed during the dog's return to its cage.

Towels and blankets

A towel or blanket that a dog is familiar with and has the dog's or owner's scent on it can be comforting to a dog and reduce its fear when handled.

Towels or blankets can be used to cover the dog's head to facilitate grasping the neck for head restraint. They can also be rolled into a bulky soft collar to go around the neck for mild restraint of the head. An aggressive dog can be distracted with towels or blankets and allowed to bite them while the handler's other hand approaches from the rear to capture and restrain the dog.

When using a towel or blanket over a dog's head, the scruff hold should not be attempted. It is safer and more effective to grasp both sides of the neck (two-hands neck hold) just behind the ears with thumbs on the back of the head and fingers underneath the mandible.

Tables and table covers

Tables that place a dog at the handler's waist height will eliminate the leaning position, which is intimidating to dogs. A slick table top, in addition to the height, reduces most dogs' desire to escape. Tables with surfaces that provide traction can embolden some dogs to struggle to jump off that they would not try otherwise. Slick top tables are also easier to clean and disinfect and therefore best for general use.

Some non-aggressive dogs may feel too insecure on a slick table and need a washable pad on the table that provides traction and insulation and can be easily sanitized after use. Sanitation should never be compromised by using a table surface that provides traction and warmth but cannot be sanitized after each use.

Whenever a dog is on a table, someone's hand or hands must always be on it to prevent it from trying to jump off. Grooming tables with a grooming arm (a table attachment for a leash) should have a neck loop and quick release to prevent strangulation if the dog falls or jumps off the table. Dogs should never be encouraged to jump onto or off of an exam or grooming table. Jumping off a table will encourage future attempts to jump. If steps or a ramp are used to allow dogs to walk up onto tables, the surface of the steps or ramp should be skid-proof but easily sanitized.

Tables with four corner legs are much more stable that a single pedestal table or scissors-action variable-height table. Pedestal tables should be bolted to the floor to prevent tipping with a heavy dog when the dog is not properly centered on the table.

Muzzles

Although muzzles can provide a degree of safety from being bitten by a dog during handling, the use of muzzles on dogs can make dogs more fearful of handling. They can be dangerous to the dog when used on older dogs or dogs with respiratory or digestive problems. Muzzles should be used selectively and not as standard policy.

Muzzles will not prevent a handler from being injured by a dog. Dogs wearing a muzzle can cause painful injury by bruising the bones of the hands or face when attempting to bite a handler. Fortunately, dogs often become more submissive and easy to handle if a muzzle is applied.

One muzzle shared by several dogs could be a highly effective fomite (object that transmits disease). They can also cause injury to the dog when improperly used. Muzzles should be clean, sanitary, and smooth where it touches the dog's face. It should be determined that the fasteners work easily before attempting to use a muzzle. A muzzle should not impinge on the dog's eyes. The dog should not be allowed to paw at the muzzle, as injury to the face or removal of the muzzle may occur.

Styles are open-ended ("sleeve") and basket muzzles. Open-ended muzzles are open at the end. Dogs should be able lick their nose but not open their mouth any further (**Figure 4.8**). Panting or drinking

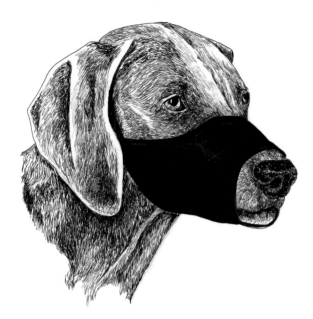

Fig. 4.8 Open-ended muzzle.

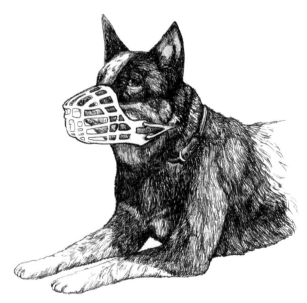

Fig. 4.9 Basket muzzle.

water is not possible. Basket muzzles are closed on the end and allow the mouth to open (**Figure 4.9**). They are made of plastic or wire. Basket muzzles allow dogs to pant and to drink water.

Dogs that have recently vomited or have respiratory distress should not be muzzled. Brachycephalic (short-nosed) dogs are better restrained by a rolled towel around the neck and behind the ears than by a muzzle. Dogs with an open-ended muzzle cannot pant and therefore cannot cool their bodies if their mouth is held shut, and so will overheat. If they vomit, the vomitus will be inhaled into the lungs and can cause fatal pneumonia. A muzzle should never be left on longer than necessary for handling, and a dog should never be left unattended with an open-ended muzzle on.

Commercial muzzles

Commercial muzzles are strong, pre-shaped, and easy to apply and fasten. Their disadvantages are cost, difficulty in sanitizing, and the need for multiple sizes if many types or ages of dogs are being handled. Commercial muzzles are made of leather, wire, plastic, or nylon. Leather, plastic, and wire muzzles go on more easily than nylon because non-fabric muzzles maintain their shape. Leather muzzles are fastened by buckles that are relatively slow to fasten. Cloth (fabric) muzzles are often fastened by a belt snap, which is faster than buckles, but cause a snap noise near the dog's ear when fastened.

Muzzles should be cleaned, and if possible sanitized, before each use. Plastic, nylon, and wire muzzles can be sanitized with common disinfectants. Leather muzzles cannot be easily sanitized. Untreated leather muzzles are porous and can trap microorganisms. Leather will also dry out and crack. Therefore, before their first use, leather muzzles should be treated with linseed or similar oil appropriate for leather, allowed to dry, and then rubbed with a beeswax for leather treatment. This treatment will inhibit absorption of microorganisms and permit rinsing and drying between each application of the muzzle. Regular re-treatment of the leather with oil and wax is based on the frequency of use of the muzzle, but four times per year should be the minimum. A properly maintained leather muzzle will also become more pliable and comfortable for the animal.

Tractable dogs or dogs that have been trained to accept a muzzle can be muzzled by one person with a commercial muzzle from behind. The muzzle straps are held in each hand with the muzzle below the dog's throat. The muzzle is then quickly and smoothly brought up and over the dog's nose. Approaching the dog from directly in front of its nose with a muzzle will cause most dogs to resist.

If the dog is not trained to accept a muzzle, commercial muzzles are best applied by two handlers. One handler should have the dog restrained in the sitting position or in sternal recumbency. The other handler approaches from the side or behind. Holding the straps on each side of the dog's head and with the muzzle cuff below the dog's mouth, the cuff should be brought up in a smooth, rapid swooping motion over the muzzle and then pulled back. The straps are fastened behind the head, below the ears. Putting treats in a muzzle to encourage acceptance can be dangerous to handlers holding the muzzle in a manner to invite exploration. This is also dangerous to the dog, who may inhale the treat, and is unsanitary unless the muzzle is thoroughly cleaned and sanitized between each use.

Another muzzle application method involves one handler holding the dog's head from behind with the handler's thumbs behind the dog's ears, palms restraining side movement of the neck, and index and middle fingers beneath the jaws to keep the jaw from being lowered. If necessary, the hands may be partially protected by leather gloves or a towel. The other handler stands beside the dog and slips the muzzle over the dog and fastens it.

Gauze muzzles

Non-stretch, 2-in (5-cm) gauze can be used as a convenient, effective, inexpensive, and sanitary temporary muzzle. The advantages of gauze muzzles are that they are portable, disposable, inexpensive, soft and non-injurious, and fit all sizes of dogs. A roll of gauze can easily be carried in a pocket and is sanitary, since after a portion is used as a muzzle, the portion can be discarded. Stretchy gauze is not a safe restraint for the handler and should not be used.

Among the disadvantages are that more skill is required to apply a gauze muzzle and application is slower than with commercial muzzles. Since gauze muzzles hold the mouth closed in the same manner as commercial open-ended muzzles, gauze muzzles also have the same disadvantages as open-ended muzzles (inability to pant or drink). They could be inappropriately applied so tightly by unskilled handlers that they cause pain and injure the skin around the muzzle.

Safer application of a gauze muzzle requires two handlers. One handler restrains the neck and jaw from behind with a two-hand head restraint hold (both hands on the neck, fingers below the jaw, and thumbs behind the ears). While gripping the head, the handler presses down on the dog's neck and shoulders with wrists and forearms to make it more difficult for the dog to lift a front leg and rake the facial area. The other handler, the one applying the muzzle, stands in front of the dog.

When preparing to apply a gauze muzzle, the length of gauze needed is the length of the handler's arms spread wide apart (about 5 ft [1.5 m]) for small and medium-sized dogs and twice that distance for large dogs (**Figure 4.10**). More than enough length should be chosen because if the length is too short to tie and the effort is aborted, the dog will be taught that escape is possible. The handler's hand should

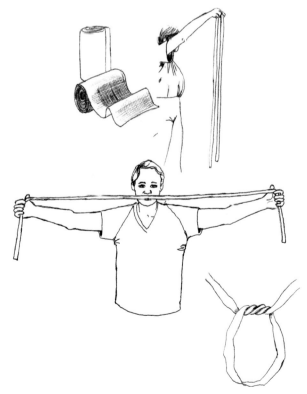

Fig. 4.10 Preparing a gauze muzzle.

never get closer than 6 in (15 cm) from the dog's muzzle while applying the loops and pulling the ties down. The first loop is made with a double overhand knot, put over the muzzle, and pulled down firmly with a knot on top of the muzzle. The double overhand knot will spread out the loop, making it easier to get over the muzzle, and when pulled down, it will hold its place better while the second knot is readied. Another loop is quickly made above the dog's nose with a simple overhand knot, flipped under the muzzle, and pulled down below the dog's lower jaw. An overhand knot is then made behind the head and under the ears, and then tied with a slip knot (a bow knot) (**Figure 4.11**).

Short-nosed dogs, such as boxers, may have their nostrils collapsed by gauze muzzles, so the top tie on the muzzle should not be pulled tight. After the tie has been made behind the head, one end of the gauze is placed under the top muzzle tie. The final tie is made on top of the dog's head to keep the gauze from being too far down on the dog's muzzle (**Figure 4.12**).

To remove a gauze muzzle, the handler's hands should not get closer than 6 in (15 cm) from the dog's mouth. The head should be restrained by one handler from behind while the other handler unties the slip knot and then quickly pulls the muzzle in a straight line parallel to the dog's muzzle. The conical shape of a dog's jaws allows the gauze to pull off easily without risking being bitten while trying to loosen the ties first.

Makeshift muzzles
Emergency makeshift muzzles can be created from ties, shoelaces, cords, or long strips of any cloth.

Walking dogs
Dogs are traditionally walked on the handler's left side. The command for trained dogs is to "heel." This is an advantage for a handler leading a horse at the same time as a dog, for a right-handed person carrying a hunting rifle, and for a handler to be positioned between the dog and traffic when walking along a road on the left side facing traffic.

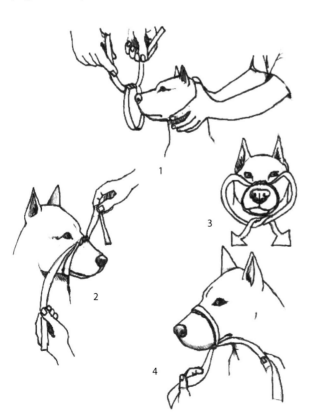

Fig. 4.11 Application of a gauze muzzle.

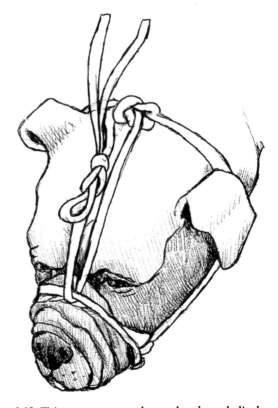

Fig. 4.12 Tying a gauze muzzle on a brachycephalic dog.

A dog should always be on a short leash when in crowded surroundings.

Dogs trained to heel are taught to walk off if the handler steps off with his left foot, the nearest foot to the dog. If the handler wishes the dog to remain still, he steps off with his right foot. Signals to stay in place are done with the handler's left hand and signals to heel are reinforced by moving the right hand.

Whenever a small dog does not follow on a leash, it should be picked up and carried. Dogs should never be dragged by a leash.

Lifting and carrying dogs

Lifting of all sizes of dogs from the floor should be done with knees bent and back straight. One person in good health and physically fit can lift dogs of up to 50 lb (22.5 kg).

Under 50 pounds

When picking up a small dog, a slip leash should be applied first. The leash is pulled forward slightly to prevent the dog from being able to turn its head to the side quickly. The other hand then reaches under the dog's chest and abdomen and supports the body while being lifted. Although common practice in dog shows to avoid disturbing their grooming, small dogs should never be picked up by their tail and a hand under the chest owing to risk of injuring the tail.

When carrying a small dog, its head should be held next to the right side of the handler's body with a left hand under the neck, fingers on the side of the neck just behind the jaw, and its body supported with the right forearm and wrist under the chest while grasping dog's left front leg (the one nearest the handler's body) so that it cannot climb up the handler's chest or wiggle away.

To lift larger dogs in this group (35–50 lb [13.5–22.5 kg]), the left arm is wrapped around the front of the chest and under the neck while the handler's right arm is placed around and behind the dog's hind legs. The left arm can be angled upward on the side of the neck to restrain the head if needed. Alternatively, the dog can be lifted under and around the neck with the left hand and under the abdomen with the right arm, the "forklift" method. This method is the only

method that provides control of the dog's head while it is being lifted.

For fractious dogs, an assistant is needed to hold the leash while the handler wraps a rolled towel around the dog's neck or places a muzzle on the dog before lifting it.

50–80 pounds

Two people should lift or carry larger dogs that are 50–80 lb (22.5–36 kg). One handler restrains the dog's head by his right arm around the dog's neck and the left arm is placed under and around its chest. The dog's shoulders are pressed against the handler's body or the handler holds the outside front leg firmly. The second handler lifts the dog's rear portion by grasping both thighs or with an arm under the abdomen and holding the outside thigh. Lift tables are also available to assist in lifting a larger dog to table height.

Over 80 pounds

If necessary, a larger dog can be lifted as with dogs of 50–80 lb (22.5–36 kg). However, most procedures are better done on the floor rather than on a table.

Cages and runs
Placement of non-aggressive dogs in cages and runs

Dogs should be placed in cages head first. One hand should have control of the cage door. Closure of the door should begin before release of the dog with the other hand so that when the restraint hand is removed there is insufficient room for the dog to escape.

Release should be as smooth and quiet as possible since this will be the predominant memory of being handled. The dog's behavior will be influenced primarily by how the dog was released from the last handling when it must be next removed from the cage. Struggling during the release will result in greater struggling when recapture is later needed. Removal of a slip lead before placing the dog in the cage prevents having to struggle with the dog in the cage to remove the lead. When placing a small dog in the cage, controlling it can be done with the restraint hand under its chest.

Aggressive dominant dogs should be kept in lower cages to avoid direct eye contact while lifting such a dog and to prevent providing the dog with a more elevated (dominant) position.

Removal of non-aggressive dogs from cages and runs

The handler should approach the cage in a friendly manner while speaking to the dog in a calm cheerful voice. Removal should begin with using one hand to open the cage door only enough to be able to get the other hand and a slip lead in. The slip lead is then placed over the dog's head. After the dog's head is controllable with the slip lead, the cage door can be opened wider and the dog assisted by picking it up, or if in a lower cage, leading it out.

When removing a dog from a lower cage, the handler's leg can aid in blocking an escape through the partially opened door while attempting to apply the slip lead. If picking it up, the neck should first be lifted by raising the slip lead and gently pulling it so there is some control of the head before reaching under the dog to lift the body.

Trimming nails

Dogs that do not frequently walk and run on abrasive surfaces must have their toenails trimmed on a regular basis, generally every 6 weeks. If dog nails touch the floor when the dog is walking, the nails are too long. An important part of puppies' early education should include desensitization to handling of their feet by counterconditioning with food treats. This is a gentle stepwise process involving a few seconds of handling the upper aspects of each leg and rewarding lack of struggling after each leg has been handled. Subsequent sessions on following days consist of handling slightly lower aspects of each leg until the foot and nails can be handled without a struggle. After handling the feet is accepted, one nail on one foot should be trimmed and the dog should be rewarded with a treat. The next session should involve trimming two or three nails. The eventual goal is for the dog to tolerate trimming all nails on all feet in one session. Success may take a couple of days to months.

Small dogs can be trimmed using the aid of an assistant, who holds the dog in his or her lap. Large dogs should tolerate trimming in a sitting or standing position. Some may roll on their back and lie still while being trimmed.

Dogs that need immediate trimming to protect them from injury from their long nails and do not tolerate trimming with mild to no restraint can be restrained by an assistant who holds the dog in lateral recumbency (held on their side). However, lateral recumbency should not be a routine restraint for nail trimming.

HANDLING FOR COMMON MEDICAL PROCEDURES

Most handling and restraint of dogs can be and should be done without tranquilization, sedation, hypnosis, or anesthesia. However, some handling and restraint procedures should be restricted to veterinary medical professionals owing to the potential danger to the animal or handler. These require special skills, equipment, or facilities, and possibly adjunct chemical restraint or complete immobilization by chemical restraint.

Restraint of individuals or parts of their bodies
Whole body
Standing restraint

To apply standing restraint with small dogs, the handler stands on the right side of the dog and restrains the head with the right hand under the throat. The left hand goes over the dog's back and lifts the abdomen while holding the dog's body next to the handler's body. The right hand can be used to hold the mouth closed to prevent panting if someone is attempting to auscultate heart or lung sounds.

For larger dogs, the handler's right arm wraps underneath and around the neck to restrain the head (called the "bear hug" hold) (**Figure 4.13**). The left arm is placed under the abdomen to hold the rear end up. The head and abdomen are held close to the handler's body. When assisting for a rectal exam, the base of the dog's tail is held to keep the dog from sitting while also keeping the tail out of the way of the exam.

Sitting restraint

For sitting restraint, the dog is placed in a sitting position. With the handler standing on the dog's

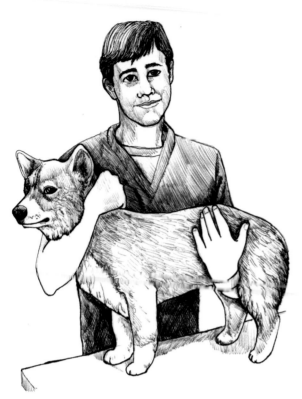

Fig. 4.13 Standing restraint.

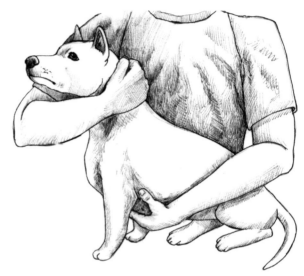

Fig. 4.14 Sitting restraint.

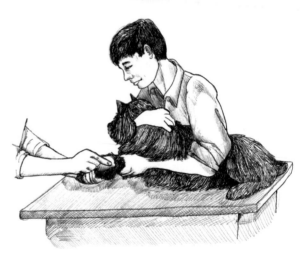

Fig. 4.15 Sternal restraint.

right side, the handler's right arm is placed underneath the dog's throat and the left arm reaches over the flank and holds the dog's body close to the handler's body (**Figure 4.14**).

Sternal restraint

With the dog in a standing position, the handler restrains the dog's head with the right hand. The left hand is placed on the rump and pushes down gently while the right hand tilts the dog's head back and up. After the dog is sitting, the handler reaches around the left side of the dog with the left hand and grasps both front legs. The dog's front legs are slid forward while the handler pushes the dog's body down with armpit and chest (**Figure 4.15**).

If handling a large dog, the handler kneels behind the dog while it is sitting and places the left arm under the neck, and the right hand grasps the front legs. The front legs are stretched forward while pressing the dog down with the handler's chest.

Lateral recumbency restraint

Lateral recumbency should be used only if there are good reasons not to use standing, sitting, or sternal recumbency. Before using this restraint, all needed materials for the procedure requiring lateral recumbency should be made ready to keep the duration of lateral recumbency as short as possible.

The dog should be in a standing position while the handler restrains its head. For left lateral recumbency, the handler stands on the dog's left side and reaches over its neck with the left hand and grasps the left front leg. The handler then reaches over the dog's flank in front of the hind leg with the right

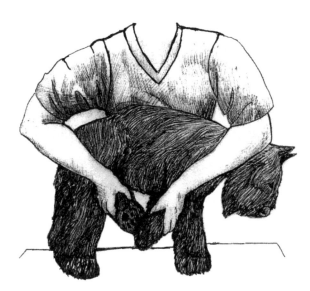

Fig. 4.16 Lying a dog in lateral recumbency.

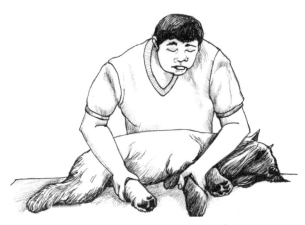

Fig. 4.17 Holding a dog in lateral recumbency.

hand. The right hand goes underneath the dog's abdomen, and grasps the left hind leg. The dog is lifted while hugging it close to the handler's body so that it gently slides down on its left side. The handler then gently restrains the dog's head with his left forearm and elbow (**Figures 4.16** and **4.17**).

Ventrodorsal restraint

A handler may hold the dog ventrodorsal (on its back) to assist with cystocentesis (urine collection by needle and syringe). A soft, padded surface such as a thick cushion or blanket should be used. Small dogs can be held ventrodorsal on a handler's lap.

Upright standing position

Examination of the lower aspects of the torso or procedures such as cystocentesis may be performed while an assistant lifts the dog's front legs and putts the dog in an upright standing position on its hind feet.

Wedging between a wall and door

An aggressive dog can be restrained for injection by pulling its leash through the space between the hinged side of a door and the door frame with the door partly open. The dog is pulled toward the angle made by the door and the wall. The door can then swing to push the dog's body next to the wall. Another handler can then approach the dog's hindquarters for chemical restraint administration, examination of its hindquarters, or intramuscular injection treatment.

Eye screw in wall and wire mesh runs

A similar method to wedging with a door can be accomplished anywhere that a large eye screw can be screwed into a wall stud at a standing dog's height. The leash is run through the eye screw and the dog's neck pulled up near to the wall. The dog's body can be pressed to the wall with the handler's leg against the dog's hip. If necessary, a portable panel (hog or sheep panel) can be used to wedge the dog's body against a wall.

Dogs in wire runs can be restrained in a similar manner by pulling the dog's leash through an opening in the wire mesh.

Head
One-hand muzzle hold

Most dogs weighing 15–50 lb (7–22.5 kg) that are not brachycephalic can be muzzled with a one-hand muzzle hold. A one-hand muzzle hold is always available, fits all dogs in the 15–50 lb range, is easily sanitized, and can be more gently applied and removed than any other muzzle.

With a slip leash on the dog, the dog is pulled to the handler's right with his right hand. The handler stands near the dog's side then hugs its body with the left hand and forearm while keeping the dog's head pulled forward with the leash using the right hand. After having the dog pressed against his body with his left hand, the handler moves his right hand to the top of the dog's shoulders. While pressing the dog's shoulders down and against the handler's body, the right hand slides alongside the dog's neck while continuing to press the neck against his body, thus preventing the dog from turning its head and reaching back. The handler's right hand continues to slide past the ear. The thumb slides over the eye and onto the top of the muzzle while the ends of the fingers slip underneath the jaw. The fingers are curled under the edge of the outside of the jawbone (mandible) into the soft space underneath and between the bones of the jaw. This hold prevents the dog from jerking back and freeing its head.

The release is a reverse of the capture. The hand on the muzzle gradually releases and slides back along the neck while pressing the neck next to the handler's body. If the dog struggles and escapes, it will be more inclined to struggle when held again.

Two-hand neck hold

To apply a two-hand neck hold, a handler quickly grasps both sides of the dog's neck just behind the ears. If the dog is aggressive, placing a towel over the dog's head first may be needed to make it possible to grasp the neck and head without being bitten. The handler's thumbs should be over the skull between the dog's ears and the index finger knuckle should be just behind the angle of the jaw and the fingers under the jaw bones. There should be no pressure on the dog's throat. Control of side movement of the dog's body is applied with the handler's forearms. Backup is blocked by the handler's body.

Mouth

The one-hand muzzle hold will restrain the head and prevent the dog from opening its mouth. To exam inside the mouth, the handler places his or her nondominant hand on top of the dog's head and muzzle. The dog's cheeks are then pressed between the premolars while carefully putting the index or middle finger of the dominant hand on the lower incisors to entice the dog to open its mouth. Care must be taken not to let the finger slip off the lower incisors and rake the lower gum.

Legs

A dog's legs can be restrained when the dog is held in the sitting, sternal, or lateral recumbent position. When paired legs are restrained, one finger should be placed between the legs during the hold for comfort of the dog and better traction for the hold.

Restraint of young, old, sick, or injured dogs

Puppies

Bitches should be separated and removed from the room if puppies are to be restrained for examination or treatments. During the first 2 weeks of life, puppies cannot see, hear well, or control their body temperature well, so they must be carefully handled and kept warm. Socialization with humans should begin at 2–3 weeks of age, but the exertion from handling should be minimal and the length of handling brief.

Senior dogs

Senior dogs should not be handled for long periods since they tire easily. Handlers should be mindful of the pain of arthritis common in older dogs. If picked up, the dog should be placed on the floor gently.

Injured or sick dogs

Normally gentle, friendly dogs will bite if they are in pain. Injured dogs should be muzzled before handling if they are not at risk of vomiting and do not have a head injury or cardiopulmonary distress. Dog crates or cardboard boxes are ideal for transporting small injured or sick dogs.

Large injured dogs should be moved on a stretcher. If a rigid stretcher is used, the dog should be strapped on it to prevent sliding or crawling off in transit (**Figure 4.18**). Two handlers holding four corners of a blanket or large towel can create a substitute stretcher, a sling, which is safer in preventing falls while transporting injured dogs than is a rigid stretcher (**Figure 4.19**). However, slings do not give adequate support if any vertebrae are fractured. Blanket or towel slings require more strength in holding the corners of the fabric than does a rigid stretcher. Commercial stretchers for dogs are available with rigid rods attached to the long sides of a sling. This wraps the dog being carried so that it cannot fall off and can be carried more securely with

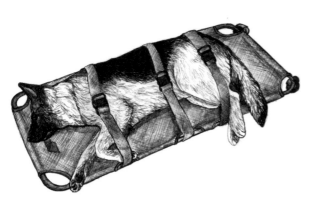

Fig. 4.18 Rigid stretcher.

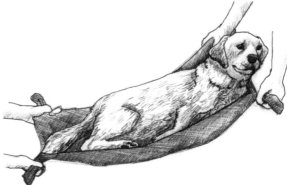

Fig. 4.19 Blanket stretcher.

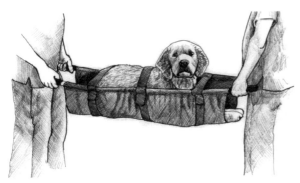

Fig. 4.20 Soft stretcher with pole handles.

just one hand at each end holding the end of both rods (**Figure 4.20**).

Gurneys, tables with locking wheels on the legs, are used in veterinary hospitals. Veterinary gurneys are available whereby the stretcher can become the top of the gurney. These are scissor-action so that the base can be raised or lowered.

Restraint of fearful or aggressive dogs

Dogs that show signs of aggression or have a history of biting should never be handled by only one handler. Each situation should be evaluated for the best way to minimize stress to the dog, protect the dog from injury, and protect the primary handler and other handlers from injury. This may require towel or blanket restraint, squeeze cage, capture pole, or chemical restraint.

Measures should be taken with puppies to prevent fear-related aggression. Use of treats when handling the puppy and socializing it to strange surroundings and various types and ages of people are important aspects of preventing fear aggression.

Injections and venipuncture

Insertion of transcutaneous needles for injection or aspiration in dogs carries the risk of slashing tissue beneath the skin, including damage to nerves and blood vessels, and breaking hypodermic needles off in the dog's body. The area in which the needle is to be inserted must be immobilized, and the dog's mouth and feet should be restrained from interfering with the procedure, especially venipuncture. The method of restraint should be comfortable, e.g. no squeezing when unnecessary, but the restraint should be firm enough if struggling occurs.

Access to veins

Venipuncture is also referred to as *phlebotomy*. It is the process of puncturing a vein with a needle and syringe to collect blood samples or to inject medications intravenously. A person who handles the needle and obtains the blood is called a *phlebotomist*.

Restraint for venipuncture of dogs requires procedures that are comfortable for the dog and do not make it feel trapped; that is, it should not be squeezed when it is not resisting the restraint. However, the method of restraint should allow the handler to immediately gain tight control if the dog resists. The dog will feel a brief sharp pain when the needle goes through the wall of the vein. The dog must not be able to suddenly move or else the venipuncture may fail. Dogs with chronic illnesses or those requiring intensive care often have many venipunctures.

Ruined venipunctures from improper restraint can result in scarred and thrombosed veins, eventually making surgical cut-downs necessary to achieve access to veins.

It is best for the handler and the phlebotomist to coordinate the withdrawal of the needle and release of the vein. Release of the vein occlusion should occur before the needle is withdrawn in order to reduce leaking of blood from the venipuncture hole. Compression should be applied to the venipuncture site after removal of the needle.

Cephalic venipuncture

The cephalic veins are located on the front of the dog's forearms. The dog should be placed in sitting position or sternal recumbency facing toward the handler's left side. The handler's left hand is placed under the dog's neck and its neck and head are hugged close to the handler's body. Restraint and proper positioning of the head are important in all cases since the sting of puncturing the vein wall may cause struggling. Additionally, curiosity makes most dogs hold their muzzle over the leg, thus obstructing the view of the phlebotomist.

To restrain a dog for a right cephalic venipuncture, the handler's right arm goes over the dog's body and the dog's body is hugged close to the handler's side with the elbow, while the right hand grasps the dog's outside elbow. The thumb of the right hand, which holds the elbow, reaches across the front of the elbow, squeezes the leg slightly, and then pulls the skin gently toward the outside (counterclockwise). This occludes and stretches the cephalic vein to facilitate venipuncture by the phlebotomist. The middle or ring finger of the right hand should be positioned behind the dog's elbow. Otherwise, it is fairly easy for the dog to pull its leg back and out of the handler's grip (**Figure 4.21**).

Large dogs may be restrained for cephalic venipuncture on the floor. The dog is put in a sitting position and the handler kneels behind the dog, holding the front leg for venipuncture with one hand and the dog's head and neck with the other.

Lateral saphenous venipuncture

The lateral saphenous veins are on the outside surface of the lower aspect of the hind legs and are seen

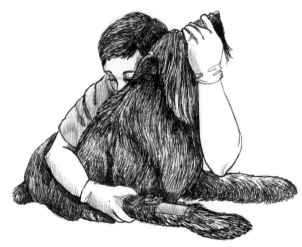

Fig. 4.21 Sternal restraint for cephalic venipuncture.

best just above the hock. The dog must be held in lateral recumbency by the handler for the phlebotomist. Occlusion of the vein is done either by the phlebotomist or a second handler (assistant). The assistant needs to use both hands on medium-size to large dogs to clasp above the stifle to occlude the vein and prevent the hind leg from flexing. One hand clasped above the stifle may be sufficient in toy to small breeds. The foot of the upper hind leg is restrained by the phlebotomist. Venipuncture of the lateral saphenous vein should not be performed with a dog in a standing position, since restraint of movement is not possible and the vein could be badly damaged.

Jugular venipuncture

The jugular veins are in the lower side of the neck on each side of the windpipe (trachea). The dog can be restrained in sitting, sternal, or lateral recumbency position for jugular venipuncture. Small dogs may be placed in ventrodorsal recumbency (on their backs) for jugular venipuncture. Large dogs (more than 80 lb [36 kg]) are best handled on the floor by putting their hindquarters in a corner and straddling the trunk of their body or kneeling behind them.

To perform a routine jugular venipuncture in an average-sized dog, the dog is first placed on an exam table. It is important to remove any collars. If a collar is left on and an attempt is made to pull it up and out of the field of the jugular venipuncture, it can compress the neck between the head and the venipuncture site. This will prevent blood from entering the jugular veins.

The dog is moved to the edge of the table and placed in a sitting position or sternal recumbency. With the handler on the left side of the dog, the front legs are held with the handler's left hand. If the dog is in sternal recumbency, both front legs will have to be held over the edge of the table and downward. Therefore, the edge of the table should be padded with a towel. The dog's head is held with the handler's right hand on the lower aspect of the jaw and its head is pointed toward the ceiling. The phlebotomist occludes the vein.

It is important to have control of the front legs. Some dogs will reach up and push the phlebotomist's hand holding the syringe away and ruin the venipuncture and possibly seriously injure the vein. This is most likely just after the wall of the vein has been penetrated if the front legs are free. If the handler cannot hold both front legs with a finger in between the legs for adequate restraint, the handler's arm should be placed around the front of the chest to block the legs from reaching up and pushing the phlebotomist away.

Because patent, uninjured jugular veins are extremely important in placing catheters in critical care, non-vital jugular venipuncture should be avoided, except in extremely small dogs with inaccessible cephalic veins.

Injections
Subcutaneous
Dogs are usually held in a sitting or standing position for subcutaneous (beneath the skin) injections. The person administering the medication or vaccination makes the injection in the upper side of the shoulder area, but not on the upper midline.

Intramuscular
Movement by a dog during an intramuscular (IM) injection can injure muscle, nerves, or blood vessels. Restraint for IM injection should involve complete immobilization of the area where the injection occurs.

The dog may be restrained in a standing or lateral recumbency position. IM injections can be given into the back of the thigh muscles (semimembranosus

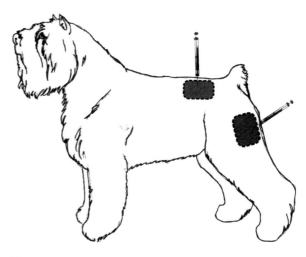

Fig. 4.22 **Most common sites for IM injections in dogs.**

and semitendinosus), the front of the thigh muscles (quadriceps), muscles above the elbow (triceps), or the lumbar (lumbodorsal) muscles. Most are given in the caudal muscles of the thigh, the semimembranosus and semitendinosus (**Figure 4.22**). Movement during the injection should be minimized by the person giving the injection by firmly holding the front of the thigh, but the dog should not be squeezed while being restrained, if possible.

Administration of oral, ophthalmic, and otic medications
Oral
Pills and capsules
If it is safe and effective, hiding medication in food is always preferable to injections. Tablets can be crushed or capsules taken apart and the medication mixed in a pasty treat such as peanut butter, soft cheese, meat-based baby foods, cream cheese, hot dogs, or tuna paste. Dogs should be trained for pilling by occasionally using small treats in which a tablet, capsule, powder, or liquid may be hidden in the future. A small portion of the food vehicle should be offered before and after the medicated portion is given.

Oral administration of medications should be done with the dog in a sitting position. If oral administration cannot be performed by hiding the medication in food, large dogs should be straddled facing out of a corner of a room to prevent them from being able to back up. If holding moderate-sized dogs, the handler straddles and kneels behind them. The handler's lower abdomen or thigh blocks their attempts to back up. Small dogs can be held similarly on an exam table, with the handler standing at the end of the table and having the dog sit with its back against the handler's abdomen.

After restraining the dog's body, the handler grasps its head and upper jaw with his left hand and presses the cheeks between the teeth while pulling down on the lower incisors with the index finger of the right hand. The thumb and middle finger of the right hand holds the tablet or capsule. When the dog's mouth is open, the handler places the medication on the back part of the tongue and closes the mouth (**Figure 4.23**).

Swallowing can be encouraged by holding the nose up while stroking the throat or blowing on the nose. The dog should be observed for signs of swallowing or of licking its nose, which also suggests swallowing the medication. A liquid (water, broth, tuna juice) should be administered afterwards as

counterconditioning and to reduce the risk of the medication lodging in the esophagus.

A pet pill gun or pill syringe can be used. These are syringe-like devices with a rubber end that entraps the pill and a plunger to dislodge the tablet or capsule after it is placed over the hump of the tongue when the mouth is open. Pill guns should be thoroughly washed and allowed to completely dry after each use.

Liquids

Oral administration of liquids should be carried out using a syringe. The dog is restrained in the same manner as for tablets or capsules but with its head held up with the mouth closed. The syringe is placed in the dog's cheek pouch, and the medication is injected slowly enough to permit the liquid to run back past the teeth and for the dog to swallow the liquid without difficulty (**Figure 4.24**). Liquid should never be injected over a dog's tongue with its mouth open because of the risk of it entering the larynx. Irritation of the larynx or aspiration pneumonia may result.

Ophthalmic

To medicate the eye, the handler must usually restrain the dog in a sitting position and hold its head and front legs while the person administering the medication holds the upper and lower eyelids apart.

A less desirable method requires just one person. The handler stands behind the dog and grasps its muzzle with one hand and places the heel of the other hand on top of the dog's head while holding

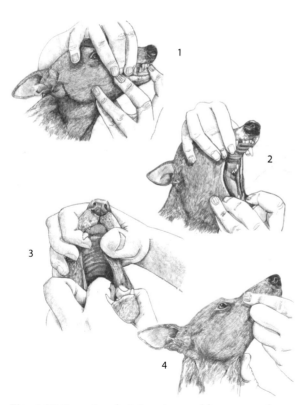

Fig. 4.23 Steps in administering a tablet or capsule orally to a dog.

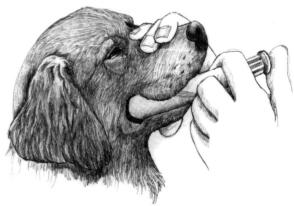

Fig. 4.24 Administering a liquid into the cheek pouch.

the medication to be applied to the face or eyes. A finger of the hand on the muzzle pulls the lower lid down and the thumb of the hand on the top of the dog's head can pull the upper lid up.

Otic

To medicate an external ear canal, a handler restrains the dog in a sitting position while the person administering the medication holds the ear flap (pinna) upward and outward as the heel of the hand is positioned on top of the dog's head. Docile dogs with non-painful ears will allow examination and treatment by one person with little restraint required.

Cystocentesis

Cystocentesis is collection of urine using a needle and syringe to collect the urine by puncturing the abdomen, entering the urinary bladder, and aspirating the urine. Restraint positions should be ventro-dorsal or upright standing. These positions stretch the body and limit torso movement. Standing in a horizontal, quadruped position or lateral recumbency permits too much movement if struggling occurs during the procedure.

SPECIAL EQUIPMENT

Head collars

Head collars (halter-type collars) are used for training dogs not to pull on a leash. Head collars have straps that go behind the head and over the nose just in front of the eyes; the leash attaches to a ring below the throat (**Figure 4.25**). Pulling on the leash applies pressure to the back of the head, pulls the nose down, turns the head, and closes the mouth. The effect is based on a dominant dog's method of grasping the muzzle of a subordinate dog to establish or reassert its higher social rank. The movement insists on attention to the handler. The pulling power of the muzzle is much less than the pulling power of a collar on the neck. To be effective, more detailed fitting is required than for other collars. To properly use a head collar, tension on the leash should be steady. Jerking and releasing the leash is not appropriate. These are not true restraint devices and should not be left on when not attached to a hand-held leash.

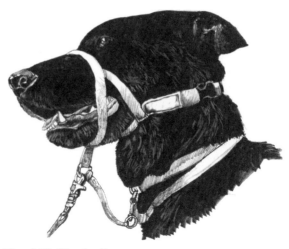

Fig. 4.25 Head collar.

Compression jackets

Compression on the trunk of the body by a snug jacket may alleviate anxiety in dogs. However, adaptation or desensitization will occur with a loss of effect in about 20 minutes. Compression jackets have been particularly advocated for dogs with thunderstorm anxiety.

Capture poles

Capture poles (inappropriately called "rabies poles") are hollow metal handles with a rope or wire cable that is fixed at the catching end, forms a loop there, and then goes through the handle to the handler's end (**Figure 4.26**). The loop is used to catch dangerous dogs by the neck and can injure the trachea (windpipe) if used with too much force. The loop is a coated cable, and so should be checked each time before use to ensure no wire strands have become frayed by prior use and, having become exposed, could injure the animal's neck. The loop is spring released by a knob on the handler's end. The recoil can cause the cable to whip at the handler's end. The handler must take care not to get whipped by the wire, or whip a bystander, when the loop is released. The handler should hold the release knob with his or her first two fingers and the wire with the last two fingers and heel of the hand to control the wire and prevent it from whipping when the loop is released. Dogs (or any other animal) should never be lifted by the neck alone using a capture pole because severe

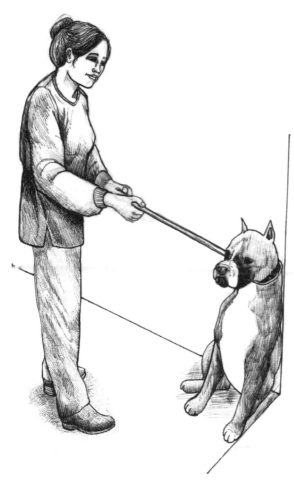

Fig. 4.26 Use of a capture pole stabilized by pushing the end into a corner.

damage may occur to its trachea and struggling when dangling could break its neck.

To apply a capture pole loop, the handler must restrict the evasive movement of the dog as much as possible. It is important to have a slow, deliberate, and persistent approach with the pole. The dog's head should be approached slowly with the loop to reduce the risk of bumping its head, eyes, or teeth with the end of the pole. Dogs often will bite at the pole, which should not be withdrawn when this happens owing to the possibility of injuring the dog's teeth and seeming submissive to the dog's actions. If the pole is not withdrawn when the dog bites, it will eventually ignore it. Some dogs learn to lower their head to the floor as an evasive maneuver. The handler must be patient and slowly continue to get

the loop to slip over the nose and then the head. Once the dog has been captured, the dog end of the pole should be pushed into a corner to control its body movements. Dogs should not be led or dragged by a capture pole.

Leather gloves with gauntlets

Gloves with forearm covers (gauntlets) can sometimes be useful in handling small dogs that bite. However, care must be taken not to restrain a small dog too tightly while wearing gloves. Gloves can reduce the sensitivity of the handler's hands to the amount of pressure being applied. Gloves should be large enough that the handler's fingers do not extend to the end. The extra length likely to be bitten by a dog can reduce danger to the fingers.

Restraint gloves are difficult to clean, and the odors from previously restrained dogs on gloves and gauntlets may increase the stress and apprehension of some dogs.

Head movement-limiting devices

Elizabethan collars are named for the large collars on dresses that were made fashionable by Queen Elizabeth I in the 1550s. Elizabethan collars for dogs are cone-shaped collars that fit around the neck with the outer edge toward the dog's nose. The head is surrounded 360 degrees on the sides, top, and bottom by the collar, preventing the dog from chewing most of its body, although it may still reach its front feet. However, peripheral sight and hearing are impaired by the collars. Some dogs cannot reach food and water with Elizabethan collars, and the collar must be removed often to allow eating and drinking. Collars are bulky and will catch on doors, furniture, scrubs, and other objects. Poorly made or poorly fitted collars can injure the neck with sharp edges. Any rough or sharp edge should be well padded with layers of medical adhesive tape.

Spherical semi-opaque (globe-shield) collars that encapsulate the head and have an opening in front for breathing and vision are commercially available as a means to protect handlers from bites. Spherical collars do not allow drinking or eating and must be frequently taken off and put on, which could increase the risk of being bitten.

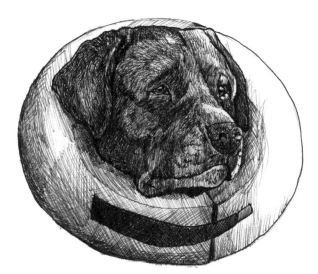

Fig. 4.27 Pneumatic movement-limiting collar.

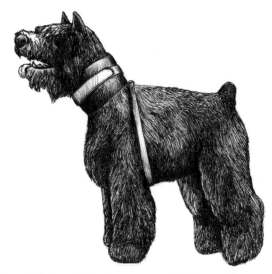

Fig. 4.28 Broad band movement-limiting collar.

Thick, broad collars wrap snugly around the neck like a human cervical collar to limit the dog's ability to reach areas of its body. Some are pneumatic (**Figure 4.27**). A retention strap is run from the top of the broad band around the lower aspect of the thorax behind the front legs (**Figure 4.28**). Broad band neck collars permit better peripheral vision and hearing and do not catch on objects, as does the Elizabethan collar. Eating and drinking are not blocked. However, access to most of the front legs is still possible.

Shock collars

Shock collars are electronic collars with metal contact points that press on the skin of the neck. A remote control operated by the handler activates a shock when desired. Shock collars often cause aversive behaviors in dogs. Vibration warnings before a shock and adjusting the voltage before use are proposed safety features. However, warning vibrations are ineffective if an association with a following shock is not first established. In addition, when a shock is delivered, the voltage is not quickly adjustable to the situation, as is use of a choke chain. Dogs that get wet during training can get a higher than intended voltage. For these and other reasons, shock collars should never be used on puppies.

Shock collars are often viewed by inexperienced handlers as a shortcut to training or a quick fix for bad behavior. The use of shock collars should be limited to experienced trainers, as a tool to consider if traditional methods are not effective at improving a seemingly incorrigible adult dog's bad behavior. In selected cases, proper short-term use of a shock collar by an experienced trainer may salvage a dog from being relinquished to a shelter or euthanized.

Vibrating, spraying, and ultrasonic collars

Vibrating collars work with a remote control similar to shock collars, though without the risk of pain to the dog and aversion. They are not reliable training tools. Some dogs can become desensitized to the vibration and ignore the stimulus. However, they can be helpful in providing command signals to a deaf dog.

Collars that emit a spray of citronella or an ultrasonic noise are also available. Typically, these are used to discourage barking. They are activated when any dog within sensor range barks, delivering a spray or ultrasonic burst to an innocent dog wearing the collar.

Blindfold caps

Blindfolds of sheer fabric attached to a dog's head and eyes like a cap have been purported to have a calming effect on dogs. Blindfolds are effective in horses, but dog caps for blindfolding dogs are not opaque and dogs do not depend as much on their sight for assessing potential threats as do horses. Evidence of the effectiveness of dog blindfold caps is only anecdotal, but dimming the light with a translucent blindfold, or otherwise, may have calming effects on some dogs in a quiet environment with no strange odors present. However, they may also exacerbate startle responses.

Mobility assistance

Dogs with an inability to control their hind legs (paraparesis) or move their hind legs (paraplegia) require assistance in walking, which can be provided with either a rear or body harness or a support sling. When neither is at hand, a towel or belt can be used as a support sling under the abdomen. Two-wheeled carts that support the dog's mid-section and hindquarters permit mobility even when the dog cannot otherwise stand on its hind legs due to paralysis or paresis.

TRANSPORTING DOGS

Dogs are transported more than any other pet animal. Most transportation of dogs is by car or truck. Some dogs are transported by airlines. Amtrak only allows service dogs to travel. Regulations on interstate, international, and air travel change frequently and must be rechecked each time a dog is to be transported.

To travel to the U.S., dogs must be more than 3 months old, vaccinated for rabies, and free of signs of infectious diseases. Livestock dogs must be evaluated for the tapeworm genus *Echinococcus*. For interstate travel, proof of current rabies vaccination and a current health certificate should accompany the dog. Travel to Hawaii and Guam, which are rabies free islands, has more restrictions.

International travel should be researched at least 120 days in advance. Requirements for importation of dogs are stringent in the United Kingdom, Sweden, Norway, and Australia. Current requirements can be obtained from the destination's embassy or consulate. A list of foreign embassies and consulates in the U.S. is available from the U.S. Department of State: http://usembassy.state.gov/

Import, export, and interstate transportation information on privately owned dogs is available at www.aphis.usda.gov/aphis/pet-travel

Regardless of the means of travel, there is always the risk of a medical emergency or escape. A chest harness or collar should be worn with an ID tag that includes the owner's name, address, and cell phone number. A landline phone number while traveling is much less useful. Dogs that travel should be tattooed with the owner's cell phone number in their ear flap or inner surface of a hind leg. Tattoos may fade and need to be refreshed before travel to be easily read. Unlike a tattoo, an embedded microchip is not immediately able to be read by someone who may try to rescue an escaped dog, but a microchip is a good second choice to ensure an escaped dog's return. A chest harness is more secure and prevents escapes better than a collar. A travel tag should also be attached to the harness or collar that provides the destination and destination contact information.

Travel by car or trucks
Cars and truck cabs

If transporting by car or truck cabs, dogs should ride in a back seat and be restrained in a restraint harness fastened to a seat belt buckle or in a crate that is strapped to floor anchors. This protects dogs from airbag injuries and the driver from interference with driving (vision obstruction, interference with braking) or being injured by a dog becoming a missile in an accident. More information on travel restraints is available at the Center for Pet Safety: www.centerforpetsafety.org.

Dogs should be desensitized to car travel by experiencing frequent short trips by car to a pleasurable destination with no adverse events during their primary socialization period (6–12 weeks of age), or as soon after that as possible.

If they will be transported in a carrier, pre-trip training should include free access in and out of the carrier, being fed in the carrier, and sleeping in the carrier to develop of feeling of security while in the carrier.

The handler should stop every 2–3 hours for the dog to exercise and eliminate. If the weather is hot, water should be provided in the shade in plastic water bowls that cannot tip over.

If the temperature is over 72°F, dogs should not be left in cars. At 72°F, the inside of a car can reach 100°F in 30 minutes. Temperatures below 55°F may be too low for some dogs.

A dog should not be allowed to ride in a car with its head out of a window. They may become excited and jump, which is hazardous to the dog and to traffic. Eye injury from flying insects or other flying objects are common in dogs that stick their head out car windows.

Pictures should be carried in case of the need to search for an escaped dog. Food, water, and any needed medications should also be available during the trip.

Interstate travel must meet federal requirements. These include a certificate of veterinary inspection, provision of adequate shelter from all elements and protection from injury, sufficient cleanliness to avoid contact with urine and feces, protection against hazardous temperature extremes, uncontaminated and nutritious food at least once per day, and a program of parasite control.

Travel by pickup truck beds

Dogs should not be loose or tethered in pickup beds owing to the risks of being thrown out, injured by sliding around or by shifting cargo, getting eye, ear, or mouth injuries from wind or debris and, if tethered, choking. An estimated 100,000 dogs die per year in the U.S. by jumping or falling from truck beds. Burns may occur from sun-heated metal.

Dogs can be safely transported in commercial kennels (also called boxes) for pickup trucks that are properly shielded, insulated, and ventilated.

Air travel
Preparing for air travel

Travel should be booked with the airline as early as possible, as the number of animals per flight are limited. In temperate weather, early morning nonstop flights should be chosen whenever possible. In hot weather, early or late flights are safest; in colder weather, a midday flight is preferable. Regardless of the season, it is best to avoid holiday periods for shipping dogs by air. The airlines should be contacted and asked about restrictions for dog breeds or sizes. Federal restrictions prevent air travel for dogs if less than 8 weeks old or not having been weaned for at least 5 days.

All dogs should undergo a veterinary exam for age and health-related restrictions. Most airlines require a certificate of veterinary inspection (health certificate) signed within the last 10 days. Some airlines require an acclimation certificate from a veterinarian. This is a form that will waive the airline's requirement that they prevent exposure to less than 45°F for more than 45 minutes during ground transfer or for more than 4 hours if in a holding facility. However, an acclimation certificate cannot waive airline requirement that the dog cannot be exposed to more than 85°F for more than 45 minutes on the ground or 4 hours in a holding facility or for providing a pressured cargo area for flights above 8,000 feet altitude.

On the day of travel, the dog should be walked outside the terminal to permit it to eliminate. Tranquilizers are not recommended as they can impair the dog's ability to maintain normal body temperature and to keep its balance during travel. Tranquilizers can also exacerbate heart or respiratory problems.

Travel crates

Travel crates approved for air travel by the Federal Aviation Administration must be big enough to allow the dog to stand and turn around. Carriers for dogs traveling in the passenger section are soft-sided. Clamshell plastic crates are used for travel in cargo holds. There can be no interior protrusions. The crate should have handles or grips and a leak-proof bottom with absorbent bedding or a pad. Soft toys or an old shirt or sock of the owner may be placed in the carrier to add to the dog's feeling of security. The crate should be ventilated from both sides. Labels should be attached that provide the owner's name, home address, phone number, and destination contact information, and a sign with lettering at least 1 in (2.5 cm) high stating "Live Animal" and arrows denoting the upright position. Containers for food and water need to be accessible from outside and secured inside. Leashes must be transported with the handler because they cannot be stored inside the crate or attached to the outside of the crate.

The dog should be fed a light meal at least 6 hours before travel. Water can be provided in the carrier without danger of spilling during the initial stages of travel by freezing the water in the carrier's water bowl prior to travel. If travel may extend to more than 24 hours, a plastic pouch of dry dog food inside a cloth or mesh bag should be attached to the crate to allow handlers to feed a small meal, if indicated.

SELECTED FURTHER READING

American Veterinary Medical Association. Model Bill and Regulations to Assure Appropriate Care for Dogs Intended for Use as Pets: www.avma.org, www.avma.org

Case L (2008). Perspectives on domestication: The history of our relationship with man's best friend. *Journal of Animal Science* 86:3245–3251.

Cooper JJ, Cracknell N, Hardiman J, et al. (2004). The welfare consequences and efficacy of training pet dogs with remote electronic training collars in comparison to reward based training. PloS ONE 2014;9;e102722: doi;101371/journal.pone.0102722

De Keuster T, Lamoureax J, Kahn A (2006). Epidemiology of dog bites: A Belgian experience of canine behaviour and public health concerns. *Veterinary Journal* 172:482–487.

Drobatz K, Smith G (2003). Evaluation of risk factors for bite wounds inflicted on caregivers by dogs and cats in a veterinary teaching hospital. *Journal of the American Veterinary Medical Association* 223:312–316.

McMillan FD, Serpell JA, Duffy DL, et al. (2013). Differences in behavioral characteristics between dogs obtained as puppies from pet stores and those obtained from noncommercial breeders. *Journal of the American Veterinary Medical Association* 242:1359–1363.

Patronek GJ, Slavinski SA (2009). Animal bites. *Journal of the American Veterinary Medical Association* 234:336–345.

Patronek GJ, Sacks JJ, Delise KM, et al. (2013). Co-occurrence of potentially preventable factors in 256 bite-related fatalities in the United States (2000–2009). *Journal of the American Veterinary Medical Association* 243:1726–1736. (Response in Letters to the Editor, Raghavan M, et al. (2014) *J Am Vet Med Assoc* 245:484.)

Raghaven M, Martens PJ, Chateau D, et al. (2012). Effectiveness of breed-specific legislation in decreasing the incidence of dog-bite injury hospitalizations in people in the Canadian province of Manitoba. *Injury Prevention* 19:177–183.

Sacks JJ, Sinclair L, Gilchrist J, et al. (2000). Breeds of dogs involved in fatal human attacks in the United States between 1979 and 1998. *Journal of the American Veterinary Medical Association* 217:836–840.

Shuler CM, DeBess EE, Lapidus JA, et al. (2008). Canine and human factors related to dog bite injuries. *Journal of the American Veterinary Medical Association* 232:542–546.

Taylor SM (2010). *Small Animal Clinical Techniques.* Elsevier Saunders, St. Louis.

Yin S (2009). *Low Stress Handling, Restraint and Behavior Modification of Dogs and Cats.* CattleDog Publishing, Davis.

Yin S (2007). Simple handling techniques for dogs. *Compendium on Continuing Education for the Practicing Veterinarian* 29:352–358.

The domestic cat (*Felis catus*) has been valued as guardian of grain stores and human dwellings against vermin (mice and rats) and small reptiles (snakes and lizards) for at least 9,500 years. Humans began to grow and store grain, which attracted vermin and reptiles, which in turn were food for cats, and thus cats were brought into proximity with humans. Cat domestication about 3,500 years ago coincided with the practice of storing grains in the fertile areas of the Middle East.

The domestic cat is currently believed to have evolved from the African wildcat (*Felis silvestris libyca*). The first recorded domestication was with the Egyptians circa 3,500 BC, who worshiped and protected cats, viewing them as symbols of fertility and strength. By 1,500 BC, the penalty for killing an Egyptian cat was death. Phoenician trading ships brought cats to Europe around 900 BC. Cats subsequently became a symbol of liberty in Roman times. They were a valued form of pest control on farms until the Middle Ages, when the Catholic Church associated them with Satan worship. Many cats, especially black cats, were killed. This slaughter of a natural predator of rats may have contributed to the spread of Black Death in Europe during the 14th century, which killed more than one-third of the human population in Europe.

The domestic cat is not indigenous to the Americas. It was imported with European settlers, often being carried aboard ships to control rats and mice. Now it is the most numerous companion pet in the U.S., although fewer households have cats than dogs. Among all domestic animals, humans have done the least amount of selective breeding with cats. The domestic shorthair cat is remarkably free of genetic diseases, although recent specialty breeds are not.

Male cats are called *tomcats*. Female cats are *queens*, and young cats are *kittens*.

NATURAL BEHAVIOR OF CATS

Feral and domesticated cats are highly social, nocturnal, territorial, semi-arboreal, solitary predators. They prefer to sleep 16–18 hours a day. Females are more social than males, and are the organizers of the colonies. Males have much larger hunting territories than females. Cats will live in large groups (called *clowders*) if their food source is limited in the number of available sites yet adequate in quantity, as is often the case in urban environments. However, if they have sufficient natural prey (rodents) over a broad region, they prefer not to live in mixed groups. The basic social unit is a queen and her kittens. Tomcats may kill kittens that are not their own.

Cat to cat aggression is often carried out by each walking on their toes as they pass each other while staring at their opponent. Suddenly there will be an attempt by one or both to grab the other cat by the back of the neck. If successful, this hold protects the cat holding the other's neck against being bitten or raked with front claws. If grabbing the back of the neck is unsuccessful, both cats will lie belly to belly while attempting to claw and bite each other until one cat retreats. This type of aggression may be directed toward a handler when he or she tries to rub a cat's abdomen. Efforts to rub a strange cat's abdomen should be avoided even if the cat seems to be inviting it.

Cats are genetically highly accomplished predators. A bell should be attached to a collar of a cat that is aggressive toward other cats or that could have the opportunity to kill songbirds or hummingbirds.

The core environmental needs of cats are to hunt, play, and scratch territorial objects.

Body language

Cats use body language and vocalizations to communicate. A relaxed attitude is demonstrated by the cat lying on one side or sitting while its tail moves slowly. A cat's tail hangs down if walking with a relaxed attitude. *Kneading* of soft surfaces is a sign of contentment. Kneading is also one of the methods that cats mark their territory or possessions. When inquisitive or greeting an unthreatening animal or human, a cat's tail is carried up.

A cat on alert is characterized by assuming a frozen sitting or lying posture, rapid flicking of the tail, and dilated pupils. Walking tiptoe with head down is an aggressive posture. Aggressive body language also includes a slight piloerection of the back, with ears erect but swiveled to the side or back against the cat's neck.

Fear is expressed by flattened ears, crouching, arching the back, salivation and spitting, and dilated pupils.

Vocalizations

Purring is a sign of contentment. Cats will often chatter their teeth, also called chirruping, if they are excited by the sight of prey. Meows are to call the attention of other cats or their handler.

Marking territory

Cats instinctively scratch objects to mark their territory and to clean and sharpen their nails. Soft wood is preferred. Scratching trees makes a visual marker, but pheromones from the cat's paws also provide an olfactory marker.

Both males and females will mark territory by spraying urine. Males spray to mark territory; females spray while in heat to attract males. Urine spraying of territorial objects is intensified with the introduction of a rival cat, and territorial aggression is often triggered by another cat's odor. Clean (deodorized) cat-handling jackets should be worn when handling an aggressive cat to avoid a territorial aggression response.

Cats rub with their cheeks (called *bunting*) when objects stimulate a gape (the equivalent of the flehmen response in horses) or when a subordinate greets a dominant cat. Scent glands next to a cat's mouth produce chemicals that are smeared on objects, including handlers, that the cat claims as its own by this facial marking.

SAFETY FIRST

Handler safety

Most domestic cats are inherently friendly. A few cats are always ill-tempered. If they are in good health, all are agile, extremely quick, and capable of causing serious injuries to handlers. Minimal restraint for the procedure to be done is the best means of handling cats.

Domestic cats have a wide variety of temperaments, but most cats are docile if socialized early and handled gently with minimal restraint.

The most frequently reported behavior problem of cats is aggression toward its owner. Most often, the cause is poor socialization of the cat as a kitten and poor handling techniques of owners, in particular excessive restraint and rough play.

Cat bites are more common in veterinarians and veterinary technicians than dog bites. Aggressively defensive cats do not pose a risk to human life; however, they can inflict serious injuries that may lead to impaired use of hands or loss of vision. Their first line of defense is their front claws. Besides causing painful injuries to arms and hands, cats will use their claws to strike at an opponent's eyes. Even superficial scratches can introduce bacteria, such as the bacteria for cat-scratch disease, or a subcutaneous fungus called *Sporotrichum*. Lab or clinic coats with long sleeves should be worn when handling cats as a means of protecting against cat scratches. Back claws are a source of injury to handlers when holding a cat near the handler's body if the cat attempts to escape.

Cats bite very quickly and let go quickly. They then will bite quickly again if the threat does not retreat. The bites are deep penetrating wounds that can injure and infect joint capsules, tendon sheaths, and bones, particularly of the hands. Permanent disabilities of the hand can result from cat bites.

Socialization with humans involves handling and playing with cats, but play should not involve using hands as simulated prey. "Fishing" play with cats using a rod, string, and feathered object is much safer.

> The risk of infection from a cat bite is more than five times higher than from a dog bite.

Domestic cats are very independent, especially if threatened. Their first reaction to a threat is to run and hide with no regard to where other cats are running or to other potentially dangerous things going on in the same area. In other words, cats run first and think later. Once hidden as well as they can, which may just be cowering in the back of a cage, they often will issue warnings (low rumbling growls, hisses, and rapid strike and retreat) to threats that continue to approach.

Cats telegraph their aggression more consistently than do dogs. Dominance aggressive cats may do little cowering or hissing before striking, but they will have a fixed stare toward their opponent, dilated eyes, and ears pulled back. They will stand confidently. The tail will move back and forth to the sides with a flicking movement at the end of the tail. The hair on the back will be raised. Their whiskers are elevated to a position where they stick straight out to the sides.

Fearful aggressive cats are more vocal and will flattened their ears and arch their back before striking, usually from a crouching position. They do not stare directly at the opponent and may present their side to what they perceive as danger.

Cat safety

Cats that are socialized to people have less resistance to being handled and restrained. As a result, they are safer from self-inflicted or inadvertent injury from attempted escapes when being handled.

Kittens should be socialized to other animals and humans outside the immediate family during the sensitive period for cats of 2–7 weeks of age. Brief daily handling and being spoken to during this period are important, although periodic handling and other human interaction needs to continue for the remainder of the cat's life. Inter-cat socialization

is particularly important during 12–14 weeks of age. It is during this period that their focus shifts from social play to predatory hunting practice. Kittens should begin their routine vaccinations 10 days prior to beginning the first socialization event with other cats, and they should have tested negative for feline leukemia virus (FeLV) and feline immunodeficiency virus (FIV). If adopted from a shelter, a kitten should be kept in its new home for 2 weeks before socializing with other cats. Kittens should not socialize with other cats that are sneezing, coughing, vomiting, or having diarrhea.

Key zoonoses

(*Note:* Animals that appear ill should be handled by veterinary professionals or others under their supervision. Precautionary measures against zoonoses from ill animals are more involved than those required when handling apparently healthy animals, and such measures vary widely. The discussion here is directed primarily at handling apparently healthy animals.)

Apparently healthy domestic cats pose little risk of transmitting disease to healthy adult handlers who practice conventional personal hygiene. The risks of physical injury are greater than the risks of acquiring an infectious disease. However, there is much overlap. Up to 80% of cat bites become infected (*Table 5.1*).

The most suitable pets for young children are dogs and cats because the risks of injury and infection are better known and more easily controlled than in other animals.

Direct transmission

Directly transmitted zoonotic diseases from cats can result in signs of disease systemically or primarily in the respiratory, digestive, or skin (integumentary) system of humans.

Systemic disease

Many zoonoses from cats can cause generalized (systemic) illness. Nearly all are described as "flu-like symptoms". None are common in adult handlers of healthy appearing cats.

Cats are the primary host for a protozoan parasite called *Toxoplasma gondii*, the cause of toxoplasmosis

Table 5.1 Diseases transmitted from healthy appearing cats to healthy adult humans

DISEASE	AGENT	MEANS OF TRANSMISSION	SIGNS AND SYMPTOMS IN HUMANS	FREQUENCY IN ANIMALS	RISK GROUP*
Bites and scratches	–	Direct injury	Bite and scratch wounds to hands and arms. Infection from cat bites, especially from *Pasteurella multocida*, is much higher from cat bites than from dog bites	All cats are capable of inflicting bite wounds and, if not declawed, scratch injuries	3
Cat-scratch disease	*Bartonella henselae*	Direct by scratches	Usually mild transient illness with enlarged regional lymph nodes	Occurrence high in young cats	2
Ringworm	*Microsporum canis*	Direct and indirect from fomites	Ring of skin inflammation with red border	Most cats carry *M. canis*	2
Visceral larvae migrans	*Toxocara cati*	Direct from soil; fecal-oral	Abdominal pain Inflamed liver	Most kittens have *T. cati*	2
Toxoplasmosis	*Toxoplasma gondii*	Direct from soil, water, or litter; fecal-oral	Usually mild transient illness in an adult; of greatest concern for pregnant women and the fetus		2
Echinococcosis	*Echinococcus multilocularis*	Direct, fecal-oral	Lung cysts that cause shortness of breath and coughing	Can occur in cats allowed to eat wild rodents in northern states of the U.S.	4

* Risk groups (National Institutes of Health and World Health Organization criteria. Centers for Disease Control and Prevention, *Biosafety in Microbiological and Biomedical Laboratories*, 5th edition, 2009):
1 Agent not associated with disease in healthy adult humans.
2 Agent rarely causes serious disease and prevention or therapy possible.
3 Agent can cause serious or lethal disease and prevention or therapy possible.
4 Agent can cause serious or lethal disease and prevention or therapy are not usually available.

Cats are the only species to normally pass *Toxoplasma* in their feces, although dogs that eat infected cat feces can mechanically and briefly pass the parasite in their feces. Toxoplasmosis is primarily a danger to pregnant women who have no immunity developed in earlier life to the parasite. If acquired first during pregnancy, toxoplasmosis can cause abortion. However, humans usually acquire toxoplasmosis from inadequately cooked meat. The cat is a low-risk source of the disease because the feces are not infective until after 1–5 days outside the host, and the organisms are passed for only 2 weeks after the cat becomes infected. Shedding of oocysts is not prolonged by FIV or FeLV infections or the administration of glucocorticoids. Still, it is advisable that litter boxes be cleaned daily, but not by a pregnant woman. Litter boxes should not be placed in a dining room or kitchen. The hair of normal cats is too dry and cats are too fastidious to allow the organism to remain for 1–5 days on the hair coat and become infective. Pet cats pick up the organism by hunting and eating prey. They should not be allowed to hunt or scavenge or be fed raw or undercooked meat products. About 30% of cats allowed to kill and eat prey will have antibodies indicating exposure to the *Toxoplasma* organism.

Cat-scratch disease (bartonellosis) is significant, affecting more than 20,000 people per year in the U.S. Up to 50% of normal cats have or previously had *Bartonella henselae*. It is more often carried by kittens and is transmitted to cats by fleas, as well as cat bites and scratches. Declawing kittens, when allowed by law, that will be in contact with children, the elderly, or others with impaired immunity is advisable, as is control of fleas. Cat-scratch disease is carried for months by kittens without clinical signs. Transmission can be by scratch, bite, or cat saliva contaminating an open wound. Young children should be closely supervised if allowed to handle cats to encourage gentle handling and minimize the risk of scratches, bites, or exposure to cat saliva. All handler's hands and scratches or bites should be thoroughly washed after handling cats.

Echinococcosis is a disease caused by a tapeworm (*Echinococcus multilocularis*) of cats that are permitted to eat wild rodents, such as voles, shrews, and lemmings, and is acquired by ingesting cat-feces-contaminated materials. Echinococcosis typically causes cysts in the lungs in humans.

Capnocytophaga canimorsus, a potentially fatal bacteria in cats' oral cavity, is a risk for humans with impaired immune systems, such as from chemotherapy, cancer, AIDS, or splenectomy. *Capnocytophaga* is less common in cats than in dogs.

Listeriosis can cause generalized disease in immunosuppressed humans that includes an atypical pneumonia. Transmission is generally via uncooked or undercooked foods.

Plague is a disease of cats that hunt and eat rodents in the southwestern U.S. Transmission to humans can occur from ill cats by their coughing, sneezing, or breathing onto a human's face, or by being bitten by a plague-carrying flea from an ill cat.

Rabies is a fatal viral infection transmitted by bites or through saliva-contaminated wounds. Cats are vaccinated against rabies less commonly than are dogs, even though most rabies cases in domestic animals in the U.S. are in unvaccinated cats.

Visceral larvae migrans, ocular larvae migrans, cutaneous larvae migrans, and acquired toxoplasmosis are serious diseases of young children. These diseases are acquired after incubation and hatching or sporulation outside an animal's body. Exposure occurs indirectly via environmental contamination by cats. Young children should be kept from playgrounds and beaches where cats are allowed to defecate. Handling cats without fecal contamination of their hair coat is not a risk for transmission of these diseases.

Coxiellosis (Q fever) is a bacterial disease transmitted by inhalation of dust contaminated by the body secretions of animals (urine, milk, feces, etc.) that are infected with *Coxiella burnettii*. Cats from farms with livestock are most likely to transmit Q fever in placental fluids.

Respiratory disease

Pasteurellosis (*Pasteurella multocida*) is a respiratory bacterial infection that can be acquired from cats, but these bacteria in humans usually require an impaired immune response to become severe or prolonged infections. *Pasteurella* is also the most frequent cause of wound infection from cat bites. Cat respiratory or oral secretions can be a source of infection in immunosuppressed humans through *Bordetella bronchiseptica*, *Chlamydophila felis*, plague (*Yersinia pestis*), and tularemia (*Francisella tularensis*). However, based on reported cases the risks of these appear low in immunologically immature children. Young children should not be permitted to kiss cats or expose themselves to pet respiratory or oral secretions. Plague and tularemia can also be transmitted by infected ticks that may be carried to humans by cats.

Digestive tract disease

Ingesting fecal-contaminated materials is required to acquire the bacterial diseases campylobacteriosis or salmonellosis from cats. Of these, campylobacteriosis is the most common, although the source is generally from kittens with diarrhea. Salmonellosis is rare in cats. The most common tapeworm (*Dipylidium caninum*) of cats can be acquired by humans, if they swallow the intermediate host, fleas. Giardiasis has been listed as a potential zoonosis from infected cats, although the status of giardiasis as a zoonotic disease from cats has been questioned.

Zoonoses that are passed in the feces in the infective form and could be acquired from exposure to the rectum are salmonellosis, campylobacteriosis, cryptosporidiosis, yersiniosis (*Yersinia enterocolitica*), and perhaps giardiasis. Among these, campylobacteriosis is the greatest risk from cats, although the risks are still small if no clinical signs (diarrhea) are present and hands are washed after handling cats.

Skin disease

Ringworm is a fungal infection of the upper layers of the skin. Cat handlers may develop transient infections by contact, often by infected hair being caught under a sleeve or collar and rubbed against the skin, or caught under the fingernails and scratched into the scalp. The zoophilic skin fungus *Microsporum canis* is a common cause for ringworm, particularly *tinea capitus* (ringworm on the head) in young children. It is often carried on cats' hair coat without clinical signs and transferred to the scalp of children by contamination of a child's hands and fingernails. Young children should have their hands washed and fingernails cleaned after handling cats to reduce the risk of acquiring ringworm. Ringworm is the most commonly reported zoonosis along with bites and scratches in small animal veterinarians.

Mange mites (*Notoedres cati, Cheyletiella blakei*) can be transmitted transiently to handlers and cause chigger bite-like itchy bumps in the skin, but transmission by animals without clinical signs of disease is highly unlikely.

Staphylococcus intermedius may be carried by cats but much less commonly than by dogs. This species of *Staphylococcus* is not typically the type that is found in people (*S. aureus*).

Sporotrichosis is caused by a fungus (*Sporothrix schenckii*) that can grow in puncture wounds. Cats with sporotrichosis in their wounds have concentrated populations of the fungus. Humans handling cats with sporotrichosis lumps and draining sores on their skin are at risk of acquiring the disease by cat scratches or by contaminating cuts on their hands or arms.

Vector borne

Tularemia is a bacterial infection that can be transmitted by deer flies and ticks. Cats may carry the bacteria in their mouth if allowed to eat rabbits or other prey that are infected with tularemia. They can also carry ticks into a household, but this is unusual.

Pets with fleas and ticks may carry disease agents to young children. Ticks from cats could transmit plague or tularemia. Children should not handle cats with fleas or ticks, and cats should be routinely examined and treated for external parasites.

Sanitary practices

Persons handling cats should wear appropriate dress to protect against skin contamination with hair and skin scales or saliva, urine, and other body secretions. External parasites such as fleas and ticks should be controlled. Rabies vaccinations in cats should be kept current. Basic sanitary practices should be adhered to, such as keeping hands away from eyes, nose, and mouth, when handling cats and washing hands after handling them. Cat handlers should be vaccinated against tetanus every 10 years.

Special precautions are needed if sick cats are handled, and sick cats should be isolated from apparently normal cats. New household or cattery members should be quarantined for at least 2 weeks to reduce the risk of transmitting a disease that new animals could be incubating before introducing to the rest of the clowder.

When handling more than one cat from different households or catteries, proper sanitation is required to prevent the spread of disease from carriers without clinical signs. Cats from different origins should not be confined in the same cage or group area. Other basic procedures are for handlers to wash their hands and to clean and disinfect table tops and cages used in handling. Restraint equipment such as blankets, muzzles, capture poles, grooming equipment, collars, cat bags, and slip leashes should be disposable or cleaned and disinfected. Leather gloves should be kept as clean as possible and used infrequently.

Companion cats should be kept exclusively indoors. Remaining indoors virtually eliminates the risks of toxoplasmosis, plague, rabies, and many other zoonotic diseases. Rough play should be avoided with kittens for behavioral reasons and to reduce the risk of diseases from bites or scratches. Gloves should be worn when handling cats if there are any open wounds on the handler's arms or hands. A cat should not be allowed to lick an open wound on handlers. Outdoor cats should not be allowed access to children's sandboxes or to gardens.

APPROACHING AND CATCHING

The cat's attitude should be observed before attempting to capture it. Most cats can be classified as non-aggressive or fear-aggressive. Most non-aggressive cats will nonetheless be resentful of restraint and will respond best to an unhurried approach and loose gentle restraint.

Non-aggressive cats

The handler should move slowly but with confidence, and use a calm assuring voice, and lower his or her body near the cat with the side of the body toward it. Small bits of food treats can be used if needed to lure the cat closer to the handler. Cats should not be stared at or leaned over.

A friendly approach by a cat is with its tail held up and with its hind legs slightly extended. Purring may be audible. It will almost touch anyone it approaches with its nose and may rub its face and head on the handler. Rolling over and exposing the belly is not a submission sign in cats. It is rather an invitation to play, but touching the abdomen may trigger a playful bite.

An apparently friendly cat should be allowed to approach the handler's extended index finger, which mimics another cat's nose, to smell it. The handler can then quietly and slowly move his hand to stroke the cat's head. Cats are not threatened by extended fingers and will not suddenly bite as dogs may do. Stroking a friendly cat's back results in arching of its back to press more firmly against the stroking hand, a signal of invitation for more petting. A slip leash should be applied and then the cat moved so that it is in front of the handler facing the handler's right side. The handler's left hand reaches over the cat's back and grasps the cat's right front leg. Holding the front leg prevents the cat from escaping the handler's support or climbing up the handler's chest. The left wrist is then under the cat's juncture of the abdomen and thorax for support of its body.

The right hand holds the slip leash and is kept near the cat's head to pet it as it is carried and to grasp the scruff of the neck if struggling occurs. Lifting the cat should be done without squeezing its chest. The handler's right hand is used to comfort and distract the cat while being carried. Distraction techniques include gently rubbing the cat's head and ears, scratching the ears or throat and chin, gently and rhythmically tapping the cat's head or face, blowing softly on the nose, and stroking or wiggling the cat's foot or leg.

Aggressive cats

The body language of an aggressive cat is that of piloerection, arched back, tail down with its tip flicked slowly, and ears erect and pointed forward. If approached, it will flatten its ears back, bat with its paws, and lean away from the threat, vocalizing.

Aggressive cats must be handled by two people. The handler has to concentrate on only the restraint. The other person performs the examination, administration of medications, or other procedures needed.

The surroundings should be prepared for a possible escape attempt. All doors, windows, and cabinet doors must be closed. Access to vents, backs of refrigerators, chimneys, or any other escape or hiding area that will impede efforts to recapture the cat if it escapes must be blocked. Anything breakable or spillable on countertops should be removed.

If a cat is in defensive posture but does not attempt to strike and retreat, a loop from a slip leash should be dropped over the cat's head to provide a means of gently moving the cat toward the handler. The handler can then either stroke and pick the cat up, or if necessary use additional capture means (wrap in a towel, pull into a transport crate or box, or administer chemical restraint). Using a thick towel to begin the stroking and gradually wrapping its body from the neck back may be effective. Wearing thick leather gloves with gauntlets to protect the wrists and forearms is an alternate but less desirable approach.

Fractious cats that will attack when capture is attempted in a cage should be entrapped by a capture pole, cat tongs, nets, or a cat loop on a flexible rod. Cats can wiggle, roll, and spin in a net; therefore, gloves or towels may need to be used to hold the cat down to administer medications or sedatives.

Feral cats may be caught in humane traps, which are commercially available, and transferred to a squeeze cage for chemical restraint to be safely handled.

HANDLING FOR ROUTINE CARE AND MANAGEMENT

Basic equipment

Tractable cats require no equipment for handling, but slip leashes should be used on cats whenever they are outside a cage to aid in positioning the cat to be picked up and to increase security against an attempt to escape. If additional restraint is needed, particularly for cats that have not been declawed, towels and blankets are basic equipment.

Slip leashes

A slip leash is a rope, cord, or flat woven strap with a metal ring honda or tied honda knot used for routine handling of cats. Flat-strap slip leashes should not be used owing to their inability to maintain an open loop when being placed over the cat's head and neck. A slip leash serves as a sliding collar and lead rope in one piece.

Slip leashes should not be used on cats with breathing problems. If an alternative does not exist, the loop should be placed around the neck with one front leg through it to prevent pressure on the trachea.

Cats should never be tied and left unattended with a slip leash because either escape or strangulation may result.

Towels and blankets

Towels can be used in the same manner as cat restraint bags. The first wrap should be around the neck, and then the rest of the body is swaddled to restrict movement of the cat's legs, euphemistically called making a cat *kitty burrito* (**Figure 5.1**). A leg can be withdrawn for venipuncture, or the cat can be held on its back with the head extended for jugular venipuncture.

Another method of swaddling cats for restraint is to fold a blanket in half while making sure there is enough remaining to easily wrap the cat. While standing behind the cat, the handler drops the blanket over the entire cat, including its head. Then, the handler quickly entraps the cat using both forearms to sweep in and *taco shell* capture the cat, pressing

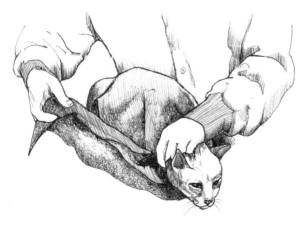

Fig. 5.1 Towel wrap restraint.

the blanket edges under the cat's legs. Rear escape is blocked with the handler's torso, and forward escape is blocked by the towel over the cat's head. The wrap is then used to immediately swaddle the cat in a burrito-style wrap.

Tables and table covers

Cats prefer elevated positions to rest, but stainless steel exam tables are not well tolerated. The time handling a cat on a table should be kept to a minimum and avoided when possible. Covering the table with a pad or towel will provide traction and insulation, but allowing a struggling cat traction for its feet may be a disadvantage for the handler. Whether or not to cover a table should be determined on an individual basis depending on the actions of the cat on an uncovered table.

Table covers should be cleaned and sanitized after each use. Warming table towels has been recommended, but the added benefits to handling cats by using warmed towels has not been objectively assessed.

Moving
Carried in arms

When a handler carries a cat, the cat should have a slip leash applied first and then be picked up with the handler's right palm under the cat's chest with an index finger between the front legs at the junction with the chest (**Figure 5.2**). The left hand, while holding the slip leash, is placed lightly on back of the cat's neck and top of its shoulders. If distraction techniques (petting, scratching) are insufficient to control the cat, the cat can be scruffed with the left hand.

An alternative hold is to allow the cat's sternum to be supported by the right wrist while the left front leg is grasped with the right hand. Both restrains prevent the cat from climbing up the handler's chest.

Transport in crates

Transport crates are useful in securing cats when they are moved. When confined to a strapped-down crate in a vehicle, cats are prevented from escapes during loading or unloading or through open windows. They also cannot become a distraction to driving or a missile during a collision.

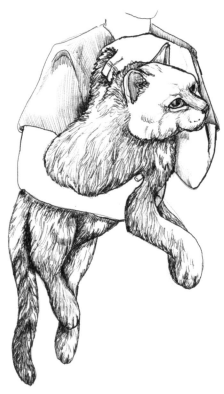

Fig. 5.2 Restraint for carrying a cat.

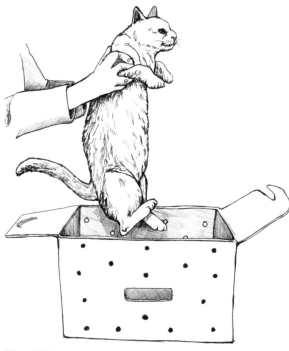

Fig. 5.3 Inserting a cat in a travel crate.

Cats in crates in veterinary hospitals are protected from harm from other animals and from doing harm to other animals or humans. However, the cat will still be stressed by the near presence of other cats and dogs and should be kept from viewing them by covering the crate with a towel. Harsh lighting should be avoided and the crate kept off the floor by placing it securely on a table or other elevated surface.

Crates may be made of cardboard or plastic. Cat crates should have a top opening. Air holes should be present on at least 10% of the surface area of the crate. Absorbent bedding should be provided. Food and water should be considered, depending on the length of time in transport.

Inserting the cat

Docile cats that have been previously acclimated to eating and resting in a crate should be given a chance to walk into a crate to seek seclusion and be offered a food treat. Putting a towel in may be an added lure, especially if the towel has been rubbed by the cat's owner, on a buddy cat, or on the cat to be crated itself.

Failing a voluntary entrance to the crate, the cat should be picked up and placed in transport crates through a top opening, rump first (**Figure 5.3**). After the cat stands in the crate, the handler's hand should remain on the cat's neck and shoulders as the other hand closes the top against the handler's forearm. The restraining arm can then be slipped out of the crate and the top opening closed. If a top-loading crate is not available, the front of a front-opening crate can be tipped up. The cat is lowered, rump first, into the crate. After closing the crate door, the handler should gently set the crate in normal position.

Removing the cat

The removal of the cat should be done in a closed room with all exits and hiding areas blocked. The top lid should be gradually opened while gaining control of the cat with one hand. If the cat is tractable, it can then be lifted out using both hands (**Figure 5.4**).

If the cat is agitated, it should be gently scruffed with one hand and its body supported with the

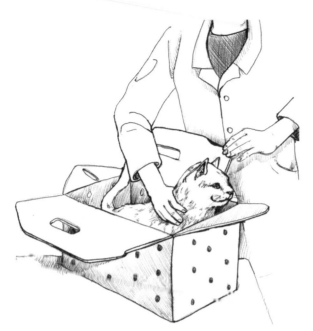

Fig. 5.4 Removing a cat from a travel crate.

other hand. If the cat is aggressive, a towel can be slid across the top door of the crate or between the top and bottom halves of a clamshell crate as a shield and visual barrier to the cat while the handler grasps the cat with the towel. Nets or gloves should be avoided, if possible.

The cat should be lifted out rather than allowing it to jump out on its own, and it should never be dumped out or scared out by thumping on the crate. If the crate does not have a top opening, the handler can turn the front door end up, or if it is a clamshell crate, the top half can be taken off of the carrier.

Cages and runs
Placement of non-aggressive cats in cages
Cats should be placed in cages head first. The slip leash should be removed. One hand should have control of the cage door. Closing the door should begin before the release of the cat with the other hand, so that when the restraint hand is removed there is insufficient room for the cat to escape.

Release should be as smooth and quiet as possible, since this will be the most persistent memory of being last handled when the cat must later be removed from the cage. Struggling during the release will result in greater struggling when recapture is later needed. Controlling the cat when placing it in the cage can be done with the restraint hand under its chest.

Removal of non-aggressive cats from cages
The handler should approach the cage in a friendly manner while speaking to the cat in a normal tone. Removal should begin with using one hand to open the cage door only enough to get the other hand and a slip leash in. Place the slip leash over the cat's head. After the cat's head is controlled, the cage door can be opened wider and the cat assisted by picking it up. Gently lift the cat's neck by raising the slip leash so there is some control of the head before reaching under the cat's torso to lift it.

Trimming nails
Cat nails are sharp and curved for easy hooking penetration of the skin. They are dangerous in their ability to cause serious physical injury and potential for producing infected wounds. Cat-scratch disease can be life-threatening in immunosuppressed people or children with immature immunity. Trimming the nails every 2–4 weeks has been proposed as an alternative to onychectomy (declawing) by an experienced veterinary surgeon. If successful, trimming nails of a house cat may reduce damage to furniture, but attempting to trim some cats can put the handler at greater risk of clawing injury or infection. Trimming is required more often in cats than in dogs because only a small portion of the nail can be safely trimmed in cats compared with dogs.

If trimming nails is considered the best means to prevent scratch injuries, infections, and destruction of property, trimming can be attempted by one or two handlers. In either case, minimum restraint should be used. A cooperative cat can be held in the handler's lap with the handler's forearms blocking the cat's movements. One hand restrains a foot, with the index finger on a claw's digital pad while the thumb gently pushed the top of the nail to extrude it from the nail fold. The other hand uses a nail trimming instrument.

A second method is done with the cat on a table. The assistant handler holds the cat in sitting or standing restraint while the primary handler holds a foot and the extrudes and trims the nails.

HANDLING FOR COMMON MEDICAL PROCEDURES

Most handling and restraint of cats for medical procedures can be and should be done without tranquilization, sedation, hypnosis, or anesthesia. However, some handling and restraint procedures should be restricted to veterinary medical professionals because of the potential danger to the animal or handler. These require special skills, equipment, or facilities, and possibly adjunct or complete immobilization by chemical restraint.

Restraint of individuals or parts of their bodies

Whole body

Standing restraint

Standing restraint of a cat is used for general physical examinations and occasionally intramuscular injections performed by another person. The handler puts the cat on a table and gains control of the cat's head by putting a thumb under the cat's collar or slip leash and cupping his or her fingers around the cat's chin and neck. At nearly the same time, the handler reaches over the cat with the other hand and lifts and hugs the cat's abdomen against his or her own abdomen so that the cat cannot sit.

Rectal temperatures can be done by one handler with the cat in standing position. The cat's body is held between the handler's left elbow and side with the cat's head directed toward the rear of the handler. The cat is restrained gently with the left hand by the base of its tail.

Sitting restraint

This is done as with dogs, except that the head is restrained with a hand under the jaws and throat rather than an arm around the neck. The other hand gently pushes the rump down. The sitting restraint position is often used for cephalic or jugular venipuncture and for oral administration of medications.

Sternal restraint

Sternal restraint is used for ear or eye treatments, administration of oral medications, and subcutaneous injections. It is also used for cephalic or jugular venipuncture.

The handler begins with the cat in standing position while restraining its front with the right hand under the neck and in front of the cat's chest. The left hand is placed on the rump and pushes down gently while holding the front of the cat's chest. After the cat is sitting, the handler reaches around the left side of the cat with the left hand and grasps both front legs and gently slides them forward while pushing the cat's body down with his armpit and blocking lateral movement with the forearms (**Figure 5.5**).

Restraint for subcutaneous injections can be sternal recumbency. The handling assistant presses down on the top of the cat's shoulders and lower neck while pushing the pelvis down with the other hand.

If the cat is to have jugular venipuncture, the cat's front legs must be held over and below the level of the edge of the table. The edge of the table should be padded with a towel.

Gentle cats can be administered oral medications if put in sitting or sternal position on a handler's lap with the cat facing the handler's knees. The handler's elbows and abdomen block sideways and backward movement. The handler's non-dominant hand is used to restrain the cat's head and to arrest forward movement, leaving the handler's dominant hand free to administer oral medications. If additional

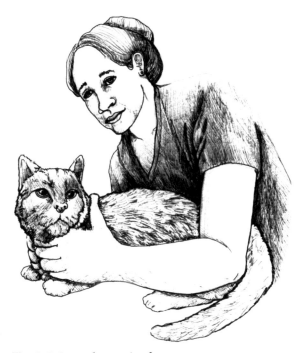

Fig. 5.5 Sternal restraint for cats.

restraint is needed, the cat can be wrapped in a towel or put in a cat bag.

Lateral recumbency

Cats should be restrained in lateral recumbency only when they cannot or should not be restrained in a standing, sitting, or sternal position. Its duration should be as short as possible. To restrain a docile cat in lateral recumbency, a handler begins with the cat in standing position. With the right arm, the handler reaches over the cat's neck and grasps both front legs while placing a finger between the legs. With the left arm, the handler reaches over the cat's flank and grasps both hind legs with a finger between the legs. A finger between the legs is very important for the comfort of the cat and to maintain a grip on each leg. The cat is lifted while hugging it close to the handler's body so that it gently slides down on its side. The handler gently restrains the cat's head with his or her right forearm.

Many cats will not tolerate being held in lateral recumbency. To prevent injury to the handler or the cat from struggling, lateral recumbency is often best done while the cat is in a cat bag. Attempts to use lateral recumbency without a cat bag will expose the handler's hands and arms to possible injury.

Lateral recumbency is generally used to provide access to the medial saphenous vein on the inside of the hind legs. It is also used to administer intramuscular injections and perform claw trimming in fractious cats.

Ventrodorsal restraint

A handler may hold the cat ventrodorsally (on its back) to do cystocentesis (urine collection by needle and syringe). If performed with the cat on a table, a soft, padded surface should be used, such as a thick cushion or blanket. Alternatively, cats can be held ventrodorsal on a handler's lap.

Scruff-and-stretch hold

If a cat is expected to strongly resist restraint, it can be restrained without a cat bag for a short procedure by stretching it out. One hand grasps the cat's skin on the back of the neck, and although all fingers are used to grasp the skin, the thumb and index finger should gather the skin at an imaginary line connecting the back of each of the cat's ears. Grasping the neck skin an inch or two back of the imaginary line between the ears would leave the head with enough mobility for the cat to turn its head and bite. The other hand grasps the hind legs with the index finger between the legs. The cat is stretched out with its back slightly arched by pressing the shoulders and back with the heel of the hand holding the skin of the back of the neck (**Figure 5.6**).

Scruffing is not universally accepted as an appropriate means of restraint, but it may be the best approach in some situations to protect the cat from greater injury or untreated disease, to reduce stress compared with alternative restraints, and to immediately protect handlers. In addition, scruffing does not affect the cat's ability to breathe, whereas wrapping a cat's neck or torso with a towel for restraint can cause respiratory difficulty. Scruffing is most often used to administer chemical restraint injections. The need to scruff a cat should be explained to owners as a brief restraint that is not injurious if properly done and does not cause tissue damage or pain. Stress to the cat must be weighed against the advantages and consequences of alternative methods. Scruffing should never be the primary means of restraining cats. Scruffing should never be used to lift a cat without another hand to support the body.

Proper release of the cat from being scruffed is directly related to the ease or difficulty in handling

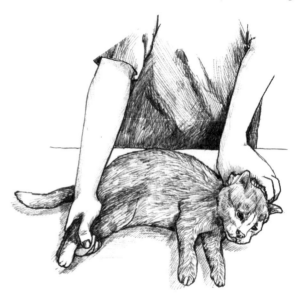

Fig. 5.6 Scruff-and-stretch restraint.

the cat again. Release should be done only during a period when the cat is not struggling and be followed by stroking and offering small bits of food treats. If release is uneventful, subsequent handling may be easier, rather than harder, in the future.

Restraint for bathing

Domestic cats do not like being submerged or having running water on their body. If a wire screen is put in the bathing tub, cats with claws will often hold onto the screen rather than try to jump out or climb up the handler's body. Alternately, mesh restraint bags may be used to reduce the risk of scratches and of the cat climbing onto a handler during a bath. Regardless of the method used, cats protest with a mournful meow during a bath.

Head

Restraint of a cat's head without risk of being clawed by either front or back claws requires a cat bag, a cat declawed on all four feet, or a very tolerant cat.

One-hand head hold

The one-hand head hold is used after the body is restrained. The most common reason for this hold is to administer oral medication. To perform this restraint, the handler's non-dominant hand is used to hold the head. The head is grasped on top of the head with the middle finger and the thumb holding the zygomatic arches (cheek bones) and pressing the back molars area. This grasp permits restraint of the head while being able to press the jaws open with pressure on the back of the jaw with the non-dominant hand and on the lower incisors with the dominant hand.

Two-hand head hold

The handler grasps both sides of the cat's neck just behind the ears. Placing a towel over the cat's head first may allow the head to be grasped with less risk of being bitten. The handler's thumbs should be over the skull between the cat's ears and the index fingers should be just behind the angle of the jaw and the other fingers under the jaw bones. No pressure is applied to the cat's throat. Control of side movement of the cat's body is attained with the handler's forearms.

Restraint of young, old, sick, or injured cats

Kittens

Queens should be separated and removed from the room if kittens are to be restrained for examination or treatments. During the first 2 weeks of life, kittens cannot see, hear well, or control their body temperature well, so they must be carefully handled and kept warm. Socialization with humans should begin at 2–3 weeks of age, but the exertion from handling and length of handling should both be brief.

Older cats

Older cats should not be handled for long periods since they tire easily. If they are picked up, when they are released they should be placed back on a floor gently.

Injured or sick cats

Normally gentle, friendly cats will scratch and bite if they are in pain. Injured cats should be handled with towels to prevent a handler from being bitten. Crates or cardboard boxes are ideal for the transport of injured or sick cats.

Injections and venipuncture

Insertion of transcutaneous needles for injection or aspiration in cats carries the risk of slashing tissue beneath the skin, including damage to nerves and blood vessels, and breaking the hypodermic needle off in its body. The area in which the needle is to be inserted must be immobilized, and the cat's mouth and feet should be restrained from interfering with the procedure, especially venipuncture.

Access to veins

Access to veins is needed for collection of blood samples and to administer medications intravenously. Restraint for venipuncture requires a method that is relatively comfortable for the cat and does not make it feel trapped, e.g. it should not be squeezed when not resisting the restraint. However, the method of restraint should allow the handler to immediately gain tight control if the cat resists. A sharp pain is often felt when the needle goes through the wall of the vein. This is not the time for the cat to move and cause the venipuncture to fail. Cats with chronic illness, or those requiring intensive care, often have many venipunctures. Ruined venipunctures from improper restraint can result in scarred and thrombosed veins and eventually require surgical cutdowns to achieve access to veins.

It is best to coordinate withdrawal of the needle by the phlebotomist and release of the vein occlusion by the handler. Release of the vein occlusion should occur before the needle is withdrawn to reduce the leaking of blood from the venipuncture site. Compression should then be applied to the venipuncture site.

Cephalic venipuncture

Cephalic veins are on the front of the forearms. Sitting or sternal restraint is used to position cats for cephalic venipuncture (**Figure 5.7**). If the cat is facing the handler's left side, the handler's left hand is placed under the cat's neck and its neck and head are held close to the handler's body, while the right hand goes over the cat's body. The cat is held close to the handler's side with the handler's elbow. The right hand grasps the cat's outside elbow with a middle finger or ring finger behind the elbow to keep the leg from escaping the hold. The thumb of the right hand holding the elbow reaches across the front of the elbow, squeezes the leg slightly, and then pulls the skin gently toward the outside. This occludes and stretches the cephalic vein to facilitate venipuncture by the phlebotomist.

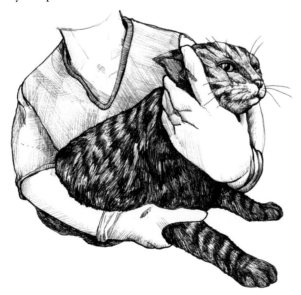

Fig. 5.7 Cephalic venipuncture restraint.

Medial saphenous and femoral venipuncture

The femoral vein is located superficially on the surface of a thigh, and one of its branches, the medial saphenous vein, is superficial on the medial surface below the stifle. Preferred restraint methods for femoral or medial saphenous venipuncture are the lateral restraint hold for docile cats and, for resistant cats, a towel wrap (burrito wrap) or a cat restraint bag.

To perform a venipuncture on the medial saphenous without a cat bag, a handler must restrain the cat in lateral recumbency. The phlebotomist grasps the paw of the lower hind leg and extends the leg. With one hand restraining the front of the cat, the handler's hand on the hind legs shifts to hold the upper hind leg in a flexed position exposing the medial surface of the lower leg. The heel of the handler's hand on the upper hind leg can then press and occlude the femoral vein near the cat's groin for the phlebotomist to visualize the vein.

Jugular venipuncture

The jugular vein is used to administer large volumes of fluids into the bloodstream or collect large volumes of blood. In adult cats, it should be reserved for critical care and emergencies. It is the preferred site for blood collection from kittens because of their size.

Jugular veins are in the lower side of the neck on each side of the windpipe (trachea). The first step in restraint for jugular venipuncture is to remove the collar. If it remains on and is pulled up out of the way, it will press on the upper aspect of the neck and prevent blood from entering the jugular veins when venipuncture is performed. The cat should be moved to the right edge of the table and placed in a sitting position or sternal recumbency. The handler holds the cat's front legs with the right hand (**Figure 5.8**). If the cat is in sternal recumbency, both front legs will have to be held over the edge of the table and downward. The edge of the table should be padded. The handler then holds the cat's head with the left hand on the lower aspect of the jaw and points the cat's nose toward the ceiling. A cat muzzle may aid in calming the cat and assist the handler's grip on the cat's head. The phlebotomist occludes the vein for the venipuncture.

It is very important to have control of the front legs. If the front legs are free, some cats will reach

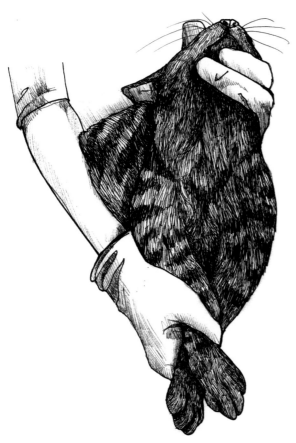

Fig. 5.8 Restraint for jugular venipuncture.

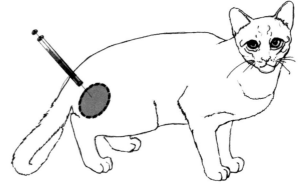

Fig. 5.9 Intramuscular injection site in cats.

Injections

Intramuscular

Intramuscular (IM) injections can cause serious injury. If the cat struggles during the injection, the needle will slash surrounding tissue. Therefore, a handler should not try to administer IM injections without assistance.

The cat may be restrained in a standing or lateral recumbency position. IM injections may be given into the caudal muscles of the thigh (semimembranosus and semitendinosus), cranial muscles of the thigh (quadriceps), or lumbar (lumbodorsal) muscles. Most IM injections are given into the caudal muscles of the thigh (**Figure 5.9**). Movement during the injection must be minimized to avoid needle trauma to the tissues, but the cat should not be squeezed with restraint, if possible.

Subcutaneous

Subcutaneous (SC) injections can be administered under the skin of the upper half of the body in the caudal aspect of the neck to mid-thorax while a handler restrains the cat in sitting or standing restraint. Injections should not be administered on the dorsal midline. Fractious cats may require a scruff hold, scruff-and-stretch hold, or towel wrap, whichever is considered to be the safest with the least stress to the cat.

Because of the risk of vaccine-induced tumors in cats, the American Association of Feline Practitioners recommends that feline panleukopenia, herpesvirus-1, and calicivirus vaccines be given below the right elbow; rabies vaccine below the right

up and push the phlebotomist's hand holding the syringe away and thus ruin the venipuncture, particularly just after the wall of the vein has been penetrated.

Lateral recumbency can also be used to access to the jugular vein. Adequate restraint in cats for jugular venipuncture in lateral recumbency requires a towel wrap or a cat bag.

Another restraint for jugular venipuncture is to place the cat in ventrodorsal recumbency (lying on its back) on a handler's lap with the cat's head toward the handler's knees. The cat's hindquarters and pelvic area are restrained with the handler's left forearm and elbow while the right hand holds both front legs with a finger in between. The left hand holds the neck with the thumb used to occlude the jugular vein. The phlebotomist holds the cat's chin and head with the non-dominant hand and performs the venipuncture with the dominant hand.

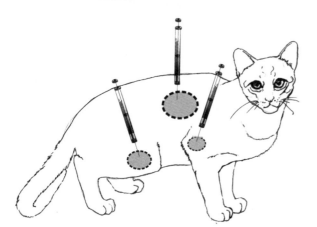

Fig. 5.10 Subcutaneous injection sites in cats.

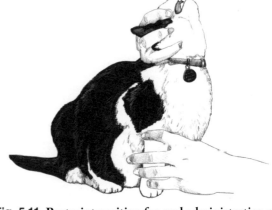

Fig. 5.11 Restraint position for oral administration of solid medications.

stifle; and feline leukemia vaccine below the left sti-fle. These areas can be amputated if otherwise inoperable tumors occur. The risk of vaccine-induced tumors is less than one per 10,000 doses of vaccine (**Figure 5.10**).

Administration of oral, ophthalmic, and otic medications

Oral administration can be facilitated by training as a kitten. Giving small amounts of crunchy treats or pieces of kibble with a pill gun and liquid treats with a syringe for liquid medications can desensitize the cat to better tolerate their use to administer medications in the future.

Oral

Tablet or capsule medication

Hiding solid medication for oral administration in food is always preferable to forcing oral medication into a cat's mouth. A small amount of a pasty, moldable cat-preferred treat should be offered, such as a paste of tuna, crushed crackers, or mayonnaise. If readily eaten, another small amount of a treat with hidden medication is offered. Capsules should be opened and sprinkled in the paste, and tablets should be crushed before adding to the paste unless medication instructions prohibit it. After the cat consumes the medicated treat, it should be given a small portion of an unmedicated treat. If hiding the medication in food is not successful in medicating the cat, restraint for oral administration is necessary.

Administering a capsule or tablet may require restraint using a bag or towel. Sitting restraint is used for oral administration of medications. An assistant holds the cat's rump against his or her abdomen while gently holding the cat's front legs to prevent forward movement and raising of the paws. Alternatively, a rolled towel can be wrapped around the front of the neck to block the front legs from reaching up and forward.

The person administering the oral medication restrains the cat's head with the one-hand head hold. The cat's head is tilted back (**Figure 5.11**). The tablet or capsule is held between the handler's right index finger and thumb, and the tip of the middle finger on the right hand is used to push the lower incisors down, while the left thumb and fingers press the cheeks inward, thus aiding in opening the jaw. The tablet or capsule is pushed into the mouth. If necessary, the eraser end of a pencil can be used to push the medication back over the hump of the tongue. A syringe of 2 ml of palatable liquid, such as tuna juice, should follow to reduce the chance of medication lodging in the esophagus and to counter-condition the cat to oral administration restraint.

Rather than using the eraser end of a pencil to push a tablet or capsule further down the throat, a pill gun can be used (**Figure 5.12**). These syringe-like devices have a rubber end that entraps the tablet or capsule and a plunger to dislodge the medication after it is placed over the hump of the tongue when the mouth is open (**Figure 5.13**). The gun should

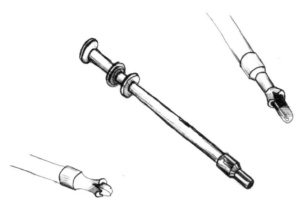

Fig. 5.12 Pill guns can deliver tablets or capsules.

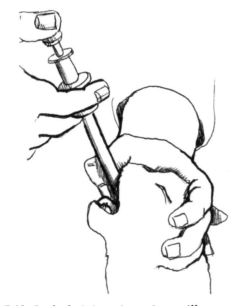

Fig. 5.13 Oral administration using a pill gun.

be rinsed and allowed to dry after each use. A cat's tolerance to pill guns may be improved by occasionally using the pill gun to deliver a special food treat.

Liquid medication

Any oral medication can be aspirated and cause respiratory problems, but the risk is particularly high with oral liquids. Oral liquid medications should never be administered to a cat with its mouth open. The medication should be aspirated into an oral syringe. The cat's body should be restrained, in the same manner as administering solid medications. However, the mouth is held closed and the liquid medication slowly injected through the corner of the upper and lower lips, into the pouch between the cheek and teeth. By injecting slowly and holding the head pointed upward slightly, the medication will run around the dental arcade and be swallowed safely. Unpalatable liquids can be diluted in beef or chicken broth, clam juice, or tuna juice to improve taste without altering the effects of the drug.

Ophthalmic

To medicate a cat's eyes, a handler is generally needed to restrain the cat's head and body. The handler holds the cat in sitting position with its rump against the handler's chest or abdomen while holding the front legs at the shoulder. The examiner holds the cat's upper and lower eyelids apart for an examination.

Medication can be administered to a gentle cat by putting it in sitting position, facing away from the handler. The handler restrains the cat with a forearm and elbow pressing the cat against the handler's side. The hand of the restraining arm restrains the head. The middle finger of the treatment hand pulls the lower lid down, and the ointment or eye drop bottle is held with the index finger and thumb. The medication is dropped into the gap between the sclera and lower lid created by pulling the lower lid down.

Otic

To medicate a cat's external ear, a handler is often needed to hold a cat in sitting position and restrain its front legs in order to administer ear medication. Gentle cats may be restrained in sternal position in a handler's lap for ear canal examination and administration of ear medications. The head should not be restrained by holding the ear flap. The cat's head should be restrained with a hand on the back of its neck and fingers and thumb behind the jaws. The head and neck are turned, as needed, for the ear canal exam or administration of medications. Fractious cats may need to be wrapped in a towel or placed in a cat bag.

Cystocentesis

Cystocentesis is collection of urine using a needle and syringe. Urine is obtained by puncturing the abdomen, entering the urinary bladder, and aspirating the urine. Restraint positions should be ventrodorsal or lateral recumbency. These positions permit stretching the cat's body while limiting torso movement.

SPECIAL EQUIPMENT

Cat restraint bag

Canvas or nylon cat bags tend to calm cats after they are zipped in. Bags provide excellent restraint without the need to tightly restrict movement, as with hand holds or towel wraps. Zipped leg openings permit access to leg veins for venipuncture. Restraint by an assistant is minimal, and safety is high for cats and handlers. However, bags are for cats that may resent a procedure such as venipuncture, and not overtly aggressive cats or cats already distressed.

Cats should be relatively quiet and handled gently in being placed in the bag properly. To put a cat in a restraint bag, the handler opens the bag and places it on a table. The cat is then placed on top of the bag. The neck portion of the bag is first clasped around the cat's neck, after which the bag is placed around the cat (**Figure 5.14**). It is important to zip the bag with one or two fingers under the zipper to prevent the cat's hair from getting caught in the zipper. Smaller zippered ports are present for access to legs (**Figure 5.15**).

A cat in a bag should never be left unattended. Although, once in the bag, a cat usually does not struggle to move, they still should be continuously supervised to ensure they cannot roll off a table. After the procedure is completed, the cat should be slowly removed and stroked in stages when it is quiet to prepare it for a possible need to use a restraint bag again in the future.

Loose-fitting mesh restraint bags with a pull string opening for minor restraint may be of value in handling cats during baths, brief transport, or administering medication.

Muzzles

Leather, nylon, or cloth cat muzzles are open-ended muzzles designed to cover the eyes (**Figure 5.16**). Cloth muzzles pose less risk for injuring the eyes.

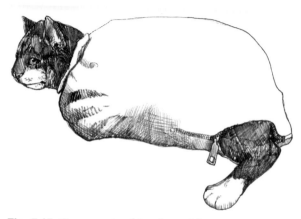

Fig. 5.15 Cat restrained in a bag with access to a hind leg.

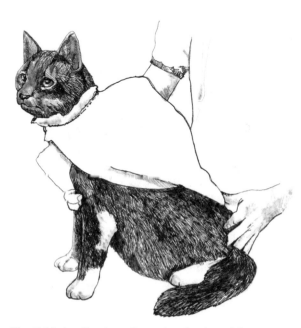

Fig. 5.14 Application of a cat bag begins with fastening it around the neck.

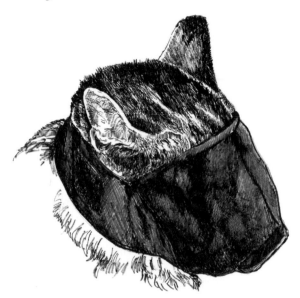

Fig. 5.16 Cat muzzle.

Cats are often quieted by being blindfolded with the muzzle. However, if the cat resists the muzzle, its feet must be well restrained. A one-hand hold restraint of the head may be easier to maintain with the traction provided by a muzzle.

Gloves with gauntlets

Leather gloves with gauntlets are excellent protection against scratches, but some cats can bite through them. If there is danger of biting, the hand should be partially inserted in the glove. The empty fingers of the glove can then be offered as a distraction, while the cat is captured by other means. However, leather gloves may carry stressful odors and exacerbate a cat's anxiety. Gloves also desensitize the handler's hands to the pressure being exerted for restraint, which can contribute to the cat escaping restraint or being injured by excessive restraint.

Loop on a flexible rod

Leads with slip rings can be placed over the head to capture a cat by the neck to control the head while a hand is used to scoop up the body. A commercial loop on a flexible rod is made for capturing cats. The loop on a flexible rod works well for quietly placing a slip leash on a cat's neck and gently pulling it snug on the neck, similar to the Mongolian urga used to capture horses. The flexible rod should not be used to bend the leash and snap on the cat.

Nets

Opposing nets on metal frames attached with pivot points are available to restrain cats. They create a giant salad-tong-like restraint tool that can be used to entrap a cat in a cage and remove it. With support under the cat's body while it is still in the netting, it can be transported short distances. The netting can also restrain a cat for administering medications or chemical restraint. It is more effective when the cat is entrapped in a standard cage at the handler's chest height. It is not effective for capturing cats in the open on the ground or a floor.

Commercial hoop nets on long poles are available for capturing and restraining cats. Nylon mesh laundry bags can also be used. The size of the mesh in the netting should be sufficiently small (¼ in [0.64 cm] or less) to prevent entanglement and injury.

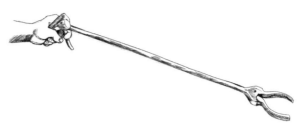

Fig. 5.17 Cat capture tongs.

Capture tongs

Cat tongs are long-handled clamps for capture and restraint of vicious cats by the neck. (**Figure 5.17**). The tongs are used to clamp the neck and restrain the head just before other means of restraint are applied. The pressure on the neck applied by tongs is difficult to control when a cat is struggling, and if the body is not controlled at the same time the tongs are used, a struggling cat could break its neck.

Cage shield

A cage shield is a wooden or metal frame the same height and width of the inside of a cage, covered with wire mesh and with a center brace and a centrally placed handle. The shield is slid into a slightly opened cage door and used to push a fractious cat against the back of its cage to administer chemical restraint.

Squeeze cage

Wire cages are available with a sliding partition that permits a cat to be compressed inside a cage so that minor procedures can be performed or chemical restraint administered (**Figure 5.18**). The use of squeeze cages should be restricted to the most vicious cats and preferably for a one-time use on a cat.

Head movement-limiting devices

Elizabethan collars are applied as with dogs (**Figure 5.19**). If tolerated by the cat, the collar will restrain it from chewing on its hindquarters. They can also provide the handler with some protection from being bit while handling or restraining the cat. Elizabethan collars must be removed to allow eating and drinking.

Spherical, semi-opaque (globe-shield) collars that encapsulate the head and have an opening in front

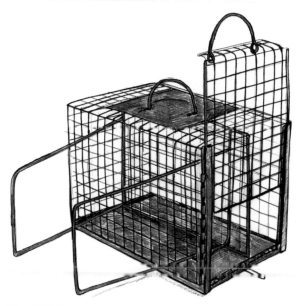

Fig. 5.18 Squeeze cage.

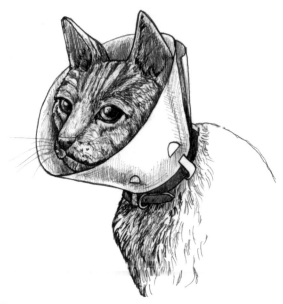

Fig. 5.19 Elizabethan collar.

for breathing and vision are commercially available as a means of protecting handlers from bites. Globe-shield collars do not allow drinking or eating and must be frequently taken on and off, which could actually increase the risk of being bitten.

Thick, broad collars wrap snugly around the neck like a human cervical collar to limit the cat's ability to reach areas of its body. A retention strap is run from the top of the broad band around the lower aspect of the thorax behind the front legs. Broad-band cervical collars permit better peripheral vision and hearing and do not catch on objects as does the Elizabethan collar. They also allow eating and drinking. However, access to most of each front leg is possible. Cervical collars for movement limitation can also be pneumatic (**Figure 5.20**). Heavy canvas construction is needed for protection from cat claws.

Pinch-induced behavioral inhibition

Two-inch paper clip binders, bent to reduce the pressure applied, have been recommended to be used on the loose skin of the upper neck as a "twitch" to distract difficult to handle cats in the same manner as scruffing. It is theorized that the pinching simulates being carried as a small kitten by the queen. However, freezing from fear may be another possibility. Similar commercially produced clips for cat restraint are also marketed.

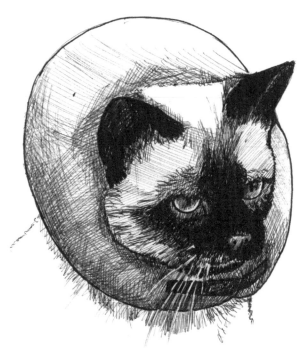

Fig. 5.20 Pneumatic movement-limiting cervical collar.

TRANSPORTING CATS

Regulations on interstate, international, and air travel change frequently and must be rechecked each time a cat is transported.

To travel to the U.S., cats must be more than 3 months old, vaccinated for rabies, and free of signs of infectious diseases. For interstate travel, proof of current rabies vaccination and a current health certificate should accompany the cat. Travel to Hawaii and Guam, which are rabies-free islands, has more restrictions.

International travel should be investigated at least 120 days in advance. Current requirements can be obtained from the destination's embassy or consulate. A list of foreign embassies and consulates in the U.S. is available from the U.S. Department of State: http://usembassy.state.gov/

Import, export, and interstate transportation information on privately owned cats is available at https://www.aphis.usda.gov/aphis/pet-travel

Regardless of the means of travel, there is risk of a medical emergency or escape. A chest harness or collar should be worn with an ID tag that includes the owner's name, address, and cell phone number. A land-phone number while traveling is much less useful. Cats that travel should have an identification microchip embedded in case the cat escapes. A chest harness is more secure and prevents escapes better than a collar. A travel tag should also be attached to the harness or collar that provides the destination and destination contact information.

Travel by car

If transporting a cat by car or in truck cabs, cats should ride in a back seat and be restrained in a crate that is strapped to floor anchors. This protects cats from airbag injuries and the driver from interference with driving (vision obstruction, interference with braking) or being injured by a cat becoming a missile in an accident. More information on travel restraints is available at the Center for Pet Safety: www.centerforpetsafety.org

Cats should be desensitized to car travel by experiencing frequent short trips by car to a pleasurable destination with no adverse events during their primary socialization period (2–7 weeks of age), or as soon after that as possible.

If a cat is to be transported in a carrier, pre-trip training should include free access in and out of the carrier, being fed in the carrier, and sleeping in the carrier to develop a feeling of security while in the carrier.

If the temperature is over 72°F (22.2°C), cats should not be left in cars. At 72°F, the inside of a car can reach 100°F (37.8°C) in 30 minutes. Temperatures below 55°F (12.8°C) may be too low for some cats.

Pictures of the cat should be carried in case a search is needed if an escape occurs. Food, water, and any needed medications should also be available during the trip.

Interstate travel must meet federal requirements. These include a certificate of veterinary inspection, provision of adequate shelter from all elements and protection from injury, sufficient cleanliness to avoid contact with urine and feces, protection against hazardous temperature extremes, uncontaminated and nutritious food at least once per day, and a program of parasite control.

Air travel
Preparing for air travel

Travel on an airline should be arranged well in advance of the intended travel date, as the number of animals per flight is limited. In temperate weather, it is best to choose early morning non-stop flights whenever possible. In hot weather, early or late flights are preferable; in colder weather, midday flights are best. Travel during holiday periods should be avoided.

Before making travel arrangements, a veterinary exam for age and health-related restrictions should be performed. Most carriers require a certificate of veterinary inspection (health certificate) signed within the last 10 days. Some airlines require an acclimation certificate from a veterinarian. Acclimation certificates waive the airline's requirement that they prevent exposure to less than 45°F (7.2°C) for more than 45 minutes during ground transfer or for more than 4 hours if in a holding facility. An acclimation certificate does not, however, waive the airline's requirement that the cat cannot be exposed to more than 85°F (29.4°C) for more than 45 minutes on the ground or 4 hours in a holding facility.

Only light feeding and access to water should be provided about 3 hours before departure. Tranquilizers are not recommended as they can impair a cat's ability to maintain normal body temperature and to keep its balance during travel. Tranquilizers can also exacerbate heart or respiratory problems.

Travel crates

Travel crates for air travel should be big enough to allow the cat to stand and turn around. There should be no interior protrusions that could injure the cat. The crate should have handles or grips and a leak-proof bottom with absorbent bedding. Both sides should be ventilated. Labels should be attached that provide the owner's name, home address, phone number, destination contact information and a sign stating "Live Animal" and arrows denoting up. Containers for food and water need to be accessible from outside and secured inside. If a collar is worn by the cat, it should be a break-away collar to prevent the risk of strangulation. Carriers for travel in the passenger section should be soft-sided. Rigid clamshell crates are needed for travel in cargo holds.

SELECTED FURTHER READING

Babovic N. Cayci C, Carlsen BT (2014). Cat bite infections of the hand: Assessment of morbidity and predictors of severe infection. *Journal of Hand Surgery* 39:286–290.

Gruen ME, Thomson AE, Clary GP, et al. (2013). Conditioning laboratory cats to handling and transport. *Lab Animal* 42:385–389.

Rodan L, Sundahl E, Carney H, et al. (2011). AAFP and ISFM Feline-Friendly Handling Guidelines. *Journal of Feline Medicine and Surgery* 13:364–375.

Scherk MA, Ford RB, Gaskell RM, et al. (2013). 2013 AAFP feline vaccination advisory panel report. *Journal of Feline Medicine and Surgery* 15:785–808.

Taylor SM (2010). *Small Animal Clinical Techniques.* Elsevier Saunders, St. Louis.

Tuzio H, Edwards D, Elson T, et al. (2005). Feline zoonoses from the American Association of Feline Practitioners. *Journal of Feline Medicine and Surgery* 7:243–274.

Yin S. 2009. *Low Stress Handling, Restraint and Behavior Modification of Dogs and Cats.* CattleDog Publishing, Davis.

CHAPTER 6

OTHER SMALL MAMMALS

In addition to dogs and cats, there are other small mammals that are domesticated or tamed and kept as pets or used in research. Since common tame species can be confused with similar non-tame species, small mammal names are often rendered more specific by reference to their Latin genus–species name, such as the house mouse (*Mus musculus*). The most common of these other small mammals are mice, rats, hamsters, gerbils, guinea pigs, chinchillas, degus, sugar gliders, African pygmy hedgehogs, rabbits, and ferrets. None are domesticated to the point of enjoying being handled by humans as much as most dogs and cats do. Handling is stressful to these other small mammals and should be kept to a minimum. Frequent brief duration and gentle handling during their juvenile socialization periods can reduce the stress of handling experienced during later life. Rats and mice are the most common laboratory animals in biomedical research. They are also raised as food for captive reptiles and birds of prey. Ten percent of U.S. households have small mammal pets, often referred to as *pocket pets*. Rats, rabbits, and guinea pigs are the easiest small mammal pets for new pet handlers. Rabbits are the most popular of the other small mammal pets in the U.S. They are also the most common pet relinquished to animal shelters, after dogs and cats, in large part due to owners being unfamiliar with the necessary handling, restraint, and nutritional needs of rabbits and all other small mammals. In March 2016, the state of New York passed legislation to require retailers of small mammals and reptiles to provide new owners with written instructions on the proper care of these animals.

NATURAL BEHAVIOR OF SMALL MAMMALS

The natural behavior of small mammals depends on whether they are prey or predator. Most are prey and so have similar characteristics. The only domesticated small mammal other than dogs and cats that is strictly a predator is the ferret. Rats are primarily prey, but in some situations they can be a predator.

Determining the gender of small mammals is important to prevent mixing groups that are incompatible. For example, if not raised together, adult male mice or male rabbits will fight each other, and adult female hamsters will fight each other. Gender determination of small mammals is often not easy. Male rodents have open inguinal canals, which enables them to pull their testes from the scrotum into the abdomen. Therefore, lack of external (scrotal) testes cannot be relied on as evidence the animal is a female.

Anogenital (AG) distance is the length from the urinary papilla to the anus. AG distance is longer in males than females, and the external genitalia in a male is somewhat circular while a female's is more like a slit. Measuring the AG distance can be used to determine gender for most small mammals. For guinea pigs and young rabbits, however, sexing requires gently pressing on each side of the genital orifice in an attempt to extrude the penis.

Small prey mammals

All small prey mammals need a dark area to hide in. Hiding is an inherent need that helps relieve the stress of constantly being on guard for dominant aggression of other members of the group or for predators. This characteristic of seeking a hiding area makes it fairly easy for most of them to be coaxed into an opaque plastic cup or a small bin for capture and transport.

The vision of small prey mammals is good for detecting movements but poor for detail. Small prey mammals have excellent senses of hearing and smell. Hearing is enhanced by being able to detect sound vibrations from the ground. Handlers should wear plastic or rubber gloves to diminish the smell of predators that the handler may have recently touched or the smell of perfumes from hand soap. Gloves are also indicated for handler protection from infectious disease and allergens from small mammals.

With the exception of hamsters, small prey mammals need the security of others of their species. However, new members must be carefully introduced to an established group. Small mammals mark their territory and possessions by rubbing a part of their body on the object to be marked. Others with a different smell are rejected. Introduction of a new member involves placing the new member in a nearby separate cage within sight and smell of the group. Over a period of days the new member cage is moved closer to the group cage. Next, the most docile member of the group is put into a third cage near the new member's. When the docile group member and the new member appear adjusted to each other, they exchange cages so that each acquires the smell of the other. After sufficient time to acquire the smells, the two should be able to be put in the same cage. If they accept the presence each other, they can usually join the main group.

Small mammals need opportunities to exercise and stimulate mental activity. Since most small mammals instinctively have a need to gnaw, objects for gnawing (kiln dried pine wood, cardboard tubes or boxes) should be offered. Most small mammals also burrow and enjoy exploring PVC pipe in the size appropriate for the species. Exercise wheels are popular enrichments for small mammal enclosures, but care must be taken that the construction of the wheel is safe for the small mammal species that will use it. Environmental enrichments, called cage furniture, should be removed before attempting to capture small mammals to avoid accidental injuries.

Most small domestic or tame mammals are nocturnal and unable to tolerate wide ranges of temperature. They should be allowed undisturbed rest during daylight hours in quiet surroundings. Their enclosures should not be exposed to drafts or direct sunlight.

The greatest stress a prey small mammal experiences is the sight, sound, or smell of a predator. All small prey mammals should be segregated at all times from dogs, cats, large birds, ferrets, and reptiles.

Predatory small mammals

Like small prey mammals, ferrets need social interaction with others of their species, long periods of undisturbed rest, and when awake lots of opportunity for exercise and exploration. Much of the waking hours are spent in mock predator activities, such a wrestling with other ferrets, exploring burrow-like structures, and marking territory and possessions with their body scent. Ferrets should never be housed within sight, sound, or smell of possible prey animals.

SAFETY FIRST

Handler safety

All small mammals may bite when restrained. Rodents have incisors that angle backward. If bitten and the animal does not release its bite, the handler should replace it in its cage or box, where it will probably release its bite. Rabbits can, and on occasion, will bite. Scratching from claws on the hind feet is typically the greatest risk to handlers from rabbits. Plastic gloves should be worn whenever handling rodents because allergies to saliva, dander, or urine are common.

Small mammal safety

All small mammals are handled on tables, and all will attempt to jump off, resulting in injury if restraint outside of its cage is not constant.

Mice, rats, and gerbils can be restrained by grasping the base of the tail. They should not be held by the last two-thirds of the tail. Holding them by the distal aspect of the tail can allow them to turn and bite the handler, or spin in an effort to escape and deglove (rip) the skin from the tail. While suspended by the end of the tail, rats can climb their tail to bite handlers. Gerbils are especially prone to tail degloving during handling. Only the base of their tail can be safely held.

If capturing to perform a grooming or medical procedure, all materials should be readied prior to capture to reduce stress to the animal from prolonged restraint.

Plastic gloves should be worn when handling nursing small mammals, especially rodents and rabbits. The young should be rubbed with used bedding after handling and before being returned to their enclosures. Otherwise, human scent may cause the mother to shun the babies.

Key zoonoses

(*Note:* Apparently ill animals should be handled by veterinary professionals or under their supervision. Precautionary measures against zoonoses from ill animals are more involved than those required when handling apparently healthy animals, and such measures vary widely. The discussion here is directed primarily at handling apparently healthy animals.)

Apparently healthy, captive-raised small mammals pose little risk of transmitting disease to healthy adult handlers who practice conventional personal hygiene. The risks of physical injury are greater than the risks of acquiring an infectious disease (*Table 6.1*).

Direct transmission

Systemic disease

Wild rodents and rabbits are potential sources of infection of humans with hantavirus, babesiosis, leptospirosis, Lyme disease, lymphocytic choriomeningitis, plague, Rocky Mountain spotted fever, and tularemia. Captive-born, properly housed (away from ticks and wild animals) rodents and rabbits do not typically carry these diseases.

Sin Nombre hantavirus is a virus transmitted by aerosol of body secretions, especially wild mouse and rat urine. The house mouse, common rat, and lab rodents have not been associated with the virus. Sin Nombre hantavirus can infect the lungs, become systemic, and be fatal to humans. The Seoul hantavirus infects rats without signs of disease. Infected humans may develop headache, muscle pains, and nausea. In rare circumstances, a hemorrhagic fever and renal syndrome may occur.

The virus that causes lymphocytic choriomeningitis, a viral disease of the brain, is carried by wild house mice and transmitted in their urine, but has also been reported in pet hamsters and guinea pigs exposed to wild mice, the reservoir for the virus. Infected wild mice and hamsters carry the virus without signs of disease.

Wild rodents can transmit leptospirosis, a bacterial disease that predominately affects the kidneys and is shed in the urine.

Coxiellosis (Q fever) is a bacterial disease that is transmitted by inhalation of dust contaminated by the body secretions of animals (urine, milk, feces, etc.) infected with *Coxiella burnetii.*

Rat-bite fever is a bacterial disease (*Streptobacillus moniliformis*) that causes fever and sore joints in humans. It is transmitted from healthy appearing rodents to humans by bites or exposure to rodent urine, feces, or other body fluids.

Monkeypox has caused an outbreak in the U.S. after it was introduced by Gambian rats and spread to owners of pet prairie dogs that were exposed to the rats. Monkeypox can be carried by rodents, rabbits, and squirrels. In people, it causes symptoms similar to smallpox infection.

Encephalitozoonosis (*Encephalitozoon cuniculi*) is a fungal infection of rabbits and less commonly other small mammals that is transmitted in body fluids, particularly urine. Infections in humans are limited to those who are immunocompromised.

Respiratory disease

Pasteurellosis from rodents or rabbits and bordetellosis from guinea pigs or rabbits are zoonotic respiratory bacterial infections. Humans usually require an impaired immune response to develop severe or prolonged infections.

Ferrets are susceptible to human influenza. The risk of transmission is greater from humans to ferrets than from ferrets to humans. The disease is also more pathogenic in ferrets than in humans.

Digestive tract disease

Ingesting contaminated fecal materials is a way to acquire the bacterial disease scampylobacteriosis and salmonellosis from ferrets or hamsters. Of these, campylobacteriosis is the most common, although the source is generally from small mammals with diarrhea, not healthy appearing animals.

Yersiniosis (*Yersinia enterocolitica*, also known as *Y. pseudotuberculosis*) causes bloody diarrhea and can be transmitted by guinea pigs that may have no clinical signs of disease.

Skin disease

Ringworm is a fungal infection of the upper layers of the skin. A common organism carried by small

Table 6.1 **Diseases transmitted from healthy appearing captive-bred small mammals to healthy adult humans**

DISEASE	AGENT	MEANS OF TRANSMISSION	SIGNS AND SYMPTOMS IN HUMANS	FREQUENCY IN ANIMALS	RISK GROUP*
Bites	–	Direct injury	Bite wounds to face, arms, and legs	All small mammals are capable of inflicting bite wounds	3
Rat bite fever	*Streptobacillus moniliformis* and *Spirillum minus*	Direct from bites or infected urine	Fever and joint pain	Uncommon in captive-bred rats	2
Pasteurellosis	*Pasteurella multocida*	Direct from rabbit or rat bites	Systemic illness signs: fever, inappetence; joint infections	Common in rabbits	2
Ringworm	*Trichophyton mentagrophites*	Direct from contact with infected skin, scale, or hair; indirect from fomites	Scaly skin sores and hair loss with or without crusts or redness	Common in guinea pigs and rabbits	2
Lymphocytic choriomeningitis	*Arenaviridae* virus	Direct from body fluids or inhalation	Flu-like signs, stiff neck, abortion	Occasional presence in rats, mice, guinea pigs, and hamsters	4
Yersiniosis	*Yersinia enterocolitica*	Direct, fecal-oral	Bloody diarrhea	Occasional in guinea pigs	3
Cheyletiellosis	*Cheyletiella parasitovorax*	Direct and indirect from fomites	Itchy chigger-like bites on the skin	Common in rabbits	2
Salmonellosis	*Salmonella enterica*	Direct, fecal-oral	Diarrhea	Occasional in guinea pigs, sugar gliders, hedgehogs, and ferrets	3
Scabies	*Sarcoptes scabiei, Trixacarus caviae*	Direct from contact with infested skin	Itchy chigger-like bites in the skin	*T. caviae* is common in guinea pigs, *S. scabiei*	2
Seoul virus	Hantavirus	Direct contact with body secretions, bites; indirect from aerosolized dried feces	Fever, headache, back and abdominal pain	Carried by wild rats, rarely by domesticated rats	2

* Risk groups (National Institutes of Health and World Health Organization criteria. Centers for Disease Control and Prevention, *Biosafety in Microbiological and Biomedical Laboratories*, 5th edition, 2009):
1 Agent not associated with disease in healthy adult humans.
2 Agent rarely causes serious disease and prevention or therapy possible.
3 Agent can cause serious or lethal disease and prevention or therapy possible.
4 Agent can cause serious or lethal disease and prevention or therapy are not usually available.

mammals is *Trichophyton mentagrophytes*. Rodent and rabbit handlers may develop transient infection by contact with infected hair or skin scales being caught under a sleeve or collar and rubbed against the skin, or caught under the fingernails and scratched into the scalp. Rabbits also may carry a skin mite, *Cheyletiella parasitovorax*, which will cause itchy skin sores similar to chigger bites in handlers.

Vector borne

Lyme disease (borreliosis), which causes a variety of systemic signs and symptoms, is carried by wild mice and transmitted by ticks. Rocky Mountain spotted fever is a blood platelet disease transmitted from ticks that wild small mammals could carry into a human's environment. Plague ("Black Death") is a disfiguring and potentially fatal bacterial disease carried by wild rodents and rabbits in the south-western and western U.S., which is transmitted by their fleas. Tularemia is a bacterial infection of wild rodents and rabbits that can be transmitted to humans by deer flies and ticks. Humans can acquire babesiosis, a blood parasitic infection carried by wild mice, but the transmission requires the bite of a tick.

Sanitary practices

Basic procedures are for handlers to wash their hands and to clean and disinfect table tops and cages used in handling. Restraint equipment should be disposable or cleaned and disinfected.

Special facilities and training are required to safely handle small mammals. The typical small mammal handler should only handle captive-bred, appropriately housed small mammals. Sick small mammals should be isolated from apparently normal animals. Rodent cages should be kept clean and in a well-ventilated area and never located in food preparation or eating areas. Persons handling small mammals should wear appropriate dress to protect against skin contamination by hair and skin scales or saliva, urine, and other body secretions. Basic sanitary practices should be adhered to, such as keeping hands away from eyes, nose, and mouth when handling small mammals and washing hands after handling the animals. Handlers should not eat food or smoke while handling small mammals. Use of plastic gloves in handling all small mammals is advisable.

Small mammals should be prevented from any direct or indirect contact with wildlife, particularly wild rodents. All food should be kept in rodent-proof containers. Wild rodent feces should be wiped with damp paper towels wetted in a solution of chlorine (one-quarter cup bleach in 1 gal [3.8 L] of water).

While wearing gloves, handlers should clean small mammal enclosures and all enclosure contents on a regular basis (at least weekly). Gloves should be changed between cleaning separate enclosures. Enclosure and enclosure contents should be cleaned outside the primary family dwelling.

Ferret handlers should maintain current influenza vaccinations.

MICE

The mouse (*Mus musculus*), also called the house mouse, originated in Asia and has spread throughout the world. They were first domesticated by royalty in Japan and China who selectively bred them for atypical colors.

White mice have been selectively bred in captivity for use in research and as pets. Some have been selectively bred for variously colored (called "fancy") hair coats. Few mice are comfortable being held gently in a handler's hand and will bite to escape. They are more likely to bite than domestic rats and are not a good choice of pet for children.

Male mice are called *bucks*. Female mice are *does*, and young mice are *pups*.

Natural behavior of mice

Mice are nocturnal and prefer to hide. Adult males fight each other. Dominant males may chew the hair off some submissive members of their group. This activity is called *barbering*.

Sexing can be accomplished using the AG distance. In males, the distance between the anus and external genitalia is much larger than in females. Also, in females nipples emerge after about 2 weeks, and the scrotum in males should be readily visible when the testicles are everted. Most small mammals housed alone are more anxious about being handled than those kept in groups.

The vision of mice is poor, but sound, smell, and movement are well detected. To attempt to avoid detection of their movement, cats remain still for long periods and advance slowly in spurts when stalking mice. Mice mark exploration paths with secretions from the soles of their feet and occasionally with urine and use their sense of smell to retrace paths.

Approaching and catching

The primary defense of mice is to seek a dark, quiet area to hide. Thus they may be captured by providing a cup, called a rodent recreational vehicle (RV), for hiding and then entrapping them for transport.

Many mice will attempt to bite if unaccustomed to being restrained or are restrained roughly. When they bite, they are often reluctant to let go. Mice are best captured from a transport cage free of water, food bowls and other moveable objects, so all feeders, water bowls, hiding boxes, and exercise apparatuses in the enclosure should be removed. All doors and windows in the handling room should be closed and possible hiding places blocked before removing a mouse from a cage. Mice will climb or jump out of boxes or cages or chew out of an enclosure, if given the opportunities.

Handlers should avoid having odors on them when handling mice, especially odors that might be associated with a predator.

Handling for routine care and management

Frequently handled pet or research mice may be handled by cupping hands around them (**Figure 6.1**). Plastic gloves should be worn for protection from allergens. More often, a handler must grasp the base of the tail and lift the mouse to a surface that it can cling to, such as the handler's shirt, lab coat arm, or a small rug on a table. The mouse will continue to try to pull away while the handler continues to hold its tail. An adult mouse can be moved short distances by the base of its tail, but if pregnant or obese, a mouse's body should be supported with the other hand.

Additional restraint can be applied by holding the tail and pressing the body down while grasping the skin on the back of the neck between the thumb and index finger (scruffing) and then swinging the body into the palm of the hand with the tail grasped between the ring and little finger (**Figure 6.2**). The non-dominant hand should be used for restraint so the dominant hand can perform examinations, write notes, and administer medications.

Young mice less than 2 weeks old can be grasped by the loose skin of the neck and shoulder with a thumb and forefinger. Plastic gloves should be worn to prevent adding odor to the babies. Mother mice will cannibalize babies having strange odors.

African (Egyptian) spiny mice are a type of mouse that are gaining popularity as pets. They are larger than domestic mice and so should not be picked up by their tail because of the risk of a degloving injury to the tail.

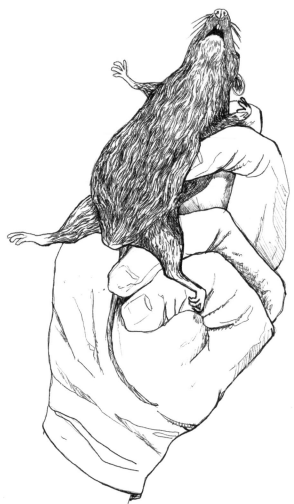

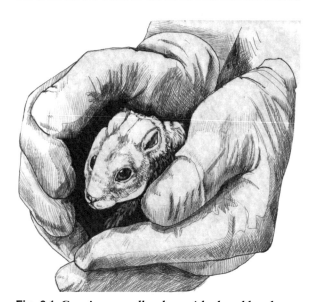

Fig. 6.1 Cupping a small rodent with gloved hands.

Fig. 6.2 Scruff-and-stretch hold on a mouse.

RATS

Pet and research rats (*Rattus norvegicus*) were derived from the Norway rat (brown rat or wharf rat), which is the most common wild rat. They were domesticated in the United Kingdom to be used in rat baiting in the 18th and 19th centuries. Rats were put in fighting pits, and wagers were made on how quickly a dog could kill them.

Rats, specifically the black rat (*Rattus rattus*), also called the roof rat, were reviled in Europe because of their association with the Black Death (bubonic plague) that killed at least one-third of the people in Europe in the 14th century. Transmission was primarily by the fleas they carried and brought into human settlements.

Many domestic rats are selectively bred for variously colored (called "fancy") hair coats. Sprague Dawley and Long Evans rats (two strains of *Rattus norvegicus*) are most easily handled and are preferred for pets.

Male rats are called *bucks*. Female rats are *does*, and young rats are *pups*.

Natural behavior of rats

Rats are smart, interactive, nocturnal omnivores. They can be prey or predator. If not overcrowded, they are clean and virtually odor free. They are less skittish than hamsters and gerbils, less likely to bite than mice, and less likely to scratch and injure a child than handling a rabbit. Rats tolerate living in mixed groups better than mice.

Rats are similar to mice in that a large AG distance is consistent with being male. Males lack nipples, and their testicles are very pronounced at all ages. The brown rat is larger than the black rat and prefers to burrow and tunnel. The black rat prefers to climb and is an excellent jumper.

Aggressive rats will arch their back, fluff out the hair on their back, and swish their tail similar to the aggressive posture of a dominance aggressive cat.

Approaching and catching

Domestic rats are generally docile if handled gently and slowly. They behave best with minimal restraint. Rat pups should be handled at weaning for socialization. They should not be startled when they are asleep or they may bite in defense. The primary defense response of rats is to hide when possible, but they will bite if cornered. The intent to bite is often signaled by a rat standing on its hindquarters and facing the approaching hand.

As with all small mammals, capturing rats is best attempted after removing feeders, water bowls, hiding boxes, or other moveable objects in the enclosure. All doors and windows should be closed and hiding places blocked before removing a rat from a cage. Capture should begin with grasping the base of the tail; a rat should not be picked up by end of its tail. Its body should be supported by the other hand (**Figure 6.3**).

The Harderian gland is located behind the rat's eyeball. Stressed or sick rats will produce a red porphyrin from the Harderian gland that looks like blood, called red tears. Porphyrin can be identified by its fluorescence using a Wood's lamp.

Handling for routine care and management

Rats like to hide, so many rats will become calm if allowed to hide in a coat pocket. They are more comfortable if allowed to move around on a sleeved arm and intermittently repositioned by grasping the base of the tail or the shoulders. Older rats often have chronic respiratory disease and can be severely

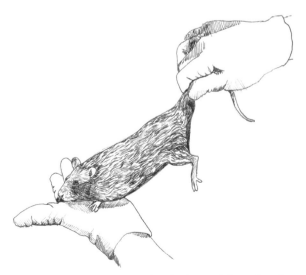

Fig. 6.3 Restraint of a rat by the base of the tail and support of the body.

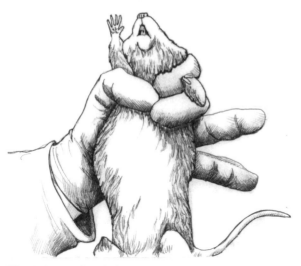

Fig. 6.4 One-handed rat restraint.

stressed by restraint. Both hands should be used to restrain rats weighing more than 200 grams.

Firm manual restraint of rats is performed by grasping the base of the tail with one hand and the rat's shoulders with the other hand, using the thumb under a front leg and the jaw. The handler's index and middle fingers restrain the front leg on the other side of the rat (**Figure 6.4**). The rat's chest or trachea should not be squeezed. If its breathing is impaired, it may panic and attempt to bite when held or when released.

HAMSTERS

The common pet hamster (*note:* no "p" in hamster) is the golden (Syrian or teddy bear) hamster (*Mesocricetus auratus*), which originated in the desert region of Syria. All golden hamsters in captivity are believed to be descendants of one male and two females captured in 1930. Not all are golden in color. New colors have been selectively bred from mutations.

Hamsters have extremely loose skin, virtually no tail, hairless feet, and large cheek pouches for storing food or hiding and transporting valued possessions, including baby hamsters. Both sexes have flank glands used for territorial marking.

Related to the golden hamster are the Russian hamsters (*Phodopus* spp.) and the Chinese dwarf hamster (*Cricetulus griseus*), which are smaller and less common than the golden hamster. Russian hamsters are usually brown or gray. All have a dorsal stripe the length of their back and hair on their feet. Like the golden hamster, Russian hamsters have cheek pouches. Russian hamsters are more social and less nocturnal.

Hamsters have been used for research on ear diseases, and because of their very short gestation period, they are used for teratogenic studies. They are less affordable for research since they need to be housed individually. Consequently, much more space is required for cages than with other rodents.

A male hamster is called a *buck*. A female is a *doe*, and young hamsters are *pups*.

Natural behavior of hamsters

Hamsters are burrowing, nocturnal desert rodents that are drowsy in the daytime and have poor eyesight, particularly in bright light. They are likely to bite, especially if startled, and are not recommended as pets for children.

In their natural habitat of the desert, adult hamsters primarily live alone in tunnels for cooler temperature and higher humidity than that on the desert's surface. They tolerate cold temperatures well and will go into pseudo-hibernation if the temperature goes below 48°F (8.9°C), and they could be mistaken as being dead during this time. In their natural habitat, hamsters have not had to evolve an ability to negotiate cliffs and ledges well. In captivity they are more likely to fall off exam tables than other small mammals. They forage for food at night and then carry it back to their burrow in their cheek pouches. Pet hamsters also like to hide food. Bedding and other areas within enclosure should be routinely checked for stashed food that is rotting.

Golden hamsters have paired glands in the skin over their flanks. The flank glands, also called hip spots, are more prominent in males, which use the gland secretions to mark their territory.

Adult hamsters prefer to live a solitary existence, except during mating. Male hamsters are much more docile than females. They should be separated after they are 6–10 weeks old. Females are larger than and dominant to males. Females are more aggressive and more likely to fight, especially if pregnant or lactating.

Sexing of hamsters is similar to that in the rat. The adult male's body protrudes more caudally owing to the testicles, and the difference is striking. The AG distance is much longer in males than in females. In dwarf species of hamsters, males possess a prevalent scent gland on the midline of the abdomen.

Approaching and catching

If attempting to sleep, hamsters bury their head under their abdomen, which impairs their ability to see, smell, or hear a handler approaching. Capture is best attempted after removing feeders, water bowls, hiding boxes, or other moveable objects in the enclosure. A handler should be sure the hamster is awake before attempting a capture to prevent startling it. To awaken a hamster, the handler should talk to it or jiggle its cage. Adult female hamsters are usually more irritable than males. A nursing female should be captured when away from her litter. Female hamsters can be extremely aggressive when they are nursing.

Gentle hamsters can be captured by cupping with both hands and then supporting their body in the handler's palm or grasping the skin on the back of the neck. They also may be induced to enter a small can or cup and moved after covering the opening.

Handling for routine care and management

For the best physical restraint, the handler must do a full-body scruff hold (**Figure 6.5**). The hamster is covered with one hand while pinning the head between the thumb and index finger. Then, without releasing the skin behind the neck, it is grasped

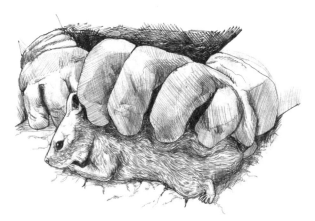

Fig. 6.5 Full-body scruff hold on a hamster.

with thumb and index finger and the skin of the back with other fingers and heel of the hand. Caution is required to not gather the skin too tightly near the head. Too much tension on the skin around the eyes can cause prolapse of an eyeball (proptosis).

When possible, restraint should be avoided if the cheek pouches contain food. Hamsters may aspirate cheek pouch materials if scruffed with their pouches full.

GERBILS

Gerbils (*Meriones unguiculatus*), also called "jirds," originated from the deserts of eastern Mongolia and northeastern China. They have thin, long-haired tails. Most are sand colored with white underbellies. Gerbils were first brought to the U.S. in 1954. They are now illegal as pets in California because of the environmental risks were they to escape into the wild. Gerbils have been used in medical research on strokes in humans.

Both genders have a ventral marking gland on their abdomen that is used to mark their territory. In gerbils, the AG distance in males is ½ in (1.3 cm), and the scrotum should be apparent after about 6 weeks. Only females have nipples.

A male gerbil is called a *buck*. A female is a *doe*, and young gerbils are *pups*. A group of gerbils is a *horde*.

Natural behavior of gerbils

Gerbils are monogamous, and pairs should not be housed separately. They live best in small groups or pairs. Gerbils are not strongly nocturnal and are usually active during the day if other activities are going on. They are gentle and rarely bite, except new cage members if introduced too rapidly to an established group. Gerbils are not as vocal as other small rodents (mice, rats, hamsters). They like to burrow in sandy soils and should be provided with deep bedding and solid-bottomed cages. Having evolved in deserts, gerbils consume little water and produce small amounts of urine. They therefore do not produce the strong urine odor characteristic of other rodents. Gerbils enjoy hiding and running through tunnels and using exercise wheels, which should have fine mesh to protect their toes. They like to chew and should not have access to plastic objects, to avoid the risk of gastrointestinal obstruction from plastic pieces. Like other desert animals, they enjoy dust baths. If stressed, gerbils will signal danger to others by thumping a hind foot. When the pups are 5 weeks old they should be separated from the mother in case she is pregnant and ready to give birth to another litter. Otherwise, she may become aggressive toward the older pups.

Male and female gerbils have an oval-shaped ventral marking gland on the abdomen. The gland is more pronounced in post-pubertal males, who use the gland to mark their territory.

Overcrowding, high humidity (more than 50% for gerbils), or other stressors in gerbils will cause porphyrin secretion in their tears. Porphyrins in tears will stain skin and hair around the nostrils and eyes a reddish-brown and irritate the skin, progressing to skin sores.

Approaching and catching

Gerbils are semi-nocturnal desert animals that are easy to handle (**Figure 6.6**). If given time to adjust to the handler's smell and voice, they may climb into cupped hands, if a handler's movements are appropriately slow. Otherwise, they may be captured with both hands or grasped in one hand using the methods used for mice; that is, carefully grasping the base of tail or scruffing the neck and shoulder skin.

> Do NOT grab gerbils by the tail, except carefully at its base. The skin could otherwise be easily stripped off during its struggling, an injury called "tail slip."

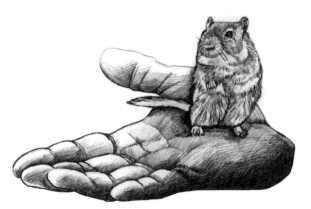

Fig. 6.6 Gerbils do not usually resist gentle handling.

Handling for routine care and management

Gerbils become stressed from handling, and many will seizure if the stress is prolonged. If firm manual restraint is necessary, a handler should grasp the body over the back with its head between the thumb and index finger or alternatively grasp (scruff) the skin on the neck and back and trap the tail with the little finger, as is done when restraining mice.

GUINEA PIGS

Guinea pigs (*Cavia porcellus*), also called cavies, are crepuscular, docile, and social animals that were domesticated as a food source about 7,000 years ago. They are from the Andes Mountains in South America, not from Guinea, but they do squeal like a pig and have the same general body shape. Guinea pigs are related to chinchillas but have no tail and no hair on their ears. They were selectively bred by the Incas from 1200–1532 AD and were brought to Europe by the Spanish conquerors in the early 1500s.

Again, the AG distance in guinea pigs is a marker for gender. However, the distances are not as distinguishable as with other rodents. A female has a Y-shaped opening made by the close proximity of the vulva to the anus. Other ways to distinguish the male is by gently pressing the abdomen to cause the penis to emerge; male nipples are less developed, and the testicles are evident in a mature male.

A male guinea pig is called a *boar*. A female is a *sow*, and young guinea pigs are *pups*.

Natural behavior of guinea pigs

Guinea pigs are rotund social rodents with short legs, small hairless ears, and no tail. Adults weigh about 30–35 oz (850–992 g). In the wild, they live in colonies (clans) of 5–10 with a dominant male in burrows or crevices in rocks. Male guinea pigs have special sebaceous glands in the skin, collectively called the "grease gland", 0.5 (1.3 cm) in above the anus, which are used to mark their territory and possessions.

They tend to freeze when startled and then scatter frantically. Panicked guinea pigs will stampede and injure smaller, weaker members of a group. A frantic attempt to escape can also lead to injury from falling if in an elevated cage or on a table. Sexually intact males will challenge each other until dominance is achieved by one. True fighting and injury of an opponent is not common. Head butting is a show of dominance, invitation to play, or irritation with the current situation.

Guinea pigs are vocal. They may whistle when alarmed or greeting a known handler who feeds them, chirp when content, and make guttural drilling sounds when agitated by a perceived threat or from pain. They purr when content and feeling secure. Teeth chattering and hissing are signs of irritation and possible aggression.

They have good peripheral vision, typical of prey animals, and very good hearing, with a frequency range up to 30,000 Hz (20,000 Hz is the upper limit for humans).

Approaching and catching

Guinea pigs are easily alarmed and will squeal loudly and attempt to evade capture by a stranger. Some will bite if restrained, but their mouth is too small to inflict severe bites to an adult handler. They have four claws on each of the front feet and three on the rear. Their primary means of defense is to either run or freeze in place.

An initial attempt to capture a guinea pig is best done using food as a lure or stroking its head and nose until calm, then grasping it with one hand underneath its chest and cupping the other under its rump. Young, small guinea pigs can be grasped with one hand. Guinea pigs have little loose skin over their neck and shoulders and attempts to scruff them can be painful to them.

Another capture method is to use one hand from above to cover its head, blocking its vision, while covering the rump with the other hand, and then reaching under it from behind. To pick up the guinea pig, the front hand is placed under the guinea pig's chest and the other hand under its rump. When being carried, they will relax if allowed to hide with its body supported by the handler's forearm and its head in the corner of an elbow.

Handling for routine care and management

Restraint of adult guinea pigs should always be two-handed (**Figure 6.7**). The thorax should be grasped

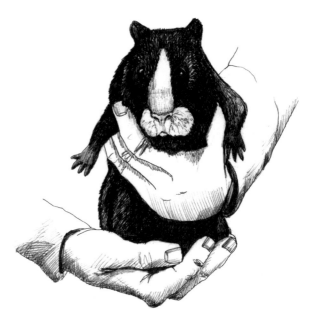

Fig. 6.7 Restraint of guinea pigs must be two-handed.

either dorsally or ventrally with one hand as the other hand supports the guinea pig's rump. They should never be scruffed. Their body weight in comparison to their musculoskeletal system strength is too great, and back or neck injuries can result.

If there is resistance to restraint, the handler should grasp the guinea pig without hesitation around the shoulders with one hand. Lift it primarily with the thumb under a leg and under the jaw (to block the animal from lowering its head to bite) and the first two fingers around the shoulders without squeezing the thorax, and then place the other hand under the body.

A guinea pig's nails need to be trimmed every 8–12 weeks. To assist nail trimming, a handler supports the guinea pig against his or her chest and holds it behind the front legs with one hand, the other hand cupped under the rump. This has the guinea pig positioned in a "C" position.

CHINCHILLAS

Chinchillas (*Chinchilla lanigera*) are soft, odorless rodents and rarely bite. They are indigenous to the Andes mountains of South America at 10,000–15,000 ft (3,000–4,500 m), living in groups of up to 100 individuals. Their native environment is high-altitude, dry, rocky slopes, cold but not frigid weather, and low humidity.

In the 16th century, their skins were being used to decorate the ceremonial dress of the Chincha Indians, from whom their name was derived. Europeans later hunted chinchillas to near extinction for their pelts. They were exported in the 1930s to be farm-raised for their pelts or kept as companion pets. Chinchillas have large ears with a similar structure and range of hearing as humans. Because of this, they have been used as an animal model for human ear research.

Chinchillas are sexed using the AG distance. A female has a urethral cone that resembles a penis, but it sits directly in front of the anus. In the male, there is bare skin between the anus and the urethral opening.

Chinchilla genders are simply referred to as male and female. Young chinchillas are *kits*.

Natural behavior of chinchillas

Chinchillas are nocturnal relatives of guinea pigs and have extremely dense, soft fur (**Figure 6.8**). Their fur has about 50–60 hair shafts per follicle compared with 10–15 in most dogs and one per follicle in humans. Their hair coat is virtually impenetrable to water. Chinchillas clean themselves by fine dust bathing. *Fur slip*, tufts of hair being pulled from their follicles, is their primary means of defense besides hiding. Other means of defense are bluffing by standing on their hind legs, chattering, barking, spitting, and urinating directly at their perceived threat. Their dense coat provides good protection against cold even below freezing. Temperatures above 80°F (27°C) can cause heat stroke. Their broad ear flaps aid in dissipating heat.

Chinchillas have strong hind legs and are very good at leaping. Young ones can jump over 6 ft (1.8 m) high and have no fear of heights, but this characteristic puts them at high risk for falling injuries.

Chinchillas sit on their rump and eat using their forepaws. They eat primarily at night and pass most of their feces at night. Like rabbits and some other rodents, they eat cecotropes (special nutrient feces) in the mornings to supplement their nutrition.

Approaching and catching

Chinchillas have a rounded body, large mouse-like ears, a long furry squirrel-like tail, and short legs. They are curious animals that with patience can often lead them to be easily captured, although they are quick and can jump distances several times their body length. If feeling threatened, they will try to urinate on a handler. Care must be taken not to startle them since they may leap hazardously and fracture their back. They usually like to be petted, but even well-tamed chinchillas do not relax when being held. Chinchillas love raisins, which can be used as a lure to catch them. However, more than two raisins a day may cause diarrhea.

Previously handled chinchillas can be cupped with both hands and swept toward the handler's body. Grabbing their hair coat will cause fur slip. Fur slip areas require at least 6–8 weeks to regrow and may come back a different color. Holding the base of the tail to prevent jumping while supporting the body is acceptable. They should never be lifted by their tail or ears or scruffed. For greater restraint, the handler should grasp the shoulders with one hand and hold the hind legs with the other hand in the same manner as holding a guinea pig.

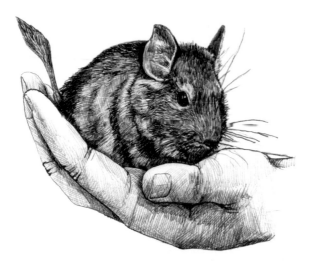

Fig. 6.8 Chinchillas have very dense hair that can be easily pulled out during some restraints.

NEVER grasp a chinchilla by its fur or the tip of the tail, as either may slip off.

Handling for routine care and management

The handler can hold the base of the tail to prevent jumping and support the body with the other hand. Examination table surfaces should be covered by a towel or other non-slip material. Further restraint can be achieved by wrapping in a small towel.

DEGUS

The degu (DAY-goo; *Octodon degus*) is from semi-arid regions of north central Chile. Their ears are large to aid in heat dissipation. They are also called "Chilean squirrels" and "brush-tailed rats." They hold food with their forepaws similar to North American squirrels. Degus are related to guinea pigs and chinchillas (in the parvorder Caveomorpha), have long-haired tails, and look like large gerbils. They have been used as a research model for development and aging. Degus are illegal as pets in California, Georgia, and Alaska. Elsewhere, pet shops that carry degus for sale and breeders of degus must be licensed by the USDA.

Female degus do not have a gap between the anus and urinary cone, while in males there is a gap. The urinary cone is not the penis.

There are no special names for degu genders. A male degu is simply called a male, and a female, a female. Young degus are *pups*.

Natural behavior of degus

Degus are social, diurnal (active during daytime) rodents that are coprophagic. They are good jumpers. They like to live in groups in burrows and clean themselves with dust baths as do chinchillas.

Approaching and catching

Although active, curious, and willing to approach humans, degus do not like a lot of handling. When possible, they should be picked up with one hand supporting the hindquarters and the other supporting the thorax just behind the front legs. They should never be picked up by the tail to avoid the risk of degloving.

Never restrain a degu by its tail since its tail may deglove (the skin may strip off).

Handling for routine care and management

If socialized as juveniles, degus can be handled in the same manner as guinea pigs (**Figure 6.9**). Restraint by wrapping with a towel may be used, if necessary.

SUGAR GLIDERS

Sugar gliders (*Petaurus breviceps*) are small (5–7 in long [13–18 cm]) tree-living (arboreal), nocturnal marsupials from Tasmania, Indonesia, New Guinea, and eastern Australia. They became a popular pet in the U.S. in the 1980s. Export of sugar gliders from Australia has been banned since 1959. They are illegal in California, Pennsylvania, Hawaii, and Alaska to prevent biopollution.

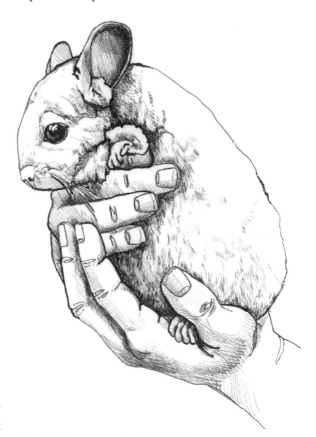

Fig. 6.9 Degus are handled similar to guinea pigs.

There are no special gender names for sugar gliders. They are called male and female sugar gliders. Young sugar gliders are *joeys*.

Natural behavior of sugar gliders

Sugar gliders are nocturnal, so all their activity occurs at night. Females have pouches on their abdomens. Males have a bald spot, which is a scent gland, on their heads. Males use their head glands and similar scent glands on their sternum and near their cloaca to mark other gliders and their territory. If frightened, male and female gliders will express their paracloacal scent glands. The secretion has a spoiled fruit odor. They also mark their territory with their urine. They are very protective of their territory, and new sugar gliders not marked by the colony's dominant male will be attacked.

Sugar gliders have 40–46 teeth. Two incisors are large and point forward, and are used to penetrate the bark of trees. They are able to glide over 100 ft (30 m) between tree limbs by a spreading their legs and using a fold of skin, the *patagium*, between their front and hind legs like a parachute and using their tail as a rudder (**Figure 6.10**). They have five digits on each foot. The inner digit on the hind feet is bulbous, without a claw, and opposes the others like a human thumb, allowing them to easily grasp tree limbs. The second and third digits on the hind feet are fused together and aid the glider in grooming its hair coat.

In the wild, sugar gliders live in colonies of 10–15 individuals in trees, nest in hollows of trees, and feed on insects and plant nectars. Their principal predator in the wild is the owl. As a result, sugar gliders become very stressed when in the presence or sound of birds.

Vocalizations include chattering for attention, yapping like a small dog when alarmed, and high-pitched crabbing when startled.

Approaching and catching

Sugar gliders should not be awakened to be caught, as this causes them significant stress. When awake, those that have been socialized to humans as juveniles may stay in a handler's open hand (**Figure 6.11**). If they must be caught, they can vocalize many different sounds when disturbed, and they can inflict a bite or gouge with their incisors.

The neck can be grasped with the handler's thumb and middle finger and the index finger on top of the head. Cloth bags can be everted over the handler's hand. After grasping a glider, the cloth is folded back over the glider, leaving its head exposed. Towels can be useful aids in capturing gliders, but looped cloth should not be used, nor cloths or towels with loose threads. Sugar gliders' feet can easily be caught in loops or loose threads, causing serious

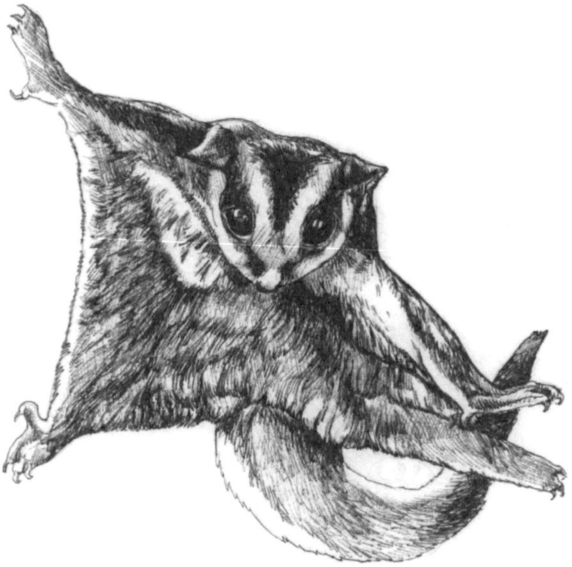

Fig. 6.10 Sugar gliders can glide long distances by spreading their patagium.

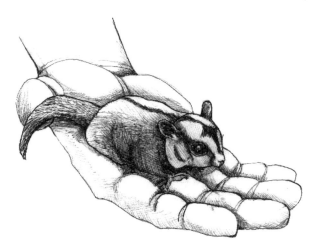

Fig. 6.11 Sugar gliders can be handled if socialized early and handled quietly.

injuries. Increasing the light in the capture room or using a flashlight may cause them to freeze long enough to use a towel for capture.

Handling for routine care and management

Safe physical restraint of sugar gliders is difficult. Scruffing the loose skin of the back can be done for restraint, although this will elicit loud crabbing from the glider. Most procedures require chemical restraint. Care should be taken to prevent their claws from getting caught in the handler's clothing fabric. If a toe is caught, freeing it may inadvertently injure the toe, wrist, or ankle. Their nails may need to be trimmed periodically.

AFRICAN PYGMY HEDGEHOGS

African pygmy hedgehogs (*Atelerix albiventris*), also called the four-toed or white-bellied hedgehog, are solitary, territorial, nocturnal, insect-eating mammals from the southern Sahara desert that prefer to live alone. Most of their body is covered by ¼ to 1 in (0.64–2.5 cm) long spines (quills). The spines are used for defense and to cushion falls. African pygmy hedgehogs are not able to fling their spines.

Foot (or hoof)-and-mouth disease is a viral disease of cloven-hoofed farm animals that has been reported in hedgehogs. Imported hedgehogs can also carry anthrax and could survive as feral animals after escape or abandonment in the southern U.S. As a result, African hedgehogs cannot be imported legally and they cannot be legally owned in some states (California, Hawaii, Arizona, Georgia, Pennsylvania, Maine, and Vermont) and several cities.

Natural behavior of African pygmy hedgehogs

Hedgehogs in the wild live in a variety of environments, including in rock crevices, brush, or burrows. They are solitary living except at breeding time. Hedgehogs grunt when foraging for food. This hog-like vocalization and a preference to forage along hedgerows were how the small marsupial got its common name. They are sensitive to strange sounds and have an excellent sense of smell, which they use in foraging for food, but their vision is weak. Tactile sensations are perceived by touching with their spines and vibrissae (whiskers). Typical vocalizations are grunting, clicking, snorting, and sniffing, but hissing will occur if it feels threatened. Screams occur if distressed. When feeling endangered, they will elevate the spines on their forehead and curl into a ball. They are good at digging, climbing, and swimming. They are resistant to many venoms, including those of many snakes, bees, beetles, and spiders. They have small teeth and will bite if irritated or threatened.

Females have five pairs of nipples and a very close AG distance. The male's AG distance is much larger, and the penis is located near the mid abdomen.

Approaching and catching

Capturing a socialized hedgehog requires slowly scooping it underneath its belly with one or two hands (**Figure 6.12**). Their bellies are covered with soft fur, but their backs are covered with short, prickly spines. If fearful or hungry, hedgehogs may bite.

Socialization of hedgehogs with handlers is best begun when the hedgehog is 6–8 weeks of age. Handling young hedgehogs with bare hands will accustom them to the handler's odors. Use of perfumed hand soap or lotions should be avoided. Additional positive conditioning to be handled can be provided with treats, such as mealworms, while the hedgehog is being handled.

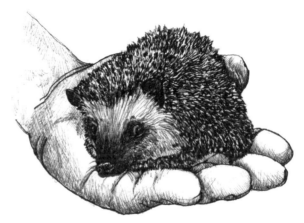

Fig. 6.12 African pygmy hedgehogs require minimal restraint.

Latex or light leather gloves or a towel should be used to handle strange or untrained hedgehogs. Although their spines are not barbed, they may penetrate a handler's skin. When excited they spread a thick frothy saliva on their spines ("anoint" them), which can cause skin irritation in some handlers. Gentle handling is needed to prevent them from rolling into a defensive ball and making a hissing sound.

Handling for routine care and management

Properly socialized hedgehogs can be held in cupped hands. Difficult hedgehogs can be scruffed by the skin between the ears. Alternatively, a hind leg can be grasped. Attempts to forcefully uncurl a hedgehog that has rolled into a defensive ball should be avoided because of the risk of injury to the hedgehog.

RABBITS

Rabbits (*Oryctolagus cuniculus*) captured on the Iberian Peninsula of Europe were domesticated by the Phoenicians about 3,000 years ago. By 100 BC, Roman armies kept rabbits as a source of food, introduced them to the British Isles, and confined them in walled pens. If they escaped and became pests, the Romans hunted them with ferrets, which could follow the rabbits into their burrows. Ferreting rabbits is still a means of rabbit hunting in some countries where rabbits burrow and live in groups (warrens), such as the United Kingdom. Rabbits were selectively bred as a farm animal in Europe during the Middle Ages by monks. By the 16th century, rabbits were kept as pets along with being a source of meat and fur. Ships kept rabbits as a source of fresh meat on voyages. They were introduced to Australia and New Zealand in the mid-19th century, where they became feral and a pest for agriculture. Rabbits were raised in the U.S. as a primary source of fresh meat for civilians during World War II.

Rabbits and hares are lagomorphs, not rodents. Hares are larger with black ear tips. Rabbits are born blind, naked, and helpless in dens. Hares are born in the open with open eyes, fur over the body, and able to run within minutes. Rabbits are kept as pets and common laboratory animals; hares are not.

Male rabbits are called *bucks*. Females are *does*, and young rabbits are *kits* or *bunnies*.

Natural behavior of rabbits

European (domesticated) rabbits (*O. cuniculus*) have different behavior from that of the North American eastern cottontail rabbit (*Sylvilagus floridanus*). Cottontail rabbits do not burrow and do not tolerate the presence of other rabbits. European rabbits, the ancestor of domesticated rabbits, are social prey animals that live in burrows of up to 30 individuals.

Rabbits like to explore and forage for food, interact with other members of their group, and huddle together when resting. Self-grooming and mutual grooming of others is frequently performed in a European rabbit warren. Failure to groom can be a sign of disease. They are herbivorous, crepuscular, and nocturnal, and like to burrow in soft, sandy dirt. They are born without hair and with their eyes closed. Immediate acceptance and care from the mother is essential to survival. Adult size ranges from 2 lb (0.9 kg) to more than 15 lb (6.8 kg). Their bones are fragile compared with other animals of the same size. Their teeth grow continuously and are normally worn down if allowed to gnaw abrasive food or objects. Rabbits are coprophagic and consume cecotrophs directly from their anus about 3–8 hours after eating. They may thump a hind foot if agitated and may spray urine. Rabbits are prey for many predators, such as dogs, cats, coyotes, ferrets, large birds, and snakes.

Sexually mature rabbits are quite territorial. They assess and claim their territory and possessions by odor. They have glands on their chin and in their perineum, which they use to rub on possessions. Both males and females will seek their highest possible role in dominance of others. Sexually intact male rabbits can be territorially aggressive and will vocalize (growl, grunt), charge, and claw with their front feet, particularly if threatened by a child, small dog, or cat. Females can be aggressive if their young are perceived to be in danger. Adulteration of the doe's pheromones on her kits from handling the kits without gloves can lead to the mother's rejection of her babies.

Young rabbits should be separated by gender at 3 months to prevent early matings. In males, the testicles are the most obvious gender determining structure. Males will need to be housed individually if not neutered.

Neutered male rabbits, called *lapins*, are more interactive and easy to handle, and therefore better pets for children. Neutered males also are less likely to attempt to mark territory with urine and feces.

Approaching and catching

Handlers should grasp the skin behind the rabbit's neck while the other hand scoops up the rump (**Figure 6.13**). The rabbit should be turned so that its head is tucked under the handler's arm while the handler maintains a grasp on the neck and supports the hindquarters. This is called the football hold (**Figure 6.14**). Some rabbits will bite, so care must be taken to avoid putting fingers near their mouth.

No effort should be made to restrain or stroke the head. Rabbits will strongly resist manipulation of their head, and attempted restraint of the head could lead to a broken neck. Chemical restraint is necessary for examining or treating the head or neck.

Heavy gloves should be worn for protection from scratches if trying to separate fighting rabbits.

Handling for routine care and management

Rabbits will try to twist and kick when resisting restraint, which can cause back injuries, including fractures. Rabbits have thin, light bones and very powerful hind legs. If they kick with suspended hind legs, they can fracture their spine and damage their spinal cord. In addition, they have sharp claws that can injure the handler if allowed to kick during handling. Slick floors can also endanger rabbits as there is the risk of back injury.

> Rabbits should never be given an opportunity to kick while being restrained or released.

The ear flaps of rabbits are important to their hearing and contribute to heat dissipation. They are delicate structures that should never be used for restraint.

A safe means of restraint is to gently scruff the skin on the back of the neck. If using a scruff hold, the hind legs must be supported and restrained. Lifting a rabbit by a scruff hold alone is likely to result in the rabbit fracturing its back by kicking. The safest way to move a rabbit is in a travel crate or to support it with both of the handler's arms.

Most routine procedures can be performed on rabbits while they are in sternal restraint on a table. A non-slip mat should be placed on the table. Otherwise, rabbits may struggle, kick frantically and

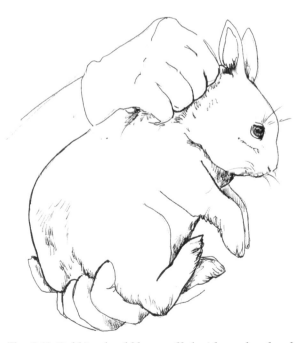

Fig. 6.13 Rabbits should be scruffed with one hand and their hindquarters supported with the other hand.

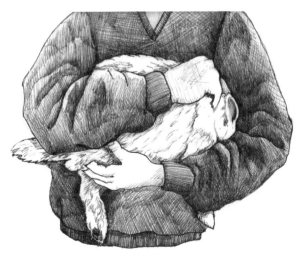

Fig. 6.14 The football hold on a rabbit.

fracture bones. The handler should keep at least one hand on the rabbit at all times. If holding with one hand, the rabbit's rump should be pushed against the handler's abdomen while one hand presses down on the top of its shoulders. If restraining with two hands, one hand presses down on the shoulders and the other on the rump. Nails can be trimmed with the rabbit in sternal position by lifting one foot up at a time. Addition restraint can be applied with towel wraps, as used with cats.

Examination or treatment of the ventral aspects of the body can be performed by grasping the rabbit's front legs with one hand, turning the rabbit over and supporting the hindquarters with the other hand. The rabbit's body should then be in a "C" shape.

Special care is required in handling baby rabbits. Handlers should wear plastic gloves and rub the babies with nest bedding when returned to the nest, to keep human odor off the babies.

Rabbits should be removed from cages rump first to prevent feet from getting caught in a wire mesh floor. To place a rabbit into a cage or box, it should go in rump first facing a side wall or facing outward. This prevents it from kicking back and spraying litter out of the box and scratching the handler's arms. The handler should ensure that the rabbit's legs are resting on the surface and ready to support its weight before releasing by pressing the rabbit down and then releasing with both hands at the same time.

> **Rabbits should be placed into and taken out of cages and boxes rump first.**

FERRETS

European ferrets (*Mustela putorius furo*) evolved from domestication of the European polecat (*M. putorius*). Ferrets have been domesticated since the days of the ancient Roman Empire (300 BC), when they were used to hunt rodents that endangered Roman grain stores. Later, the Romans used ferrets to control an overpopulation of rabbits. Rabbit hunting with ferrets was common practice in Europe and Asia during the Middle Ages. To protect the rabbit pelt and meat, ferrets were selectively bred for their ability to be handled and burrow for flushing skill. Some

also wore a harness with a long leash, a muzzle, or a bell. Ferrets would flush the European rabbits from their burrows, and they would then be caught with nets or by trained dogs or falcons. In the mid-19th century, ferrets were bred for their fur, and in the 20th century they were used to run lead wires and cables during building and airplane construction. They became popular in the U.S. as a companion pet in the late 1960s.

The black-footed ferret (*Mustela nigripes*), which is indigenous to North America, is a different species and not domesticated. Domesticated European ferrets have been in North America for 300 years. They are illegal in some states (California and Hawaii), territories (Puerto Rico), and cities (New York City and Washington, D.C.) due to concern that they would become prolific and prey on indigenous wildlife if some became feral. This biopollution has occurred in the Shetland Islands and New Zealand.

Domestic ferrets were selectively bred for white hair coats during the Middle Ages so that they could be more easily located. However, ferrets with predominately white hair coats often have Waardenburg syndrome, an inherited trait causing a broadened skull and partial or total deafness. Ferrets are also an animal model for research on human influenza.

Male ferrets are referred to as a *hob*, females as a *jill*, spayed females as a *sprite*, castrated males as a *gib*, and vasectomized males as a *hoblet*. Immature ferrets are called *kits*.

Natural behavior of ferrets

Ferrets are approximately the same size as domestic cats, with a longer body and shorter legs. Males are substantially larger than females. They have nonretractable claws, which should not be removed but require frequent trimming. Their anal sacs are used like the scent glands in skunks. Most body odor comes from sebaceous glands that are stimulated by male hormones.

Ferrets hunt prey in burrows and are fearless, with short attention spans. They are also extremely curious and will explore every aspect of their environment, especially holes, ducts, rugs, blankets, and tunnels. Their fearless aggression is most evident in 3–4-month-old males when they play bite each other to establish their group hierarchy and practice their predator skills. Females are more independent and more likely to aggressively bite than males.

Unlike their more solitary wild cousins, domesticated ferrets like living in groups with established familiarity. A group of domesticated ferrets is called a *business*. New members to the group must be introduced slowly and carefully because ferrets are territorial. Adult males use perianal scent gland secretions, body oils, and sometimes urine and feces to mark their territory and possessions. They will also groom themselves with their urine to attract jills.

Ferrets are crepuscular, most active at dawn and dusk, although they can become imprinted with more diurnal activity during their critical socialization period with humans (4–10 weeks of age). They are nearsighted and depend more on detection of odors and their hearing to sense changes in their environment. They search their surroundings by sniffing the ground, and often sneeze. Their vision adapts slowly to sudden bright light or darkness. Their pupils are horizontal, in contrast to the vertical pupils of cats. Horizontal pupils may aid seeing prey (rabbits) with hopping gaits, while vertical pupils may aid tracking of prey (mice) with flat horizontal movements. They like to chase bouncing hard rubber balls and Ping-Pong balls. Balls should be hard enough to keep the ferret from eating pieces of them and large enough not to be swallowed whole, to prevent intestinal obstruction. The sound range best heard by ferrets is high frequency, 8 kHz to more than 16 kHz, which is the vocal range of their prey.

Food odors are important in olfactory imprinting in young ferrets. Food preferences are developed during their socialization period between 60 and 90 days of age. They will hide ("ferret away") food or favorite toys in an area in their territory that seems the most inaccessible to other animals. The word ferret comes from Latin (*furittus*) for "little thief."

When awake, ferrets are boundlessly energetic, but it is normal for them to sleep 12–16 hours per day. They like to sleep in enclosed areas or piled with group members. If excited and happy and wanting to play, ferrets will perform the "dance of joy," jumping in differing directions in a whimsical manner like that of a baby goat, bumping carelessly into objects.

A similar excitement, the "war dance," will occur with the tail hair fluffed out.

Vocalizations include the "dook" (also called chuckling) to express excitement. If angered or frustrated, they may make a hissing sound, arch their back, and fluff out hair on their tail. If endangered, they will scream. Barking, chirping, or squeaking is used when a ferret is frightened and defensive.

Approaching and catching

Approaching a ferret is similar to the method of approaching cats. Pastes of food treats on a tongue depressor will attract and distract a ferret for a short time during an acclimation period to a handler. They particularly like fish-oil-flavored pastes. Gentle ferrets can be captured and picked up like a cat (**Figure 6.15**). They often like to hide in a large pocket or bag when carried.

When approaching a ferret for the first time, the handler should keep fingers curled when reaching toward it. If unsure of the ferret's disposition, the handler can use a thick towel to cover the ferret and block its vision before capture. To gain control of a resistant ferret, a handler should scruff the ferret and lift it off its feet. This usually has a calming effect and will cause it to yawn. After the skin on the back of the neck and shoulders is scruffed, the second hand is placed under the rump to support the weight of the body during restraint.

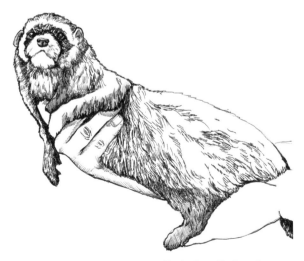

Fig. 6.15 Pet ferrets can usually be handled in the same manner as a cat.

Domesticated ferrets have retained the predatory characteristics of their wild ancestors: constant searching for prey and aggressive play, including play biting. For this reason, a ferret's face should never be held near a handler's face. Ferrets are generally docile and receptive to the gentle handling used on dogs and cats, but if scared they can inflict severe bites out of fear. If bitten, a handler should not put a ferret down immediately or it will develop a habit of biting to be released. Because of the risk of bites to the face or fingers, babies and other young children should not handle or be left alone with ferrets. Ferrets do not bare their teeth before biting.

Ferrets practice their fearless aggression in play fighting with each other. During play fighting, they may bite, hold on, and shake their head right and left. Ferrets, particularly younger ones, may bite a handler as an expression of play aggression. Other causes for bites are from being startled, territorial aggression of toys, fear-based aggression from previous poor handling, and maternal aggression. Congenital deafness occurs in some ferrets with white in their hair coat. Deaf ferrets are more easily startled than normal ferrets. Odors on the handlers hand, such as hand lotion or tobacco, may also stimulate a ferret to nip.

Controlling nips and bites should include frequent quiet handling and positive reinforcement of good behavior, beginning during their juvenile period. Removing kits from their mother too early and a lack of maternal discipline can result in a lack of respect for other animals and rougher play aggression. The reaction to bite or nips should be to briefly place the ferret in a special cage or crate (not its normal sleeping cage or crate), without toys or food for a time out, deprived of attention or reward.

If ferrets are allowed to escape during handling, they will seek safety in very small spaces. Therefore, all possible exits, cabinets, drawers, etc., must be blocked prior to beginning a handling session. A ferret should wear a collar with a bell to help locate it if it escapes.

Handling for routine care and management

Distraction with food treats is sufficient for minor examinations. Greater restraint than simply picking a ferret up and carrying it involves grasping the ferret firmly with one hand around the shoulders and neck. Ferrets are well muscled and require a firm grip. The handler's thumb and index finger should be positioned beneath the jaw to prevent it from turning its head to bite.

Ferrets can be scruffed with the skin on the neck while their hind legs are held to mildly stretch the ferret out, in the same manner as a scruff-and-stretch hold for cats. Precautions need to be taken so the ferret cannot fall. They should never be scruffed and held above the floor, since they may escape the restraint grip and fall. Instead, they should be held over a table with a padded surface. Ferrets have muscular necks, unlike other small tame animals. Although they must be held more tightly than other small animals, excessive force will cause greater struggling and should be avoided. Towel wraps provide greater restraint when needed.

Nail trimming is needed every 2 weeks. This can normally be done while the ferret is being gently held in a handler's arms or lap, especially if the ferret was gently handled and desensitized for nail trimming as a juvenile.

HANDLING SMALL MAMMALS FOR COMMON MEDICAL PROCEDURES

With few exceptions, small mammals should be moved and housed with group members to reduce stress. Although any other member of an established group may be helpful, observant handlers may notice certain members may have preferred friends within the group. Including a close friend with the individual needing medical procedures is best. Having a companion or companions along with a small mammal can also facilitate the return of all to the larger group.

Since most small mammals have been used in medical research laboratories, special restraint equipment has been developed for them. Plexiglass restraint tubes are commonly used to contain and restrain mice and rats. The tubes have a variety of access ports for different procedures. They also have a slot in the top so that a mouse can be restrained by the base of the tail and dragged backwards into the tube. Similar restraint tubes can be created using

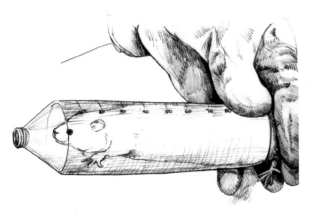

Fig. 6.16 Large injection syringes can be modified and used as a small rodent restraint chamber.

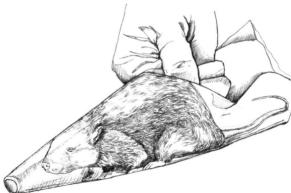

Fig. 6.17 Clear plastic cones can be used to restrain rats.

the plastic casing for large syringes with breathing holes cut into the blind end (**Figure 6.16**). Rats can also be restrained for medical procedures using a sheet of transparent plastic rolled into a cone or a cake-decorating cone bag. The rat is placed in head first and can be held in the cone by one hand (**Figure 6.17**).

Guinea pigs are large enough that they need to be handled with both hands. A towel or mat should be provided on the exam table for traction and warmth.

Plexiglass restraint boxes, similar to rodent restraint tubes, are available for rabbits. Rabbits can also be restrained by wrapping in a towel or being placed in a cat bag. Rabbits are very uncomfortable on a slick table, which could lead to violent kicking and possible back injury. Therefore, a mat or rug should be placed on rabbit handling tables. Pressing down on their shoulders while they lie sternal on a table will usually provide sufficient restraint for most procedures.

Injections and venipunctures

Insertion of transcutaneous needles for injection or aspiration in a small mammal carries the risk of slashing tissue beneath the skin, including damage to nerves and blood vessels, and breaking hypodermic needles off in its body. The area in which the needle is to be inserted must be immobilized, and the animal's mouth and feet should be restrained from interfering with the procedure, especially venipunctures. The method of restraint should be comfortable; that is, no squeezing when unnecessary, but the restraint should allow immobilization if struggling occurs.

Access to veins

Venipuncture is necessary to withdraw blood for various analyses or to inject intravenous solutions.

In mice, rats, and gerbils, venipuncture is best done from the lateral vein of the tail while the rodent is in a restraining tube. Lateral saphenous veins are a second choice. The jugular vein may be used in anesthetized rats.

Since hamsters and guinea pigs do not have tails, the lateral saphenous vein is used for venipuncture. Access to other veins, such as the cephalic veins and ear veins in guinea pigs, usually require chemical restraint.

The lateral saphenous vein is the most accessible in chinchillas, and only very small blood samples can be taken from cephalic, lateral saphenous, or ventral tail veins. The jugular vein is the best site for larger volumes of blood, but anesthesia is needed.

Venipuncture in degus generally requires chemical restraint. The cephalic and lateral saphenous veins are accessible, but degus become stressed from the restraint needed to perform venipuncture. Access to their jugular veins requires anesthesia. Venipuncture of the lateral tail vein is possible, but there is risk of degloving the tail.

Venous access in hedgehogs is via the jugular vein during anesthesia.

The lateral saphenous veins are the most accessible in rabbits, but marginal and central ear veins can be used. Required restraint for each is through the rabbit being held in an assistant's arms using the football hold.

The jugular, cephalic, and medial saphenous veins are accessible in ferrets, with the restraint methods used on cats.

Injections

Subcutaneous

Subcutaneous (SC) injections are the safest route for injections, but some injectable materials, including all oil-based medications, must not be given SC. SC injections can be given in the loose skin of the neck in all small mammals that can be scruffed for handling. The loose skin of the flank is also a possible SC injection site in rats, chinchillas, and ferrets. Fur-slip may occur in chinchillas if the skin is lifted (tented) to administer an SC injection.

Intramuscular

Intramuscular (IM) injections are undesirable in small mammals due to the risk of muscle, vascular, or nerve damage. In situations where IM injections are unavoidable, the front muscles of the thigh (quadriceps) are preferable (**Figures 6.18** and **6.19**) The leg receiving the injection should be immobilized by the person administering the IM injection with the muscles gently pinched and feeling the location of the femur to help avoid hitting the bone. An assistant handler is needed to provide routine head and body restraint of the animal. The epaxial lumbar muscles are occasionally used for IM injections in chinchillas, rabbits, and ferrets.

Intraperitoneal

Intraperitoneal injections (IP) are given into the belly cavity to administer fluids to sick rodents or administer substances for research. Small rodents are given IP injections while scruffing the rodent and holding the tail with the little finger. Mice, gerbils, and hamsters are injected into the right caudal quadrant. IP injections in rats are administered by a veterinarian or technician, with the rat being restrained by a handler who uses one hand to grasp the rat's shoulders with fingers under the jaw. The handler's other hand supports the rat's body and restrains the hind legs. Rats are injected into the left caudal quadrant.

Intraosseous

Intraosseous (into bone marrow) injections are used to deliver fluids to the blood stream when venipuncture is impossible. Intraosseous injections are not feasible in small rodents, but may be performed in large rats, chinchillas, guinea pigs, rabbits, and ferrets using the femur bone.

Administration of oral medications

Mixing medications in drinking water is a very unreliable means of medicating small mammals. Undermedication and overmedication can result, and if drinking is completely avoided due to the adulterated taste of the water, the animal will become dehydrated. Mixing powdered or liquid medication in small amounts of highly palatable food that can be consumed only by an individual animal may suffice

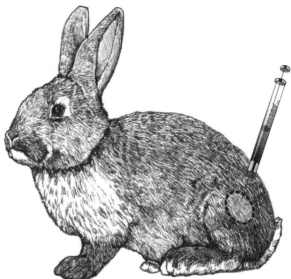

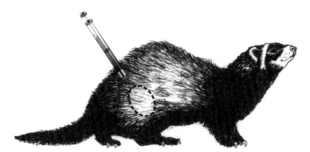

Fig. 6.18 IM injection site in a ferret.

Fig. 6.19 IM injection site in a rabbit.

if the mixing does not adversely affect the medication's actions and the mixture is readily consumed. Possible foods for mixtures can include bread, banana, peanut butter, raisin paste, and fruit-based baby food.

If oral administration of liquid or soft pasty medication using restraint is needed, the animal should be held vertically, head up, with the head movement minimized by scruffing or towel or cloth wraps around the neck. Small rodents may be medicated with a gavage needle (curved and blunted) and syringe. Larger small mammals may be administered liquids in the corner of the mouth with an eyedropper.

SELECTED FURTHER READING

Ballard B, Cheek R (2017). *Exotic Animal Medicine for the Veterinary Technician*, 3rd edition. Wiley-Blackwell, Ames/Oxford.

Bays, TB, Lightfoot T, Mayer J (2006). *Exotic Pet Behavior*. Saunders, St. Louis.

Bennett B (2009). *Storey's Guide to Raising Rabbits*, 4th edition. Storey Publishing, North Adams.

Campbell KL, Campbell JR (2009). *Companion Animals*, 2nd edition. Pearson, Upper Saddle River.

Judah V, Nuttall K (2016). *Exotic Animal Care and Management*, 2nd edition. Cengage Delmar Learning, Albany.

Warren DM (2015). *Small Animal Care & Management*, 4th edition. Cengage Delmar Learning, Albany.

CHAPTER 7

COMPANION BIRDS

Birds have been kept in cages for their beauty and companionship for more than 4,000 years. Ancient Egyptians kept doves, pigeons, and parrots as pets, and ancient Greek aristocracy kept mynahs and parakeets. Egyptians and Persians used homing pigeons to carry messages 3,000 years ago. Royalty and the very wealthy kept companion birds during Medieval and Renaissance Europe. In the 15th century, canaries were bred in captivity, and eventually were used in underground mines to detect poisonous gasses.

When the Aztecs were conquered by the Spanish in 1521, the Palace of Moctezuma I (Montezuma) in Tenochtitlan (Mexico City) had a caged bird zoo and one for birds of prey. Other cities in the Aztec empire also had birds in zoos.

There are about 9,000 known species of birds. The largest order is Passeriformes, containing the perching birds (canaries, finches, mynahs). Passerines have three front toes and one back toe on each foot. They are also known as song birds for their ability to vocalize melodies. The order Psittaciformes contains the most popular companion birds (parrots, cockatoos, macaws, lories, and budgerigars). Psittacines have two toes in front and two back toes on each foot. Their beaks are hooked, which they use for climbing, breaking nuts, and defense. Toucans are the only common companion birds in the order Piciformes. Toucans have large, pointed bills which can be as long as their body. Pigeons and doves are in the order Columbiformes. This order is characterized by small head and beak, large wings, and a bobbing movement of their head. They have excellent flying ability.

Caged companion birds include a wide variety of birds. Some can learn to mimic the human voice, such as budgerigars, cockatiels, African Grey parrots, and Yellow-naped Amazons. Some birds, such as canaries, like to live alone, while others, such as finches, prefer living in small groups.

Since common tame species can be confused with similar untamed species, companion bird names are often rendered more specific by reference to their Latin genus-species name, such as cockatiel (*Nymphicus hollandicus*).

Budgerigars (also called parakeets, *Melopsittacus undulatus*) and cockatiels are the easiest birds to manage for new bird owners. Both are very social and need frequent interaction with other birds or humans. Budgerigars are the most popular companion birds. They are smaller and less expensive to own but more flighty and willing to bite when irritated.

Popular passerines are canaries and finches. Canaries prefer to live alone. Finches prefer to live in small groups. Neither canaries nor finches tolerate handling well.

Many popular caged companion birds are exotic to the U.S. The budgerigar and cockatiel came from Australia. The canary came from the Canary Islands. African Grey parrots are from west and central Africa. The Rosy-faced Lovebird is from the Namib Desert. The Common Hill Myna comes from south and southeast Asia, and the Common Myna is from India and Australia. The Wild Bird Conservation Act of 1992 prohibits importation of most exotic wild birds into the U.S.

Wild-caught parrots cannot be imported into the U.S. or Europe. Export of all native birds of Australian has been banned since 1960. Some wild-caught Central and South American parrots are still smuggled into the U.S. from Mexico.

NATURAL BEHAVIOR OF COMPANION BIRDS

Birds are social animals that preferably live in groups (flocks). Flocks provide added protection, more efficient scouting for food sources, and mutual grooming in areas of the body not reachable to groom unassisted. Small nomadic species, such as budgerigars, congregate in large groups for protection from predators. Pair bonding is weaker in nomadic birds than in larger species that are more territorial, as with South American parrots. Conversely, attempts to establish dominance over others is less intense with small nomadic species compared with large territorial birds.

Vision and taste are birds' predominant senses. Vocalization can be very complex. Vocalization helps coordinate activities such as foraging for food and announcing time to roost and aids in locating mates, establishing territories, and alerting to danger. Birds that make loud noises, such as screams, are species that will mingle with other avian species in the wild. Birds that do not mingle with other avian species are quieter.

Birds clean and align their feathers by preening, using their mouth to stroke their feathers. They also coat their feathers with an oil from the uropygial gland near the tail while preening. The oil helps waterproof their feathers. Preening occurs after bathing and eating. Social birds may *allopreen*, i.e. preen each other.

Other than mutual grooming, birds do not normally use physical force for interactions among each other. Communications, including dominant aggression, involve vocalizations, posturing, blocking access to resources, and position within the immediate surroundings. Apprehension is often indicated by an open beak while leaning away from an object or handler. Fighting is reserved primarily for territorial disputes. Play activities build combat and mating skills and assist in determination of social rank.

Birds do not possess a diaphragm. Their lungs are always filled with air. Air sacs are able to move air in and out. Some of the air from air sacs is delivered to the bones, providing some distributed warmth in cold weather, dissipation of heat in warm weather, and adding buoyancy when in water for water birds. Heat stress causes panting as a last resort and, in some species, rapid fluttering of the throat. Exposure to cold weather leads to fluffing of feathers to trap insulating pockets of air and sitting on their feet to keep their feet warm.

Bird mannerisms include alternating pupil dilation and constriction and flaring tail feathers when excited. Wings are spread when acting secure. Puffing out its feathers momentarily or wagging its tail signals a greeting.

The major activities are being on alert for predators and foraging for food. Although both can be stressful, these activities are important in maintaining normal mental health and behavior.

SAFETY FIRST

Many companion birds may enjoy interactions with humans, but none enjoy being restrained. A handler should always reassess the need for a bird to be handled and restrained before subjecting it to those stresses.

Hooked beak birds such as parrots are generally more tolerant of being handled. There are many species of parrots (psittacines). Small-sized parrots include budgerigars, lovebirds, lories and lorikeets, small conures, caiques, *Pionus* and *Poicephalus* species, and cockatiels. Large-sized parrots are cockatoos, Amazons, the African Grey and Eclectus parrots, large conures, and macaws. They can be socialized with humans and may bond with a human family member if socialized while young. Birds that are hand-raised are imprinted with humans and require more human attention for a feeling of security.

Handler safety

Companion birds use their beaks to balance going from perch to perch. Most only aggressively bite as a last resort when frightened. They also use their beaks and tongues to investigate their surroundings by touch and taste. Large psittacines may make biting a game if they can evoke a reaction from a bitten handler.

Small, straight-billed perching birds (finches, canaries) resent being handled and will defensively stab or bite. Parakeets, parrots, other psittacine birds may also bite, and since large parrots can crack walnuts with their beak, they can just as easily break a finger. Raptors (birds of prey) primarily use their talons to attack. Pigeons and doves are not aggressive and pose no physical threat to handlers. When handling any bird, a handler must expect to be defecated on and should wear appropriate outer clothing. Ear protection is advisable if handling a large psittacine screamer. The sense of sight in birds is excellent, and like most animals, they are very inquisitive. Handlers who wear bright colors or shiny jewelry invite being pecked when handling birds.

Birds demonstrate their dominance over other birds by assuming higher perch positions. Allowing a bird's head to be above the handler's eye level by the bird resting on the handler's head or shoulders gives the bird the impression it is dominant to the handler. Furthermore, allowing a parrot to perch on a shoulder positions them in a way that the handler cannot control them well and invites bites to the handler's ears, neck, lips, and possibly to the eyes. The lack of control from shoulder perching can also increase the risk of serious injury to the bird if it becomes suddenly startled. A handler should not hold a parrot higher than the handler's mid-chest level.

Attempts to bite should be reprimanded by either being startled, such as suddenly dropping the hand the bird is perched on a short distance, or human attention should be taken away by isolating the bird for a short period.

Bird safety

Most birds will resist being handled and will endanger themselves trying to escape from this. For most species of birds, restraint of the wings is the first objective for handlers. Bird bones are very light and break easily, particularly wing or leg bones. Handlers must remain mindful that it is easy to restrict a bird's respiratory movements by holding them too tightly, which can cause unnecessary struggling and lead to shock. The sternum's movement must not be restricted, otherwise they cannot breathe. Their tracheal rings are complete and relatively resistant to collapse when birds are held by the neck.

> Birds do not have a complete diaphragm and the lungs are associated with the chest wall. Slight compression around the chest during restraint can severely limit their ability to breathe.

Feathers trap air and provide efficient insulation. However, when birds are handled the insulation of their feathers can predispose them to becoming overheated. Physical restraints should be used for the shortest period possible to reduce the risk of the bird overheating.

Birds are very susceptible to pneumonia caused by chilling or exposure to drafts; therefore, a bird should never be placed near an open window or air conditioner vent. Damage to flight feathers may endanger birds, such as pigeons and raptors, that are released for sport. Birds should never be left unsupervised with dogs, cats, ferrets, reptiles, or children. Banding young birds can put them at risk of constricting the leg during growth or being caught on objects by a loose band.

Companion birds should not exercise freely in a house. The dangers are numerous and include the risk of eating poisonous plants or household pesticides, pecking electrical cords, eating carpet, being injured by a fan, being burned by heaters and stoves, becoming entangled in terry cloth towels, getting caught in open toilets, inhaling ammonia from cleansers, being injured or killed from attack by predator pets, and escaping through open doors or windows.

Key zoonoses

(*Note:* Apparently ill birds should be handled by veterinary professionals or under their supervision. Precautionary measures against zoonoses from ill birds are more involved than those required when handling apparently healthy birds and vary widely. The discussion here is directed primarily at handling apparently healthy birds.)

Apparently healthy captive-bred, caged companion birds pose little risk of transmitting disease to healthy adult handlers who practice conventional personal hygiene. The risks of physical injury are greater than the risks of acquiring an infectious disease (*Table 7.1*).

Direct transmission
Systemic disease
Many zoonoses from birds can cause generalized (systemic) illness. Nearly all are described as flu-like symptoms. None are common in adult handlers of healthy birds.

Table 7.1 **Diseases transmitted from healthy appearing caged companion birds to healthy adult humans**

DISEASE	AGENT	MEANS OF TRANSMISSION	SIGNS AND SYMPTOMS IN HUMANS	FREQUENCY IN ANIMALS	RISK GROUP*
Bites, nail, or talon injuries	–	Direct injury	Bite wounds to face, hands, or arms	All birds are capable of inflicting bites or wounds	3
Salmonellosis	*Salmonella typhimurium*	Direct, fecal-oral	Diarrhea, systemic infections	Common in birds	3
Psittacosis	*Chlamydia (Chlamydophila) psittaci*	Direct, fecal-oral and respiratory secretions; indirect from fomites and bird mites	Pneumonia	Fairly common in birds	3
Avian tuberculosis	*Mycobacterium avium*	Direct, fecal-oral, respiratory secretions	Pneumonia	Avian TB is rare in caged birds. Most TB in caged birds is from infected humans	3
Avian influenza	Type A H5N1	Direct, respiratory secretions	Mild conjunctivitis and respiratory distress to possible death	Outbreaks in domestic birds in 15 U.S. states in 2014–15	4

* Risk groups (National Institutes of Health and World Health Organization criteria. Centers for Disease Control and Prevention, *Biosafety in Microbiological and Biomedical Laboratories*, 5th edition, 2009):
1 Agent not associated with disease in healthy adult humans.
2 Agent rarely causes serious disease and prevention or therapy possible.
3 Agent can cause serious or lethal disease and prevention or therapy possible.
4 Agent can cause serious or lethal disease and prevention or therapy are not usually available.

Avian influenza (fowl plague) is an influenza A virus that is able to mutate to a form that can affect humans. The disease in birds is highly contagious, affecting fowl, turkeys, pheasants, ducks, and many wild species, but rarely waterbirds or pigeons. Clinically, there is a short course of disease and very high mortality. Birds that survive have a nasal discharge, white spots on the comb and wattles, and swelling of the head and neck. Some strains, notably H5N1 and H7N7, have emerged as the cause of fatal, but rare, human infections. Precautions include keeping caged companion birds and wild birds separate and promptly reporting any possible cases of avian influenza to state agriculture and public health authorities.

Respiratory disease

Psittacosis (from *Chlamydia*, formerly *Chlamydophila*, *psittaci*) and avian tuberculosis (from *Mycobacterium avium*) are two respiratory diseases that can be acquired from birds by nasal secretions and feces, but the risks are low in captive-bred, properly housed, caged companion birds. However, infected birds may not show clinical signs.

Psittacosis is a bacterial disease transmitted by parrots, macaws, cockatiels, and budgerigars. Canaries and finches are less commonly infected with psittacosis. It is transmissible to humans as a respiratory disease. In birds with clinical signs, psittacosis is a systemic infection and signs include diarrhea and ocular and nasal discharge. Pigeons, doves, budgerigars, cockatiels, and cockatoos are less likely to show clinical signs of disease, while parrots, lorikeets, mynahs, and canaries are more susceptible to illness from psittacosis. Psittacosis is more common than avian tuberculosis, but fewer than 50 cases in humans are reported annually in the U.S.

Avian tuberculosis occurs most often in parrots and occasionally in toucans, finches, and pigeons. Parrots with tuberculosis are more likely to appear ill, while infected pigeons are more often carriers of the disease without signs of illness. Transmission to handlers can occur from contact with infected birds' feces.

Several systemic fungal diseases, such as histoplasmosis and cryptococcosis, are associated with birds, but transmission is from soil or bedding contaminated with bird feces, not direct transmission from birds.

Newcastle disease is caused by a virus and manifests as respiratory and neurologic symptoms. In general, affected birds appear ill and most die. However, Amazon parrots can be carriers without signs. In humans, Newcastle disease can cause mild conjunctivitis and influenza-like respiratory symptoms.

Digestive tract disease

Salmonella bacteria are often carried by birds. Since birds eliminate their feces indiscriminately and their eggs pass through a cloaca, if these are contaminated, birds can easily expose handlers to *Salmonella*. Salmonellosis in humans causes severe diarrhea, and the bacteria can enter the bloodstream and cause abscesses in various organs. Yersiniosis is due to a bacteria that causes diarrhea and abdominal pain that can mimic appendicitis. Campylobacteriosis is a common cause of diarrhea in people that can be acquired directly by fecal-oral exposure from birds, but eating uncooked poultry is a much more common source of exposure. *Cryptosporidium* species in birds do not cause cryptosporidiosis in mammals.

Skin disease

Red mites of birds (*Dermanyssus gallinae*) can cause skin irritation in humans, but they require birds to reproduce. Infestations in humans are usually transient. It is a major parasite of domestic fowl but also occurs on other birds, including aviary and wild colonies. Infested birds usually have signs of excessive preening, restlessness, and ruffling of feathers.

Vector borne

Equine encephalomyelitis viruses and West Nile virus are carried by birds and transmitted by mosquitoes.

Sanitary practices

When handling birds from different households, proper sanitation is required to prevent the spread of disease from carriers without clinical signs. Birds from different origins should not be confined in the same cage. Other basic procedures are for handlers to wash their hands and to clean and disinfect table tops and cages used in handling.

Persons handling birds should wear appropriate dress to protect against skin contamination through feathers and skin scales or fecal droppings. Basic sanitary practices should be adhered to, such as keeping hands away from eyes, nose, and mouth when handling birds and washing hands after handling birds. Immunocompromised handlers should not clean cages.

Handlers should not kiss birds. Stressing birds should be avoided. Stress can cause dissemination of psittacosis and other diseases. The origin of birds should be verified to prevent buying illegally imported birds. Legal importation requires a quarantine period and prophylactic treatment for psittacosis. Dust from bird enclosures and feathers should be controlled. A face mask should be worn when cleaning cages and floors. After cleaning, cages should be disinfected with 1:100 solution of bleach to water (2 tablespoons/gal [3.8 L]).

Special precautions are needed when sick birds are handled. Sick birds should be isolated from apparently normal birds. New group members should be quarantined for at least 2 weeks to reduce the risk of transmitting a disease that new birds could be incubating before introducing them to the rest of the group.

APPROACHING AND CATCHING

Companion birds need to be handled for socialization with humans, environmental enrichment, and to determine their body condition. Feathers obstruct the visual assessment of loss of muscle mass or the development of abdominal enlargement. Early detection of diseases requires palpation of the bird's body.

Before attempting to capture a caged companion bird, the room and the cage should be prepared. Light from windows should be blocked with shades or blinds to reduce the chance that an escaped bird will try to fly through the glass. Heaters and fans should be turned off. Vents, windows, and doors should be closed. Bowls, toys, and other objects in

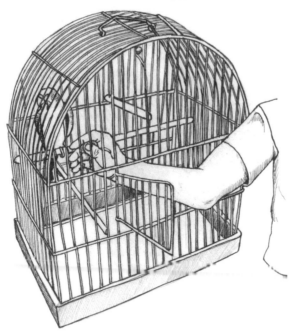

Fig. 7.1 Objects unattached to the cage should be removed before capturing an untamed bird.

the cage that are not attached to the bars should be removed from the cage (**Figure 7.1**).

Handlers should wash their hands before handling each bird for sanitation and to reduce odors of other birds or predators (dog and cat odors).

The handling of birds is greatly facilitated if the bird is properly socialized and handled between 4 weeks and 3 months of age. Young birds should be desensitized to handling with towels and trimming of nails and flight feathers. Mirrors in cages may reduce bonding with handlers and should be avoided. Pet birds tolerant of handling (primarily hooked-bill birds) should be handled daily and allowed to exercise outside their cage. At least 10 hours of quiet sleep is important. Bad behavior, nibbling fingers, biting, or screaming should be ignored. Bird behavior is not altered by reprimands. Some may be emboldened by getting reactions from handlers by exhibiting bad behaviors.

Catching socialized companion birds is not difficult. A slow approach and offering a small food treat before handling can be helpful in reducing resistance. The handler should present a horizontal index finger slowly toward the bird's breast, and the bird will step onto the finger. Birds will step up onto

a finger but usually not over or down onto a finger. To ask a bird to step off of a finger, it should be presented to the perch at its breast level.

If a small bird to be captured has not been trained to step up onto a finger, it must be caught barehanded from behind. It should be grasped around its neck from behind with an index finger and thumb while cupping the remaining fingers around the wings and chest. After positioning the hand for capture near a small bird, having an assistant briefly turn off the room lights to distract the bird and impair its vision can facilitate the final capture.

Untamed birds in small cages may be better approached using a towel over the handler's capture hand. The bird is captured from behind with fingers around its neck and cupping the body loosely. The towel is folded back off its head after capture. In a large cage or aviary, a net may be necessary for capture. After net capture, the bird's neck is grasped from behind and the net is carefully removed while retaining control of bird's neck and holding the wings close to the bird's body without squeezing its chest.

HANDLING FOR ROUTINE CARE AND MANAGEMENT

Basic equipment
Nearly all handling of birds is manual. Restraint tubes, muzzles, squeeze cages, etc. are not used in bird handling. The basic handling equipment for birds is an angular (square or rectangular) cage and towels.

Restraint of individuals or parts of their bodies
Whole body
A bird's body is restrained by holding the wings against its body and controlling movement of the head. It is important not to impair the ability of its chest to easily expand. A handler's fingers should be separated when handling birds to reduce compression on the thorax and the ability to breathe. Care is also needed to avoid damage to the plumage.

Towels can be used, but looped thread cloth should be avoided because the loops can catch the bird's nails. Gloves should not be used, except for raptors (hawks and owls). Capturing the bird should be done by approaching it from behind and placing the towel over the bird's head and grasping around its body and wings. The cloth over the head is then folded back as if removing a hood from a monk. The restrained bird should be held close to the handler's body to provide a better feeling of security in the bird. Macaws may protest loudly enough that ear protection is advisable.

Commercial avian straight jackets are available that fold over the wings and wrap around the body with a velcro closure. The bird requires little to no further restraint after the wrap is applied. However, commercial jackets require two handlers for birds that resist restraint and are applied more slowly than towel wraps.

Head
A bird's head is typically restrained by a hand with the palm behind the head with either an index finger and thumb, or an index finger and middle finger, positioned on each side of the neck and under the jaw, restraining head movement. This is the same neck collar hold used on rodents.

Wings
The escape of companion birds by flying out of opened doors and windows can be reduced by trimming one-half to one-third of the ends of their primary flight feathers, which are 4–10 feathers on each wing. Trimming is not pinioning. Pinioning is an amputation of the wing at the carpal joint. Trimming is performed by extending a wing and clipping the ends of the feathers with sharp, unsprung scissors. Birds that have not been trained when young to accept restraint and wing extension may need to be wrapped in a towel by an assistant and to have a wing extended. Clipping flight feathers can also eliminate or reduce the risk of flying into closed windows, onto hot cooking ranges, or into the blades of fans. Aggressive birds may need to be clipped to protect owners, handlers, or other animals. Wing clipping should not be performed until fledglings learn to fly to prevent behavioral disorders associated with a lack of confidence.

Although wing clipping can be a safety precaution, it can render the bird more vulnerable to other dangers such as being stepped on or injured by other pets. Mild wing clipping or strong wind currents outdoors can enable many birds to still fly, but their ability to control a landing may be impaired and result in injury. Clipped wings should be bilaterally symmetrical or the bird will be imbalanced when attempting to fly and may injure itself. Clipping so closely that any ability to fly is lost can cause injury to the sternum (keel bone) if the bird attempts to fly or falls from an elevated position. Wing clipping should be done in increments to allow the bird to adapt to the inability to fly and the different coordination needed to maintain balance. It should never be severe enough to prevent the bird's ability to glide to the floor. The regrowth of feathers should be checked 6–8 weeks after a trim to determine if re-trimming is due.

During the molting season, new growing feathers have an abundant blood supply and are referred to as blood feathers. Blood feathers should not be trimmed or significant blood loss may result.

Mouth
Birds that are not given sufficient opportunities to grind down the growth of their beak require trimming of the beak. Use of cuttlebones, concrete perches, or other abrasives in the cage usually eliminates the need to trim beaks.

A hand-held rotary grinder is often used to achieve a normal-shaped beak. The noise of the running grinder should be introduced at a distance to the bird for short training periods, and based on signs that the bird has become desensitized to the noise, the grinder is moved closer until it can be used briefly on the beak. With repeated brief use, the duration of use can be increased. Alternatively, an emery board may be used.

The mouth is not specifically restrained. The bird's head is restrained while the beak is trimmed.

Legs
Nails can also overgrow if normal opportunities for abrasion of the nails do not exist. Providing one cement perch in addition to wooden perches will usually eliminate the need to trim nails. Training for nail trimming should begin when birds are in their socialization period. Only the tip of the nail should be clipped or ground down.

Restraint of a leg during nail trims is done by grasping and extending the leg while the body is held with a neck collar hold and fingers cupped around the wings and chest. Larger birds are held by an assistant while the person trimming the nails extends and holds the leg with the nails to be trimmed. Depending on the size of the bird, nails may be trimmed with human nail clippers, dog nail trimmers, or hand-held rotary grinders. The same restraint is used to apply identification leg bands, but embedding a microchip into the left pectoral muscle of the bird is preferred by most handlers for identification.

Handling variations for various bird sizes and types

Small birds (budgerigars/parakeets, canaries, finches)

If full-body restraint is needed, a towel can be placed over the handler's hand to mask the hand approaching. However, handling small or medium-sized birds with towels or cloths may cause them to become overheated.

The neck is grasped between an index and middle finger or the index finger and thumb. The chest is held loosely with fingers spread apart to aid in avoiding restriction of chest movements (**Figure 7.2**). The bird's feet may be allowed to grasp the handler's little finger. An alternative grip is to hold the neck between the thumb and middle finger with the index finger on the top of the head.

Medium-sized birds (pigeon to hawk-sized: cockatiels, cockatoos, conures, parrots)

The bird's body must be grasped with both hands, but respiration cannot be restricted. The wings and chest are held gently on both sides by two hands with fingers separated. Alternatively, the head is restrained by using the handler's thumb and index finger on the neck while holding the wing tips (distal reminges) and the legs (tibiotarsal bones) (**Figure 7.3**). A firmer and more comfortable grip on the legs is with the thumb and middle finger around the legs and the index finger between the tibiotarsal bones.

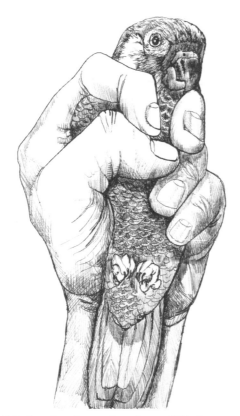

Fig. 7.2 One-hand restraint of a small bird.

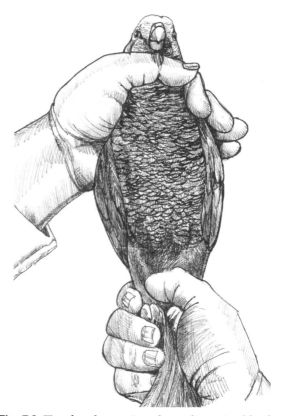

Fig. 7.3 Two-hand restraint of a medium-sized bird.

Large birds (Amazon, African Grey, macaw, cockatoo parrots)

Large birds can be dangerous to handlers. For example, macaws can have a wing span of up to 4 ft (1.2 m) and with their extremely strong jaw strength can inflict severe bites.

Parrots defend themselves primarily with their beaks, so their heads must be secured first. Towel restraint should be used if the bird is resistant to being handled. Gloves should not be used. Approaching slowly from the front will cause less distress in the bird. A handler wraps the towel over the head and around the wings (**Figure 7.4**). The neck is grasped between the thumb and fingers with the tips of the fingers beneath the lower aspect of the jaw (**Figure 7.5**). At the same time, the bird's feet are grasped with the other hand and then the bird is held next to the handler's body. A non-toxic wooden stick can be offered for the parrot to bite as a distraction, if needed.

Raptors/birds of prey (hawks, owls, eagles)

IMPORTANT: A State Rehabilitator license is required to care for and rehabilitate sick or injured wildlife, and a Federal Special Purpose Rehabilitation Permit is needed in order to care for and rehabilitate migratory birds and endangered or threatened species of wildlife such as raptors. To keep a raptor, a handler must serve a 2-year apprenticeship, pass a written exam, build acceptable facilities, and maintain thorough records of care.

Raptors use their talons for primary defense, so their feet must be secured first. A handler should never take off leather gloves with gauntlets when handling a raptor. Low lights in room for diurnal birds (hawks) and bright lights for nocturnal birds (owls) can create an environment more conducive for quiet handling.

Permanently captive raptors usually have jesses (leather straps attached to grommets in leather anklets with around the legs) for easier leg restraint.

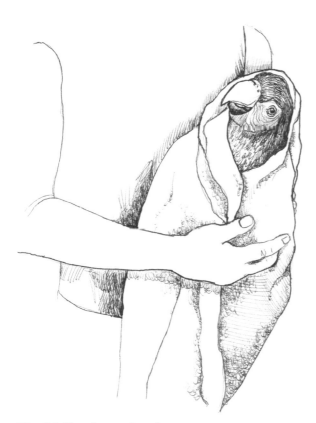

Fig. 7.4 Towel restraint of a parrot.

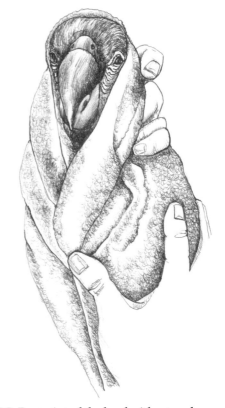

Fig. 7.5 Restraint of the head with a towel.

If the handler approaches from behind, the wings, body, and legs are grasped together, and if the handler approaches from the front, the legs are grasped first. Appropriately thick leather gloves should be used. One gloved hand should be kept between the bird and the handler's face as protection and a distraction while the bird's feet are grasped with the other hand by placing an index finger between the feet. Raptors will occasionally bate; that is, attempt to escape, flip over, and hang by the jesses.

Releasing in a cage

A bird should be returned to its cage after removing all toys, perches, bowls, and other cage materials. It is then placed on the cage floor and the door is closed against the handler's arm that restrained the bird. The arm should be carefully withdrawn while keeping the door closed on it until the door can be latched. Then, while opening the door a minimal degree, cage materials are returned to the cage as quietly as possible.

HANDLING FOR COMMON MEDICAL PROCEDURES

Most handling and restraint of birds can be and should be done without tranquilization, sedation, hypnosis, or anesthesia. However, some handling and restraint procedures should be restricted to veterinary medical professionals because of the potential danger to the animal or handler. These require special skills, equipment, or facilities, and possibly adjunct chemical restraint or complete immobilization by chemical restraint.

Injections and venipuncture

Insertion of transcutaneous needles for injection or aspiration in birds carries the risk of slashing tissue beneath the skin, including damage to nerves and blood vessels, and breaking hypodermic needles off in its body. The area in which the needle is to be inserted must be immobilized and the bird's mouth and feet should be restrained to prevent interference with the procedure, especially venipunctures. The method of restraint should be comfortable; that is, no squeezing when unnecessary, but the restraint should be firm if struggling occurs.

Venipuncture

Venipuncture is performed to collect blood for diagnostic analyses or for intravenous injections. Blood samples are usually collected from the right jugular vein in small birds. The left jugular is much smaller. The crop should be empty to reduce the risk of regurgitation and aspiration.

In larger birds, the preferred veins for venipuncture are the brachial veins underneath the wings near the body, the ulnar veins underneath the wings more distal to the body, and the medial metatarsal veins on the legs.

Birds can be restrained for venipuncture from the jugular vein or leg veins with a restraint jacket, which has a flexible back with two straps that attach in front of the keel with Velcro.

Injections
Intramuscular
Intramuscular injections are typically given into the ventral area of a pectoral muscle (**Figure 7.6**).

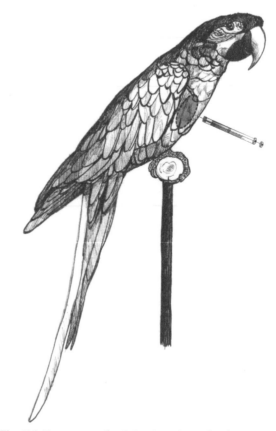

Fig. 7.6 Intramuscular injection site in birds.

Subcutaneous

Subcutaneous injections are administered into the inguinal skin fold immediately in front of a leg or the axillary area under a wing.

Intraosseous

Intraosseous injections are used only for fluid administration. Intraosseous injections require sedation or anesthesia. In small birds, intraosseous injections are given into the proximal tibiotarsal bone below the stifle joint. The distal and proximal ulna can also be used in large birds.

Intraperitoneal

Intraperitoneal injections should never be administered to birds because a needle could rupture the air sacs.

Administration of oral medications

Adding medication to food and water is the least stressful method of oral administration, but it is also the most unreliable for delivering the desired dose. Medications may be unstable in water or they may make the drinking water unpalatable. Direct administration is more reliable for accurate dosing.

To directly deliver oral liquid medication, the handler should put the tip of the syringe or dropper with medication into the corner of the bird's beak and direct the tip toward the other side of the mouth, not toward the throat. While talking quietly to the bird, the handler should deliver the medication slowly, providing sufficient time for swallowing. The tip of the syringe or dropper should be maintained inside the mouth at the corner of the beak until done. A treat should be offered while continuing the restraint until the bird is quiet. Then, it is released slowly.

Oral medication can also be administered with crop tubes. When using a crop tube, the handler elevates the bird's beak, places the feeding tube into the esophagus and stopping after it is in the crop. This is determined by the end of tube being just below the base of the neck. The required distance should be determined and the crop tube marked prior to placement in the bird.

SPECIAL EQUIPMENT

Special handling equipment for procedures on birds includes gloves and gauntlets, bags, tubing, lighting, harnesses, and leg and beak bindings.

Bags

Bags for restraint of birds include stockings, pillowcases, and other cloth bags.

Cardboard tubing

Toilet paper or paper hand-towel cardboard tubes can be placed around appropriate-sized birds for temporary restraint. The purpose is to impair movement of the wings and legs but not compress the breathing movements of the thorax.

Lighting

Diurnal birds are quieter if deprived of bright lighting. Diurnal birds of prey (falcons, hawks, eagles) are kept quieter with hoods. Nocturnal birds (owls) are quieter in bright lighting.

Harnesses

Bird harnesses are used with a leash for exercising birds. The harness has a loop that goes over the bird's head and is connected to a loop that goes around their body behind the wings.

Beak binding

Beak binding can aid in the restraint of straight-beaked birds. Toucans and other large, pointy-beaked birds can be aggressive with their beaks. While wearing a face shield and leather gloves, the handler grasps the bird's bill. The bill is then taped shut or bound with elastic bands. In addition, a large cork or a tennis ball with a slit cut in it should be pushed on the point of beak.

Restraints for raptors
Hood

Hawks are diurnal hunters that depend on their vision. Hooding them quiets their activity, reduces their startle reactions, and allows them to be carried without exciting them.

Gloves and gauntlets

Gloves and gauntlets are made of leather, and typically are used for handling raptors. Gauntlets are heavy gloves that extend beyond the wrist and protect the forearm.

Leg bindings

Jesses are leather straps about 8–9 in (20–23 cm) long that are strapped to each leg. A leash is a leather strap about 3 ft (1 m) long that can be attached to the jesses. Bewits are leather strips that tie bells to the feet of raptors. A creance is a long, lightweight line that is tied to the perch on one end and the jesses on the other for teaching a raptor to fly from the perch to the handler's gloved fist.

SELECTED FURTHER READING

Ballard B, Cheek R (2017). *Exotic Animal Medicine for the Veterinary Technician*, 3rd edition. Wiley-Blackwell, Ames, IA/Oxford.

Bays, TB, Lightfoot T, Mayer J (2006). *Exotic Pet Behavior*. Elsevier Saunders, St. Louis.

Campbell KL, Campbell JR (2009). *Companion Animals*, 2nd edition. Pearson, Upper Saddle River.

Judah V, Nuttall K (2016). *Exotic Animal Care and Management*, 2nd edition. Delmar, Cengage Learning, Albany.

Warren DM (2015). *Small Animal Care and Management*, 4th edition. Cengage Delmar Learning, Albany.

CHAPTER 8

REPTILES

Reptiles are animals with scales or scutes for a body exterior that lay eggs and are cold-blooded (ectothermic). Reptiles include chelonians (turtles, terrapins, and tortoises), lizards, snakes, and crocodilians (crocodiles and alligators). No reptile can be domesticated. Some chelonians, lizards, and snakes can become semi-tame; crocodilians do not.

Many reptiles are docile and can be kept as pets, although they do not tolerate, nor can they endure, much handling. The reptiles that are commonly kept as pets are in the orders Chelonii (or Testudines) (turtles, terrapins, and tortoises) and Squamata (lizards and snakes). More than 7 million reptiles are currently kept as pets in the U.S. It is estimated that 50–90% die in the first year of captivity, in large part due to owners being unprepared to provide a proper environment, housing, and diet. Of those reptiles that survive, many will escape or will outlive their owners, leading to abandonment. Some will be abandoned from lack of interest or from management expenses.

Among reptiles, the snake has occupied a special place in human history and religion. In Egyptian history, the Nile cobra adorned the crown of the pharaoh. Snakes were worshiped as one of the gods and were used to kill adversaries and to commit ritual suicide. Cleopatra is believed to have committed suicide through the bite of an Egyptian cobra. The Ancient Greeks also held snakes in high esteem, believing that by being able to shed their skin, snakes had healing powers. As a result, snakes are part of today's medical symbols; for example, the bowl of Hygieia (pharmacy), the Caduceus (U.S. Medical Corps), and the Staff of Aesculapius (practice of medicine).

There are more than 10,000 species of reptiles, which include 400 species of chelonians and the much larger order Squamata (snakes and lizards). There are 3,400 species of snakes (suborder Serpentes) and more than 5,600 species of lizards (suborder Sauria).

The most popular pet turtles in the U.S. are the red-eared slider (*Trachemys scripta elegans*), eastern box turtle (*Terrapene carolina carolina*), western painted turtle (*Chrysemys picta bellii*), map turtle (*Graptemys geographica*), and wood turtle (*Glyptemys insculpta*). The most popular pet snakes are the ball python (*Python regius*), corn snake (*Pantherophis guttata*), California kingsnake (*Lampropeltis getula californiae*), rosy boa (*Lichanura trivirgata*), and gopher snake (*Pituophis* spp.). Popular pet lizards include the bearded dragon (*Pogona vitticeps*), gold-dust day gecko (*Phelsuma laticauda*), leopard gecko (*Eublepharis macularius*), crested gecko (*Correlophus ciliatus*), and blue-tongue skink (*Tiliqua scincoides intermedia*).

NATURAL BEHAVIOR OF REPTILES

All reptiles are "cold-blooded" (*poikilotherms*, ectotherms); that is, they do not have a fixed body temperature, but they do have a preferred body temperature for maximum activity. They normally have a relatively low metabolic rate and eat infrequently compared with mammals. The preferred body temperature range enables the most activity, optimum reproductive functions, and the ability to digest food. The immune system is also most responsive at the preferred body temperature. It is important to provide an environment that is appropriate for the species, which can vary from rain forest to desert.

With the exception of some lizards, most reptiles cannot outrun a predator. Because of this, their first means of defense against a perceived predator is to hide.

Defense methods among reptiles are varied. Coloration of their body aids in hiding in their natural habitat. Chameleons and anoles are able to vary their coloration to become less conspicuous. Reptiles can move quickly but only for short periods of time. They have little capacity for prolonged exertion. If unable to hide, snakes and lizards will attempt to rush to a nearby safer location. Tortoises and some turtles can retract their head and legs into their shells for defense. If capture is imminent, many snakes and lizards will use a rolling maneuver to evade capture. Many lizards and a few snakes are also able to shed the end of their tail, and the lost portion will continue to wriggle to distract an attacker. Some snakes (eastern hog-nosed snakes and grass snakes) will fake death to avoid attackers. Tail waving can be a distraction for predators from a snake's head and body to allow a biting strike by the snake to be more successful. Large snakes may regurgitate to distract a potential predator while the snake tries to escape. Lizards and turtles often urinate or secrete musk odors when picked up to distract a perceived predator, the handler.

Hearing and sight are not a reptile's primary means of determining threats. Reptiles have a low respiratory rate, which does not move air quickly enough to smell odors in the way that mammals smell. Instead, reptiles assess their environment primarily by smell using their tongue. Snakes and lizards flick their tongue to be able to deliver odors to the vomeronasal organ rapidly for the perception of smell.

Lizards have ear drums, but snakes and chelonians do not. Snakes and chelonians hear by sensing vibrations from the ground or in water and transmitting the information to their inner ears. Lizards have upper and lower eyelids. Snakes have a transparent spectacle (eye covering), which clouds their vision during shedding.

Adult male reptiles usually do not tolerate each other, particularly during breeding seasons. They associate rapid movement with aggression. Chelonians and lizards are more territorial than snakes. Aggression and defense are demonstrated in lizards, snakes, and some chelonians by an elevated body, open mouth threats, vocalizations, tail flicking, and head bobbing. Resentment of invasion of personal space or territory can cause eliminations, such as urine or foul-smelling musk.

Chelonians

Turtles live most of their lives in or near water. They have webbed feet with long claws. Tortoises are terrestrial and have thick elephant-like feet with stubby claws. Terrapins are semi-aquatic, hard-shelled chelonians. The term *terrapin* is ill defined. It is derived from a Native American word used by the early European colonists in North American for edible turtles.

Turtles move faster than tortoises. Both protect themselves by hiding, when possible. A unique form of defense for chelonians is to draw a portion or all of their feet, head, and tail within their shell. Coloring to match environment colors provides some additional protection. Bottom dwellers, like alligator snapping turtles, have spikes on their *carapace* (upper shell) to catch algae for camouflage.

Snakes

Snakes will usually attempt to avoid perceived danger by hiding. If this is not an option or is ineffective, some species will fake death, secrete foul odors, make threatening noises, flick or shake their tail, or inflate their body with air or spread the skin on their head to appear larger. For example, hog-nosed snakes when frightened can inflate their bodies, flatten their necks, raise their head, and hiss, appearing like a cobra. Some snakes are usually gentle, such as ball pythons, corn snakes, western hog-nosed snakes, and gopher snakes. Kingsnakes may or may not be gentle. Other snakes may be typically bad-tempered, such as water and bull snakes.

A snake's tongue is located in a sheath in the front of the mouth. It is flicked to obtain chemical particles and deposit them in the vomeronasal organ in the roof of the mouth to determine the smell of the particles. Flicking the tongue indicates alertness.

Vision is best in arboreal snakes, which is especially required for them to hunt birds. Burrowing snakes have poor vision. Snakes do not have ear canals or ear drums. Low frequency sound vibrations are transmitted via their body, particularly their jaw when it is on the ground, to the columella in their inner ear.

All snakes are carnivorous. Most eat rodents. They swallow their food without chewing. Food that is three times the diameter of a snake's head can be swallowed because they can disarticulate their jaws. The limiting factor in size is how much the mouth and throat can stretch. Digestion of whole food is a slow process (2 or more days) in their GI tract. The trachea opens just behind the tongue sheath in the front of the mouth. This allows the snake to breathe when has its mouth full of prey and is involved in the slow swallowing process.

Lizards

Lizards also prefer to hide for defense. Lizards that cannot hide may resort to aggression. Bobbing of the head up and down is a warning of possible aggressive defense. When threatened, a bearded dragon will flare out the skin of its throat, gape its mouth, and bob its head up and down to bluff its threat to move away. Some lizards have autonomous tails that can be released while making an escape. A regrown autonomous tail is off-color from the lizard's body color. Horned lizards can constrict the muscles in their neck to elevate their blood pressure enough to rupture small blood vessels near their eyes. The result is squirting blood from their eyes toward their perceived threat. Chameleons move very slowly. Rather than hurrying to hide, they change their body color in an effort to hide.

Lizards shed skin in patches. Failure to shed skin completely (*dysecdysis*) can allow the drying dead skin to constrict around the toes and end of the tail. Normal shedding (*ecdysis*) takes 5–7 days. Dysecdysis can be caused by lack of sufficient humidity or poor nutrition.

SAFETY FIRST

Handler safety

No reptile is domesticated. Some tolerate being handled, but all prefer not to be handled and persist in seeking escape. Chelonians can inflict tissue-crushing bites with the horny plates of their beaks but, with the exception of snapping turtles, most do not. Snakes and carnivorous lizards have teeth, and their bites produce penetrating wounds. Their teeth slant back toward their throat and will either tear

tissue if the victim jerks away, or the reptile's teeth will dislodge in the wound. Non-venomous snakes have 2–4 rows of teeth.

> Handlers of reptiles must become sufficiently familiar with various species to recognize aggressive species (rock pythons, anacondas, Tokay geckos, and iguanas) and poisonous species (Gila monsters, Mexican beaded lizards, rattlesnakes, copperheads, cottonmouths [water moccasins], and coral snakes).

Safer handling of chelonians

Chelonians do not have teeth, but they have a beak with serrations that can inflict injury and many have sharp claws. Tortoises generally hide in their shells and are not aggressive. Turtles (especially snapping turtles) can be aggressive.

Snapping, softshell, and mud turtles have long necks, dangerous bites, and bad dispositions. If restraint is absolutely necessary, a handler should hold these species by grasping the shell between the hind legs or grasp the top shell edge above the head and hold the base of tail. They should not be picked up by their tails.

Safer handling of Squamata

Some snakes and lizards can grow to longer than 6 ft (1.8 m) and become a physical danger to handlers. Constricting snakes longer than 8 ft (2.5 m) and venomous snakes are inherently dangerous.

Snakes and lizards should be moved to a separate quiet, warm enclosure with no substrate to eat. Food should never be presented by hand. When taking the lid off any enclosure of an aggressive lizard or snake, the lid should be opened on the off side (away from the handler) and the lid held in front of the handler as a shield. Opening the side next to the handler may invite a strike or escape attempt toward the handler.

When a calm lizard or snake is held, it should be given a chance to hold onto the handler's hands and arms more than the handler holds onto the lizard or snake. The goal should be to allow the lizard or snake being held to have the illusion of being free while protecting it from falling and preventing its escape. Squeezing the body and attempting to prevent it from moving risks the lizard or snake trying to escape and the handler being bitten.

Snakes

Corn snakes and ball pythons are docile and popular pets. Ball pythons are nocturnal ground snakes with a calm disposition. Arboreal snakes, such as corn snakes, are more rapid moving than ground snakes. However, it is easier to accidentally drop a ground snake since they do not hold on to a hand or arm as well as arboreal snakes.

About 2 weeks before shedding, a snake produces a cloudy liquid between layers of the skin. This is most evident in the cloudy appearance of the eyes. During this period, snakes become irritable and are more likely to bite.

Snakes that cannot hide protect themselves by biting. Slowing of the flicking rate of the tongue and a stiffened body signals an impending strike. Snakes hunt for food by smell. Handlers should always wash their hands before handling snakes. If a snake smells rodent or rabbit odors on a handler's hand, it will be more likely to bite the handler. The odors of fingernail polish or hand lotion may elicit a defensive response from a snake unadapted to the smell. A handler should never allow any snake near his or her face. Some snakes may strike just from smell of food on the handler's breath. Snakes that eat other snakes, such as kingsnakes, may bite if they smell other snakes on a handler's hands. Feeding a snake in its primary enclosure may cause the snake to become aggressive whenever approached. Food should be offered only in a separate enclosure dedicated for feeding. Handling of snakes should be done at random times. If all handling is at the time of feeding only, snakes will associate hands with food and may become aggressive when handled.

Snake mouths contain many harmful bacteria, and all snakes are carnivorous with sharp teeth. The teeth angle inward, toward their throat, to aid in preventing the escape of their prey. If a handler is bitten on the finger or hand and the snake does not let go, the snake's head must be pushed forward while prying the jaws open to reduce tearing bitten skin further. Alternatively, a bitten handler may put a wooden spatula or plastic credit card in the snake's mouth and push between the handler's skin and the snake's teeth. Submerging a snake's head in water to stimulate it to release is unreliable since snakes have air reserves in their air sacs and can hold their breath for a long time. Teeth are typically small, except the long, backward-curving teeth of *boids* (boas and pythons) for holding their prey while they constrict their body around it.

The fangs of venomous snakes are long to penetrate the skin of their prey or adversaries and deliver venom through a canal in the fangs or along a groove in the surface of the fangs. Only four types of snakes are venomous in North America: rattlesnakes, copperheads, water moccasins, and coral snakes. Poisonous snakes in captivity are more dangerous than those in the wild because captive snakes will store more venom than those that must hunt and kill their prey.

Constricting snakes constrict to kill food and may constrict a perceived predator, including a handler. A constrictor snake should never be put around a handler's neck. That position puts the handler's face and neck vulnerable to being bitten. If a snake constricts the handler's neck, it is very possible that the handler will be unable to remove it by him- or herself, especially if the snake is more than 6 ft (1.8 m) in length. Boids will bite the victim, anchor the tail on a stationary object, which prevents the victim from unwrapping the snake, and constrict the victim. Struggling and an increased respiratory rate will intensify the snake's strength of constriction. Large constrictor snakes can kill within a few minutes without the human victim being able to call out for help. The chance of surviving the bite of most venomous snakes is greater than surviving a large constrictor snake attack. If help is available, the snake must be unwound from the tail since pulling on the snake's head will cause more struggling and increase the strength of constriction. When larger snakes are handled, an assistant handler should be present for every 5 ft (1.5 m) of the snake's length.

Lizards

Lizards defend themselves by biting, clawing, or slashing with their tail when they cannot escape what they perceive as a threat. Some have sharp dental plates for plant diets, and others have sharp teeth for eating insects or animals. All lizards may bite, some have long talons, and some have muscular tails that can inflict serious injury. Iguanas have long, sharp claws and long tails that they lash with for defense. Monitors will bite and hold while thrashing with their bodies. The Gila monster and Mexican beaded lizard are the only poisonous lizards in North America.

Popular pet lizards are bearded dragons and leopard geckos. Leopard geckos are nocturnal, gentle, and quiet, especially during the day. Bearded dragons, particularly males, can be aggressive to other bearded dragons, but they are docile to humans and easy to handle.

Lizards, like snakes, should not be fed in their primary enclosure to reduce the problem of aggression in anticipation of food each time a hand enters its main enclosure.

Reptile safety

The international illegal wildlife trade is more lucrative than drug smuggling, because of easier bribery of wildlife and customs officials in many countries than drug enforcement officials and the ease of altering of documents, such as faking captive breeding. The risks of being caught are low and existing fines are insufficient deterrents. The preferred animals for smuggling are reptiles since most are small, resilient, and require infrequent access to food and water. Rare species command very high prices.

> The safety of many reptiles is adversely affected by the illegal international trade in reptiles.

Pet reptiles have an extraordinary ability to escape, and many that do not will be abandoned by their owners. Several states, particularly in the southern U.S., are trying to deal with the problem of exotic reptiles escaping or being abandoned and released into the environment. For example, in southern Florida 26% of all fish, reptiles, birds, and mammals are exotic. Feral Burmese and reticulated pythons are particularly a problem. They are ambush predators that have a bad disposition and survive well in environments like the cypress swamps of southern Florida.

In 2012, the U.S. Fish and Wildlife Service listed the Burmese python, yellow anaconda, and Northern and Southern African pythons as injurious invasive species under the Lacey Act. This makes it a federal crime to import these snakes or transport them across state lines. Thousands of pythons, a non-indigenous species, have been removed from the Everglades National Park, but they remain prevalent.

Chelonian safety – turtles, terrapins, tortoises

Aquatic chelonians have smaller *plastrons* (lower portion of the shell) compared with terrestrial species and are often unable to completely withdraw their head, neck, and legs into their shell. To compensate for this, aquatic chelonians, such as soft shell turtles and snapping turtles, are aggressive and capable of inflicting severe bites.

Squamata (scaly reptiles) safety – snakes and lizards

Snakes

Snakes should not be handled within 24–48 hours of feeding. Otherwise, they may regurgitate as a defensive tactic and become malnourished.

Live food (mice and rats) should not be released in a box with a snake because the snake may be injured, especially if it is in the process of shedding its skin. Feeding of live prey to snakes is illegal in some European countries. Rodents as food should be humanely pre-killed and from captive colonies that are disease and parasite-free. Snakes should also not be fed in groups since competition for the food may cause injuries. Tongs should be used to provide the food to keep human scent separated from the snake's thoughts of food.

Young snakes shed their skin about once per month. This frequency decreases with growth, and adult snakes shed about twice per year. Snakes should not be handled when their eyes are clouded by shedding skin. They do not eat, cannot see well, and will become agitated during shedding. Shedding in snakes begins by stretching the mouth open, and typically the entire body from front to back will shed in one piece. The new skin of snakes just following shedding is fragile and can be damaged.

Handlers should never restrain a snake by its tail since there is risk of muscular injury to the snake. Ball pythons and corn snakes are bred strictly for unusual colors by some breeders, using inbreeding and subsequently weakening the species. Snake diets should also be assessed since brittle bones from malnutrition are common and require gentle handling to avoid fractures.

Lizards

Before handling lizards, handlers should be familiar with their species, their temperament, and their diet. *Metabolic bone disease* (demineralized bones that fracture easily) caused by poor diets often occurs in pet lizards. In addition, most lizards have explosively quick movements that can put them in danger of being dropped during handling. Proper handling restraint and handling over tables can minimize the risk of the lizard being dropped and possibly breaking bones from the fall.

Live insect prey should not be left in the feeding enclosure. If the lizard loses interest, the insects may cause eye damage to the lizard by feeding on eye moisture.

Key zoonoses

(*Note:* Apparently ill animals, including reptiles, should be handled by veterinary professionals or under their supervision. Precautionary measures against zoonoses from ill animals are more involved than those required when handling apparently healthy animals and vary widely. The discussion here is directed primarily at handling apparently healthy animals.)

The risks of zoonoses from wild-caught reptiles are much greater than from captive-bred reptiles (*Table 8.1*).

Other than bites and claw wounds, the only zoonotic disease of great significance from captive-bred reptiles is salmonellosis. There is a high degree of risk of acquiring salmonellosis from reptiles, including those that appear healthy. The morbidity and mortality of salmonellosis can be high, particularly in humans who are young, elderly, or otherwise have impairment of their immunity. Reptiles captured in the wild, particularly if the reptile is an exotic species, can have many other zoonoses.

Reptiles can carry salmonella bacteria (*Salmonella enteritidis*) in their digestive tract without symptoms. Infected humans can have diarrhea, vomiting, and fever if it is confined to the gastrointestinal system. Invasion of the blood stream may occur and

Table 8.1 **Diseases transmitted from healthy appearing captive-bred reptiles to healthy adult humans**

DISEASE	AGENT	MEANS OF TRANSMISSION	SIGNS AND SYMPTOMS IN HUMANS	FREQUENCY IN ANIMALS	RISK GROUP*
Bites and clawing	–	Direct injury	Bite wounds to face, arms, and legs	All reptiles are capable of inflicting bite or claw wounds, or both	3
Salmonellosis	*Salmonella arizona, S. marina, S. enteritidis,* among others	Direct from handling reptiles; indirect from fomites (cages, bowls, cage toys)	Diarrhea, systemic disease and abscesses	Common	3
Edwardseillosis	*Edwardsiella tarda*	Direct from handling reptiles; indirect from fomites (cages, bowls, cage toys)	Diarrhea and wound infections with gangrene	Common	3

* Risk groups (National Institutes of Health and World Health Organization criteria. Centers for Disease Control and Prevention, *Biosafety in Microbiological and Biomedical Laboratories*, 5th edition, 2009):
  1 Agent not associated with disease in healthy adult humans.
  2 Agent rarely causes serious disease and prevention or therapy possible.
  3 Agent can cause serious or lethal disease and prevention or therapy possible.
  4 Agent can cause serious or lethal disease and prevention or therapy are not usually available.

result in sepsis, abscesses in various organs, and meningitis.

Children younger than 5 years old should not handle reptiles, and households with children under 1 year old should not keep reptiles in the house. The U.S. Centers for Disease Control and Prevention estimate that more than 70,000 people in the U.S. acquire salmonellosis from reptiles each year. Pet reptiles may be the cause for 5–11% of human salmonellosis in the U.S. Transmission is by direct contact with the reptile or objects or surfaces that they have touched. Salmonella can remain infective on objects and surfaces for days and even longer in wet wooden enclosures. The risk of salmonellosis is greatest with aquatic reptiles that defecate in water. Federal regulations ban the sale of turtles with shells less than 4 in (10 cm) in length owing to the risk of transmitting salmonellosis, especially to small children.

Edwardseillosis is a disease of handlers' skin or digestive tract that can be acquired by exposure to reptile feces or feces contaminated water. Carrier reptiles can appear normal.

Campylobacteriosis can be transmitted to humans from reptiles, but there is no evidence it can be transmitted to healthy adults with a normal immune system.

Pentastomiasis (tongue worms) is a disease caused by respiratory worms of large exotic snakes. The worms pass eggs in snake feces and respiratory secretions which, if ingested by humans, will penetrate the intestines, become encysted, and calcify. Eating underprepared snake meat can also be a source of infection. The incidence is primarily in wild-caught snakes in foreign countries.

Sanitary practices

Reptile enclosures should not be located in or near human food preparation or storage areas. Enclosures should be spot cleaned daily with a thorough cleaning on a regularly scheduled basis. Cleaning should include disinfection with 5% bleach (sodium hypochlorite) followed by thorough rinsing before reintroducing the animal. Phenol or pine scent disinfectants should be avoided. All cleaning equipment such as sponges, buckets, and sinks should be cleaned and disinfected. Cleaning reptile enclosures should not involve soaking in bathtubs, basins, or laundry sinks. When cleaning reptile enclosures, gloves and protective glasses or goggles should be worn. Reptiles should not be allowed to roam freely in a home or living area, and they should be kept out of food preparation areas.

Persons handling reptiles should wear appropriate dress to protect against skin contamination with skin scales or saliva, urine, and other body secretions. Reptiles should never be fed by hand nor allowed near a human's face. Hands should be washed after handling any reptile or objects touched by the reptile. Handlers should not eat or drink while handling reptiles.

Young children, the elderly, pregnant women, and people with immunosuppressive diseases or who are on immunosuppressive medications should not handle reptiles due to risk of salmonellosis.

TURTLES AND TORTOISES (CHELONIANS)

Approaching and catching

Small chelonians can be captured by grasping the sides (bridge) of their shell from above with the handler's thumb between the front and hind legs on one side and the first three fingers on the other side between the other side's front and hind legs (**Figure 8.1**). Putting a wrap of self-adhering elastic bandage material around the shell can provide a better gripping surface, if needed.

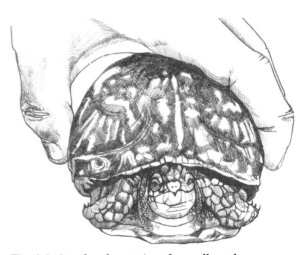

Fig. 8.1 One-hand restraint of a small turtle.

Large chelonians can be captured with two hands by the handler placing his/her thumbs on each side of the carapace (the upper shell) and other fingers under the plastron (the lower shell). Towels should be used to handle aquatic species for protection against their long claws.

Common snapping turtles (*Chelydra serpetina*), alligator snapping turtles (*Macroclemys temmincki*), and soft-shelled turtles can extend their head a long distance (two-thirds the length of their shell) to inflict a bite. These can be grasped by their tail for initial control. To lift the turtle, its tail is firmly held and its body supported by grasping the edge of the carapace (upper shell) behind the neck or with a hand placed under the back part of the plastron. Small biting turtles can be grasped and lifted by holding the back portion of the shell along with both hind legs.

Soft-shelled turtles will scratch and are difficult to hold without injuring them. Handlers should wear light gloves to protect themselves from scratches.

Handling for routine care and management

If a turtle needs to be turned over for examination, inversion must be done slowly to reduce the risk of intestinal torsion. Other than for brief examinations, handlers should not hold a turtle or tortoise upside down or its head lower than its heart. Either of these positions makes it difficult for the chelonian to breathe properly.

If examination of the chelonian's head is needed, the handler should gently pull on a front leg or prod near the rectum to cause the head to come out and then the head can be quickly grasped with the handler's fingers behind the jaws. The head may also be lured out by offering fresh fruit, especially berries.

Some tortoises and some turtles can retract their head and feet so effectively into their shells that chemical restraint is needed to handle these body parts for examination or treatment.

SNAKES

If pet snakes have been raised in captivity and handled gently while young, they are usually easily handled with little restraint. Garter snakes, kingsnakes, hog-nosed snakes, and gopher snakes caught in the wild are sometimes kept as pets, but these are more intolerant of handling, susceptible to stress, and may have diseases and parasites they acquired in the wild.

Snakes kept as pet should not exceed 6½ ft (2 m) in length. Constrictors more than 8 ft (2.4 m) in length are so strong that they are considered inherently dangerous. Many escape or are released when they become a burden or bore to their owner, resulting in endangerment to the snake's health and survival, to indigenous wildlife, or to unsuspecting humans.

Approaching and catching

A handler should make sure the snake is aware of his or her presence and move at slightly slower than normal speed. Snakes bite in self defense or a feeding frenzy. Handlers need to make efforts not to threaten snakes or to interfere with their feeding.

A tame snake is picked up by placing a hand toward the snake's side with outstretched fingers and sliding it under the first one-third of the snake's body. As it is picked up, the remainder of the body should be supported with the handler's other hand. The handler's fingers should be spread to provide wider support (**Figure 8.2**). The snake's head should not be reached for first nor the body held so tight that it cannot keep moving.

Young snakes, shedding snakes, and snakes expecting food are more likely to bite. Arboreal snakes will try to progress up the handler's arm which, if permitted, can allow proximity to the handler's face and neck. This should not be allowed.

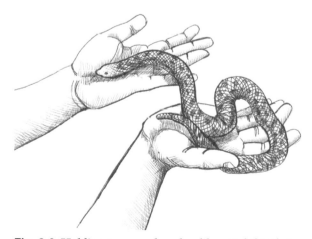

Fig. 8.2 Holding tame snakes should not inhibit their movement.

Handling for routine care and management

Snakes are typically supported with their movement directed, and not held in a manner to inhibit their movement. Holding them tightly stimulates the snake to attempt to escape from a predator. This can also seriously damage their muscles and cause death days later. They should be given the illusion that they are free to escape when they want. As they are loosely held, a "rolling hands" technique of holding them gives them the illusion that they are not trapped. They are allowed to move from one hand to the next, and then the hand they left becomes the next hand they move to. Immobilizing types of restraint should not typically be used. When holding a snake, it should never be held near the handler's face.

The most likely time for a handler to be bitten is when reaching into a snake's enclosure. The handler may startle the snake because of the movement of his or her hand. The risk of being bitten is exacerbated if the handler's hand has an odor of food, such as recently held mice. When reaching into an enclosure for an unfamiliar snake, the handler should block the snake's head with one hand held flat with fingers together. The purpose is to create a barrier over the snake's head while reaching for the body with the other hand. A flat hand is more difficult to bite.

Handling should not be attempted if there is a food smell on the handler's hands or if the snake has recently eaten. Handling a snake soon after it has eaten may cause the snake to regurgitate. This is common in ball pythons.

If a snake is possibly dangerous, a snake hook should be used first to lift the snake and then grasp its body. For those that are known to be dangerous, the head should be immobilized before picking the snake up. The basic hold for snake head restraint is to grasp the base of the skull between the thumb and middle finger with the index finger on top of the head. A snake pinning hook to pin the neck down on a soft surface may be needed to limit movement until the snake's head can be grasped for manual control. The snake's body should be restrained and supported after capturing the head to prevent thrashing and breaking its back. The snake's head should

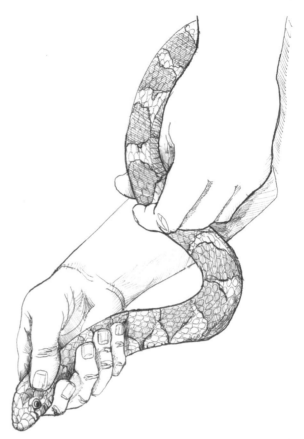

Fig. 8.3 Dangerous snakes must be held by their head and their body supported with the handler's other hand.

be held firmly without being squeezed (**Figure 8.3**). Approximately one handler is needed per 5 ft (1.5 m) of snake to control boids.

Snakes have musk glands near their cloaca that they may use to excrete a malodorous secretion, which also is distasteful to their predators.

Special equipment

Lifting hook

Snake hooks can be used to move snakes a short distance such as into a transport bag. The hook is worked under the snake between the first one-third to one-half of the snake's length to pick it up. The snake will remain still, trying to keep its balance. Snake hook poles should always be tilted down, away from the handler. Otherwise, the snake may slide toward the handler. Hooks can also help in guiding the movement of snakes on the ground or floor.

Pinning hook

A pinning hook is a Y-shaped stick with tubing for padding that can be used to introduce a handler's presence and, if necessary, pin a snake's head. Pinning hooks should be used when the snake is on a padded surface to reduce risk of injury to the snake. A strap of elastic extends from one of the ends of the Y to the other. The head can be immobilized by pressing the elastic band just behind the head, pushing the head down and trapping it until the head can be grasped by a free hand. Two pinning hooks may be necessary for difficult snakes. The base of the head is then grasped between the thumb and middle finger with the index finger on the top of the head and the hook removed.

Shields and squeeze box

Plexiglass or wire mesh shields with handles can be used to pin snakes until the head can be restrained. Properly fitted ventilated plexiglass or wire mesh lids on a box can be used to contain the movement of the snake while the shield descends into the box to squeeze it for administering injectable medication or chemical restraint. The bottom of the squeeze box should be padded.

Capture pole

A capture pole can be made with a 3-foot-long (1 m) wooden pole, eye screw, and a long cord. One end of the cord is tied to, or otherwise fixed to, the end of the pole. The other end of the cord is run through an eye screw placed 1 in (2.5 cm) from the end of the pole where the end of the cord is fixated. A capture loop is then recreated between the fixed end and the eye screw. The loop is dropped around the snake's neck and the loop closed on the neck by pulling on the cord. The risk of injuring the snake is greater than with a hook, but if gentle pressure is applied with the loop and restraint is short, a capture pole can be safe and effective.

Capture tongs

Capture tongs are long-handled metal grasping instruments. It is difficult to gauge the pressure being exerted with tongs, so the risk of injury to a snake can be significant. Tongs can make a snake thrash and bite itself. Capture tongs should not be the sole means of restraint of a snake, but tongs can be useful to assist with handling with a hook.

Tongs should be used in presenting food to large snakes and in moving environmental enrichment objects in a snake enclosure.

Transparent, flexible tubes

Bad-tempered snakes, such as small reticulated pythons, with a history of inappropriate biting should be handled in the same manner as poisonous snakes. Aggressive snakes can be moved to a large plastic bucket with its transport bag or with a snake hook. As the snake investigates a possible escape route upward and out of the bucket, a flexible, preferably darkened, tube can be placed over the snake's head and down part of the front of its body. A snake hook can help guide the head, if needed. Use of a cone to guide the snake into the tube is another method.

The tube should be just large enough to accommodate the thickest part of the snake's body so that it cannot turn around in the tube and long enough to keep the handler's hand on the tube, out of danger. Tubes work best for pit vipers owing to their broad triangular head. When the snake has entered one-third of the tube's distance, the snake and tube are grasped to entrap the snake (**Figure 8.4**). If the first tube seems too large in diameter, a smaller tube can be slid down the open end to the snake for it to enter. The snake and small tube can be grasped and then the larger tube removed. Releasing the snake back into the bucket, transport bag, or enclosure is done by allowing it to move forward through the tube and out the other end.

LIZARDS

Common pet lizards include central bearded dragons, anoles, skinks, iguanas, chameleons, and geckos.

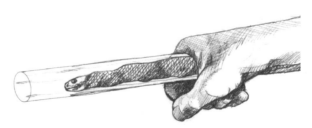

Fig. 8.4 Tube restraint for dangerous snakes.

Leopard geckos and bearded dragons are the easi-est lizards for new owners of lizards to handle and manage. Green iguanas (*Iguana iguana*) are com-mon lizard pets even though they are territorial and aggressive, have long claws, will bite, and have a long muscular tail that they use to lash handlers if excited. Only experienced handlers should handle large iguanas.

Approaching and catching

Small to medium-sized lizards (geckos, bearded dragons, uromastyces) accustomed to being handled can be grasped from above their body. The handler should move his or her hand slightly slower than normal to capture lizards. A lizard's shoulders and the pelvic area should be supported and restrained as needed to prevent the lizard from lashing and damaging its vertebrae. Subdued lighting is helpful. Many lizards will become more difficult to handle and aggressive if in natural sunlight.

Well-handled iguanas may tolerate moderate handling without resistance. Handlers must exercise special care to control an iguana's long muscular tail. A defensive position they may take is to bend in a U shape to ready the tail to slash in defense. The cap-ture of a defensive iguana involves grasping the base of the tail with one hand, lifting the hind legs off the floor, and then grasping the neck and shoulders with the other hand. Immediately after picking the iguana up, the handler should trap the tail between his or her forearm and body. In some cases, snares may be used to gain control of the head. When this is done, the tail must be quickly grasped as soon as the head is snared to prevent thrashing, which could break the iguana's neck.

Handling for routine care and management

Lizards are most comfortable if they can continue to move, or think they can move, at their own will. Holds that primarily provide support while the han-dler directs their continuing movements are most successful. Small, calm lizards are best held loosely and letting the lizard move from one hand to the other in a rolling hand movement. Lizards are easily stressed by firm restraint and can be injured by tight restraint.

A blanket or towel to cover the lizard's head may be used to assist in its capture and immobilization. Lizards used for research may be restrained with small clear-plastic tubes for brief physical restraint similar to restraint tubes for rodents.

Small lizards

Small docile lizards can be easily picked up and held in a palm and on an arm without any restraint (**Figure 8.5**). Care must be taken, since small lizards that are not handled often may attempt to jump off the handler's hand. Tiny lizards such as anoles and small geckos can be easily injured even with care-ful handling. Unnecessary handling and restraint should be avoided whenever possible.

When additional restraint is needed, a small lizard should never be restrained by its tail, which will break off, a reaction called *tail autonomy*. Most lizards are very fast and should be grasped around the shoulders and pelvis. This can be done with one hand for smaller lizards.

Iguanas and other large lizards

Arboreal lizards, such as green iguanas, have long claws to help them climb. Their claws can inflict serious injuries to handlers if the restraint applied does not prevent them from being able to rake their claws on the handler.

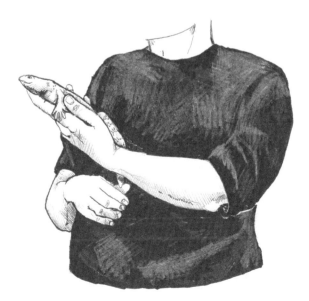

Fig. 8.5 Small lizards can be held loosely.

If handled often, an iguana can be picked up by sliding a hand underneath its body and between its legs. The front end is supported with a hand below the thorax between the front legs, and the rest of the torso rests on the handler's forearm. The lizard's tail is restrained under the handler's arm and against the handler's body. A slow, quiet approach is best. If the iguana becomes excited, it will grab whatever it can and hold on to prevent being picked up.

Another restraint for medium-sized to large lizards is to grasp them from above their back. The thumb and index finger are placed on the lower neck and three fingers behind one shoulder. The other hand restraining the pelvis is positioned with an index finger in front of a hind leg, the thumb behind the other hind leg, and three fingers on the base of the tail.

Leather gloves with gauntlets and a jacket with long sleeves should be used if a lizard has long talons. Towels can be used as hoods and wraps for capture when needed. A noose can be made of thick cord to snare a lizard that quickly evades hand capture. Nets can be used for capturing difficult cases.

Any time a large lizard is captured, consideration should be given to trimming the nails to reduce risk of handler injury with further restraint. A blinder wrap can be helpful in trimming nails. The wrap is created by padding the eyes with cotton balls and wrapping the head with self-adhering elastic bandage material.

Many lizards will not release after biting someone, such as the handler, and their bite will intensify if the victim struggles. If being quiet and calm does not result in the lizard ending its bite, it should be placed on the floor, with the victim lowering his or her body, if necessary. The lizard's attention should shift to letting go and attempting to escape or assuming a defensive posture in an attempt to scare the victim away. Defensive posturing can include tail whipping, head bobbing, opening the mouth wide, standing higher on all four legs, standing broadside, and extending their dewlap forward. Other deterrent maneuvers by lizards include spraying musk or urine and feces from the cloaca.

HANDLING OF REPTILES FOR COMMON MEDICAL PROCEDURES

Most handling and restraint of reptiles can be and should be done without tranquilization, sedation, hypnosis, or anesthesia. However, some handling and restraint procedures should be restricted to veterinary medical professionals owing to the potential danger to the animal or handler. These require special skills, equipment, or facilities, and possibly adjunct chemical restraint or complete immobilization by chemical restraint.

Most medications are given to reptiles by injection rather than by mouth. Injections are preferred in larger reptiles, considering the danger to handlers when handling a reptile's head and mouth. Routes for injections are intramuscular, subcutaneous, intracoelomic, intravenous, and intraosseous. For injections other than intravenous to be effective, the animal must be well hydrated and at a preferred temperature for normal activity for its species.

Injections and venipuncture

Insertion of transcutaneous needles for injection or aspiration in reptiles carries the risk of slashing tissue beneath the skin, including damage to nerves and blood vessels, and breaking hypodermic needles off in the body. The area in which the needle is to be inserted must be immobilized, and the reptile's mouth and feet should be restrained from interfering with the procedure, especially venipuncture.

Venipuncture
Chelonians
Veins that can be accessed in chelonians include the jugular vein, brachial vein, dorsal and ventral coccygeal (tail) vein, femoral vein, and subcarapacial (beneath the shell) vein, found on the midline just under the carapace (upper shell) above the retracted head of the turtle. The jugular vein on the right side is preferred for turtles and the dorsal vein of the tail is preferred for tortoises. The head must be captured and extended to access the jugular vein.

Snakes
The vein used for venipuncture in snakes is the ventral coccygeal vein caudal to the vent on the midline

of the tail. Chemical restraint may be necessary. In anesthetized larger snakes, the palatine vein in the roof of the mouth can be accessed.

Lizards

Restraint for venipuncture in lizards may be assisted by using cotton balls over a lizard's eyes and using self-adherent elastic bandage loosely wrapped around its head to hold the cotton in place.

The ventral coccygeal (tail) vein is often used and accessed with the lizard held ventrodorsally (on its back). However, using the ventral coccygeal vein can be hazardous when restraining lizards with autonomous tails. The tail may pull off or spontaneously be shed if the ventral tail vein is routinely used. The ventral (central) abdominal or jugular vein can be accessed after chemical restraint and ventrodorsal positioning, but hematomas often occur afterwards.

Injections
Intramuscular

Intramuscular (IM) injections are the most common method of drug administration to reptiles. It has been traditionally believed that IM injections given in the hind legs or tail are absorbed and carried to the renal portal system, resulting in more rapid elimination from the body and uneven distribution in the body. Injections in the front half of the body of reptiles have been preferred. Although evidence is lacking for clinically significant first-pass elimination of drugs by the renal portal system of all injectable drugs in reptiles, most veterinarians will give IM injections in the front half of the body of reptiles.

In chelonians, IM injections are usually given in the upper (proximal) front leg (**Figure 8.6**). Although less convenient, the pectoral muscles at the junction of neck and front leg can also be used. The hind legs may be used, but the medication dosage may need to be increased.

Snakes are administered IM injections in the dorsal muscles of the back in the front one-third of the body (**Figure 8.7**). No restraint or hand restraint of the head may be needed. When full body restraint is needed, a squeeze box can be used. A squeeze box for snakes is a box with a removable top. To administer IM injections, the standard top is temporarily replaced with a slightly smaller wire mesh top with handles that can be slid down the box, pressing the snake on the bottom. An alternative to a wire mesh treatment top is 0.5 cm plexiglass drilled with multiple holes. In addition to breathing and injection access holes, treatment tops need a center handle. The bottom of the treatment box for squeezing snakes from above should have a firm but non-rigid bottom, such as foam rubber. Injections should be performed by angling the needle toward the head and inserting the needle underneath scales, not through them.

The deltoid muscles of the shoulders are preferred for IM injections in lizards (**Figure 8.8**). The forearm muscles of large lizards may also be used. Chameleons and small geckos do not have sufficient muscle for IM injections.

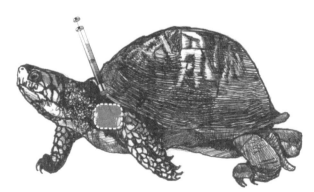

Fig. 8.6 Intramuscular injection site in turtles.

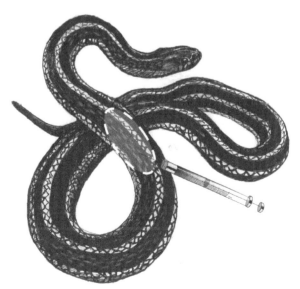

Fig. 8.7 Intramuscular injection site in snakes.

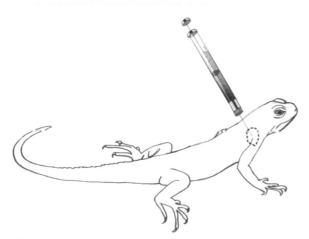

Fig. 8.8 Intramuscular injection site in lizards.

Subcutaneous

Subcutaneous (SC) injections are not often administered to reptiles. When they are, the injection in chelonians is given in the ventral neck flap or under the skin cranial to the fore- or hind legs. In snakes, the injection is given in the cranial one-third of body in an epaxial (dorsolateral) area. As with IM injections, the needle should be angled toward the head and the injection made underneath, not through, the scales. Lizards are given SC injections in an epaxial thoracic area.

Intracoelomic

Intracoelomic (IC) injections are uncommonly used in reptiles. Reptiles do not have a diaphragm, so their body cavity is unlike the chest and abdominal cavities of mammals. IC injections can cause compression of their lungs, and there is risk of puncturing or cutting an internal organ with the injection needle.

When IC injections are given to chelonians, they are administered through the caudal skin folds where they attach to the bridge (junction on their sides between the upper and lower shell). In snakes, IC injections are given in the lateral part of body just dorsal to the ventral scales and in front of the cloaca in the caudal one-fourth of its body. Lizards are placed in ventrodorsal recumbency (on their back) with their head tilted downward. The injection is given in the caudal one-third of the body. The midline should be avoided because of the risk of penetrating the ventral abdominal vein.

Intraosseous

Intraosseous (IO, inside a bone) injection should be done in reptiles only after they are radiographed to check bone density. If they have metabolic bone disease, an IO puncture is likely to fracture the bone.

Injections in chelonians are given either at the junction between the plastron and carapace just cranial to a hind leg or into the tibial crest. IO injections are not possible in snakes. In lizards, IO injections are given into the proximal femur (entered between hip joint and greater trochanter) or the distal femur (entered at stifle joint). The proximal tibia may be used in larger lizards. The point of injection is at the tibial crest.

Administration of oral medications

Giving drugs to reptiles by mouth can be hazardous to handlers because of the risk of being bitten, or difficult owing to the resistance of the reptile, particularly chelonians. Oral medication is used more often in lizards than in snakes or chelonians. If possible, the best method of oral medication for reptiles is to apply the medication on or in food. The amount of food should be limited to ensure the likelihood that the reptile will consume the medicated food. In some cases an oral syringe with a metal ball-tipped gavage needle or rubber feeding tube can be placed in the corner of the mouth and the medication delivered slowly.

Oral administration of medications with a lubricated feeding tube can be safe for the reptile, if care is used to open a reptile's mouth with a wooden spatula or popsicle stick. In some cases, the lower neck flap (dewlap) can be pulled gently to open the mouth. It is relatively easy to avoid the glottis (opening to the windpipe). The glottis in snakes is located in the front of the mouth. This allows the snake to have its mouth stuffed with a meal and still breathe. It is at the base of the tongue in lizards and chelonians.

If a feeding tube is inserted too far, the stomach may be reached, which can be hazardous to the reptile. The length from mouth to stomach should be estimated beforehand. In snakes, the distance is one-third of its body length. In lizards, it is one-half the body length, and in chelonians it is the distance from the nose to the junction of pectoral and abdominal shell plates, or *scutes*.

TRANSPORTING REPTILES

Chelonians and lizards

Opaque plastic storage boxes or tubs are the best means of transporting chelonians and lizards. If the chelonian is an aquatic species, it should have a moist towel under it and over it. Transporting lizards should be in plastic containers with tight lids and sufficient holes or slits for adequate ventilation.

Snakes

When moving snakes, a double-lined bag should be used to contain the snake, and the bag placed in a plastic box. The bag should be canvas or cotton to allow ventilation. Pillowcases (breathable cotton) will suffice for most non-poisonous snakes. Seams should be double stitched to prevent the snake's head from pushing a hole through a seam. Gentle snakes can be simply lifted into a transport bag. Transport bag openings should be tied off and the bag lifted and carried by the end of the knot to reduce the risk of being bitten through the bag.

For added safety in bagging aggressive or poisonous snakes, the bag's neck can be placed through a triangular metal hoop at the end of a pole. This will hold the bag open without putting the handler's hands at risk. A snake hook is used to place the snake in the bag. The bag is removed from the hoop and the bag neck tied tightly with a cord.

Having a double bottom or stitched-cornered bag will protect the handler's hand from a bite if the bottom of the bag is grasped while removing the snake. The handler locates and grasps the snake's head using the bag as a shield. Then, the handler reaches into the bag, grasps the base of the head, and uses the other hand to lift the body as the snake is removed from the bag. Aggressive snakes are released from a head hold by the handler removing the thumb and middle finger while the snake's head is pressed down with the index finger, which is then immediately removed to complete the release.

SELECTED FURTHER READING

Ballard B, Cheek R (2017). *Exotic Animal Medicine for the Veterinary Technician*, 3rd edition. Wiley-Blackwell, Ames/Oxford.

Bays, TB, Lightfoot T, Mayer J (2006). *Exotic Pet Behavior*. Elsevier Saunders, St. Louis.

Campbell KL, Campbell JR (2009). *Companion Animals*, 2nd edition. Pearson, Upper Saddle River.

Clancy MM, Davis M, Valitutto MT, et al. (2016). Salmonella infection and carriage in reptiles in a zoological collection. *Journal of the American Veterinary Medical Association* 248:1050–1059.

Holz P, Barker IK, Crawshaw GJ, et al. (1997). The effect of the renal portal system on pharmacokinetic parameters in the red-eared slider (*Trachemys scripta elegans*). *Journal of Zoo logical Wildlife Medicine* 28:386–393.

Judah V, Nuttall K (2016). *Exotic Animal Care and Management*, 2nd edition. Cengage Delmar Learning, Albany.

Warren DM (2015). *Small Animal Care and Management*, 4th edition. Cengage Delmar Learning, Albany.

Woodward DL, Khakhria R, Johnson WM (1997). Human salmonellosis associated with exotic pets. *Journal of Clinical Microbiology* 35:2786–2790.

RANCH, FARM, AND STABLED ANIMALS

CHAPTER 9

CONTAINMENT FOR RANCH, FARM, AND STABLED ANIMALS

Good animal handling begins with safe and secure containment of the animal. Safety of the animal and of the handler depends on appropriate, well-maintained enclosures. It is true that "good fences make good neighbors" (from the 1914 poem *Mending Wall* by Robert Frost). However, otherwise excellent fencing contractors who do not have animal handling experience often build highly attractive, but unsafe, fencing for horses and livestock. It is essential to understand the strength and typical behavior of animal species to construct appropriate enclosures for them. Animal owners, animal handlers, and veterinary professionals should evaluate planned enclosures and inspect construction in progress to ensure enclosures are built firstly to ensure the safety of the animals and their handlers, and secondly for esthetics

All domestic animals have basic needs that should be provided by good handlers: adequate and accessible food and water; room to stand and to raise their head, stretch, turn around, move forward, lie down, roll, and groom themselves without restriction; regular exercise; and social contact with people and other animals of their own species.

Containment (and handling) of farm animals used for federally funded research in the U.S. requires oversight by an Institutional Animal Care and Use Committee that ensures compliance with the Public Health Service Policy and Animal Welfare Regulations. The welfare of farm animals in research is guided by the Federation of Animal Science Societies' Guide for the Care and Use of Agricultural Animals in Research and Teaching.

> Public knowledge of how livestock are contained and handled is the major motivation for finding improved methods for raising and handling livestock.

The oversight of containment and handling of livestock for food production varies by state welfare laws and the extent of their enforcement. The most effective approach to achieving good animal handling for livestock depends on a team approach to solving problems that includes consumers (the public), members of the food marketing chain, and the livestock producers. The best assessment for the quality of handling requires audits of animal health and behavior by objective criteria compiled and evaluated by trained observers of normal animal behavior without conflicts of interest. Currently, these assessments are voluntary, and those who do not value animal handling quality do not volunteer to undergo objective, independent opinion. The expectations of informed consumers are the driving force for improved livestock handling and containments.

CONFINEMENT AND BEHAVIOR

Confinement should not produce avoidable physical or mental injury to animals. Intentional and unintentional excesses in the degree of confinement of production animals and horses are among the most common forms of animal abuse in the U.S. Some livestock producers who overly confine animals or provide little or no mental stimulation for them claim that this should be acceptable because the animals continue to breed, grow, or produce milk, eggs, or fiber. The ability to grow and be productive in some respects, however, does not rule out physical or mental abuse.

There is a difference between conscience-based welfare and economic-based welfare, although they frequently, and should, overlap. The only way to assess whether animal confinement is acceptable to the average person's conscience is to learn the normal behavior and physical being of animals in natural or near natural confinement, and for knowledgeable third parties without a financial conflict of interest to objectively compare and score the behavior and physical condition of the confined animals, as has long been advocated by the international consultant and author on livestock welfare, Temple Grandin.

Areas of confinement for domestic or wild animals should be large enough to permit normal move ment, mental stimulation, frequent interaction with other living beings, and a zone of personal space. Confined animals should be monitored for abnormal aggression, self-mutilation, and stereotypic behaviors. Factors other than confinement can cause aggression, self-mutilation, or stereotypic behaviors in random animals, but additional room in the confinement area should be considered if these abnormal behaviors exceed the level considered to be beyond random significance, which is 2% of the animals.

CONTAINMENT AND STRESS

Most stresses to domestic animals are caused by their handlers. Stress can be physical or psychological. Containment should be safe from injury and provide protection from weather extremes to eliminate physical stresses. Animals can often adapt to continued physical stresses, but not to continued psychological stresses. Psychological stress can be the result of something fearful in an animal's environment or from the lack of sufficient mental stimulation.

Stabling horses without turnout pens or time at pasture, keeping sows in gestation crates, and confining chickens in battery cages are all mentally sterile environments. The absence of adequate mental enrichments often leads to weaving, pacing, self-mutilation, pawing, kicking, and cribbing in horses; bar biting, head weaving, and tongue rolling in sows; and feather picking in birds.

Stress is associated with greater transmission of disease, including salmonellosis. In addition to providing safety from injury and temperature extremes, good containment eliminates or minimizes exposure to fearful stimuli, such as harassment by predators and overcrowding and bullying by more dominant herd members. Good containment should also be as large as feasible with other enhancements to provide sufficient species-appropriate mental stimulation.

Raising herd animals in isolation can lead to psychological stress in the animals from the loss of psychological security that a group provides. Isolation causes an unrelenting need to be on alert for possible threats. However, very young or very old, pregnant, or sick animals may require segregation for safety or because of their frequent need for care by handlers.

CONTAINMENT AND LIABILITY

Containment injury to animals

Failure to provide or maintain adequate enclosures can subsequently cause injury to animals while they are contained. Sources of injury can include protruding nails, exposed metal edges, weak boards, faulty wire attachments to fencing, and holes or gaps in flooring. Containments should always be examined for potential hazards prior to each use.

Animal escape consequences

How an animal may have escaped from containment should not be discussed until after a complete investigation. Possibilities, even if wrong, could invite allegations of negligence.

Animal endangerment

Livestock, especially horses, are a danger to themselves when they escape. They can get hit by moving vehicles, attacked by dogs, fall in holes, become lost and starve, or be stolen, among other dangers.

The most useful means of identifying escaped horses that will assist their return is having good quality, recent photographs of the horse and close-ups of its markings. In addition to photographs, stabled horses should have ID plates on their halter or dog tags with the owner's name and phone number. Lip tattoos can be useful for pastured horses that may escape. Tattoos inside the upper lip are used on race horses and recorded on their registration papers. Microchips and retinal identification are good identifiers that may aid in the return of escaped horses, but both require special equipment for detection and are best used along with halter tags or plates or tattoos rather than in place of these more obvious identifiers.

Injury to humans

Owners and handlers of animals are responsible for human injuries resulting directly or indirectly from escaped animals. For example, a handler can be liable for injuries to another person from an escaped bull that was in the handler's care. The other person's injuries can be crushing by the bull or breaking a leg by jumping a fence to escape the bull.

Prevention of escape

Preventing escapes necessitates double checking gates and doors that should be closed. Stall doors should be double latched. Gate hinge pins should be oriented to prevent gates from being lifted off the hinge pins. Gates adjacent to public roads should be locked. Perimeter (secondary) fencing should be created around pastures, especially horse pastures, located near busy roads or highways. There should be a regular schedule of checking the condition of fences, ideally daily, and as soon as possible after thunderstorms and ice storms. Fence strength and height should be appropriate to the species, as well as the age and condition of the animals enclosed and the size of the enclosed area.

> Reasons for a desire to escape should be reduced or eliminated. Always provide adequate food and water, sufficient exercise and companionship, and prevent harassment (dogs, trespassers, herd bullies).

Escape is often motivated by lack of food or water or being frighted. New members to a herd should be introduced slowly and at times when the herd is distracted by a new food source to prevent bullying. When sorting out a member of a herd to provide treatment for an illness or injury, at least one known preferred herdmate should be kept with the animal. Horses should be put in stalls before thunderstorms. Dogs should be prevented from chasing horses.

Response to escaped horses and livestock

Escaped livestock, including horses, can be a life-threatening danger to themselves and to humans, but despite the urgency needed to return them to confinement, excitement or disorganization in the efforts to contain them can worsen the situation. If the animal is off the handler's property, law enforcement should be contacted for notification of potential personal or property damage that could be done by the loose animal. Neighbors should be contacted and requested to contact the handler if they see a loose animal.

When possible, animal access to roads should be blocked and a temporary enclosure created. Horses escape enclosures more often than other livestock. Primary reasons are fear, hunger, thirst, or sex drive. The response to a loose horse should include gathering a halter and lead rope, grain in a bucket, and a flashlight, if night is near. If the animal's location is not known, a spiraling circle should be walked to look for tracks. Places where other horses are kept should be checked as well as where food or water might be found, because a common cause for horses to try to escape enclosures is inadequate access to food or water. In some cases, enlisting the aid of a drone may be the best way of locating an escaped horse.

When possible, the horse(s) should be lured into containment. Herd members do not like to be separated from the herd. If not all of the herd members have escaped, the best lure is to tie other well-mannered horse(s), but not stallions, inside pastures or pens and open the gates to lure a loose horse or horses into the enclosure. Another way of using herd members as a lure is to lead another well-mannered horse (not a stallion) as encouragement for a loose horse to follow. Grain in buckets may be used as a lure if only one horse is loose. Using food for a lure for more than one loose horse is too dangerous for the handler.

The handler of the loose horse should discourage anyone else, including law enforcement officers, from attempting to catch the horse, to prevent likelihood of injuries to an inexperienced handler and stirring up the animal(s). These assistants can be helpful by positioning themselves between the animals and a roadway to try to prevent animals going into traffic and endangering motorists. Assistants should block any other exits as much as possible. Simple portable rope corrals created with poles and mesh fencing, construction netting, or one to three strains of ropes may assist in containing loose horses until an appropriate handler calms and catches individual horses. Several people are required to keep the corral line stretched out.

The approach to a loose horse must be done quietly with confidence, preferably by a handler known to the horse. The portable corral can be used to herd the horse into a fixed enclosure (pen or pasture) or to slowly shrink the corral to enclose the horse so that a handler can approach the horse without it fleeing. Like most fences, a portable corral is a psychological enclosure, not a physical enclosure. If frightened enough or aggressively approached, a horse will challenge the enclosure and try to either run through it or jump it. After a successful capture, the horse should be kept in relatively close confinement such as a stall until the excitement of its adventure has subsided.

FENCES AND GATES

Construction and maintenance
Definitions
Fences are used for enclosures of various sizes. There are perimeter fences and pasture fences. *Perimeter fences* are usually on the edge of the owned property with a 15 ft (4.6 m) alley to the pasture fence. Perimeter fences along a road may be referred to as an exterior fence. If the perimeter fence is between two adjacent landowners, it may be called a *divisional fence*. Double fencing (perimeter with a pasture fence) helps protect horses from escape and any resulting liability risks as well as risks to people attempting to interact with a horse over a single fence line. Because people will put themselves at risk in trying to interact with horses, horses are considered an attractive nuisance liability. *Pasture fencing* consists of a boundary fence and may also include temporary cross fencing for more efficient grazing. Cross fencing can be two or three strands of electric wire or rope. Pastures are larger enclosures for grazing and exercise.

All large animal enclosures should include a small catch pen for feeding, watering, and checking the condition of livestock or horses. *Pens* are fenced areas at least twice the size of a typical stall for fresh air. *Runs* are narrow pens for fresh air and are usually attached directly to a stall. *Corrals* are square or round pens approximately 50 ft (15 m) in diameter

for exercise or training. *Paddocks* are small pastures of half an acre or more for exercise. *Alleyways* between paddocks aid in moving horses and preventing play and fights over a fence.

Improper fencing
The price paid for a fence does not indicate its ability to contain and protect animals. Human error (poor construction or maintenance) is the most common cause for fence failure. Although some areas may have regulation on the placement and appearance of farm fencing, there are no regulations on the quality of farm fencing. It is incumbent on owners and contractors to know the proper fencing to contain different species safely. Unfortunately, contractors without proper animal-handling knowledge may recommend and build improper fences and gates. Members of the American Fence Association are pledged to adhere to a code of ethics. To become a Certified Fence Professional, they must pass a certifying exam and attend continuing education courses. Proper animal fencing requires knowledge of specific needs based on species, age, breed, sex, and production system. Proper fencing should last 25–50 years.

Fencing is an expensive investment. Often, improper fencing is selected because it is less expensive; barbed wire for horses, for example. Conversely, fencing may be selected because it is more expensive with an assumption it is best for a situation, although in reality its use is inappropriate, such as pipe fencing for goats. Typical relative costs (from lower to higher) are barbed or high-tensile wire, polyester braided electric rope, wire mesh, wood, vinyl, and pipe.

How fences work
Fences are intended to keep animals from escaping and, in many cases, to keep intruders out. Fences for horses and cattle are often assumed to physically keep them from escaping, but that is not true. Common fences for horses and cattle are more psychological barriers than physical barriers. Field fences are psychological barriers. Horses or cattle can go through them or over them, but they must not think they can. Desire to escape is increased by fear or the insufficiency of food or water.

Fences for large animals must either deter them from rubbing on the fence or be built in a manner to withstand the weight and pressure of a cow, bull, or horse rubbing against the inside of the fence. Nails and staples are to keep boards or wires from falling on the ground. Fence posts provide the strength of the fence. For strength, boards and wires should be on the inside of the fenced enclosure (**Figure 9.1**). If the animal presses on, rubs, or runs into the horizontal planks or wire, the pressure should be absorbed by the posts, not the nail heads or fence staples.

The suitability of fencing varies with the size, sex, age, and disposition of the animals to be contained and the density of containment (animals/square yard). The height of fences and gates depend on the enclosure size, number of animals, and type of animals to be contained. Smaller enclosures (corrals, paddocks, runs), large herds, stallions, or horses trained to jump require fences of greater height than standard pasture fence height.

New enclosure considerations

If creating a new pasture, what the land was previously used for and what physical or toxic hazards might be present should be investigated. Outdoor containments for large animals should be located on higher ground with good drainage. Pastures for horses should be cleared of burrowing varmints (moles, prairie dogs, groundhogs, and badgers). Burrow holes pose a risk to horses that could break a leg.

Access to water is essential, but ponds and lakes can be dangerous drinking water sources during winter weather. If they freeze, animals can slip, fall, and break bones or fall through ice in an attempt to reach drinking water. Horses that have not been

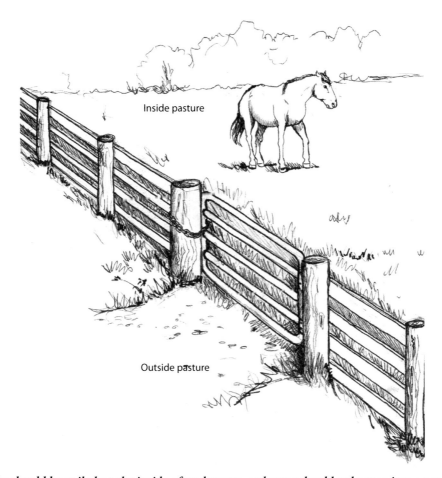

Inside pasture

Outside pasture

Fig. 9.1 Planks should be nailed on the inside of enclosures, and gates should only open into a pen or pasture.

raised in pastures or on a range are at greatest risk of making bad decisions with ice. All livestock should be provided access to drinking water from running streams or heated water troughs during icy weather and barred from access to ponds and lakes due to the risk of slips and broken bones, and break-throughs and drownings. Snow should never be relied on as a source of drinking water.

Square corners for enclosures should be avoided, whenever possible, if groups of animals will be contained. Square corners discourage large animals from moving when driven into right-angle fence corners. Hogs tend to pile on each other and overheat in corners, and submissive horses are more easily trapped in corners by dominant horses attempting to bite and kick them. Rounded corners can be built or horizontal boards can be applied diagonally across square corners to eliminate the risk of submissive animals being trapped in corners by bullies.

Vegetation should be mowed under and outside of fences to prevent livestock and horses from reaching through the fence to eat the "greener grass" on the other side and breaking down the fence. The fence line should be set back from the property line to ensure that an outside strip can be mown. Keeping vegetation mowed under fencing is also important to prevent electric fencing from shorting out on wet vegetation. A perimeter fence surrounding the primary fence should be considered when busy roads are near to prevent escape and keep livestock or horses away from possible discarded trash from vehicles.

Safety and routine care

Safe, effective fencing does not have to be expensive, and expensive fencing is not necessarily safe or effective. Furthermore, fencing that is built to be safe does not remain safe without appropriate routine care. Fences should not have any protruding nails or loose wire. Possible sources of injury inside fence enclosures, such as old farm equipment or other junk that could cut or otherwise injure enclosed animals, should be removed, as well as noxious weeds. Trees should be fenced. Horses may strip the bark, causing the tree to die, and this might result in the tree falling on the boundary fence. Dead limbs on standing or fallen trees can also cause penetrating wounds in horses.

Fence materials should be as visible as possible so that animals, especially horses, can easily see their boundaries and not run into the fence. When light colors cannot be used for horizontal portions of the fence, streamer ribbons (*fladry*) should be tied to the fence to increase visibility.

New herd members must be introduced gradually, otherwise dominant herd members will chase the new member into, through, or over a fence. New herd members need to be introduced across a fence by keeping them in adjacent pens and later together in a pasture or large pen that allows personal space to not be violated until social adjustments are made. The introduction of a new herd member is facilitated by providing a single gentle companion at first and slowly adding more members of the herd. Diversions at the time of initial entry of a new member, such as moving the herd to a fresh pasture, also aid in the acceptance of the new member.

Gates

Gates are used to provide access for humans, animals, or machinery. Gates for a man or a horse should be at least 4 ft (1.2 m) wide. Gates for trucks and small tractors should be 12 ft (3.7 m) wide, and for larger farm equipment 16 ft (4.9 m) wide.

Each pen or pasture should have at least two gates. Latches should be able to be opened with one hand but secure against animals opening them. Horses can learn to open simple latches with their lips, and cattle will open them with their tongues.

Upper hinge pins (pintles) for gates should be positioned pointing downward so that horses or cattle cannot lift the gate up and off its hinges with its nose or neck or rubbing it with its rump. The lower hinge pin should point upward.

Posts that long gates attach to should be buried at least 4 ft (1.2 m) deep. Gaps between gates and adjacent posts should not be more than 3 in (8 cm) to prevent hoofs from getting caught when rearing (**Figure 9.2**).

A "man gate" or "pass through" is an opening that will only accommodate humans. A simple one is created with a triangle made with three posts in a fence line. It creates a 90-degree turn that most livestock or horses cannot maneuver through.

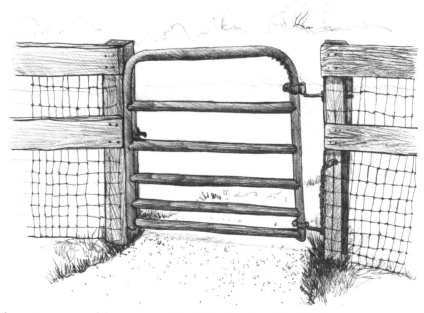

Fig. 9.2 Vertical gaps in gates and fences posts should be less than 3 in (8 cm).

Gates have to be as secure as the adjacent fence. If mesh wire extends to near the ground on the fencing, the mesh on the gate should also do so. If chicken wire is buried on the outside of the fence, it will discourage dogs or other predators from digging underneath if it is also buried on the outside of the gate.

Gates should open only to the inside of the pen or pasture and be located in well-drained areas.

Gates for livestock should be located in a corner of a pen or pasture to help move the animals along the fence line and out the gate. Corner gates are not recommended for horses. Horses congregate around gates. A gate in a corner may thus be a risk for a subordinate horse being trapped in the corner to be bitten or kicked. Therefore, gates for horse enclosures are best located along the fence line, not in a corner. If a gate will be left open at times, it should fold against the fence rather than form an acute angle to trap a horse being chased by another.

Gates to pastures separated by an alleyway should oppose each other and swing open across the alleyway in different directions. When they are opened, the gates can form a channel for animals, usually horses, to move freely from one pasture to the other while still being contained.

Children should not be allowed to swing on gates. Sagging gates become dysfunctional. A short post, called a toe block, at the latching post can be a support for the swinging end of the gate when the gate is closed and aid in preventing sag. Diagonal brace wires from a hinge post to the end or middle of a gate should not be used for horse enclosure gates owing to the risk of a horse's head getting caught in the wire and gate angle. For the same reason, cross braces should not be used on gates because they may trap feet and legs.

Gates should be located 40–60 ft (12–18 m) from a road to permit parking without obstructing the road while opening the gate.

Fence materials

Fence materials for ranch and farm animals include wire strand (barbed wire), electric, woven mesh, rail (including pipe or buck fence), plank, and panel.

Wire strand

The most common farm fencing material in the U.S. is barbed wire. Barbed wire is two or more twisted strands of regular or high-tensile wire with

2–4 wire barbs with sharp points added every 5–6 in (13–15 cm). It can be put up on wood posts or steel T-posts set in the ground 8–20 ft (2.5–6 m) apart.

Barbed wire fencing is relatively inexpensive. It was developed in 1867 by a New York blacksmith, Michael Kelly, for containing cattle. The design was improved by Joseph Glidden. There is now 52 billion miles of barbed wire fence in the U.S. Barbed wire works relatively well for cattle because of their behavior and thick skin. However, barbed wire fencing is unacceptable for any other species. Because of the injuries it can cause to animals other than cattle, it has been called the "devil's rope." A minimum of four wires of 16½ gauge should be used for cattle containment.

Barbed wire fencing is suitable for cattle ONLY.

Barbed wire should never be electrified. An animal caught in barbed wire will struggle violently if also being electrocuted and become severely lacerated. In some states, electrifying barbed wire is illegal. A strain of electrified smooth wire on offset insulators mounted on the pasture side of the fencing can be used to augment a barbed wire fence. This can be particularly helpful if keeping a bull separate from heifers.

High-tensile, smooth-wire fence is 11–14 gauge. High-tension wire is a better choice than barbed wire for cattle, especially if it will be electrified, but high-tension wire is more expensive. Thick wire that is strung tight is an effective barrier without being electrified. High-tension wire requires heavy corner braces for proper stretching and strength to withstand a cow bumping or pushing into the wire. Brace wires for corners should be placed on the outside of the fencing to prevent entrapment of a leg. Tension fences need braces at corners and every 1/8 mile (1.3 km). Standard high-tensile wire has 3–5 strands with posts every 10–12 ft (3.1–3.7 m).

High-tensile, polymer rail (plastic straps) has the appearance of plank fence since it is made with two high-tensile steel wires joined by a 4–6 in (10–15 cm) sheet of vinyl.

Electric

Electric fences have been used since the 1930s and are suitable for all mammalian farm animals. Advantages include relatively low expense, low maintenance, easily modified, little to no skin damage, deterrent to trespassers and predators, and portability, which is useful in subdividing pastures and pasture management. Electric fencing is for enclosing pastures. It is dangerous for animals and handlers if used on small enclosures because of the increased risk of an animal touching it, becoming agitated, and having limited room to move away.

Electric fence consists of a fence charger, conducting line (9–14 gauge smooth wire, rope with copper or steel strands, conducting tape or conducting mesh), and insulators for posts. Insulators prevent a metal post or wet wooden post from shorting out the fence. Fiberglass and plastic fence posts may not need insulators.

Grass and weeds underneath older electric fences should be kept trimmed to prevent shorting out when wet. Modern low-impedance models do not short out from contact with wet vegetation or cause fires during droughts, as older models can. However, vegetation should also be regularly trimmed under newer electric fencing since if vegetation touches it some of the effectiveness of the fence will be drained.

Electric fences use very little electricity. Chargers (also called "controllers" or "energizers") are plug-in, battery, or solar powered. Plug-in chargers are more dependable and less expensive in the long-run than battery-powered units. Solar-powered chargers have the highest initial cost. Under some circumstances solar chargers are adequate, but solar chargers are not as powerful as AC chargers. For the safety of animals and humans, the charger should pulsate at a rate of about once per second.

Chargers need to be grounded using 6–8 ft (1.8–2.5 m) steel or copper rods driven into the ground at least 4 ft (1.2 m), or however deep the constant moisture level is in the soil. Ground rods need to be at least 10 ft (3.1 m) apart and connected by copper wire and at least 50 ft (15 m) away from other ground rods or grounded metal objects, otherwise stray voltage problems may occur. Additional ground rods are needed every 3,000 ft (915 m). If lightning is common, additional ground rods should be placed at least every 150 ft (46 m) to minimize damage to the fence and risk of electric strike reaching livestock. Because livestock have a horizontal posture with four legs on the ground, they are more likely to die from lightning strike than humans. Charger output is measured in pulses of joules. One joule will charge a strand of electric fence 6 miles. Because of their hair coats, animals are better insulated from electric shock than humans.

Ground wires will permit a charge delivered when the ground surface is dry. This is important in droughts, when animals may be trying to feed under a fence after the pastures are depleted. One wire is used for temporary confinement to a grazing area, as in subdividing a pasture. One electric wire is also sufficient as a barrier on the animal containment side to reinforce otherwise weak non-electric fencing. However, one electric reinforcement wire may be ineffective during dry weather due to inadequate grounding.

Multiple wire fences should contain at least three wires with alternating hot (live) wire and ground wires. If four wires are used, the second wire from the top should be the ground wire. If five wires are strung, the second and fourth wire should be grounds. Multiple-wire electric fences can be effective for long distances and in dry areas, and they can help control predators. Electric fences should be marked with public warnings every 200–250 ft (60–75 m). An electric wire 6–8 in (15–20 cm) off the ground can be helpful in stray dog control. At least 5,000 volts on the fence line is required to keep predators out. To deter horses, 2,000–3,000 volts are recommended. Ruminant livestock require 2,000–5,000 volts, and possibly more for bulls.

Standard steel or aluminum wire can be used. Aluminum is rustproof and conducts electricity better than steel, but the conductivity of aluminum is only about 60% of copper, which is the best for conduction. Steel only has 10% of the conductivity of copper. Electric tape adds increased visibility, but tape flutters in the wind and can get weighed down with ice. Fluttering can be reduced by twisting the tape between fence posts. Polyester rope with interwoven copper or steel threads can function both as an electric and a physical containment system.

The number of strands needed for primary fencing should be sufficient to keep livestock from putting their heads between the strands and then getting shocked. The electric shock on their neck may cause them to jump forward, sending them into the fence and destroying it. Only one strand may be sufficient for perimeter fencing or cross fencing. One strand of electric fence can also be used to supplement other fencing, such as inside mesh fencing for horses to prevent the horses from pushing on the mesh to scratch themselves, or along the bottom of a hog fence to prevent hogs from rooting under the fence. An electric stand along the bottom of a fence can also be a deterrent to roaming packs of dogs or wild predators.

Electric fences have the disadvantages of possibly losing power, and the visibility of the wire may be low. However, fladry (strips of fabric) tied to electric strands can enhance the fence's visibility. Electric fencing is not very effective for thickly coated animals or animals in powder snow because of the insulating effect of hair and snow. Barbed wire or mesh wire should never be electrified. The danger of being caught and shocked at the same time could have disastrous results. Lightning is a common cause of electric fence failure. People should never stand by an electric fence in a thunderstorm because of the risk of transmitted lightning strike.

Wire mesh

Wire mesh affords the best protection from escape and from entry of predators other than raptors. Mesh fencing is preferable for small ruminants, poultry, and mares with foals. The size of mesh openings should be appropriate for the species. Cattle mesh, also called field mesh, is often 4 × 4 in (10 × 10 cm) spaces, or larger, and is economical and effective for cattle but the large openings are dangerous for other species. Cattle mesh should only be used to contain cattle.

Mesh may be welded wire or woven. Woven wire mesh is tied in the corners of each space, not spot welded. It is relatively expensive but is the best choice for strength. Woven wire is sold in 20-rod rolls (330 ft [100 m]) made of aluminum or galvanized steel. Vertical wires are called *stay wires* and horizontal wires are *line wires*. A tag with the code 10-47-6-9 means 10 horizontal wires, 47 in (119 cm) tall, 6 in (15 cm) between stay wires, and 9 gauge wire (top and bottom wires are thicker). Adult cattle require 9 gauge wire, and chicken wire is 20 gauge. Horse or ruminant mesh should be woven. It can have square, rectangular, or V-shaped openings. Poultry wire is welded with hexagonal openings. Galvanized wire, which is dipped in hot zinc oxide, is more resistant to rust. All fasteners should be galvanized at class 3, the heaviest galvanized coating. During fence construction, mesh wire should be stapled on the contained animal side of the fence posts. Maintenance should include keeping fence line free of weeds and vines.

Enclosures of mesh fencing should have mesh gates. Mesh gates are safer than tube gates. They are less likely to allow legs to get caught and are necessary to continue the predator control that mesh fences provide.

Chain-link ("cyclone," "hurricane") fence is relatively expensive and is neither welded nor tied at junctions. The wires run vertically and hook around the adjacent wire, creating a diamond pattern. The tube posts and top tube rails of residential chain link fencing are too weak to withstand pressure from large animals. The mesh, peaks of the diamonds, usually project above the top tube railing, which could snag halters, ear tags, neck chains, or other body attachments.

Rail or pipe

Welded steel pipe fence provides the greatest strength and is often used for stallion pens. It is unforgiving if bumped into, and if rail spacing is too wide, a head or leg can become caught. Component pipe fence is galvanized steel with horizontal rail connections that swivel to accommodate changes in terrain and be simple to install, but expensive. Another form of steel rail is interlocking steel pipes that run through holes in wooden posts. Repair of pipe fencing requires welding skills. Aluminum rails are commercially available but may not have sufficient strength for livestock.

Virginia rail fence is zig-zagged rails. Split rail requires chiseled holes in posts to hold horizontal rails. No post holes are required.

A *buck fence*, also called a jackleg fence, is a rail fence. It is used in terrain with frozen, rocky, or soggy ground because post holes do not have to be dug. Four or 5 in (10 or 13 cm) diameter poles are used. The fence supports are 5–8 ft (1.5–2.5 m) poles called "bucks." Two buck posts are joined together in an X-shape. The crossed buck posts are joined by a 10 ft (3 m) horizontal top rail, three to four outside horizontal rails, and one inside (rub pole) horizontal rail (**Figure 9.3**).

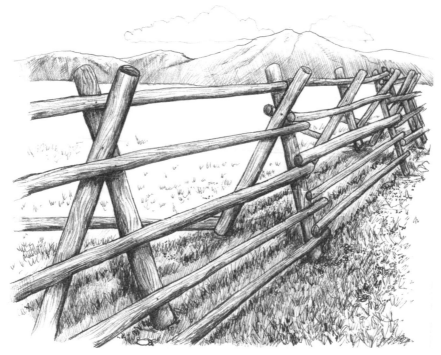

Fig. 9.3 Buck fences do not require posts in the ground.

Plank (board)

Plank fencing can be made of wood or vinyl, or a combination. Wood plank fencing is the most traditional horse fencing in the U.S. It is also the most expensive plank fencing and requires the highest maintenance.

Wood plank is oak or treated pine or poplar. Pressure treatment of soft woods with copper compounds will provide some resistance to rot. The quality of pressure treatment and duration of resistant to rot varies.

Planks are 1–2 in (2.5–5 cm) thick and 4–6 in (10–15 cm) wide. Horses will chew pine planks, and all wood planks have to be repainted on a regular basis. They may bow or crack and break (especially if horses can rub on them), and there is a potential nail hazard. Wood plank fencing often requires use of an electric wire with offset insulators added to the top rail to ensure the horses' respect for the fence. To enhance a wood fence's strength, horizontal poles or planks should span three posts. Therefore, horizontal planks on a fence with posts 8 ft (2.5 m) apart should be 16 ft (5 m) long. Nailed plank ends and middles should alternate going up or down a post. Wood planks should be spaced wide enough to prevent trapping an adult animal's head and small enough to prevent escape of young animals. Nailing a top board flat on top of the posts enhances the fence's stability and reduces chewing damage to the fence. Wood plank fencing can be painted or stained. White paint is most visible at night.

Vinyl (PVC) plank is lower maintenance than wood, but will develop mildew, particularly on the north side, and will have to be power-washed with mildew-removing chemicals. Vinyl plank fence is expensive. Horses that rub on the fence can break or pop the planks out of the posts. If kicked, vinyl planks can break, splinter, and leave sharp edges that are dangerous. An electric barrier wire is generally needed on the inside of the top rail. There is a variety of vinyl fencing, and not all vinyl fencing is strong enough for horses. Hollow plank is not strong enough to withstand pressures that horses exert on fences. Vinyl plank with internal ribs may be strong enough for some horses. Vinyl-clad (polymer-coated) plank is wood plank that has been dipped in vinyl. It is much stronger than hollow or ribbed vinyl plank but can warp with age. Vinyl used for fencing must contain a UV inhibitor, or it will become brittle and crack with exposure to sunlight.

All broken wood or vinyl plank fencing must be repaired immediately, or the enclosed animals removed to another area of containment. Not only is escape possible when planks break, broken planks can become spears that can impale animals.

Concrete can be impregnated with wood colors and poured in molds that produce a surface texture of wood. Concrete plank fence is durable but dangerous to animals that run into it.

Panels

Panels are welded steel rods 8–16 ft (2.5–5 m) long. Their primary advantage is portability. Panels are used for quickly assembled pens for cattle, horses, and hogs. Panel heights vary depending on the intended species: cattle panels are 50 in (127 cm) tall, horse panels are 60 in (152 cm) tall, and hog panels are 34 in (86 cm) tall. Panels are used for equine training pens and for isolation of sick, new, or injured horses. Square openings in the panels should be appropriate for the species. Feedlot panels have shorter height openings as they approach ground level, which reduces the risk of a hoof getting caught or a piglet's head getting through and caught.

Fence posts

Posts can be wood, steel, plastic, fiberglass, stone, or concrete. Steel, fiberglass, and plastic posts are usually driven in the ground. Stone, concrete, vinyl, or vinyl clad must be hand set in dug holes. Wood posts can be driven or hand set. Wood posts set with hydraulic post-hole drivers are the most stable.

Wood posts that resist rot and insect infestation include cedar, cypress, redwood, and pressure-treated pine or fir. Wooden line posts are typically set 8 ft (2.5 m) apart (in straight stretches of level ground up to 15 ft [4.6 m]), are 3 ft (1 m) deep (depending on the locality frost-line), 4 in (10 cm) in circumference, and at least 4½ ft (1.4 m) high. Fence posts in pens should be 5–6 ft (1.5–1.8 m) tall. Posts for high tensile wire or electrified rope can be up to 30 ft (9 m) apart. Posts for corrals or round pens should be 6 ft (1.8 m) apart.

Wood corner and gate posts are typically buried or driven 4 ft (1.2 m) deep or buried one-third of their length, whichever is deeper. They should be at least 8 in (20 cm) in diameter for corner and gate posts, and brace posts should be 5 in (13 cm) in diameter, or greater. Line posts are usually 4 in (10 cm) in diameter. Livestock will chew the edges of square posts if the posts are on the animal's side of the fence. Round posts that are faced or half-round allow a more secure attachment for mesh fencing and are without the edges that the animals can easily chew on.

Steel T-posts for horses should be topped with mushroom-shaped caps to reduce the risk of impalement. Wooden line posts should be used every 50–75 ft (15–22.5 m) of T-posts to keep T-posts from bending if pushed on by cattle or horses.

Species considerations

Horses

Fence materials

Fencing for horses must be easily visible and high enough to discourage attempts to jump it. It must be strong enough so that when horses scratch their rump by pushing and sitting on the fence or leaning into it to get to the "greener grass" on the other side, the gate will not open or the rails pop off. Horse fencing should have some flexibility on impact to reduce the risk of injury from horses running into it in play, fear, or attempted escape from a bully. There should be no vertical openings large enough to entrap a hoof (more than 3 in [8 cm]), and no sharp edges or projections.

> Of the large domestic animals, horses are the hardest on the maintenance of fencing, and poor fencing can be a significant danger to horses.

The best fence types for horses are electric rope, woven wire, pipe, or plank and post. Each has its advantages and disadvantages. Therefore, a horse containment should have more than one type of fence based on their strengths in a particular situation. For example, electric rope works well for pastures for economy and effectiveness, woven wire for smaller enclosures when wanting to keep children and dogs out of enclosures, and pipe or plank and post for smaller enclosures, particularly those needed for stallions. Three strands of electric fence or three planks can be sufficient for mares and geldings, while colts and stallions may need up to five strands or planks.

If horizontal planks are nailed to the outside of a fence, vertical face boards should be nailed over the boards. This extends the connection to the post and significantly increases the strength of the fence when challenged by horses inside the fencing. The space between horizontal planks should be too small for a horse to put its head through sideways and possibly get stuck.

Quiet-mannered adult horses in a closed herd may be contained without incidence in barbed wire, chain link, or high-tensile wire pastures, but all these enclosures are very hazardous for young horses, hot-tempered horses, or herds that may occasionally have new members, or for any horses that are crowded. It is best to avoid barbed wire, chain link, and high-tensile wire in all instances for containing horses, since the type of horse that may be enclosed in the future may change. Barbed wire is the leading cause for lacerations in horses. Cattle mesh is unsatisfactory for horses because the openings are too large, 4 in² (26 cm²) or more, which can catch horses' hooves. Welded wire comes apart when rubbed on or kicked by horses. Chain link can catch horseshoes and halters, and the top edge of the mesh can cut a horse's neck.

Woven wire 2 × 4 in (5 × 10 cm) mesh or diamond-shaped mesh is safe for horses and aids in keeping predators out of enclosures. A sight board or pipe should be used at the top edge of mesh fences to make the fence more visible. Sight boards also deter horses from reaching over and smashing a fence down to graze. The bottom of mesh fencing should be flush with the ground.

Electric fences are particularly effective for horses. Horses have short hair coats and thin skin. Some wear metal shoes. These factors facilitate the effectiveness of electric shock. Unlike with other fences, electric fences are not used as scratching posts and chewing rails for cribbing by horses.

If run into by a panicked horse, electric fences cause few to none of the injuries that are common with other fences. The introduction of a horse new to an electric fence should be supervised. It takes at least 700 volts to get the respect of horses. Because of the short pulse of the charge, it does not cause burns or abnormal heart rhythms. Typically 4,000–5,000 volts are used for horses.

Layout of fences

Horses cannot stand in mud for long periods without developing hoof and leg problems. Horse facilities should have a dry lot (an all-weather or sacrifice paddock) at a well-drained area to allow hooves and pasterns to occasionally dry out in wet weather. There should also be a 12 ft (3.7 m) wide, all-weather lane from stables to turnout areas.

Curved corners in pens, paddocks, and pastures help submissive horses to escape from an attack by another horse. Enclosures with right-angle corners can be blocked with one or two diagonal boards as another means to aid an escape from herd bullies.

Fence height

The height of horse fencing depends on the size of the enclosure and type of horse. Smaller pens or crowded pastures require higher fences. For mares, foals, and geldings, most pens should be at least 5 ft (1.5 m) high. Most pasture fences should be at least 4½ ft (1.3 m) high. Pens should be at least 6 in (15 cm) above withers height. Stallion pens and gates should be 7 ft (2.1 m) high. Horses that are trained or have learned to jump should be kept in 9 ft (2.7 m) high pens. Donkeys should be enclosed with at least 5 ft (1.5 m) fencing since they are able jumpers. A perimeter fence should be as high as the withers of the tallest horse (usually 54–60 in [137–152 cm]).

Stallions

Mature stallions should not be kept on the other side of a single fence from other horses. The pens for other horses should be separate with a distance of at least 12 ft (3.7 m) between the enclosures. To improve stallion behavior when not breeding, stallion pens should have different gates for use when breeding and when being taken out for other reasons. Perimeter fencing is advisable wherever stallions are kept.

Foals

The lowest panel, board, or wire should be 12 in (30.5 cm) or less from the ground if foals are present to prevent them from rolling underneath a fence. Otherwise, the space from ground to the bottom of the lowest horizontal part should be more than 12 in (30.5 cm) to aid in mowing, trimming, and reduction of the risk for adult leg injuries. When electric fence is used, a strand of electrified wire, rope, or tape should be at foal nose level.

Gates

Gates should be 2 in (5 cm) 14-gauge, or stronger, tubular steel. Aluminum gates are not strong enough to withstand the pressures exerted from horses. Gates with diagonal or Z-bars can leave narrow corners that can trap heads and legs and therefore should not be used for horses, nor should support cables. A toe block or gate rest is a block of wood on which the end of the gate rests when fully open and fully closed, reducing the strain on the hinge posts. Gates that open and close with one hand are safer when leading horses and only one hand is free.

Slinky-type spring gates are not appropriate for horse gates because they will catch horses' tails. Bungee-type retractable rope gates are safer.

If on a major road or a residential area, a small (24 × 24 ft [7.3 × 7.3 m]) catch pen should be built to go through to the pasture gate to prevent other horses from escaping when moving horses in or out. When an alleyway exists between pastures and gates are opposite each other and both open into the alleyway, they can become a channel between pastures.

Introduction to new pen or pasture

Handlers should always walk a horse around the inside perimeter of a new pen or pasture in both directions before turning it loose for the first time in that enclosure. If the fence is electric, it should be turned off and fladry should be tied to the top fence strands for increased visibility until the new horse is accustomed to its new surroundings. Water troughs should not be located close to electric fences.

If the current reaches the water by mishap, the horse may get shocked and avoid ever drinking from that trough afterwards. Hay should not be tossed over electric fences. Horses may try to pick pieces off the fence. Pastures for horses should be checked routinely for rocks and animal burrows that could injure horse hoofs or legs. Farm or ranch equipment should not be stored or discarded in horse pastures. Pastures should be inspected for potentially poisonous plants. State Agricultural extension offices can provide information on the identification of poisonous plants common to the region.

Cattle

Pens for cattle should be made of dense wood or metal and be high enough to discourage animals' attempts to jump over the fencing. For cattle, handling pens should be at least 5½ ft (1.7 m) high, and the lowest board should be close enough to the ground to prevent attempted escape underneath. Pressure-treated pine fence posts in pens should be 6–8 in (15–20 cm) in diameter. Osage orange or black locust fence posts, which are stronger than pine posts, may be 4–6 in (10–15 cm) in diameter. A pasture fence should be at least 4 ft (1.2 m) high with the lowest clearance and no more than 1 ft (0.3 m) from the ground to keep calves in and still allow mowing or trimming underneath.

Barbed wire was developed specifically for cattle and is commonly used. At least 4 strands should be used to contain cattle. Wire mesh is better than barbed wire, but more expensive. Wire mesh with square or rectangular openings of 4 in (10 cm) or more should be used only for cattle. High-tensile smooth wire that is not electrified is inadequate since cattle do not respect it and will reach through for vegetation on the other side, eventually breaking the fence down.

Electric wire can be used as a temporary barrier for another type of fence that needs repair or to subdivide pastures for rotational grazing. Electric boundary fence should be 5–6 strands. This will ensure that cattle touching the fence will be shocked on the nose or ears; these areas are sensitive enough to cause cattle to be deterred in challenging the fence.

Cattle panels are welded-mesh wire prefabricated fencing modules that are 52 in (132 cm) high and 16 ft (4.9 m) long. Horizontal wires are closer together at the bottom to prevent calves from catching their head in the fence. Utility panels are 4 × 4 in (10 × 10 cm), extra heavy gauge rod mesh 4–6 ft (1.2–1.8 m) high and 20 ft (6.1 m) long.

Bulls, especially during the breeding season, are most likely to challenge a fence. Some will learn to push down posts. In this case, an electric fence or exceptionally stout fence must be used. If escapes continue, the bull must be sold for slaughter. Electric fences are adequate to contain bulls in large, isolated pastures. At least 2 × 6 in (5 × 15 cm) plank fence with 6 × 6 in (15 × 15 cm) posts every 4 ft (1.2 m) or welded pipe rail fence should be used for bulls contained in small pens or near populated areas and busy roads.

Small ruminants

Pastures for sheep and goats should be woven wire with 4 in (10 cm), or smaller, square openings to prevent them from putting their heads through the fence and getting caught. Supplemental electric strands may be needed in addition to mesh fencing for goats to keep them from climbing out and to serve as an additional deterrent to predators. Temporary fencing can be made with electric wire, cord, tape, or net and step-in plastic or fiberglass posts. Strong soft steel cable with electricity can also be used as temporary fencing. Corner posts for pastures should be at least 6 in (15 cm) in diameter and braced. A barbed wire fence is inappropriate for small ruminants.

Chicken wire can be buried on the outside to discourage dogs from digging under pen fences. One strand of electric wire at the bottom can aid in discouraging predators from entering pastures but be difficult to keep wet vegetation from touching the wire and draining the charge.

Sheep

Pasture fencing should be at least 4 ft (1.2 m) high for sheep. Woven wire is best. Smooth wire electric fencing can be effective if at least 5 strands are used. Training to respect electric fencing requires shearing of the sheep and confining them in a training enclosure with a live strand. Low-tensile aluminum wire will whistle in the wind, making sheep more aware of the boundary. Sheep panels (prefab fence module) are similar to cattle panels, but shorter (34 and 40 in [86.4 and 101.6 cm] high).

Goats

Fencing that is 4 ft (1.2 m) high may be sufficient for adult does, but climbers and jumpers, particularly kid goats, may require fencing to be 6 ft (1.8 m) high, or more. Fencing for bucks should be 5–5½ ft (1.5–1.7 m) high. Goats will climb on sloping braces at fence corners, so braces should be constructed outside the pen or access to the braces blocked. Water troughs in pens with kids should not have more than 14 in (36 cm) of water to reduce the risk of a kid falling or jumping in and drowning. Horned and polled goats should not be penned together.

> Adequate fencing is much more challenging for containing goats than containing sheep.

An exercise mound of dirt should be provided in the center of the enclosure at least 8 ft (2.5 m) way from the fencing. The mound should be 5–6 ft (1.5–1.8 m) high. Exercise yards for goats should be 25 sq ft (2.3 m²) per goat to prevent overcrowding.

The best fence for goats is woven wire with a barrier strand of electric fence on the inside at goat nose height. Horned goats often get their horns caught in large square mesh fencing, becoming susceptible to injury from their struggling, other goats, and predators. Portable electric net fencing is good for moving dehorned adult goats to new areas of containment, but horned goats and kid goats can get caught in the mesh and should not be contained in electric net fencing. Similarly, hay nets should not be used for feeding hay to kids or horned goats.

Smooth wire fencing for goats should have at least 5–7 strands. The lower strands should be 9 in (23 cm) from the ground and 9 in from each other. Higher strands can be up to 12 in (31 cm) apart. Electric fence should have hot lines about 12, 24, and 42 in (30.5, 61, and 107 cm) high.

Trees must be protected from small ruminants, especially goats. Goats prefer to nibble on the tops of plants and low tree limbs. This helps them reduce the risk of ingesting parasite larvae. Goats will learn to walk on their hind legs and eat all the leaves, limbs, and bark as high as they can reach. If the lower limbs are low enough, goats will even climb trees. At least 3 fence posts and mesh wire should be used to create a triangular fence at least 6 in (15 cm) away from the trunk of young trees in a goat enclosure. Sheep do less browsing, concentrating on grass and low weeds, but they will browse taller plants occasionally.

Tethering goats for containment puts them at risk for strangling; injured legs, ears, and eyes; attack by predators; and teasing by malicious adults or children. Kid goats should never be tethered for prolonged containment, and tethered adult goats should never be left alone. Tethering by a lead to a stake or a running tether on a long line can be done for short periods if supervised and protected from predators. Water, shade, and shelter from adverse weather must be provided. Tethering is appropriate for emergency situations and to periodically permit short-term grazing an area that is not enclosed.

South American camelids

Fencing for camelids (llamas and alpacas) should prevent camelids from jumping over a fence, putting their heads through openings, and predators from entering. Although camelids that are well fed, not lonely, or chased by dogs can be contained by 4 ft (1.2 m) fencing; safer fences should be 5 ft (1.5 m) high, 2 × 4 in (5 × 10 cm) mesh, or V-mesh, woven wire. Fences and gates to contain adult male llamas should be at least 5½ ft (1.7 m) high. Barbed wire is dangerous to camelids and should be strictly avoided.

Woven wire should also cover or be incorporated in gates to aid in preventing dogs from harassing or killing camelids and to prevent young camelids (*crias*) from crawling underneath. Horizontal sight boards are not needed, since llamas do not bolt and run into fences as horses will. The visibility of a sight board may entice some llamas to jump a fence.

Seven or more strands of high-tensile, electrified wire can be effective. Gaps between wires should be less than 10 in (25 cm), preferably 3–6 in (8–15 cm), especially if crias are enclosed, to prevent camelids from sticking their heads through the gaps. Ribbon or masking-tape tags should be put on new electric fence to entice camelids to touch the fence with their nose to learn respect for the fence. Touching an electric strand to other parts of their body is not very effective since their hair is a highly effective insulator. If board or rail fencing is used, an electric strand of wire is needed below the lowest rail to discourage dogs from entering the enclosure.

Swine

Swine are the only mammalian livestock in the U.S. commonly kept entirely indoors on concrete. Their movements are very restricted in this environment, more than the allowed movements of any other mammalian livestock. Other options for total indoor confinement on concrete exist (*Table 9.1*).

Indoor confinement on concrete

Without significant modifications, close confinement on concrete is psychologically sterile. Excessive confinement without mental enrichment can lead to stress, mutilation, and cannibalism, such as pigs chewing other pigs' tails off. Chains are often hung in enclosures to replace rooting for mental enrichment, although this is insufficient by itself. Straw bedding for hogs to root and chew provides the best mental enrichment and provides more natural bedding as well. However, straw bedding is more labor intensive and adds to biological waste. Indoor confinement for swine should include regular monitoring of ammonia levels and stereotypic behavior.

Behavior scores that involve percent of time lying, standing, dog-like sitting, and total postural changes can indicate the degree of stress. Frequency of sows sniffing piglets and piglets resting in contact with the sow indicates maternal acceptance and occurs more frequently in sows kept in farrowing pens than in individual crates.

Confinement for hogs should provide reasonable room for normal interactions with other hogs. Open door pens that permit sows to enter and exit freely reduce stereotypic behavior compared with individual crates.

Hoop barns

Hoop barns are tent-like, low-cost housing that are an alternative to total indoor, concrete confinement. Deep bedding with straw is used and natural airflow is provided with hoop barns. They have 4 ft (1.2 m) high sidewalls and are covered by tubular steel arches covered with an opaque UV-resistant polypropylene tarp (**Figure 9.4**). Concrete slabs are provided at feeders and water sources. Hoop barns can hold 75–250 hogs, which fight less than group-raised pigs raised on concrete in close confinement.

Pastures

Pasture fencing for hogs includes woven wire 26–34 in (66–86 cm) tall, attached to wooden or steel posts. If the woven wire is strung 4 in (10 cm) off the ground, a string of barbed wire can be used underneath to discourage rooting the fence up. Two or more strings of barbed wire can be strung above the woven wire to contain hogs predisposed to attempt jump over the fence.

Electric fence is comparatively inexpensive, but it the least secure for containing hogs. Hogs may be trained to respect the fence in a small secure lot. One electric line strung through the pen and near food will ensure that a hog encounters the strand and learns what it is, without a risk of the hog escaping in reaction to touching the electric line. A hog trained this way will not challenge an electric strand of fence again if it is on. If the fence charge is lost, some hogs may soon challenge the fence. A charger for electric fencing for hogs should deliver at least 2,000 volts on the fence line. The lowest strand should be a maximum 6 in (15 cm) from the ground. A total of 3 or more evenly spaced strands should be used, with the highest strand at least as high as the

Table 9.1 **Four common ways to house swine**
• Indoor concrete and/or slatted floor in individual pens
• Indoor concrete and/or slatted floor in group pens
• Hoop barns or sheds with open sides and deep litter flooring for groups
• Free range on pasture with wallows and huts

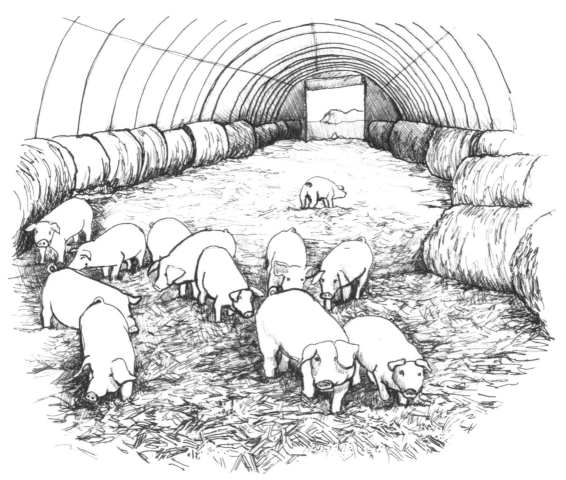

Fig. 9.4 Loose housing of swine in a hoop barn.

tallest hog's nose. More strands and a lower bottom strand are necessary if piglets are to be enclosed in the fencing.

Moveable fencing for hogs is preferable for rotating lots. Electric strands, steel mesh panels, or wooden gates may be used. Electric fences can be 2 strands: 4 in (10 cm) above the ground for pigs up to 80 lb (36.3 kg) and 12 in (30.5 cm) above the ground for pigs weighing more than 80 lb (36 kg). Steel mesh panels for hogs are 34 in (86 cm) high and 16 ft (5 m) long. They can be moved by one person and placed using 5 ft (1.5 m) steel T-posts. The bottom of the fence is most vulnerable. Hogs may root, dig, and lift the fence up to go under it.

Gates in hog pens should be used only for moving hogs in and out. Handlers entering a pen should climb over since hogs can escape with speed and force if the gate is unlatched for a handler to enter.

BARNS, STALLS, AND THREE-SIDED SHEDS

Barns are 4-sided buildings with a roof used to confine livestock. For some species, especially horses, barns are typically subdivided by stalls for individual animal separation. Three-sided (also called *walk-in, run-in, loafing*) sheds provide free access to a pen or pasture and are sufficient protection from the weather in most climates for livestock and horses. They provide some protection from insects, wind, rain, and sunlight.

There should be no protruding nails, bolts, wires, metal edges, or broken boards in barns, stalls, and sheds for livestock or horses. Flooring must be non-slip. If buildings are made of metal, the construction should include nailing the bottom edge of the metal sheets to base boards to prevent a hoof from getting under the bottom edge of metal sheeting. Feeders should be metal or rubber, not plastic. Wood panels inside barn stalls or in 3-sided sheds should be sealed against moisture for cleaning and sanitation.

A 3-sided shed opening should face south or east, away from winter's prevailing winds in North America. Sheds may be stationary or portable. Stationary sheds should be constructed on an elevated base of dirt or built up with crushed stone covered by bedding, and the pad's surface should slope toward the shed's opening to keep the interior dry. The roof should slope toward the back to help keep the entrance drier. If the shed has electricity, wiring should be in a metal conduit to protect it from birds and rodents. The shed should be located away from trees, which might come down in a storm and damage the shelter.

Species needs

Horses

Horses are herd animals that need more fresh air and exercise than any other domestic animal. When confined to a stall environment, they tend to develop undesirable behaviors (weaving and cribbing) and are at a greater risk of respiratory, intestinal (impaction colics), and musculoskeletal problems. Most horses are stalled because of anthropomorphism (treating horses as if they were human), lack of exercise space, protecting the hair coat from bleaching by sunlight, or protecting the mane and tail from traumatic hair loss from horse bites and vegetation, such as burrs and branches.

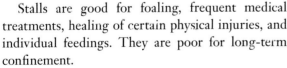

Not all horses need to be stabled, but all horses should not be stabled all the time.

Stalls are good for foaling, frequent medical treatments, healing of certain physical injuries, and individual feedings. They are poor for long-term confinement.

For the average-sized adult horse, stall dimensions should be at least 10 × 10 ft (3 × 3 m), but 12 × 12 ft (3.7 × 3.7 m) is preferable. Being square, they are generally referred to as *box stalls*. The minimum floor space for a donkey is 8 × 8 ft (2.5 × 2.5 m). The ceiling should be a minimum of 9 ft (2.7 m) to prevent head injuries if rearing occurs. Overhead lights should be at least 9 ft high and covered by a wire cage or a jelly jar (thick glass) cover. Preferably, light covers should be sealed against bugs, dust, and water as fire prevention. Stall doors should be at least 4 ft (1.2 m) wide and 7 ft (2.1 m) tall. Latches on doors should be able to be opened with one hand, but unable to be opened by horses. There should be no clutter or structures protruding into an aisle or any other area where horses will be handled or restrained. No halter hooks should be placed on stalls that could scrape, cut, or otherwise injure horses. Stall doors should slide sideways flush with the wall or swing open to the outside for handler safety. Stall doors should never swing into a stall. Horses like to chew wood edges. Wood edges that might be chewed should be protected with metal flashing or corner protection metal. Alleyways inside barns should be at least 10 ft (3 m) wide.

If a horse can kick through a wall, the results can be catastrophic. Horse stalls and 3-sided sheds must be lined with kickboards at least 4 ft (1.2 m) high of rough sawn oak, two layers of ¾ in (1.9 cm) plywood, or ¾ in plywood covered by rubber mats.

Healthy horses are very athletic, but their powerful, quick movements can be extremely dangerous to them and to their handlers if the footing is slick. Flooring should be non-slip such as textured concrete, rubber pavers, or rubber matting.

Many barns with stalls for horses are mistakenly built for human comfort with inadequate air flow for horses. Horses urinate about 2–3 gal (7.5–11.5 L) of urine per day. Hazardous levels of ammonia can be quickly produced that are injurious to horses and handlers' eyes and lungs. Horses expire about 2 gal (7.5 L) of water into the air each day. Condensation can be a problem without adequate ventilation.

Inhalation of dust from hay and bedding can also be a problem in stabled horses. Stables should prevent drafts but allow temperatures near that of the outdoors with an abundance of fresh air exchange. Horses prefer temperatures around 40°F (4.4°C). Heating of stalls is usually unnecessary and can be detrimental to a horse's health. Barns should have at least 8–10 air exchanges per hour (all air completely replaced every 6–7 minutes). Air movement required is about 2 mph, equal to the sensation of a faint breeze. Removal of wet bedding should be done as often as possible or at least twice per day.

If shavings are used, dust-free, kiln-dried pine shavings should be used for bedding. Oak has tannic acid in it that injures hooves. Walnut has oils that can cause laminitis (inflammation and separation of a layer in the hoof). Sawdust will break down and become dust that can irritate the respiratory system, eyes, and frog of the hoof if adequate stall cleaning and ventilation are not provided. If straw is used, wheat straw is preferred for bedding. It drains well and does not dry hooves.

To promote good ventilation, solid stall walls should be avoided. Mesh walls are best for stalls with foals. Fans above stalls, which blow existing stall air around the stall, do not provide good ventilation if used alone. Effective ventilation pulls air through the stall. Dutch doors allow horses to be confined indoors with their head outdoors for fresh air and socialization. Horses may like this so much that their constant leaning on the lower door can weaken the hinges, and so reinforcing boards on brackets are needed. Additional means of providing better ventilation in barns include pot vents, ridge vents, and cupolas.

Grills should be used between stalls or Dutch doors to exercise pens to allow socialization among horses. This is more important for young or insecure horses. Vertical openings between bars or grills should be less than 3 in (7.5 cm). Larger spaces will allow a jaw or hoof to be caught.

As long as other horses are present, tie (also called straight or standing) stalls can be used for short-term confinement. These are slightly wider than the width of a horse (at least 4 ft [1.2 m]), long enough for a manger at the tie ring end (at least 8 ft [2.5 m]), and separated by narrow partitions. As with box stalls, kick boards should be present and 4 ft (1.2 m) tall. Tie stalls are efficient in space and for cleaning time. These work well for temporarily containing horses that are turned out most days. Only gentle horses should be tied in tie stalls, since the handler must ask the horse to move over in order to slip past the horse after tying or before untying the horse in the tie stall.

It is stressful for a horse to be kept alone. Although almost any other animal is beneficial for companionship, a pony, miniature donkey, or goat is usually the best surrogate herd member for a single horse. If kept in stalls, the companion should be in an adjacent stall with bars between the stalls for the horse to be able to see the companion.

Three-sided sheds for horses must be stationary because portable sheds could be easily moved by the strength of horses. The confinement area of a 3-sided shed should be wider than deep to reduce risk of a dominant horse trapping a submissive horse that cannot escape being injured. The open side should be entirely open or, at a minimum, two-thirds open to avoid horses hitting their shoulders trying to get out of the shed. The minimum height for a 3-sided horse shed is 8 ft (2.5 m) and the minimum space is 100 sq ft (9 m²) per horse.

Whenever nails are used for construction or repair, a careful sweep of a magnet on a long handle should be done to retrieve any dropped nails. This is particularly important if using a contractor who is unfamiliar with horses, because such contractors tend to be more careless about leaving nails. They do not know that nails are a common cause of hoof infections and that there is a high risk of tetanus in horses.

Cattle

Adult beef cattle may require housing for protection from cold weather extremes when ill or calving. Otherwise, they cope well with wide ranges of weather as long as the pasture is well maintained and they have access to shade and protection from the wind and hail.

Dairy cattle are provided shelter in barns as free-stall housing (4 × 8 ft [1.2 × 2.5 m] stalls), loose housing (a large area with bedding), stanchion housing (individual stalls with tied or held by head stanchion), or open lots with wind shelters. Free-stall and loose-housing cattle are fed in a separate area. Cattle in stanchion housing and open lots have feed provided at the stanchions or in the lot.

Dairy cattle spend 40–65% of their time lying down. Bedding material for dairy cattle has a major influence on the health of the udder. Bedding provides cushioning when recumbent, helps preserve body heat, and facilitates cleaning. Bedding should not be palatable; otherwise digestive problems from its ingestion may occur.

Calves that will become replacement heifers are separated from the mother cow usually within the first 3 days of life. They are raised in small individual pens with hutches, which resemble large dog houses. The pens are dirt covered with straw. Hutch calves can see, hear, and smell other calves in hutches.

Small ruminants

Goats have a strong dislike of rain and mud. If not given a means of avoiding both, their attempts to escape will be greater. Goat sheds can be a 3-sided walk-in shed on runners so it can be moved like a sled. The walk-in shed should provide at least 15 sq ft (1.4 m²) of space per goat. Sheds should be located with the opening away from the prevailing wind and in a well-drained area. Mature buck goats during the rutting season should be kept in individual pens with an aisle between other bucks.

Ewes and does will often allow their desire to be with a herd to override their need to stay with their newborn lamb or kid. Small stalls called *lambing jugs* (or claiming pens) are beneficial for ewes after they have lambed to bond with their newborn lambs in a safe, clean, and dry area for 1–3 days before rejoining the flock. Pens for does and kids are called *kidding pens*. Strangers and dogs should not be permitted near a lambing jug or kidding pen to prevent unnecessary stress to the mothers. Jugs or pens can also be used as a hospital stall, if carefully cleaned and disinfected after use. They should be 4 × 6 ft (1.2 × 1.8 m), or larger, depending on the size of the breed.

Walk-in sheds are adequate shelter for South American camelids unless the weather is extreme. Although they originate from the Andean Mountains, the winter weather is moderated there by proximity to the equator. Therefore, South American camelids are not capable of tolerating extreme cold and need more complete shelter than a 3-sided shed when the temperature is less than 15°F (−9.4°C).

Swine

Barns for housing swine exclusively indoors on concrete are described in other textbooks. Containment that provides greater environmental diversity for mental stimulation, socialization with other hogs, and relief from standing and lying on concrete better meets the criteria for desirable containment of all species.

> Loose housing with straw bedding for containment is associated with less lameness, abrasions, and stereotypic behaviors in swine than total indoor confinement on concrete.

Lameness is common in stall confined sows on concrete owing to a lack of movement to nourish joints, an inability to maintain muscular tone, and the difficulty handlers have monitoring the sows' ability to move. In Europe, sows are more commonly *loose housed*: group housed in herds of 30–40 hogs per pen, and then fed individually in feeding stalls to prevent fighting over food. Straw bedding is provided for hogs to root and chew. Branches and logs may also be included in pens. Lameness, abrasions, and stereotypic behaviors are less common than in intensive indoor confinement operations. Intensive confinement in gestation stalls has been promoted to decrease inter-aggression among sows by physical separation, but the use of gestation stalls has also prevented selective breeding against aggression in sows.

The best temperature range for swine is 55–85°F (12.8–29.4°C). Hogs do not sweat or pant efficiently to dissipate overheating. They must cool themselves by wallowing in mud or with misting fans. However, they also need to stay dry when sleeping, be able to stay out of drafts, and get away from the mud when eating and other times when desired. Hogs raised outdoors must have sufficient pasture to have access to mud and to get away from it; if in a smaller area, they need slatted wood platforms to escape the mud when required. Hogs on dirt, but without a pond, will root to create a wallow if their snouts are not ringed. Hog-made wallows can be a source of infection and are difficult to manage. Artificial wallows are shallow pools in which hogs can wade, wallow, and cool themselves. The pools are constructed of metal, concrete, or pressure-treated pine. Dry lots for hogs should be sloping to prevent them from becoming exclusively mud lots during rainy seasons. Swine must always have access to shade.

A range hog house is a 3-sided walk-in shed that is on runners so that it can be moved like a sled. Usually there is no floor. Straw bedding is usually provided, although in some areas peanut hulls or wood shavings may be preferred. To provide better wind shelter, the hog house should be 8 ft (2.5 m) wide and 16 ft (4.9 m) long with a roof that slopes from the entrance toward the back. At the highest point, the entrance, the roof should be 5 ft (1.5 m) above the runners. The entrance should face east or south, away from prevailing winds. A-frame houses may be used, but these allow poor access by handlers. Hog houses should be firmly fixed to the ground when in use or reinforced by a low strand of electric wire to prevent hogs from rooting under an edge and lifting the structure.

If sows are in close confinement, farrowing crates are intended to reduce the risk of piglets being crushed or smothered by the sow. Sows are usually put in farrowing crates from one week prior to farrowing until 3–4 weeks after farrowing. The basic crate is 5 ft (1.5 m) wide and 7 ft (2.1 m) long. The middle space for the sow is 2 ft (0.6 m) wide and 7 ft (2.1 m) long with an 8–10 in (20–25 cm) space between the bottom of the inner side panels and the floor to permit piglets to escape from being crushed by the sow. Other operations use pens at least 6 × 8 ft (1.8 × 2.5 m) with guardrails around the edge 6 in (15 cm) from the wall and 8 in (20 cm) from the floor to provide a shelter for piglets to avoid being crushed. A creep area is also provided in one corner to provide additional heat to the piglets. Huts in pastures are an alternative to farrowing crates, but some handlers argue that domestic sows are larger and less nimble than feral sows and crushing is still a problem.

New gilts being added to an established group of sows should be watched for several hours because of the possibility of territorial aggression by the sows. It is safer to bring sows into a gilt pen rather than gilts into a sow pen for first introductions. Spraying sows and gilts with the same odor can help with introductions. Another option is to put them all together in a large pen with extra options for sleeping sheds. Individual feeding should be done in feeding stalls 24 in (61 cm) wide by 72 in (183 cm) deep.

Boars should be kept in pens where they can see and touch noses with sows to socialize the boar and reduce the risk of fighting when the boar is put in the breeding pen.

Gates in hog pens should only be opened for moving hogs in and out. Handlers entering a pen should climb over since hogs can escape with speed and force if the gate is unlatched for a handler to enter. Handlers should step or climb over hog pen fences.

Barn fire hazards

A barn is always a fire hazard owing to the materials it contains and the need for good ventilation for the animals, which in turn can become good ventilation for a fire. Barn fires not only destroy shelter and food for surviving animals, they also cause horrific injuries and death to entrapped animals. The national U.S. standard for fire control involving barns is the National Fire Protection Association (NFPA) 150: Standard on Fire and Life Safety in Animal Housing Facilities.

Smoking

The most important rule in reducing the risk of barn fires is that under no conditions should smoking in or near barns ever be allowed. Service people or construction workers need to be personally warned, because if they were not raised with or now own a barn, they are probably unaware of the extent of the risk. Prominent "No Smoking" signs, fire extinguishers, and a list of emergency numbers for police, fire, and hospitals should be located at all entrances.

Wiring and electrical fixtures

Heat lamps are frequently a source of barn fires, which most frequently occur in winter. All plug ins should be GFIC receptacles, and wiring should be rodent and moisture proof. Use of extension cords should be avoided, and when necessary only outdoor industrial-grade extension cords should be used. Wiring should be protected by metal conduits to keep horses and rodents from chewing into wiring. Service boxes should be in dry dust-free locations and mounted on fire-resistant materials. Electrical appliances should be disconnected when not in use. Light bulbs should be encased in thick glass to prevent contact with cobwebs and being broken by animals in the barn.

> The most common cause for barn fires in the U.S. is heating equipment and electrical wiring.

Electric motors should be dust proof. Box fans do not have encased motors and are intended for low-dust home environments. However, they are frequently used to cool stalls in barns. Box fan cords are not durable, and when used in barns they are often attached to extension cords. Stall fans should have sealed ball bearings, a thermostatic shut-off switch to shut the fan off if overheating, and a UL507-certified motor, safe for outdoor use. Extension cords should not be used.

> The main cause of horse barn fires in summer months is inexpensive box fans.

Hay and other flammables

Damp hay produces gases that are flammable on exposure to air. Barn fires from hay combustion are most likely to occur within the first 2 months after cutting and storing the hay; that is, late fall or early winter. Legume hay is more likely to catch fire than grass hay. The risk of combustion is also increased by bale size (large round bales), tightly bound bales, and high moisture content (more than 20%). Hay with an internal temperature of 150°F (65.6°C) or higher is dangerous.

> Microbes in damp hay can generate enough heat for spontaneous combustion.

Hay should be well dried before storage. Square hay bales should be loosely stacked on their sides on top of pallets to facilitate exposure to air and staying dry. The roof over hay storage should be leak proof. Storage of hay and bedding material in another location rather than the barn containing animals is preferable. Other buildings should be at least 50 ft (15.2 m) from a barn with animals. Hay lofts are particularly dangerous. In addition to quickly spreading a fire, hay storage in lofts above stalls also reduces air quality with dust and decreases ventilation. When in the same building as horses, hay should be surrounded with cinder or concrete blocks and a fireproof door to prevent drafts. Hot shoeing of horses should not be done near hay or bedding.

Electrical sparks can cause fires if dust from hay is dense. Hay dust in the air can be particularly bad if hay is stored in barn lofts. Cobwebs also burn easily and can quickly spread a fire throughout the ceilings. Space heaters can also ignite hay dust or cobwebs easily.

All gasoline motor vehicles produce sparks and should not be stored in a barn with animals. Gasoline-powered equipment, gasoline and kerosene cans, paint, and fertilizers should be stored in another building. Small flammables, such as grooming aids and insecticides, should be stored in a fire-resistant box within the barn. Oily rags, especially those with linseed oil, should be removed immediately after use and placed in a metal can. Compost piles should be kept as far away from a barn as feasible since they can generate enough heat to ignite combustible materials. Lightning rods should be placed on animal barns.

Extinguishing fires

Sprinkler systems in barns are a highly effective means of controlling or extinguishing fires, but owing to their expense, they are infrequently used. Planning for the risk of fire should include easy access for fire trucks and an adequate water source that is outside the barn. Fire extinguishers should be 10 lb (4.5 kg), ABC (A = wood, paper, plastic; B = liquids; C = electrical fires) or better. Fire extinguishers and flashlights are best placed at each entrance, the feed room, and the tack room.

Evacuation

If a fire begins in a horse barn, a handler has less than 10 minutes to get the horses out. Horses that escape could still have permanent lung damage from smoke inhalation. Evacuation is easier if each stall has two exits, an inner isle door and an exterior door to a run or paddock.

If horses are present, non-nylon halters and lead lines should be kept in a prominent location with battery-powered emergency lights or fluorescent markings for fire fighters to easily find. Nylon halters can catch fire, melt, and burn the horse's face.

Anyone who has access to the barn should be aware of the appropriate actions in case of fire. Doors to the outside should slide easily and completely open or they should swing open to the outside. Halters with leads should be within easy reach of the stall door. If halters are not easily available, a handler should use anything that can be put around the horse's neck near its head to lead it out, such as a rope, belt, or electric cord. When stalls are connected to outside runs or pens, the runs or pens should have outside exit gates to permit rescue without going through a burning barn. If the horse freezes up, the handler should try to back it toward an exit or create an improvised blindfold using a coat or shirt.

Once outside, rescued horses must be restrained by tying, holding the lead rope, or be in a secure containment. They should never be turned loose and never left alone while the barn is burning.

> Loose horses panicked by a barn fire may run back into the fire seeking the security of their usual environment.

Occasional fire drills should be run to acquaint everyone with ideal procedures. Where to contain the animals if a barn is on fire and after it is gone out should be determined in advance. An outside enclosure should be designated to confine animals during a barn fire. Shelter from weather may be important since most barn fires occur in winter.

POULTRY CAGES, AVIARIES, AND FREE RANGES

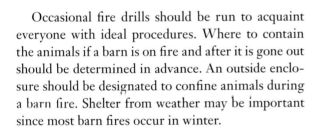

> The AVMA policy on Layer Hen Housing Systems states that "housing systems should provide for expression of important natural behaviors, protect hens from disease, injury, and predation, and promote food safety. Participation in a nationally recognized third-party audited welfare program is strongly advised."

Poultry, excluding ratites (emus, ostriches) and water-fowl, are generally housed in sheds with solid floors, in slat or wire mesh-bottomed cages, or in small group cages. Commercial chicken houses are cage housing because more chickens can be maintained with less land cost and labor involved. About 90% of layer hens in the U.S. are in cage systems, but there is a growing market trend toward cage-free eggs. International regulations have begun to restrict the use of cage housing on the grounds that the confinement is extreme and cannot be considered humane. Proponents of cage systems for their part stress the protection from selected diseases, limiting pecking injuries to only those birds within the cage, and the litter-free air quality.

Poultry housing quality should be based on the incidence of lameness, feather condition, frequency and severity of wounds, number of soiled birds, and ammonia levels. Housing should provide natural behaviors and reduce the risk of diseases, injuries, and attack by predators.

Conventional cages

Conventional cages are wire cages about the size of a filing cabinet drawer, called a *battery cage*, in which 3–8 hens live, but cannot dust bathe, walk, perch, or forage. The arrangement of cages is similar to the cells in a battery. Each bird is allowed 67 in^2 (432 cm^2) of space. In addition, they are prohibited or inhibited from flapping their wings, stretching their wings out, shaking their body, or wagging their tail. Some wire floors can cause foot damage. These have a reduced space and labor economic advantage at the expense of prohibiting natural behavior, decreasing normal bone strength, and causing stereotypic behaviors. Cage-free systems include sawdust-covered floor, a roosting area, and private nesting boxes.

Close confinement can be one cause for cannibalism, pecking injuries, and failure to eat or drink. Combs and wattles in chickens and snoods in turkeys are more at risk of injury when in close confinement or without environmental enrichment. The injuries can lead to being pecked by other birds. To eliminate that risk in close confinement operations, the comb is amputated (*dubbed*) and the two wattles are amputated (*dewattled*). In turkeys, the snood is amputated (*desnooded*).

Debeaking (partial amputation of the end of the beak) is performed on all poultry being closely confined to help control cannibalism. One-third of the upper beak is amputated in broilers, and one-half of the upper beak is removed in turkeys. Debeaking prevents birds from being able to perform the natural foraging behavior of pecking on the ground or on a floor surface.

Enriched or furnished housing

Enriched housing provides more room for behavior enrichment and may include perches, nest boxes, and scratch areas. Up to 60 birds may be housed together. Perching is a natural behavior for poultry and strengthens bones and muscles in their legs and feet. Perches strengthen leg bones, reduce pecking by more dominant hens, and reduce or eliminate breast blisters, which are caused by lying on bedding wet with urine. Litter permits the natural behavior of dust bathing and improves feather condition. It also provides an opportunity for foraging, which reduces pecking injuries. Mortality is lowest in poultry housed in enriched housing.

Nesting is a natural behavior of laying hens. Nests can be individual nests or community nests for four hens. Individual nests for hens should be 1 sq ft (0.09 m²) and 1 ft (0.3 m) high. Nests should be positioned about 2 ft (0.6 m) above the floor and have a landing board below the entrance to facilitate access to the nest. Partially covering the entrance to the nest by about two-thirds with a cloth flap will encourage birds to enter. Wire cages (1 × 2 in [2.5 × 5 cm] welded wire mesh) inside hen houses can be used in mild climates. Wire cages are typically 12 in (30.5 cm) wide, 18 in (46 cm) deep, and 16 in (41 cm) high.

Barn or aviary

Poultry barns are cage-free buildings where birds are kept on the floor with access to litter and nest boxes. An aviary is a barn with multi-tiered perches or platforms.

Free range and backyard housing

Free range is used primarily for broilers/fryers and roaster chickens. It provides housing for protection from sun and wind with access to an outdoor pen or pasture during the day.

Commercial free-range operations require one acre of range for 400–500 pullets. Range rearing is for warm weather months. Protection from the sun and wind is provided with a skid shed with a slanted roof that is moved occasionally.

Small flocks can be kept in a backyard housing. Chickens are highly social. At least 3 should be housed together. A minimum of 2–3 sq ft (0.2–0.3 m²) per chicken is needed in a coop (**Figure 9.5**).

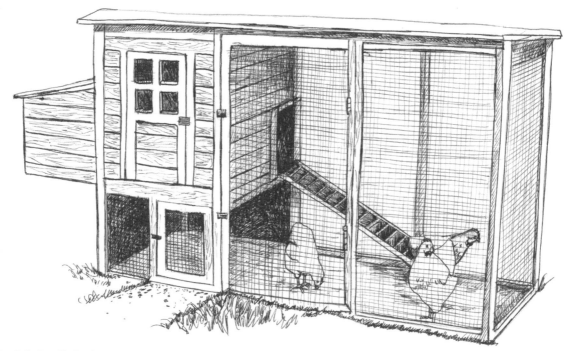

Fig. 9.5 Small chicken coup with nesting boxes, roosts, perches, and access to ground to pick and dust bathe.

Backyard coops should provide predator-proof fencing, straw bedding, a roost or elevated slatted floor, perches, nest boxes, and accessibility to dirt for dust bathing. At least 2 nesting boxes should be provided for 4 or 5 hens. The interior should be easy to clean. Supplemental heating may be necessary in winter.

Runs should have a roof to protect chickens from wild bird droppings and predators. They should provide space that is at least 4 sq ft (0.4 m²) per chicken. Small laying flocks and turkeys often have roosts or perches. Roosts may be built over wire and dropping pits, or they may be over a dropping board, which requires periodic cleaning. Roosts can injure the breasts of broilers/fryers, roasters, capons, and heavyweight breed turkeys, and so they should not be used for these birds.

Roosts are used for sleeping. A roost in a chicken coop should be as high as possible while still allowing head room for the chicken. In addition, roosts provide an area for birds to group without piling onto each other. Roosting keeps birds off the ground and out of their feces.

Poultry with outdoor access have to be secured away from attacks by dogs, cats, coyotes, skunks, weasels, foxes, owls, and raccoons, especially at night. Hawks are daytime predators of poultry. An electric wire a few inches above the ground or mesh fence extending below the ground level can help protect against predators that cannot fly. Buried mesh fencing should be curved toward the outside of the enclosure and backfilled with rocks or stone. Mesh should be attached by screws and washers, not staples. Raccoons can pull staples out.

Other poultry

Turkeys

Turkey poults up to 8 weeks of age each need 1 sq ft (0.09 m²) of floor space in brooder houses. From 8–12 weeks of age, they should have 2 sq ft (0.2 m²) for each bird. Adult turkeys should have at least 3 sq ft (0.3 m²) for hens and at least 5 sq ft (0.5 m²) for toms.

Lightweight breed turkeys can be kept on wire or slatted porches. Heavyweight breed turkeys will injure their breasts and feet and should be raised in paved or gravel yards. Community nests for five birds is acceptable.

Ducks

By 7 weeks of age, ducklings should have 2.5 sq ft (0.2 m²) and adult ducks 6 sq ft (0.6 m²) per bird in indoor confinement, and less (3 sq ft [0.3 m²] per bird) in a yard. Ducks should be housed in divided groups of three to reduce fighting.

Geese

Geese need 5 sq ft (0.5 m²) per goose if in housing with access to a yard. The yard should provide up to 40 sq ft (3.7 m²) per goose. Community nests for 3–5 breeders is sufficient.

Although adult geese can protect themselves against predators smaller than a coyote, goose eggs and goslings are susceptible to attack by raccoons and skunks and should be kept in 6 ft (1.8 m) high fine mesh fencing to keep out predators.

Ratites

Pairs or trios of ratites require about 1 acre of enclosure. Woven wire 2 × 4 in (5 × 10 cm) mesh fencing at least 5 ft high is recommended. Electrified (hot) wires should be on the outside bottom of the fence to keep predators out.

High-tensile wire at least 6 ft (1.8 m) high is also safe and effective if a minimum of 15 strands of wire is used, starting with 4 in (10 cm) off the ground and every 4 in (10 cm) for 4 ft (1.2 m) and then every 8 in (20 cm) for the top 2 ft (0.6 m). Electrified wires should be placed outside the fence to discourage predators from entering. Since feathers are poor conductors of electricity, hot wires have relatively little effect on poultry.

Chain link is not advisable as it can result in caught toe injuries. Neighboring groups should be visible. Alleyways between ratite pens are beneficial for moving birds to different pens. Three-sided sheds should be provided for protection from weather extremes; however, ratites rarely seek shelter after they are 6 months old.

INDUSTRIAL FARM ANIMAL PRODUCTION

In stark contrast to what is otherwise considered minimum space and environmental enrichments essential for other domesticated animals, chickens in battery cages, bull calves in veal crates, and sows in gestation crates are confined with little movement possible, and natural behavior is not possible for prolonged periods. These confinement situations are associated with a greater incidence of tail-biting and cannibalism in sows, tongue rolling and sucking objects in calves, and feather pecking in poultry. Lameness is more common because the lack of movement impairs normal nutrition of joints, and less variety of weight-bearing stresses weakens bone strength. Industrial farm animal production is geared toward only a few selected breeds, which weakens the genetic diversity of the species and risks creating one breed that could have unusual susceptibility to diseases. A perfect alternative does not exist, though. Free-range confinement requires greater land use and has higher risks of predation, parasite transmission, and flystrike.

Industrial farm animal production, also called concentrated animal feeding operations (CAFOs) and factory farming, was created to meet economic interests with inadequate regard to the five basic needs (freedoms) of animals. Extreme confinement of food-producing animals began with battery cages for chickens during the Great Depression as a lower-cost means of producing eggs. Gestation cages for sows were introduced in the 1960s as a lower-cost method to meet the growing demand for pork products in rapidly developing Asian countries. Battery cages and gestation crates are prime examples of industrial confinement that are considered unacceptable for housing any other birds or other mammals, including zoo animals, research animals, working animals, and pets.

Veal crates are small stalls for bull calves that will not be used for breeding. Crates for veal calves are labor- and cost-saving, but not all veal production is as restrictive as crates. Restricting movement of calves results in softer, paler veal meat. Veal crates are 2–2½ ft (0.6–0.8 m) wide, and calves are tied to the front of the crate. The floor is slatted or slanted to reduce the calf's contact with urine and manure. Calves are kept in isolation until slaughter around 16 weeks of age, without physical contact with other calves and often without visual contact. At least eight states have banned veal crates, and the American Veal Association has encouraged the elimination of veal crates.

Gestation crates are 7 × 2 ft (2.1 × 0.6 m) metal enclosures that pregnant sows weighing 300–600 lbs (136–272 kg) are confined in throughout their pregnancies. The typical sow will have on average 2.5 litters per year for 3–4 years, spending most of that time in gestation crates. Larger sows do not have room to lie on their sides and must rest on their chests. The floors are slatted to allow urine and feces to fall away into a pit. Gestation crates are illegal in at least eight states in the U.S., Sweden, and the United Kingdom. More than eight grocery, restaurant, and food service chains in the U.S. have announced plans to eliminate swine operations that use gestation crates from their supply chains.

The supposed need for gestation crates is to prevent fighting among pregnant sows, although the risk can be controlled by preventing overcrowding, providing an opportunity to root (straw bedding), and avoiding mixing new sows into an established social group. However, the alternative of either turnout stalls or group housing risks potential inter-sow aggression and environmental stresses.

The American Veterinary Medical Association's current policy on sow housing states that "sows should be provided with adequate quality and quantity of space that allows sows to assume normal postures and express normal patterns of behavior."

Cages for laying hens were introduced into the U.S. in 1931 to prevent diseases acquired from contact with dirt, to increase the efficiency of handlers, and to reduce the cost of containment through reducing the space for each bird. By 1990, 95% of all egg production in the U.S. involved battery cages. Battery cages provide insufficient space to hunt and peck for food, dust bathe, flap wings, perch, or nest. Advantages of battery cages are protection from predators, avoidance of disease vectors, and shelter from temperature extremes. Decreased aggression is often cited as an advantage of battery cage conditions, but the concurrent debeaking, restricted ability to move, and reduced lighting in battery conditions are the primary reasons that aggression to other birds is decreased. Poultry battery cages were banned in California in 2008 and Europe in 2012. The McDonalds Corporation is the largest egg buyer in the U.S. It will phase in cage-free eggs with a goal of being totally cage-free by 2025.

Between 2005 and 2008, the Pew Commission on Industrial Farm Animal Production examined how animal agriculture affects human health, animal health, the environment, and rural communities. Commissioners represented the fields of veterinary medicine, agriculture, public health, business, government, rural advocacy, and animal welfare. The commission held public meetings across the country and published several technical reports. Among the findings were "animal welfare problems, mainly as a result of the extremely close quarters in which the animals are housed."

In 2008, the Pew Charitable Trusts Commission on Industrial Farm Animal Production and John Hopkins University Bloomberg School of Public Health recommended phasing out gestation stalls and battery cages within 10 years.

SELECTED FURTHER READING

AVMA (2012). *Welfare Implications of Laying Hen Housing.* Literature Review, January 26.

Ehringer G (1995). *Roofs and Rails.* Western Horseman, Inc., Colorado Spring.

Hill C (2005). *Horsekeeping on a Small Acreage: Designing and Managing Your Equine Facilities*, 2nd edition. Storey Publishing. North Adams.

Humane Society of the United States (2005). *Making Your Horse Barn Fire Safe.* HSUS, Washington.

CHAPTER 10

ROPES, KNOTS, AND HITCHES

Ropes are essential tools for working safely with animals, particularly livestock and horses. They can save a handler's life or endanger it depending on the skill exercised in using them.

Egyptians began using ropes and simple knots to handle animals at least 6,000 years ago. Now, there are approximately 4,000 knots recorded, most of which were developed by sailors.

A famous knot in mythology was the Gordian Knot. Gordius was a peasant who became an ancient king of Phrygia, a part of the current nation of Turkey. He tied the yoke of his ox cart to a pole with a knot that no one could untie. Whoever could undo the knot was said to be destined to become ruler of all of Asia. When Alexander the Great came to Phrygia in 333 B.C. and saw the knot, he severed it with his sword. By the age of 30, Alexander ruled Asia.

"Cutting the Gordian Knot" is a phrase that means quick to make a decision in a difficult situation. Good animal handlers must, on occasion, cut the Gordian Knot, figuratively and literally. Quick knot cutting in an emergency is vital when animals become bound in ropes and struggle. All good handlers who use ropes carry a sharp, easily accessible knife for this purpose.

TERMINOLOGY AND ROPE CONSTRUCTION

Definition of terms

Ropes are more than $\frac{5}{12}$ in (1 cm) in diameter. Smaller fiber diameters are referred to as cord twine, string, or thread. Ropes are made of natural fiber or synthetic fibers. A rope that is used to handle or restraint livestock and horses is called a *lariat*. A lariat may have a running noose for catching animals or no noose for tying (tethering, picketing) animals.

Natural fiber rope

Among natural fibers, *manila* and *hemp* are the strongest plant fibers for ropes. Hemp is smoother than manila and derives from the stalk of *Cannabis sativa*, a non-drug species of the marijuana family. Hemp is the oldest rope fiber, but its use declined approximately 200 years ago because of the preference for the stronger manila rope. Until World War II, manila rope, from the leaves of *Musa textilis*, a member of the banana family, was widely used. Synthetic fiber ropes became common after WWII. Most manila rope came from the Philippines, and it derives its name from the capital of that country. Cotton and flax (both soft) are more manageable but will stretch and rot. Cotton continues to be widely used for lead ropes and is the preferred type of rope for restraining animals' legs.

Jute and sisal are less expensive, weaker plant fibers. Jute and sisal are natural fibers more commonly used for making twine. Jute is from *Corchorus* plants and sisal is from the leaves of *Agave sisalana*.

Leather was used by Spanish and Mexican vaqueros, who plaited 4–12 strands of leather into ⅜ in (0.95 cm) diameter rope called a *reata* (riata is an Americanized spelling of reata) of 50–65 ft (15–20 m) in length. The average nylon rope for catching cattle is 30–40 ft (9–12 m) long. Leather reatas are strong, flexible, and thin but with sufficient weight for long throwing. However, they require frequent treatment with tallow to prevent sunlight or water damage. They are also about 10 times more expensive than other ropes. The word *lasso* comes from the Spanish word "lazo" meaning noose or snare.

Maguey ropes are hand-made 4-stranded ropes, ⅜ in (0.95 cm) in diameter made from fibers of the maguey plant of Mexico. These have a smooth surface and are relatively firm, which aids in forming loops. They are the preferred rope of Mexican charros. The use of natural fiber ropes (made from hemp, abaca, or yucca plants) spread from Mexico northwards. Reatas and maguey ropes should be dallied (wrapped around an object) rather than tied owing to the risk of breaking if jerked with much weight.

The advantages of natural fiber ropes are a hairy-like rough surface that provides better traction and easier grip. Horses may respect the roughness (fiber ends that stick out are called "staples") more than smooth, soft ropes. Mecates are vaquero (Spanish-style) reins for training horses that were originally made of horsehair for its strength and prickliness. The disadvantages of natural fiber ropes are that they absorb water and swell, making knots difficult to untie. They can support mildew and rot, and they become brittle from strong sunlight or salt.

Natural fiber rope is always *twisted* (also called *laid*) to increase strength from alternate twisting ("laying up") of components. Prior to World War II, all rope was twisted. Fibers are twisted commonly to the right to form yarn. Three yarns are twisted to the left to form strands. Three strands are twisted to the right to form the rope. Rope with strands twisted to the right are Z-laid; S-laid is twisted to the left. Ropes have 8–22 twists per foot. Hard-twisted rope has more twists per foot and is stiffer. Three-stranded rope is plain, also called hawser-laid rope. More than 3 strands in a rope is weaker than 3 strands of the same diameter. Four-stranded rope is smoother than 3-stranded rope but harder to grip. Synthetic fiber rope is occasionally twisted. Twisted rope, with its lumpy surface, holds knots and hitches better than single-cord rope. A *splice* is interweaving sections of untwisted rope. Twisted rope can be untwisted in sections to form a loop on an end of a rope with an eye splice or to join two ropes together by a short splice of the end of each rope.

One of the disadvantages of twisted rope is that there is no protective outside layer. Every fiber twists to the outside multiple times and so is exposed to abrasion, moisture, and sunlight.

Synthetic fiber rope

Synthetic ropes vary in material and in strength (*Table 10.1*). However, because synthetic rope is generally made of continuous fibers that run the length of the rope, synthetic ropes are stronger than natural fiber ropes, which are composed of short fibers that do not extend the length of the rope. Most ranch ropes are a nylon–polyester combination for strength with

Table 10.1 **Synthetic fiber types and relative strength, in decreasing order of strength**
• Nylon (polyamide) – strongest and very elastic, but absorbs water
• Polyester – less elastic, more UV resistant, resistant to water
• Polypropylene – weaker, susceptible to UV damage, and can melt with heat from friction

moderate elasticity in a twisted pattern. Synthetic ropes are lighter, stronger, and less expensive than natural fiber ropes. In addition, they do not rot or become brittle. The disadvantages of synthetic fiber ropes are that heat, even friction, can cause them to melt, and their smoothness can cause hand grips and knots to slip.

Synthetic fiber ropes are constructed in a variety of patterns. They may be twisted, as with natural fiber ropes, *plaited* in 4–8 stranded solid plaits, or *braided* in 16 or more strands (the *mantle*) around a core of long twisted center fibers (the *kern*) (**Figures 10.1** and **10.2**). The mantle of braided rope protects the inner fibers,

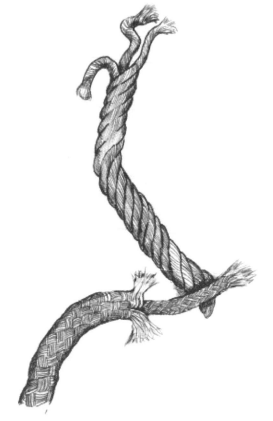

Fig. 10.1 Twisted rope (above) and braided rope (below), which show mantle and kern.

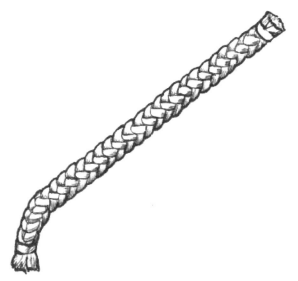

Fig. 10.2 Plaited rope.

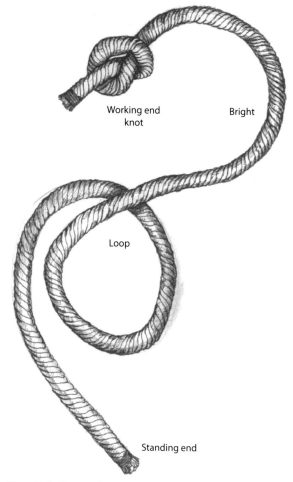

Fig. 10.3 Parts of a rope.

while all fibers of twisted or plaited rope are exposed to the elements. Braided synthetic rope is soft, strong, and flexible with various uses, including mountain climbing. Plaited and braided ropes do not hold knots and hitches as well as twisted rope.

The Shoof Vet-Rope is a marine-grade polyester, oval-shaped rope that is woven with a hollow center, which causes it to flatten with tension. It is made in New Zealand. The Shoof rope is used for leg restraint of large animals and permits greater comfort to the animal and the handler, but its construction also allows it to stretch more than conventional twisted rope, which can be disadvantageous in some restraints.

Rope parts

Ropes have a *working end*, *standing part*, and *standing end*. A 180-degree bend in a rope is called a *bight*. A circular bend is a *loop* (**Figure 10.3**).

A sliding loop (noose) can be made with a knot, called a *honda*, that forms a small fixed loop or channel for the rope's standing end to slide through. Hondas made with the rope may have a small leather wrap called a "burner" around the honda loop to reduce friction as the slip loop slides through. Hondas may also be metal (aluminum or stainless steel) or plastic. Metal hondas allow the rope to slip back and forth more easily to provide immediate pressure release when an animal stops resisting restraint. Metal hondas are also more reliable in wet conditions. Tied hondas may have a metal lining inside the tied loop

to permit better sliding, similar to a complete metal honda. Hondas may have a swivel base or be designed to allow breakaway for roping practice. If a honda is to be used around the neck of a horse, a double-overhand knot can be tied in the rope (2 ft [0.6 m] from the honda for 2-year-olds and 18 in [46 cm] for weanlings and yearlings) to prevent the loop from completely closing and squeezing the neck of young horses.

A quick release honda is a metal honda that can be opened to release a caught animal without the need to loosen the slip loop (**Figure 10.4**). Quick-release hondas have a finger latch to quickly open the metal honda. The finger latch has a hole in it so that a leather string can be grabbed to open the latch rather than putting a finger in the honda and endangering that finger if the animal moves while the finger is entrapped (**Figure 10.5**).

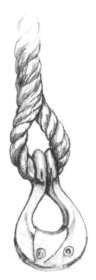

Fig. 10.4 Quick-release honda.

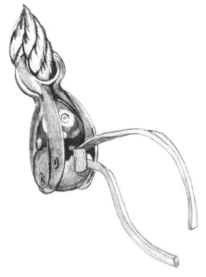

Fig. 10.5 Leather tether for opening the honda latch.

EQUIPMENT MAINTENANCE

Stabilizing the ends of ropes

The ends of ropes will fray or unravel if not fixed. A *stopper knot*, such as an overhand, figure 8, or blood knot (a multiple-wrapped overhand knot) can prevent unraveling and create a knob at the end of a rope. A stopper knot can also reduce the chance of the rope being pulled and running through a handler's grip. However, an end knot can be an impediment to tying other knots or hitches.

Unraveling the end of a twisted rope a short distance allows the strands to be interwoven back (back spliced) on the rope end to form a *crown knot*. A crown knot doubles the diameter of the rope but does not create an obstructive "knob" to the same degree as an overhand or figure 8 knot.

To create smooth ends on a twisted rope, they may be whipped, dipped, back spliced, or melted (if synthetic). Wrapping a section of rope with electrician's or duct tape, then cutting through the tape and rope together with a sharp knife, prevents the ends from unraveling until a more permanent means of fixing the ends is applied. The ends of twisted ropes can be wrapped (*whipped*) with string hiding the ends of the string underneath the wrapping (**Figure 10.6**). Natural fiber string should be used to whip natural fiber ropes, and synthetic string used to whip synthetic ropes.

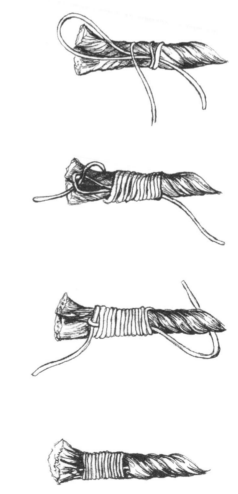

Fig. 10.6 Whipping a twisted rope end.

Nylon and polypropylene twisted, plaited, or braided ropes can be burned on the end to melt the fibers together by open flame, hot irons, or hot plates. If not melted evenly and carefully, rough or sharp strands may develop and be dangerous to the handler's hands.

Some twisted ropes are prevented from unraveling by bending a band or ring of metal, a ferrule, around the end. Ferruled ropes should not be used for animal restraint because of the risk to the animal or handler of the metal developing sharp edges. Dipping rope ends into lacquers and similar liquids that dry into a hard encasement also produces a surface that can be hazardous. Dipped end ropes should also not be used for animal restraint.

Storing ropes

Ropes not in use should be stored properly. Softer, twisted ropes are coiled, and then the coil is collapsed and tied. This is called *hanking* a rope (**Figure 10.7**). Hanked ropes prevent tangling when releasing the coil.

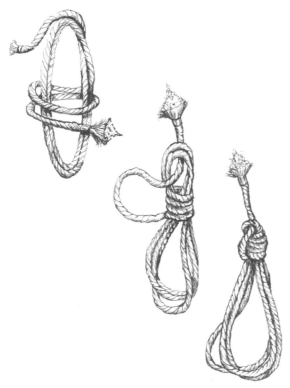

Fig. 10.7 Hanking a rope for storage.

Lariats are stiff and need to maintain their curve. These are coiled and stored as circular coils, not hanked. Ropes with strands twisted to the right (Z-twisted) need to be coiled in a clockwise direction. Valuable lariats are stored in rope cans.

Ropes cannot be sanitized, but they should be rinsed thoroughly after use, dried with a towel, and stretched out to dry before being hanked or coiled.

When hung up for storage, ropes and leather restraints should never be hung over a thin peg or nail, as this would cause a sharp bend and weaken the fibers. When hanging hanked ropes, the rope should be hung over a tack knob, a 2–4 in (5–10 cm) diameter hanger.

Leather quality and care

Leather is tanned animal skin. Most leather in the U.S. comes from cattle hide. Thick, strong leather for safe tack comes from steers with high-quality hide, not heifers, and is vegetable tanned.

Tanning makes leather more durable, pliable, and resistant to wear and rot. The most common methods of tanning are vegetable tanning and chrome tanning. Vegetable tanning produces leather that is non-corrosive to metal and non-irritating to the skin, can be carved or molded, and is strong, if thick. Vegetable tanning is used for saddle and other tack construction. The Hermann Oak Leather Company, founded in 1881, in St. Louis, Missouri, is the leading vegetable-tanned leather manufacturer in the U.S. Hermann Oak tans only steer hides.

Chrome tanning is less time-consuming and less expensive than vegetable tanning and more commonly used. It produces leather that is soft, pliable, and strong when thin. It is often used for making leather clothes. Most chrome tanning is now done in Mexico and Argentina.

Well-tanned quality leather can last generations if treated properly. It should not be constantly stretched, repeatedly soaked with water, or allowed to dry out. Leather can be shaped by wetting it to create the desired shape, but must be dried slowly with gentle ventilation. It should not be heated during the drying process.

Leather should be moisturized one to four times per year with oil, usually a variable combination of lanolin or neatsfoot oil, mink oil, cedar oil, beeswax, and a petroleum-based solvent, with beeswax then added to the surface. This lubricates the internal fibers and inhibits drying and becoming brittle. The frequency should be more often if exposed to moisture, drying, or dust.

Leather should be cleaned with a damp cloth as often as needed based on its use. Abrasion can wear the external surface of leather and small particles of grit ground into the leather can abrade internal fibers.

Leather should never be stored in a plastic bag, where it would likely mold. Exposure to extreme heat and very low or high humidity should be avoided. Exposure to air and gentle ventilation reduces the risk of mildew. Leather should not needlessly be exposed to sunlight. It should be stored in the shade or indoors when not in use.

Cleaning ropes

Animal-handling ropes cannot be sanitized, but with basic cleanliness, the same rope may be used on many healthy appearing animals with little risk of transmitting disease. Keeping ropes clean not only reduces the risk of transmitting disease but can also remove sand and other abrasives or chemicals that can break down the rope fibers.

Urine, manure, and saliva should be rinsed from natural fiber ropes with just water. The uncoiled damp rope should be laid over hay bales or tied between two objects to dry on all sides of the rope before recoiling or hanking. Synthetic fiber ropes can be washed with water and a mild soap, and then thoroughly rinsed. Synthetic fiber ropes should be air dried uncoiled, as with natural fiber ropes, before they are coiled for storage.

EQUIPMENT SAFETY

Whenever ropes are used to handle or restrain large animals, the handler should never allow a rope attached to the animal to become wound around his or her hand, arm, or leg. When tying an animal by a halter, if the tail of the lead rope is long enough to be a hazard, a *daisy chain* (chain sinnet, monkey braid) can be tied to shorten the length of the lead rope. Daisy chains are formed with a series of loops and bights.

All handling equipment should be reinspected for weaknesses that might cause breakage before each use. When using a hitch, the object tied to should be strong enough to withstand an animal pulling against it with all its force. Lead snaps are often die-cast, created in molds that permit air to be entrapped in the metal, often zinc, which weakens it. Steel or iron snaps are more reliable.

A sharp knife should always be carried by animal handlers who use ropes to free entangled animals, an assistant, or the handler. In addition, quick release hitches can be pulled tight enough by a horse that the hitch cannot be untied. The knife should be retrievable by one hand and either a fixed blade in a scabbard or an assisted-opening folding knife with a cord that extends from the handler's pocket for quick retrieval, in case one of the handler's arms is entrapped by a rope. The blade should have a partially serrated edge for cutting thick ropes.

> Handlers who use ropes when working with livestock or horses should always carry a sharp knife that can be quickly retrieved and opened with one hand.

USEFUL KNOTS, BENDS, AND HITCHES FOR ANIMAL HANDLERS

Definition of terms

A *knot* is intertwining a rope to itself. A *bend* is intertwining a rope to another rope or two ends of the same rope. A *hitch* is intertwining a rope to another object, such as a hitching ring. *Splicing* a rope is to unwind the strands of a twisted rope so that they can be interwoven with the strands of another rope or to create crown knots, halters, and other rope handling tools.

Tying knots, bends, and hitches is more difficult than it appears. Practice is required to acquire and to maintain the skills. If not used frequently, monthly practice of tying knots and hitches should be planned. Forming the knot, bend, or hitch is just the first part. For many knots, bends, and hitches, how they are pulled tight is just as important. A flip or twist in the pull down or a lack of proper pull down (tightening) can ruin a knot or hitch's effectiveness.

Each knot has a different purpose. The selection of which knot to use is based on its ability to remain secure, the speed and ease of tying and untying, and its size.

Overhand knot (thumb knot) and other stopper knots

The *overhand knot* is the simplest knot. It is used as a stopper knot to keep the end of a rope from fraying or to put knobs in the length of a rope to add traction point and prevent the ends of ropes from pulling through a handler's grip. The overhand is made by making a circle with rope and bringing one end over the top of the loop and through the loop (**Figure 10.8**).

Bulkier stopper knots may be created by going through the loop 2 or 3 times. The triple overhand knot was called the *blood knot* because it was used on

the ends of the British cat o'nine tails, a whip used to flog sailors for punishment. It has also been used to tie the ends of waist cords of monks and nuns, in part to symbolize three sacred vows.

The *figure 8 knot* is another stopper knot (**Figure 10.9**). It is formed by creating a bight at the end of a rope, twisting the bight 180 degrees, and then inserting the working end of the rope through the formed loop.

Square knot

The *square knot* is popular for tying two ropes of equal diameter together. It will not slip or jam, but it should not be used in potentially dangerous situations because it creates sharp bends that weakens ropes. It may have caused more deaths and injuries than other knots because of its popularity and misuse.

The square knot is an overhand knot tied on an overhand knot (**Figure 10.10**). It is tied right

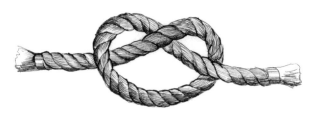

Fig. 10.8 Overhand knot.

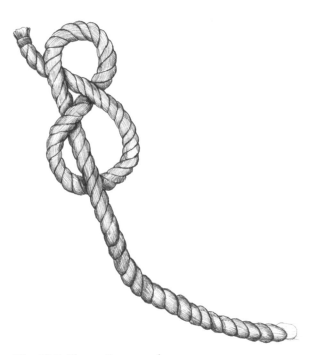

Fig. 10.9 Figure 8 stopper knot.

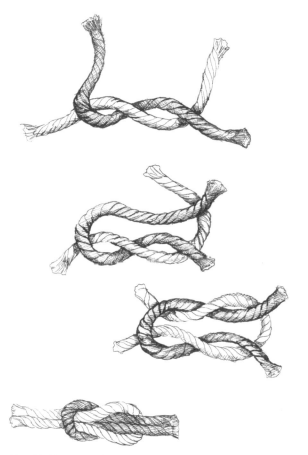

Fig. 10.10 Square knot.

over left, then left over right. When tied properly, the shorter free ends will be in line with the tied or taut lines. A double overhand knot (the working end goes around the rope twice) is the first half of a *surgeon's knot* and the first knot used in a gauze muzzle for dogs (**Figure 10.11**). A *reefer knot* (reef is a name for a type of sail) is a square knot with a bight in one of the short ends. This acts as a slip knot to quickly untie the square knot. Shoelaces are typically tied with double reefer knots.

The *granny knot* (right over right or left over left) is similar to a square knot but will slip under tension or will jam (**Figure 10.12**). Pulling on the longer ends of a granny knot will make the short free ends go out of line with the long ends to form an "X" or cross. Granny knots have no useful purpose. They are merely improperly tied square knots.

Quick release hitch (lead rope tie)

The most common *quick release hitch* is the standard lead rope tie (**Figure 10.13**). It is the most commonly used hitch for lead ropes in handling horses. This hitch allows the working end to be pulled to the side, which is the easiest direction to release a quick release hitch. This tie is performed after the end of the lead rope goes through a tie ring or around a stout horizontal post. With the end that is through the tie ring, a loop is made on the left side of the lead rope going to the horse's halter. The working end of the lead is taken over and then under the lead to the horse and then bent into a bight. The bight goes through the loop. The hitch is tightened around the lead and then slid up to the tie ring.

When horses that may untie hitches are tied, the working end of the lead rope should be dropped through the bight of the hitch to prevent pulling on

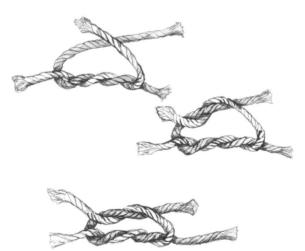

Fig. 10.11 Double overhand in a surgeon's knot.

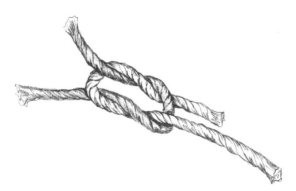

Fig. 10.12 Granny knot.

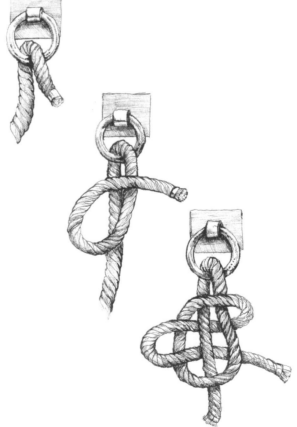

Fig. 10.13 Quick-release lead rope hitch.

the end untying the hitch. Alternatively, a bowline should be used to tie horses that untie quick release hitches.

A variation of the quick release hitch is a shoe-lace-like tie (a double reefer knot), called the halter hitch or manger tie. This variation requires pulling the working end toward the tie ring, and it is much more difficult to release the hitch in a hurry than the standard tie for lead ropes. It is not recommended as a substitute for the true quick release lead rope hitch.

The *highwayman's hitch*, also called the "draw hitch," is a quick release using a bight around the object (**Figure 10.14**). The highwayman's hitch is performed by putting a bight through the tie ring. The end of the lead is wrapped around the lead line and lead line bight and then a second bight is put into the first and the hitch is pulled down tight to the tie ring. When the hitch is untied, it has very little rope to be unwound around the tie ring or post. The advantage of this hitch is that it permits a quick tie of a very long rope and a quick release. Unlike the standard quick release hitch, which requires the length of the lead to run through a tie ring and then regrasping the lead, a highwayman's

hitch is released with a pull with one hand with the grip retained on the rope after its release from the hitch ring. The disadvantage is that horses that untie themselves from a highwayman's hitch will become completely loose, compared with untying the standard quick release tie that leaves the lead rope draped through the tie ring. Most seasoned horses, even if untied, will stand in place if the lead line is still running through the tie ring. The highwayman's (another term for bandit) hitch was reputedly used in the past by robbers to tie their horses for a quick getaway.

Honda knot

A *honda knot* is created by making an overhand knot in the end of the rope as a stopper knot and then making another overhand knot a few inches up the rope. Before tightening the second overhand knot, the stopper overhand knot in the end is put inside the loop of the overhand knot and trapped by pulling the second knot tight. This produces a small fixed loop (honda), a channel for the other end of the rope at the end of lariats for livestock and horses and in creating slip leashes for dogs and cats (**Figure 10.15**).

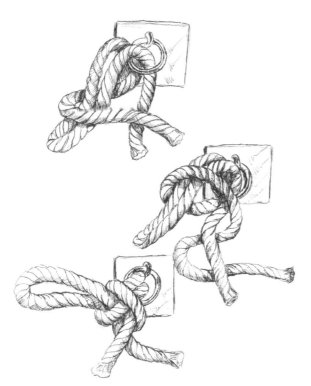

Fig. 10.14 Highwayman's hitch.

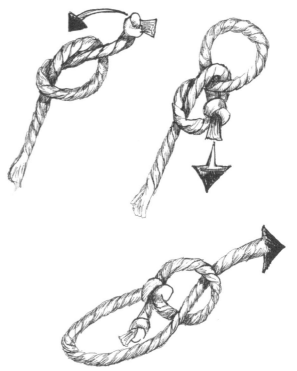

Fig. 10.15 Honda knot.

Sheet bend (weaver's knot; tail tie)

A *sheet bend* is used to tie two ropes together (**Figure 10.16**). This simple bend is secure, even if the ropes are of different sizes. It is also used to tie cords to cattle or horse tails to restrain the tail. A double sheet bend can be used to tie a lead rope to a horse halter. It is lighter, softer, and stronger than a typical metal fastener for a lead rope.

The sheet bend is created with a bight in one end of a rope while the other rope end goes through the bight, is wrapped completely around the bight, and is then trapped underneath itself where it first emerged from going through the bight. A double sheet bend is wrapped around the bight twice before going under itself.

Bowline ("king of knots")

The bowline (pronounced "BO-linn") knot has many uses since it creates a loop that will not slip, bind, and risk choking an animal if around its neck. It is the preferred knot to tie the lead line of a horse that can untie a quick release hitch. Its name comes from being used to secure the edge of a square sail toward the bow of a ship, i.e. a bow line. It is probably the most versatile knot used in handling large animals (**Figure 10.17**).

The knot can be tied with one hand, but most people learn to tie the knot by memorizing "the rabbit comes out of the hole, goes around the tree, and back down the hole." A loop is created first and twisted 270 degrees. The end of the rope goes through the loop, circles around the standing part of the rope and

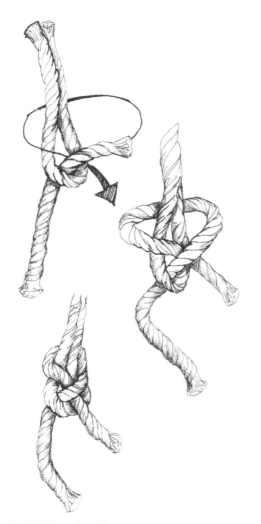

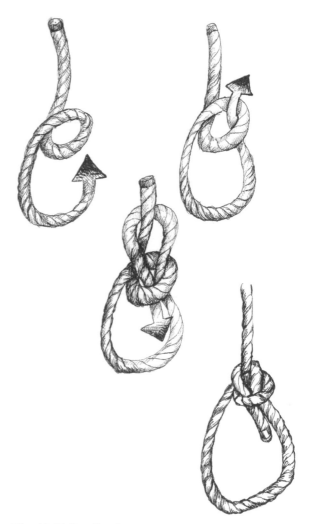

Fig. 10.16 Sheet-bend knot.

Fig. 10.17 Bowline knot.

goes back through the loop. The loop is then pulled closed finishing the bowline knot. The bowline has also been recommended for tying lead ropes since it does not bind and horses cannot untie it.

Making two loops for the "rabbit's hole" will create a double bowline that is even stronger than an ordinary bowline.

Bowline on the bight

A *bowline on the bight* knot is useful for making a rope collar in the middle of a long rope with 2 trailing lines, as needed for breeding hobbles or creating a Scotch hobble (**Figure 10.18**). The knot will not slip and choke the animal. It is easily untied even after tension has been on the knot. It has been used for *casting* (laying down) sedated horses for surgical procedures, but less commonly since the advent of newer injectable anesthetics that produce relatively smooth inductions and recoveries.

Half hitch

A *half hitch* is a quick way of tying to an object, but it is generally unreliable (**Figure 10.19**). It can be a reliable knot if tied repeatedly over itself as when tying legs on a recumbent animal or on a cattle chute cleat (then called the cleat hitch). Wrapping figure 8 knots with a rope around a cleat on a cattle chute should be done with the heel side of the hand to keep the fingers less vulnerable to being trapped in the wraps and for strength gained by that grip in pulling the rope around the cleat.

Clove hitch

The *clove hitch* works by friction and is generally unreliable for tying animals with a rope (**Figure 10.20**). If an animal rocks the rope back and forth, it will loosen a clove hitch. It is most practical when used as a tie to a second post after wrapping around a first post. This prevents a rocking effect on the hitch, which could cause the hitch to untie.

Picket line hitch

Sometimes the most convenient place to tie an animal, particularly a horse, is to a rope tied horizontally between two secure objects such as trees. This is called a picket line. Picket lines may be chest height, but overhead picket lines will reduce the risk of pulling the line down or becoming entangled. A *picket line hitch* is similar to the clove hitch

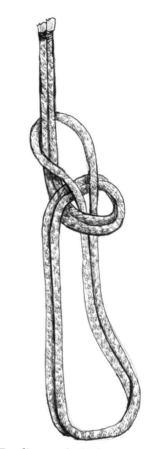

Fig. 10.18 Bowline on the bight.

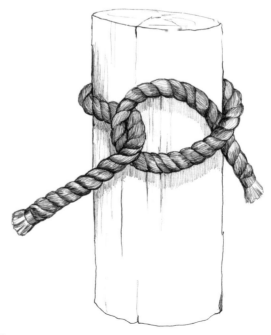

Fig. 10.19 Half hitch.

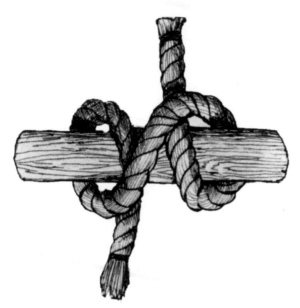

Fig. 10.20 Clove hitch.

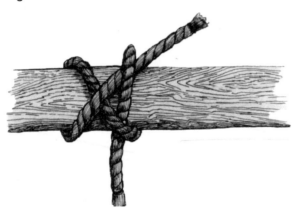

Fig. 10.21 Picket line hitch.

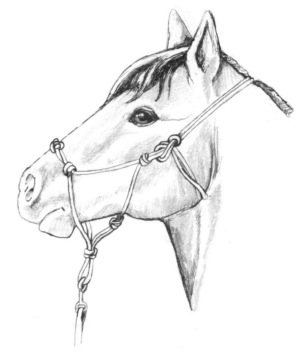

Fig. 10.22 Rope halter.

but is much more secure because the working end is trapped under itself (**Figure 10.21**).

Rope halter ties

Rope halters for horses can apply more pressure to the poll and bridge of the nose than leather or nylon band halters. As a result, a clearer correction for misbehavior can be delivered, and horses are less prone to pull or lean on the halter and lead rope (**Figure 10.22**). Rope halters also take less room to store and do not trap moisture that can promote bacterial or fungal infections, as leather halters do. The knot used to tie a horse's rope halter is a sheet bend (**Figure 10.23**). A double sheet bend can be used to attach the lead line to the halter rather than a metal clip.

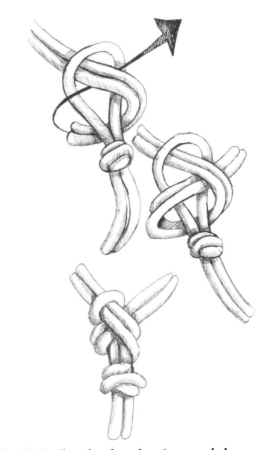

Fig. 10.23 Sheet bend used to tie a rope halter.

USING A LARIAT

Throwing a lariat loop is sometimes necessary for capturing livestock and horses. Some handlers consider lariats as the least stressful option for untrained animals, and others consider lariats as the last resort for capturing an animal. Opinions are affected by the handler's skill in using a lariat. The proficient use of lariats must be routinely practiced. The ability of the handler is the most important factor in how soon, how often, or whether throwing a lariat is used in capturing animals. The skill must be acquired by repeated practice on inanimate objects before being attempted on animals.

Poor use of a lariat can instill fear in animals of humans approaching them. Injuries to an eye can result, especially with metal quick-release hondas. A leg may be accidentally caught, increasing the risk of a broken leg or neck. On the other hand, throwing a lariat loop might be the only practical available means of capturing range cattle or untamed horses. The correct rope in the hands of an experienced roper can be less stressful on managing calves than alleys, chutes, and head catches. Cattle handling using lariats is not rodeo calf and steer roping. These sports are exciting, flashy, and sometimes inhumane events that are for entertainment only. Good cattle and horse handling with ropes is slow, quiet, and can even be boring to watch.

Throwing lariats originated with the Spanish, but two variations gradually developed separately in California and Texas. Common lariats used in Texas-style roping are stiff ropes $\frac{5}{16}$ or $\frac{3}{8}$ in (0.3 or 0.95 cm) in diameter and 28, 30, or 35 ft (8.5, 9.1, or 10.7 m) long. Roping from horseback is done with saddle horns with small diameters designed for tying. Californio-style roping is done with softer ropes at greater distances. Cattle are quietly roped from outside their flight zones. Leather reatas or Mexican maguey ropes 50–60 ft (15–18 m) long are used for Californio-style roping. If done on horseback, saddles are used with large-diameter saddle horns (gourd horn) that are more effective for dallying (wrapping the rope without tying). Dallying the rope is easier on the cattle being handled than is tying. Small loops are thrown with speed in Texas style owing to the brushy environment in south Texas and the need to catch cattle quickly. Big loops are used in California and Basin and Mountain states where the land is more open and so more suited for large, slowly tossed loops.

Throwing a rope with the handler on the ground is used to capture and sort cattle when chutes and other handling facilities are not available. It may also be used as an early tool in horse training. Before throwing a lariat from the ground, a stout stationary object should be selected as a potential dally post, and light or lightweight gloves should be worn. Smaller animals may be restrained by taking the rope behind the handler's seat (a half dally). This allows the handler to grip with the half wrap on his body and to push backwards with his legs rather than try to pull with the arms and maintain just a hand grip on the rope.

Anatomy of a lariat loop

Lariat loops (nooses) consist primarily of base, tip, honda, and spoke. The *base* is the top part of a loop and the bottom portion is the *tip*. The *spoke* is the portion of the rope that has passed through the honda and extends to the portion that is held with the base by the throwing hand. The *bottom strand* of the loop is the section of rope from the honda side of the base to the tip. The *top strand* is the section of loop from the tip to where the rope goes through the honda (**Figure 10.24**).

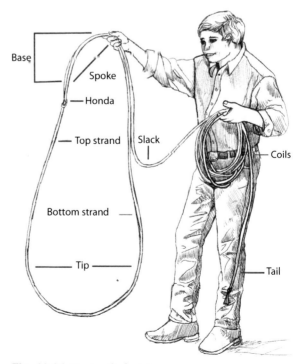

Fig. 10.24 Parts of a lariat.

Hondas on lariats should be rope, rawhide, or lightweight metal. Heavy metal hondas on ropes to be thrown can injure the animal's eyes, ears, or facial bones. Metal hondas are useful in training horses and other animals to give under pressure. When the animal quits pulling on the rope, there is an immediate release of pressure, constituting a reward. Quick release hondas unsnap, preventing the need to loosen the rope first. These hondas can be useful in restraining cattle, but they can be dangerous to handler's fingers if the handler uses his finger to unclasp the latch when freeing the animal. Rather than putting a finger in the honda to release the snap, a rawhide string to pull the snap open should be used.

The thrown loop (tossed loop)

Occasionally there is no other realistic option than roping for capture, particularly with cattle. If cattle are to be caught with a lariat, they should first be herded into the smallest holding area that is strong enough to contain a group of pushing cattle. A dally (snubbing) post should be identified and its strength inspected before attempting to catch a cow or calf.

In preparation of a catch, the group is approached at an angle quietly on foot with a loop ready and held low, dragged on the ground, and held slightly behind the right leg for a right-handed roper. The spoke should be held to extend about one-fourth down the top strand. The toss is a silent, smooth upward movement of the arm with a slight flip of the wrist. The loop should make one-half turn by the time it reaches its target, with the tip of the loop falling over the target. The honda should fall in front of the target and not hit it.

Swinging the rope before a toss will frighten cattle and must be avoided if they are not yet agitated. If the cattle are not quietly settled and run from the quiet approach of the handler, a thrown loop must have momentum to quickly get to the animal to be caught. One swing of the loop is generally enough. The longer the rope is swung around the handler the more frightened the cattle will become. As soon as the animal is caught, the handler has to pull it in a circle close enough to make a dally (loops/wraps) around the dally post. Once caught and snubbed, the animal is driven toward the dally post while the slack is taken up in the rope. If the reason for catching the animal requires that it be held for more than

a minute, a halter should be placed on the animal and tied to the post. The neck loop should then be loosened or removed to prevent the animal from choking.

Ropes with quick-release metal hondas can be tossed, but they should not be swung and thrown. The weight of the honda unbalances the loop and can cause injury to the animal if thrown with accelerated momentum.

The hoolihan

Because of their quick movements and long neck, horses can easily duck and avoid a thrown lariat loop if they see it coming directly toward their head. However, range horses that are trained to be ridden are trained to be gathered in rope corrals and stand side by side with their rumps to a wrangler (western-style horse handler) while he selects and ropes individual horses for work. This is much safer than milling among a herd of 20 or more riding horses, called a *remuda* in the Southwestern U.S. (a *cavvy* in the Great Basin states) early in the morning. The type of loop thrown to select the horses from a remuda is called a *hoolihan*, which is thrown off the index finger after swinging the loop smoothly and quietly around the roper's body. The hoolihan gently drops down over the horse's head from behind.

A right-handed roper holds the loop over his left shoulder. This allows a large loop to be held close to the body and not be dragged on the ground. The spoke should be held so that it extends about three-quarters down the top strand. The throw begins with smoothly swinging the loop clockwise around the body. The loop is released when the right hand is over the handler's head in approximate line with the left ear. The loop should make one half turn, and the tip should drop over the target. Only the best, most experienced ropers catch horses from a remuda for the other wranglers. Horses unaccustomed to ropes should only be caught with a rope in a small round pen with solid, high walls by a skilled roper.

The hoolihan loop can also be used to catch cattle in a pen. The advantage of a smooth, quiet swing to develop momentum and a large loop may be helpful in catching cattle in some situations. However, more room is needed to swing the loop around the thrower's body than required of many other thrown loops.

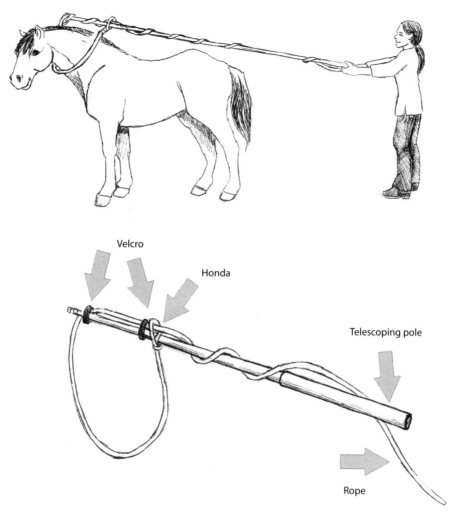

Velcro

Honda

Telescoping pole

Rope

Fig. 10.25 Improvised uurga.

Loop on a stick (uurga)

During the 13th century, the Mongolian Empire battled knights in armor using a lariat loop on a long pole called the uurga. They would catch and pull the knights off their horses to the ground, where they were more vulnerable to attack. The uurga is a traditional horse capture tool of Mongolian horsemen.

Spanish colonialists used a long-handed pole with a semicircular hocking knife on the end called a "desjarretadera" to cut the Achilles tendon to capture cattle to be slaughtered. Throwing of reatas (leather ropes not on sticks) later replaced the desjarretadera for catching most untamed livestock.

Still today, the loop on a stick, an improvised uurga, can sometimes be more effective and simpler than throwing a lariat. A telescoping pole, available at most home care stores, can be easily transported and adjusted to desirable lengths. Attaching the loop with Velcro strips will hold the loop open until quietly placed over its target (**Figure 10.25**). The pole can then be removed and the animal captured by dallies around a stout post or running the tail of the lariat through a tie ring.

SELECTED FURTHER READING

Bigon M, Regazzoni G (1982). *The Morrow Guide to Knots.* William Morrow and Company, New York.

Costantino M (2010). *The Knot Handbook.* Metro Books, New York.

Owen P (1993). *The Book of Outdoor Knots.* The Lyons Press, Guilford.

Sharp J (1966). *Knots, Hitches, and Their Uses.* Central Oregonian, Prineville.

CHAPTER 11

HORSES, DONKEYS, AND MULES

Although the horse (*Equus caballus*) was the last of today's livestock to be domesticated, among all domestic animals it has held the closest link with humans. Until the last 100 years, few dogs and fewer cats were allowed in homes. Most dogs were not trained for work. Horses had to be contained near human shelters and go through extensive training to be useful to humans. In some Middle East cultures favorite horses were sheltered in the same tents as humans. After becoming domesticated, horses provided unsurpassed mobility to humans until the development of steam engine locomotives. Horses enabled the spread of languages and cultures and the advancement of human civilization.

Humans owe horses humane, appropriate handling, at a minimum. They have served humans as beasts of burden for more than 6,000 years, beginning on the Eurasian Steppes, vast grasslands that extend from the Ukraine to southern Siberia and Mongolia. Domestic horses are believed to have evolved from the Przewalski's horse of central Asia, the Tarpan from eastern Europe and the Ukrainian steppes, and the forest horse of northern Europe. The earliest evidence of domestication has been found in Kazakhstan, where they were raised initially for food. Horses were the most abundant game in the more arid regions of the Steppes.

Horses were eventually found to expand the strength, speed, and stamina of their drivers and riders in the Middle East. Hittites became superior in military tactics by training horses to pull chariots that could carry archers. The first known text on horsemanship was the Hittites' Kikkuli text. The Scythians of central Asia and later the Assyrians used mounted archers to create faster military forces that were more mobile over rough ground than chariots. The first book on schooling a riding horse, *On Horsemanship*, was written in about 350 BC by the Greek horseman,

historian, and soldier Xenophon. Many horse-handling principles of Xenophon are still used today. Pants were invented as clothing for riding horses.

The domestic horse was brought to the New World (to the island of Hispaniola) with the second voyage in 1493 of Christopher Columbus and introduced to the Americas' mainland by the Spanish conquistadors. Hernando Cortez landed on the coast of Mexico in 1519 with 13 horses, the first domestic horses in the Americas. Small numbers of horses may have become feral soon after the Spanish settled New Mexico in 1598, but many were left behind when they were hastily driven out of the American southwest by the Pueblo Revolt of 1680. The horses were captured by the Pueblos, who began trading them with Plains nomads, resulting in the spread of horses throughout western North America. The horses that remained in the wild were called mustangs, from the Spanish word *mesteño* for "wild and free."

Civilization could not have advanced without the contributions made by the horse. Cavalry was important to the ancient Hittites, Egyptians, Greeks, Romans, and Crusaders of the Middle Ages. Horses were essential for the conquests by the Spanish empire and Napoleon. The most successful military force in history was the Mongol cavalry of Genghis Khan. His horse-mounted archers, called "the devil's horsemen," conquered more than four times the area of the empires of Alexander the Great, the Romans, and the Persians. Empires in the Americas were much smaller than those in Europe and Asia owing to the lack of the horse prior to the Spanish conquests.

The price horses have paid for being domesticated and cared for in captivity has been high. For example, perhaps the best horsemen of the American Indians were the Comanches. To contain the Comanches, Colonel Ranald Slidell Mackenzie crushed the Comanches' capacity for future war by killing more than 7,000 of their horses between September 1874 and June 1875. In 1877, after evading the U.S. Cavalry for 1,400 miles through the superiority of their Appaloosa horses, the Nez Perce Indians, led by Chief Joseph, were captured by Colonel Nelson A. Miles. All their horses, more than 1,000, were sold or killed to prevent the Nez Perce from another attempt to escape into Canada. It is estimated that 1.5 million horses died serving in the American Civil War and that more horses and mules suffered casualties than men did in the Union and Confederate armies combined. During World War I, 256,000 British and 68,000 U.S. horses lost their lives. The total loss of horses from World War I from both sides from artillery fire, poison gas, work exhaustion, malnutrition, and disease may have been more than 8 million. Today's civilization and national boundaries would not have been possible without the horse.

Adult sexually intact male horses are called *stallions*. Castrated males are *geldings*. Adult female horses are *mares*. Nursing baby horses of either sex are *foals*. *Weanlings* are horses of either sex between weaning and 1 year old. Horses between 1 and 2 years are *yearlings*. A *colt* is a young male horse, and a *filly* is a young female horse, both under 4 years of age.

NATURAL BEHAVIOR OF HORSES

The natural behavior of horses is based on how feral horses in the U.S. behave. In reality, these are not truly wild horses, but untamed feral horses. Their ancestors were selectively bred for domestication for 6,000 years. The few that descended directly from the escaped Pueblo horses of 1680 have been untamed for only about 340 years.

Unlike actual wild animals, feral horses can be re-domesticated and trained. Their selective breeding in the wild was based on survivability and have resulted in tougher, more resilient, and in some cases, smarter horses than those that remained in domestication, being selected for breeding based on hair coat color, conformation without meaningful purpose, and extremely placid dispositions that fail to protect them from natural dangers. Feral horse behavior does not always predict the behavior of domesticated horses, but the similarities are greater than those between wolves and dogs.

Horses are highly social prey animals that prefer to live in groups. Horses in the wild prefer to form small bands of 3–30 horses, usually a stallion and 4–6 mares with foals, that share a grazing territory. The sexually mature mares within a band are called the harem. Each band of mares and immature horses is led by an older dominant (*boss* or *lead*) *mare*. Dominant mares lead the band to water and grazing sites. She is also the ultimate disciplinarian. She occasionally reinforces her social position by roaming through the herd checking the deference given her. An insufficient response to move elicits controlled aggression to reassert the recognition of her role in the herd.

The band also has a dominant or *lead stallion*. The lead stallion guards the periphery of the herd and the slowest of the band against predators when the band is moving. Young stallions nearing puberty at about 2 years of age are forced out of the herd. *Bachelor stallions* follow bands at a distance. Young stallions will shadow-box (rearing and pawing at the play opponent) as part of the process of determining social rank. During breeding seasons, some bachelors will occasionally challenge the lead stallion for his position as band sire. By the time of social maturity, around 4 years of age, most fillies will leave the band to join another.

After the dominant mare and stallion, the remainder of the herd is in a linear hierarchy. Physical injury among band members is usually avoided by threatened bites and posturing as if to kick. Ignoring this body language will lead to meaningful bites or kicks. Like other animals, the rank of horses in a herd is primarily based on deference, not by actual fighting. Fights that can result in serious injury are most often between adult stallions or between a nursing mare and any perceived threat that might endanger her foal. The occasional mixing of fillies with members of different bands, along with roaming bachelor stallions eventually replacing older, previously dominant stallions, maintains the needed genetic diversity.

Boss mares can be particularly difficult to handle if allowed to control the movement of a handler or access to food, or food-possession aggression. Stallions may be more receptive to handling than boss mares if they do not feel the need to assert their social status with a human handler during breeding seasons or being handled roughly. Fillies and mares are more likely to kick; colts and stallions are more likely to bite or strike.

The opportunity to socialize with other horses, to feel the security of other horses being present, and to graze 12–17 hours per day are essential to horse mental health. Each of these opportunities beneficially affects their ability to be handled by humans. Freedom to graze in groups is a great stress reliever in horses. Another stress reliever is mutual grooming, such as standing nose-to-tail with a herd buddy, nibbling each other's withers and swishing flies away from each other's face. Devoid of companionship with other horses, some horses will develop a bond with goats, ponies, and donkeys, or other animals. If goats are used, meat breeds such as the Boer or large dairy breeds (Alpine, Saanen, LaMancha, or Toggenburg) should be selected rather than small or miniature breeds.

Horses use their nimble lips to gather grass to bite with their incisors when grazing. This ability allows many horses to learn to open latches on stalls, pick up one grain of corn from a feeder, and untie knots, among other feats of lip dexterity.

Horses main means of defense is to flee from perceived danger. Large predators of horses usually jump on the horse's back and neck, to which the horse responses with violent bucking to become free of the attack. If successful in escaping, the horse will be more inclined to buck with greater effort the next time. Analogous actions occur if young horses started under saddle are allowed to buck and especially if they are successful in ridding themselves of the rider.

Horses sleep only a few hours, most of it dozing in a standing position since they are able to fixate their legs in extension with their *stay apparatus*. If startled while dosing, they are likely to kick. The sleep time is usually in multiple short periods of approximately 15 minutes each. To achieve rapid eye movement (REM) sleep, they must lie down to sleep for an hour or two every few days, and in a herd, they typically will not lie down unless another trusted horse is near and remains standing as a sentinel to guard against predators.

The most frequent communication among horses is body language, using the ears, eyes, nostrils, position of the head and neck, pawing with front hooves, cocking a hind leg as if to kick, and swishing the tail. Vocalization is less common, including nickering, neighing (whinnying), snorting, and squealing. Smell and touch (nuzzling, grooming of each other in pairs) are other means of communication. Status in the band is reaffirmed by forcing others to move, particularly from favorite food, using body language. If the threat is unsuccessful, the more dominant horse will follow through with a bite or a kick.

Foals and weanlings play mostly by themselves in the first 3 months of life. Interactive play peaks at 3–4 months of age. Friendships with particular horses will develop later. Foals and weanlings defer to the authority of older, more dominant horses by clacking (also called snapping, clapping, or champing), a smiling, smacking action of the lips (**Figure 11.1**).

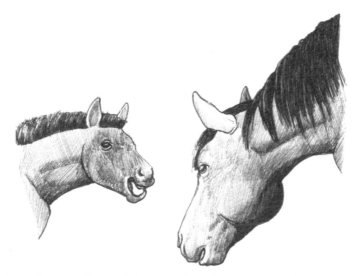

Fig. 11.1 Immature horses defer to adult rank by a smiling, clacking expression.

The temperament of horses depends much on their genetics. There are three general groups of horse breeds. The group believed to be the oldest are the *hot bloods* (Arabians, Barbs, and Thoroughbreds), which originated in hot climates and have been selectively bred for racing. Hot bloods are the most likely to be over-reactive and hyper-excitable. *Warm bloods* (Quarter horses, Morgans, Andalusians) tend to be responsive and tractable, but when they react, their reactions are more explosive. They have been selectively bred for diverse forms of work involving light draft work or under saddle tasks. *Cold bloods* (Clydesdales, Percherons, Friesians) are quiet and relatively unexcitable. Their breeding has been for their large size, quiet temperament, and ability to pull heavy loads.

SAFETY FIRST

Horses are frequently bred or purchased based on color or other physical attributes, yet owners want their horses to have good behavior, which is not directly related to color or physical attributes. Behavior is a result of genetics, role modeling by well-behaved dams and other herd members, and by proper training. A good horse can be any color, or as often said, "There is no bad color on a good horse."

Handler safety

The best way to avoid injury from horses is to understand their normal behavior, anticipate their reactions in advance, and make the appropriate adjustments to avoid the situation or deal with it safely. Horses outweigh humans 5- to 10-fold with greater proportions of muscle and respiratory ability. Handling cannot be done with force. Injury to themselves or to humans can be great due to the body size, strength, and speed of movement of horses. They can frequently find a reason for an attempt to flee, but their handler may not see, hear, or smell it. Horses that are the most likely to injure a handler are stallions, nursing mares, or sick or injured horses.

Most of the injuries to people are not due to horse aggression. They are from the inherent danger of being around horses and handler incompetence or negligence. Inherent dangers include the unpredictable nature of horses, such as their tendency to

suddenly frighten ("spook"). Horses are prey animals with a primary defense of fleeing (flight). Aggression is usually reserved for foal protection, herd control, and stallion mating rights.

Incompetence results in injuries to handlers who assume or claim a higher level of skill than the handler actually has. Forms of negligence are providing or using defective tack or other handling equipment, failure to assess surface or ground conditions that can cause a horse to fall, and failure to warn others of known dangers with a particular horse.

Leadership

Horses have an intrinsic need for leadership in order to remain safe. Leadership is established by control of resources and movement. Handler and horse safety depend on the handler becoming the appropriate leader, and this must be done without scaring the horse. Anger or excitement is neither appropriate nor effective, and the horse should not be exhausted or excessively constrained. Key components of the handler becoming the leader are if the horse wants to stop, the leader directs it to go; if the horse wants to go to the right, the leader has it go to the left; and if the horse wants to go to the left, the leader has it go to the right. Horses should be petted occasionally, but only when they do something better than the last time they were asked for a response or action. Petting should be reserved for establishing or maintaining leadership, although petting can be an appropriate reward for simple acts, such as the horse standing still when approached in a pasture.

Petting and rest should be the reward for proper actions by the horse. The use of food as a reward is unreliable and inappropriate for training horses that are ridden or perform other work in variable environments and can destroy respect for a handler's personal space. Food has been used successfully by some trainers of horses to perform tricks in controlled environments.

The goal for a relationship with a horse is for it to become the handler's working partner, not a pet. The working partnership is not equal. The handler must be the senior partner, the leader. Good partnerships require mutual trust. Some horse handlers can manage horses without getting their trust, but the horse will remain untrustworthy and potentially dangerous, especially to other handlers.

Expressions of attempted dominance aggression by a horse are pinning their ears, dropping their head, swishing their tail, and hunching their back. If the handler does not correct the behavior with appropriate timing and metered reaction, the horse will assume it has achieved a higher social rank than the handler.

Effects of environment

Changes in weather can make horses more difficult to handle. Wind reduces their ability to smell and hear. It can also blow around horse-scary objects such as plastic bags. A sudden return to more moderate temperatures will invigorate horses that were tired from heat and flies or horses that were well-rested hiding from cold winds. Unusual objects on their horizon will concern them, such as a motorcyclist on the road, a moved trash can, or a veterinary truck parked in a new location. Irritation from flies can cause distraction, stomping, and kicking. Horses kept for excessive periods in box stalls will be less attentive to the handler and more reactive when taken out to be handled.

> A misbehaving horse will agitate others in the vicinity.

Mental health of horses

Horses are happier and easier to handle if they can move readily (they were designed for continual movement including while eating), see distances, eat at will, and be with their herdmates who, in turn, re-teach them social humility and the importance of personal space on a daily basis. Providing time at pasture with other horses improves a horse's ability to be handled by humans. When horses are kept in groups in pastures and pens, their shoes, especially hind shoes, should be removed to prevent serious injury from disciplinary kicks that would not otherwise be harmful from dominant horses.

Horses that are not allowed daily opportunities to socialize with other horses or to run, roll, and graze will develop physiological and mental problems.

Excessive confinement prevents normal muscular activity, hampers venous and lymphatic circulation, and reduces the health and nutrition of joints. Stiffness, leg swelling, and lameness can result. Excessive confinement can also cause or aggravate stereotypic behaviors, such as cribbing, weaving, and stall walking.

For the best response from horses, a handler must possess confidence, firmness, patience, and kindness. Horses learn good habits quickly from pressure followed by properly timed release and being free enough to make a mistake and given appropriate correction within three seconds. After three seconds, the horse will not be able to make the connection between the action and correction.

Horses should be expected to maintain good manners. They should stand still and pay attention to the handler when being handled. They should show no attempt at dominance over the handler such as nipping, shoving, or walking on the handler. Horses should be expected to walk mannerly alongside the handler with no pulling, balking, or dragging along. They must respect the handler's personal space; that is, to stay an arm's length away from the handler unless invited closer. Excessive rubbing and scratching horses between weaning and 2 years of age can teach a horse to move toward pressure, whereas the basis of training is to teach horses to move away from pressure, such as a rein, rider's leg, or spur.

Socializing newborn foals (so-called imprinting) is believed to affect the behavior of horses for the rest of their lives, but handling foals can be overdone. Excessive handling of foals and incorrect handling of weanlings, yearlings, and 2-year-olds will not yield good results. If attempting to socialize by *imprinting*, it is recommended to begin in the first 48 hours after foaling. The mare should be caught first and held by an assistant with the mare against a wall or strong fence. The mare is rubbed and groomed for 10–15 minutes, followed by rubbing and handling all parts of the foal's body. Exposure to clipper noise and other stimuli it will encounter later in life is also recommended. The effectiveness of foal handling can be negated if the mare is distressed and becomes agitated. Her actions will supersede any rubbing of the foal by the handler.

Body language

Most communications between horses and from horses to humans are by body language. The body language vocabulary is not large. They use ear, head, and neck position, movement, pawing, and tail swishing. The essential body language for a handler of horses to know includes whether the horse's head is up, its neck tense, the ears forward, the eyes fixed on a perceived threat, and it is blowing hard out the nostrils (snorts) and lifting its tail; this all means red alert, the horse is ready to bolt. Ears held back moderately and head low can mean "I want you out of my space," but at grain feeding time, it often means "hurry up and give me food," or when working it means a sign of resolve to work hard and pay better auditory attention to the rider or handler.

When aggressive, horses pull their ears back and tightly flatten them to protect them from being bitten. This does not enhance hearing. Non-aggressive horses often turn their ears backward to focus their hearing of what is happening behind them. This is a typical ear position for horses when racing, whereas a horse preparing for a successful jump points its ears forward.

Being able to see the white part of a horse's eye is a better indication of fear or aggression than the position of their ears. Dancing or swaying on the hind feet and swishing the tail rapidly back and forth (if not being harassed by flies) means "I am dominant and my patience is gone." This is a signal the horse is ready to kick. Passive body language can be licking lips, lowering head to wither's height, blinking eyes, or cocking a hind foot over onto the front of the hoof, which means "oh, this is not as bad I as thought" or "been here, done that." Pawing the ground is a sign of impatience or frustration.

Respectful of space

Horses must be required to respect human personal space, an approximate 3 ft (1 m) radius around a handler, unless invited closer. Horses instinctively push or lean toward pressure, but they must be taught to move away from pressure (a push or an advance toward them) by tapping their shoulder or chest until they move out of a handler's space. Then, they should be immediately left alone until they invade the handler's space again. A handler should never allow a horse pin him or her against a wall or other solid object. This is dangerous and a sign of dominance with lack of respect for humans.

When it is necessary to work closely with a horse's body in a standing position, the handler should keep a hand on the horse to detect its movements and to push away, if needed. When working low on a horse's legs, a handler should not sit, kneel, or place a hand on the ground. The handler should crouch and remain on his toes so that he can immediately stand and move away quickly if the need arises.

Bad manners in horses

Wild horses digest food in small portions eaten throughout the day. They are designed to be continuously moving, traveling up to 50 miles per day to new grazing areas, occasionally socializing with other horses, and respecting their leaders. Most bad manners and vices in horses are the result of having developed a lack of respect for human dominance, excessive confinement, or a lack of socialization with other horses.

Nipping and biting

Horses bite by either by nipping (pinching) or by grasping with the mouth. Nipping with the teeth is to test dominance or to make a horse or human move. Nipping of humans almost always begins from being fed food treats by hand. Handing horses food treats gets them in the habit of associating hands and pockets with food. When the treats do not appear when it desires, the horse will invading the handler's personal space, do a body search with its nose and lips, and eventually nip the handler out of frustration.

> Never feed a horse food treats directly from a hand.

A horse opening its mouth wide to grasp a handler's arm, shoulder, or neck is a highly aggressive and dangerous act. Among the injuries to handlers from horses, 3–4.5% are from bites. A horse that attempts the grasping bite has no respect for humans. Most of these horses should be euthanized (humanely put to death) as they are a highly dangerous menace to handle and should not be bred. Stallions and some boss mares are most likely to aggressively bite and must be watched carefully.

Kicking

Horses can kick with the strength, speed, and accuracy to kill a mountain lion attempting to attack. Horses are agile and will kick with both hind legs with pinpoint accuracy when in great fear. One-leg kicks may be used to deter a nuisance, such as harassing dogs, other horses, and sometimes humans. The kick zone using both hind legs is about 6–9 ft (1.8–2.7 m).

Adult horses do not usually kick humans, except when they are startled from behind or in self-protection from fear of injury.

Horses cannot stand on three feet and do a sweeping kick to the outside as well as cattle can. However, they can hop forward raising both hind feet off the ground, twist their lumbar region and pelvis, and kick one leg sideways at head height.

Handlers should never approach a horse directly from behind. This is their blind spot, and being startled can cause the horse to kick. The horse should be spoken to in order to announce a handler's presence from a distance when approaching at an angle from behind. When a handler walks behind a standing horse, he or she should walk closely enough to brush against its rump to prevent being at peak force range for a kick. The handler should keep the closest hand on its rump so the horse knows the position of the handler and the handler can feel any tension or shifting of weight in the horse. Alternatively, the handler should walk at least 10 ft (3 m) behind the horse, outside the kick zone.

A horse should not be allowed to turn its rump toward a handler. If this occurs in a stall, the handler should make a small movement and slight noise, such as hitting a wall with a solid object, then gradually escalate this to more movement and louder noise to stimulate the horse to turn its rump away. The annoying movement and noise should cease the instant the horse moves its rump away from the handler. Over time the horse will seek the less disturbing stance toward the handler without being prompted.

Horses can go into a light sleep while standing because of a unique stay apparatus that can lock their legs and prevent them from collapsing. Lying down and deep sleep occurs when they believe they are safe and a herd sentry is on guard. Care must be taken not to startle a sleeping horse that is standing, or it may become startled and kick. The typical posture of standing sleep is head lowered, lower lip drooping, and tail motionless.

When working on an area of pain at the flank or hind legs, it is best for a handler to run his or her hands over the normal area on the other side to allow the horse to adjust to this touch and then reach underneath from the normal side to the affected side to test the horse's sensitivity to the area of possible pain.

Striking or pawing

Striking or pawing with the front legs is a sign of impatience. Horses should be trained as a yearling to stand tied for long periods to teach patience and prevent a habit of pawing. If a horse develops a destructive and possibly injurious habit of pawing when restrained, kick chains should be considered. Kick chains are leather straps fitted around the pastern with a 1 ft (0.3 m) stainless steel chain. The chain creates noise and bumps the leg if the horse paws or kicks. Kick chains do not cause harm to the horse if they are used only when the horse is in a stall. Kick chains should never be used on a horse that is in a pen or turned out in a pasture. Persistent use of kick chains is not necessary.

Dragging a handler when led

When being led, a horse should not walk with its shoulder ahead of the handler's shoulder, as some will attempt to pull a handler forward. If a horse attempts to drag the handler, the horse's head should be pulled toward the handler while pushing its hindquarters away. After turning the horse in tight circles and allowing the horse to calm down, the handler should lead the horse forward to give it a chance to behave. If it does not, the handler should repeat the circle and disengage the hindquarters as many times as needed until the horse walks forward properly without dragging the handler. Making a horse circle tightly causes its hind legs to cross over each other, which takes its pulling power away. A chain shank on a lead can be tried on difficult cases. Briskly backing a horse or turning it in a tight circle aids in re-establishing leadership over the horse.

Rearing

A longer than usual lead with a stopper knot on the end should be used if rearing is anticipated. If a horse rears, the handler should give it more length of the lead rope and move away from range of the front hooves. The end knot will reduce the risk of the lead slipping through the hand. Attempts to keep the horse down may result in it overcompensating and falling over backwards or pulling the handler in close enough to be hit by its hooves. While moving away, the handler should also move in a semicircle toward the horse's hip to make its hip begin to circle away from the handler when the horse comes down. Longeing (lungeing in the UK) it in small circles both directions immediately after it rears can eliminate any thought of a reward for rearing and discourage it from rearing again. Jerking down on a lead rope as a misguided reprimand can cause the horse to rear again.

Horse safety

The safety of horses is entirely dependent on the handling ability of their owners and who else handles them. Horses protect themselves instinctively by flight reactions. Their flight reaction occurs before thinking: i.e. run first, think later. This reaction can put the horse as well as the handler in danger. Understanding how horses monitor for possible dangers and communicate with each other can be helpful in identifying and defusing potentially dangerous situations.

A technique of exposing horses to a wide variety of new stimuli in a couple of days is sometimes used to demonstrate for entertainment how quickly a young horse can accept a saddle and rider for the first time. The technique, a form of flooding or mental exhaustion from persistent overstimulation, works well for initial acceptance of the saddle and rider, but flooding does not cause lasting effects without daily, less intense, follow-up training periods. Slower, shorter training periods are more effective, safer to horse and rider, and less stressful to young horses in the early stages of their training than flooding to exhaust them.

Senses for safety

Horses rely to a large extent on their sight for safety. They have excellent peripheral distance vision and constantly scan the horizon, but they cannot see directly behind them. Handlers who remain watchful for dogs in the distance, blowing plastic bags, and other potentially horse-scary things have a safety advantage.

Horses' sense of hearing is acute and enhanced by highly mobile ears. Handlers who use a soothing voice inflection when horses wish to flee will be at a safety advantage. Horses are relaxed by hearing sounds of normal activity. A handler trying to be too quiet or causing excessively loud noises will make horses act nervously.

Horses monitor odors for danger and social status. They greet each other by smelling each other's breath. Pecking order is begun at the first greeting. A handler should not allow strange horses to smell each other's breath while they are under his direct control. One horse may strike out when they begin sorting out the level of their social status after smelling each other.

Horses touch each other as a way of being accepted as a member of the herd and asserting social status within the herd. Handlers can reinforce horses' respect and trust by grooming them and stroking them after they perform a desired action or demonstrate a proper response. It is beneficial to establishing trust with horses for handlers to spend time milling with them, and when they do not attempt to flee, casually stroke them as they graze. A handler's presence and touch should be associated with normal herd activities and relaxation, not just being worked or receiving medical treatments.

The sense of touch is well developed in horses. The touch of a fly on their skin will cause the skin to twitch to shake the fly off. Horses have a sensitive prehensile upper lip that can pick out grains of oats from corn and pills from feed and closed latches on gates and doors. Some horses will use the tactile hairs on their muzzle to test electric fences. There are handlers who believe horses should only be rubbed and not patted because they have such a sensitive sense of touch. Yet a dominant herdmate may reprimand another horse who violates the herd's social structure by a controlled kick to the abdomen. Patting a horse is not painful, and desensitization to pats are needed for horses kept in warm, humid climates since a handler may need to slap a horse to kill horseflies on its body for the protection of the horse and the handler. Horses quickly learn to not resent a non-injurious slap that protects it from painful bites. Desensitization to pats also reduces the risk of startle reactions if accidentally bumped or slapped when tacking up or removing the saddle or when mounting or dismounting.

Vocalizations

Horses have a spectrum of vocalizations with which to communicate and assist each other's safety. A *nicker* is used to acknowledge near presence of a herd member. When calling out for the location of another herd member, a loud *neigh* or whinny is used. *Clacking* (snapping, tooth clapping or champing) is a chomping movement of the jaws with the corners of the mouth pulled back that signals submission. Clacking is used often by foals, weanlings, and yearlings around dominant herd members. If a horse is feeling good and is excited, a deep breath and *blow* are used. A *snort* is also used when excited, but is also an announcement it is ready to run. Horses that feel they are working hard or harder than desired comment with a *grunt* or groan. A *squeal* is an aggressive noise used more often by mares to startle a potential opponent. Screams are rare sounds of great fear, such as in a barn fire.

Riding safety

Most trained horses are handled for the purpose of being ridden. Riding horses can be a hazardous activity for both the rider and the horse. No license is required to ride a horse. Yet horseback riding has a greater injury rate than riding a motorcycle, which does require a license. On average an injury occurs every 7,000 hours of riding a motorcycle. Injuries occur after an average of 350 hours riding horses. Good riding is a true partnership, but many horse owners do not strive to attain this partnership because of their unawareness of its importance or how to achieve it.

Preparation for safe riding begins long before it is time to mount. No prospective adult horseback rider should attempt to ride a horse that he or she cannot catch, reasonably handle while it is on a lead rope, or saddle (tack it up) without help. If a prospective rider cannot catch the horse to be ridden, the rider should develop better horse handling skills or

realize that the current horse is the wrong horse for that rider. Teaching children or people with physical disabilities to safely ride horses requires special environments, horses, and highly skilled instructors.

> No prospective adult horseback rider should attempt to ride a horse that he or she cannot catch and saddle without help.

Veterinary professionals who work with horses may not be experienced riders, but horse owners may look to their veterinary team for basic advice. In addition, the veterinary professional needs to be able to identify riding situations that are excessively dangerous to the horse or its rider as a part of preventive medicine. No horse is a completely safe horse. Horses are 5–15 times larger, 20–40 times more powerful, and 3–4 times faster than a human. If a rider falls from horse to the ground, it will be generally be at a distance of 3½–5½ ft (1.1–1.7 m) possibly head first.

There are many styles of horseback riding. The most popular in the U.S. are western-style and English-style. Either can be made relatively safe or can be highly dangerous, depending on the training of the rider, the training of the horse, and the quality and maintenance of the tack used. It is more common for English-style riders to ride after qualified instruction, during supervision, and in more controlled environments than a large percentage of western-style riders. Because of the lack of qualified supervision, the average western-style rider may be at greater risk.

Proper rider attitude

Proper rider attitude is essential. A good rider is like an aircraft pilot who surveys the upcoming environment: the rider controls the horse's attention, speed, direction, and behavior. The rider should not be just a passenger. The horse must know that its rider is the leader, and it must trust its rider. Some self-confidence is required to ride horses, because if thoughts are persistent about falling or getting thrown off, the prospective rider should not ride. At the same time, if the rider is not aware that there is a risk of falling or getting thrown off, he or she should not ride. Fear is detrimental and dangerous, but respect for the risk is important in maintaining safety. Being nervous at times can heighten awareness and be an asset, but not if the nervousness is overt enough to be perceived by the horse. Being afraid and denying the risks of riding are both dangerous attitudes for riding horses.

Ride a safer horse

The majority of riders who get hurt are injured by horses whose training or physical abilities do not match the training and physical abilities of its rider. Inexperienced riders riding poorly trained, improperly managed, or infrequently ridden horses place themselves in danger.

Riding a horse is not like riding a motorcycle. Motorcycles can be ignored for months, if not years, and then be ridden and perform the same as the last time. A horse is a partner to the rider, and has a variable disposition and physical abilities that changes over time. Without recent favorable experiences with the rider, the partnership does not exist. Horses must be handled and ridden on a regular basis to be behaviorally reliable and physically able to be reasonably safe. When a partnership does exist, the horse is more than transportation. Unlike a motorcycle, it can use its own senses to assist the rider in safely traversing dangerous terrain and being vigilant for other possible dangers.

Properly managed riding horses spend the majority of their time in the pasture interacting with pasture mates to learn good citizenship, and they get handled every day in ways that reaffirm the handler's gentle, consistent, and firm leadership. Moreover, they are routinely exposed to new experiences in a variety of surroundings that build trust in the handler and his leadership.

Stallions can be unpredictable and should be ridden only by experienced riders with knowledge of how to handle stallions. Mares in foal, lactating mares, ill horses, and yearlings (younger than 2 years) or aged horses (older than 25 years) should not be ridden.

Assess the horse's attitude before and after each ride

A rider should catch and groom the horse he or she plans to ride. The relationship to do this successfully is important for safer riding. Grooming the horse develops a trusting relationship between the horse and the handler. The horse's attitude after riding should also be assessed. If horses become more resentful of being ridden during a ride and have an improved attitude after a few days rest, they may have had pain from the exercise, such as saddle sores or arthritic pain.

Check and maintain riding tack

Riders should check and maintain the condition and safety of their own *tack* (riding gear on horses) and saddle the horse themselves. This is just as important as skydivers packing their own parachutes. It not only helps to ensure proper tacking up, but it allows a rider to assess the horse's attitude that day. Each piece of tack should be examined, especially the reins, cinch (*cinch* is Spanish for girdle, *girth* is old English term for girdle and a term used by English-style riders), and stirrups. Chicago screws, metal rein snaps, and where leather bends around metal are the most probable sites of breakage or of coming unfastened. In addition, the string rawhide ties on western cinch latigo straps and on bridles should be checked before each ride.

Dress appropriately

Equine helmets should be worn when riding, especially if the rider is inexperienced or the horse is young. Equine helmets are designed to protect the back of the head and are different from bicycle helmets. Many bike helmets have gaps in the shell and are pointed in the back to improve air flow, but this design provides insufficient protection for a fall from a horse.

A rider should be sure that the helmet is adjusted to fit his or her head. The chin strap has a "Y" that fits over the ears which should be adjusted so that the bottom of the "V" portion of the "Y" is just below the ear. The chin strap should be snug enough to permit just one finger underneath. The visor part of the helmet should be 1 in (2.5 cm) above the eyebrows. If an impact occurs to the helmet, it should be replaced even if there visually appears to be no damage. No earrings should be worn since they can get caught in the helmet straps. Many states have laws requiring riding helmets for riders 18 years old or younger. Children should wear helmets around horses, whether or not they plan to ride.

> Riders should wear an equine helmet that meets standards set by the American Society of Testing Materials (ASTM) international and certified by the Safety Equipment Institute (SEI).

Temporary partial blindness when among horses can be dangerous. Hoods on garments should not be worn. Long hair should be kept out of the face to prevent restricted vision. Loose long hair can also be caught in tack buckles, lead chains, and lead line snaps. Goggles should be worn if working with horses in muddy conditions.

Body protectors (protective vests) are recommended for jumping events, especially cross-country jumping. They assist in preventing some bruises, abrasions, fractures, neck, and shoulder injuries. The ASTM also rates vests. British-made vests are rated by the British Equestrian Trade Association (BETA) or the European Committee for Standardization. These have three levels of protection with Level 1 being the least protective. The ASTM standard is considered to be between the European standards of 2 and 3. Some use air bag technology and have a ripcord that is attached to the saddle to activate inflation if a fall from the saddle occurs. Proper fit should permit the wearer to breathe easily and move his arms in a full range of motion.

Proper footwear is very important in riding safety. Western-style riders should wear boots larger than normal so that they are loose enough to come off easily in case of a fall. Traditional cowboy boots are designed for riding. Roper boots have short tops and lower heels. They are designed for walking and are not as safe as traditional cowboy boots to ride in. The boot should go at least half way up the calf and have large heels (at least 1 in [2.5 cm] high) and little to no tread. Boots that have crepe soles or deep treads or are lace-up are more likely to hang up in a stirrup if the rider is thrown or falls off the horse. Lace-up boots are meant to be tightened around the ankle, which is just the opposite of what is desired in a safe western riding boot.

Riding clothing should be snug but not tight. To prevent getting hung up on a western-style saddle horn, the rider should unbutton the lower buttons on jackets or slickers (raincoats for riding) to prevent the jacket or slicker from hooking over the horn and thus preventing the rider from leaning back if the horse stops suddenly. Hip-length coats could become caught behind the cantle. Waist-length coats or split knee length ("duster") coats are safer. Other clothing or accessories that might get caught on the saddle horn or cantle should also not be worn.

Riding pants or jeans should not fold or bunch on the inside of a rider's leg or have a thick inseam, especially at the rider's knee. Otherwise the friction on the inside of the rider's leg that occurs during riding will abrade the leg. Western-style pant legs should be long enough to bunch ("stack") when standing so that when straddling the saddle the ends of the pants do not ride over the top of the boots.

Pant legs should be over the top of the boots if working in brush to keep weed burrs and other debris out (Texas style) and stuffed inside the boots if working in mud or snow to keep pants dry ("buckaroo," northwestern style). For comfort, and to prevent loss of pocket contents, nothing should be carried in hip pockets. If access to pockets is needed while riding, a vest or jacket with pockets should be worn. English-style riders use knee-high riding boots that are worn over the lower aspect of their pants; these negate the problem of the pants going over the top of the boots.

Care in tacking up

Tacking up is putting the riding or harness gear on a horse. There are potential hazards in the process of tacking up, particularly in putting on the bridle, since the horse can resist by swinging its head and hitting the handler's face. Other potential hazards are being kicked when reaching underneath the horse and being stepped on during tacking up.

Saddling

The horse should always be brushed first, including under the chest where the cinch or girth will press on the skin. Each foot should be picked up and the bottom surface cleaned with a hoof pick. Packed dirt, mud, or snow can interfere with traction and act in a similar manner to sliders used to move furniture. Cleaning the feet also allows the rider to check for lameness and search for its cause. Proper use of the pick is to push dirt and debris away from the handler. Pulling the pick toward the handler may result in injury to the handler or the frog of the horse's hoof.

After the horse has been groomed and the hoofs picked out, the saddle pad or blanket is placed on the back 4–6 in (10–15 cm) further up the neck than where it should sit when the horse is ridden. The pad is then slid back slightly to get the hair underneath to lie flat. The offside stirrup is placed over the saddle seat. With one hand grasping the roll of the cantle and the other holding the horn, swell, or front of the skirt, the saddle is lifted and laid down gently on the horse's back. The front of the saddle pad or blanket should be about 1 in (2.5 cm) in front of the saddle. The saddle blanket should be lifted and tented under the gullet of the saddle to allow air to reach under the pad and prevent it from binding on the withers. Before reaching underneath the horse to grasp the cinch or girth, the horse should be forewarned by a pat on the lower chest. When reaching underneath the horse, the handler or rider should reach with the right hand and face forward relative to the horse to protect his or her head from a possible kick.

Saddling is similar to that with an English saddle, except the irons should be run up to the saddle before saddling the horse. Swinging irons can injure the rider or the horse. Unsecured irons can also catch on fences and other objects, or the horse can catch its hoof or jaw in an extended iron. After saddling, the irons can be run down and the length of the stirrups readjusted before or while the rider is in the saddle.

If a double-rigged (2 cinches) western saddle is used, it is important to connect the front cinch first and then the back cinch and breast collar, if using one. The back cinch should not be so loose that a hoof could get caught in it when kicking at belly flies or for other reasons. A loose back cinch can also allow a branch to slip under it on trail rides. There should be a cinch keeper (cinch hobble), which is a small strap that connects the front and rear cinches underneath the horse's chest to prevent the rear cinch from sliding into the flank area. Back cinches are fastened last when tacking up, and unfastened first when removing the saddle.

The front cinch should be tightened at least three times: (1) when initial saddling, (2) after the horse relaxes, and (3) after the handler has longed the horse or ridden for a few minutes. The final tightening of the girth on an English saddle can be done while sitting in the saddle. Tightening the cinch on a western saddle must be done from the ground. The final position of the front cinch should be with the front edge about 4 in (10 cm) (4 finger widths) behind the elbow. The rider should be able to slip 3 fingers under the cinch or it is too tight.

After fastening the cinches, accessory equipment that attaches to the cinch can be fastened, such as a breast collar, martingale, or tie-down. Tie-downs should always be run through a keeper in the breast collar, so that when the horse puts its head down, it cannot step over the tie-down and trap its head in that position with the tie-down under a front leg. Tie-downs should never be attached to a curb strap or chain, which could cause serious injury to the mouth or teeth. They should only be attached to a noseband.

Bridling

The bridle is put on the horse after saddling. All components of the bridle should be inspected for integrity of the leather and proper attachments. If using a snaffle bit, a chin strap (called a bit hobble) should be attached to the snaffle rings between the bit and the reins to prevent the bit from slipping through the side of the mouth.

A bridle is a headstall with attached reins, bit, chin or curb strap, and usually a throatlatch.

The horse should be untied before bridling. The halter is removed and the crownpiece is fastened around the neck. The lead rope should be draped over the neck to keep it off the ground where it might be stepped on by the horse or wrap around the handler's leg. The bit should be rubbed with the rider's hands to check for any rough or sharp spots and to check for excessive heat or cold bit temperature. The rider stands on the horse's left side just behind its ears. Split reins should be draped over the right shoulder to keep them off the ground as with the lead rope. If using romal or loop reins, the reins are put over the neck before bridling. Loop reins must never hang down in front of a horse due to the danger of it stepping through the loop and entrapping its head. Working horses are often taught to ground tie (remain stationary if the reins are dropped to the ground). Only split reins must be used for ground tying.

The rider's right hand is placed on top of the horse's upper neck. While holding the headstall with the left hand, the rider's left hand is placed on bridge of the horse's nose. The right hand is slid up the horse's neck and between its ears and then reaches down to the horse's forehead to grasp the top of the headstall (crownpiece), which is held with spread fingers. The rider's left hand is then moved down to the bit and the bit held under the muzzle.

The thumb of the left hand is placed under the bit and the other fingers used to push the chin strap away from bit. The bit is brought up the horse's mouth with the rider's hand while simultaneously lifting the crown piece with the right hand. If the horse does not voluntarily open its mouth to take the bit, the thumb of the left hand is placed in the mouth at the bars (gap) of the teeth and pushed up on the roof of the mouth to encourage the horse to open its mouth. The bit is gently put in the mouth and chin strap under the chin.

The crownpiece of the headstall is placed over the right (offside) ear and then the left ear by cupping the right hand over the ear and pushing the ear forward while lifting the crown piece over the right hand covering the ear. The same procedure is repeated to place the crown piece over the left ear. The headstall drags over the rider's hand, not the horse's ears. Care should be taken when lifting and pulling the crown piece backward over the right hand and the horse's ear that the headstall does not rub the horse's eye, particularly on the right side. The forelock should be pulled from under the browband so that it can aid in fly control of the ears and keep the head cooler. If the headstall is split ear, the ear on the side of the split is placed in the split first and then the headstall is put behind the other ear.

The throatlatch should be fastened with sufficient laxity to permit free movement of the horse's head without the throatlatch binding the throat. Four fingers should easily slide between the throatlatch and the horse's throat. Adjustment of the browband is then checked, including cheek pieces and placement of the bit in the mouth, and chin or curb strap as well as the throatlatch strap. Both the chin strap and throatlatch should have about 3 fingers width distance from the jaw and throat, respectively. If the horse gapes its mouth and rolls its tongue, the bit may have gone under its tongue by mistake.

Cavessons and *nosebands* are headstall accessories separate from the bridle in western riding and incorporated in the headstall of the bridle in English riding. A cavesson keeps the mouth from gaping open to relieve the pressure exerted on the bit. Nosebands are connected to a strap that runs through a breast collar and attaches to the cinch. Its purpose is to prevent the head from being raised beyond a desired point. Either cavessons or nosebands should cross the nose above the level of the nose cartilage with one or two fingers space underneath. A drop noseband is placed over the bridle with the noseband around the lower part of the nose in front of the bit. Drop nosebands should allow the horse to lick but not completely open the mouth.

When removing the bridle, a romal or other looped reins are placed over the neck near the ears. Split reins are placed over the rider's right shoulder. The halter or lead rope is put around the neck between the bridle and the saddle. After unfastening the throatlatch, the headstall is taken off over the left ear and then the right ear with right hand. The rider's right hand is kept between the horse's ears and the headstall slowly lowered to allow the horse to push the bit out of its mouth without banging on its teeth.

The ease in removing the bridle, particularly being gentle with the horse's ears and letting it slowly drop the bit from its mouth, sets the tone for success at the next bridling attempt.

Unsaddling is done in reverse order from saddling. That is, accessories that attach to the front cinch (chest harnesses, martingales, tie-downs) are unfastened before the front cinch is loosened. With doubled-rigged saddles, the rear cinch should be undone before the front cinch.

Safety checks before mounting

Safety checks should be performed before mounting, beginning with grooming the horse to ensure that no dirt, plant material, or other debris might be rubbed into the horse's skin with the tack. The cinch area on the lower chest is most likely to be dirty and must be carefully brushed clean. The rider's hands should be run over the entire horse to search for problems that may not be visually apparent. The rider should pick out all hoofs to remove rocks and caked mud or snow. Caked mud or snow in the hoof can cause the horse's feet to have no traction and cause falls.

Tack needs to be adjusted to fit the horse. Poorly adjusted tack can be ineffective or uncomfortable to the horse, and can adversely affect the horse's attention to the environment and to the rider.

The rider should be certain that the horse will willingly flex its neck laterally by gently pulling on a rein on the right side and then the left to ensure a one-rein stop can be accomplished. The one-rein stop, gradually circling the horse in smaller circles, is a rider's emergency brake.

The rider should longe the horse with a halter or neck rope with a cavesson and a longe line at least 15 ft (4.6 m) long to assess the horse's attitude before getting on. This can be done with the bridle on as long as the reins are securely wrapped or tied to the saddle. The rider should longe the horse in both directions and pay particular attention to how calmly the horse makes the change in direction. When the horse can make the change in direction without excitement or resentment, it can be considered to be in a proper frame of mind for being ridden. Longeing should not be done in an arena where other people are riding.

Mounting

The horse should be moved away from nearby objects that may injure rider or horse. The saddle should be gripped and rocked from side to side to spread the horse's feet slightly and become better balanced for mounting. It is best to have the horse's feet positioned so that the left front foot is slightly forward. This will facilitate mounting and reduce the horse's desire to move as the rider is mounting. The horse's mane is grasped along with the reins with the left hand. Holding the mane and reins while mounting gives the rider immediate control of the horse if needed. The left rein should be held shorter than the right in order to make the horse's hindquarters move away if the horse tries to move. The horse should be required to stand still when mounting and stay still for about 30 seconds after being mounted. If it moves while the rider tries to mount, the rider should step down and back the horse at least 20 ft (6.1 m) and then try again. This should be repeated as needed until the horse stands still to be mounted. Moving during mounting is disrespectful and dangerous.

While standing on the left side of the horse and facing its right hip, the rider's right hand holds the left stirrup and angles it to more easily place the rider's left foot in it. On a western saddle, the horn can be grasped with the rider's right hand rather than the cantle to mount, but if the horse moves its rump away as the rider attempts to mount, mounting will be difficult to impossible. If the rider grasps the cantle with his right hand to mount, he/she has three points of contact (mane, stirrup, and cantle), which allows the rider to move with the horse no matter how it moves. Mounting is accomplished by the rider hopping on his right foot two or three times, moving to the right and closer to the horse on each hop so that the toe of the left boot will not bump into the horse's side, and then a strong final hop to mount. Mounting should not be attempted by pulling up into the saddle with both hands, rather than using a strong final hop to propel the rider upward and into the saddle. The saddle could be pulled off center and control of the horse lost if mounting is improperly performed.

The needed stirrup length can be approximated by the length of the rider's arm. The rider can stand facing the same direction as the horse on the left side. The rider places his or her right hand on the middle of the saddle and lifts the stirrup to the chest with the left hand. An approximate proper length is for the bottom of the stirrup to be at the middle of the rider's chest. After mounting, the rider should be able to stand in the stirrups with a couple of inches clearance from the saddle, or if the feet are dangled, the bottom of the stirrups should be just below the ankle bones. Shorter length stirrups are needed for jumping horses. Changing the length of stirrup leathers can be done while mounted in an English saddle. Western saddles must be adjusted by the rider or an assistant on the ground.

Position in the saddle

Horses can change direction quickly, and the change cannot always be anticipated. Therefore, the safest sitting position in the saddle is the middle of the saddle (called "centered riding") without leaning. Foot pressure on the stirrups should be on the ball of the foot with the heels down and in a perpendicular line with the rider's shoulders. A few exceptions exist. If riding a colt that might stop and turn very quickly, the rider's heels can be slightly in front of her shoulders. When riding at speed and asking for a quick stop, it is best to lean back slightly with the rider's heels slightly ahead of her shoulders.

During the ride

Attention must be paid to the horse's attitude and focus of attention while riding. Its attitude should have been checked before mounting, and its predominant focus of attention should be on its feet (where it is stepping) and the rider. The rider should ride with his or her attention ahead, looking for objects or situations that might frighten or endanger the horse. Maintaining the horse's attention on the rider can be achieved by directing it in a zig-zag pattern, circling, and doing vertical flexion of its face by rhythmic gentle pulling and release of the reins when needed. The goal is to have the horse go where it should, not necessarily where it wants.

A ride should always begin at a walk or trot. The rider should circle the horse anytime it wants to go faster than the rider wants it to. It is important to keep the horse's feet moving. Attempts to keep an energized or frightened horse's feet still will cause it to feel claustrophobic and add to its anxiety and the rider' difficulty in handling the horse. After the horse is warmed up and maintaining a calm attitude, it can be loped (cantered) or galloped. If needed, the rider should ride the horse at a walk, trot, and lope in a small round pen and move to larger pens as the rider's confidence increases.

If a horse spooks, the rider should not let it stop and stare at what it is afraid of or run from it. The horse should be made to work harder by trotting in a zig-zag manner (doing rollbacks) near the object, always turning toward the object. After the horse begins to relax, it can be allowed to slow down and walk away from the object at an angle. Moving directly away from the object will put it in the horse's blind spot and heighten its anxiety again.

The horse should not be allowed to stop and eat while a rider is in the saddle. Allowing it to eat while being ridden will be an escalating problem that results in the rider losing control of the horse's attention.

Extreme care is necessary to cross pavement, especially if the horse is shod. Smooth metal shoes are very slick on pavement. Asphalt, oil spots, or light rain, which floats oil in the pavement to the surface, exacerbate the slickness of pavement.

Riding along roads is best avoided. Roadsides are often littered with glass and wire that can injure the horse's hooves and legs. If it is necessary to ride alongside a road, a rider should ride toward oncoming traffic, if permitted by state law.

> The herd instinct of horses should not be underestimated.

Another rider should never be left behind on a ride, even for short distances. A horse left behind may panic from being away from the group and race across a road or into other dangers to join up with other horses that it knows. Horses free in a pasture will usually run up to or along a fence line, which can frighten horses being ridden on the other side of the fence, especially if the pastured horses and ridden horses are unfamiliar with each other.

Emergency stops and dismounts should be practiced as a precaution against a runaway. Pulling back on both reins of a horse believed to be out of control is a common reaction by inexperienced riders but can be very dangerous. Either the horse will not stop because it can easily outpull a rider's arms with its mouth and neck, or it will stop and may then rear up and fall over on the rider. A rider that tries to jump off incorrectly may get caught in the stirrups and be dragged.

To regain control of a horse that wishes to go faster or in a different direction than the rider desires, the *one-rein stop* is an emergency brake that must be applied slowly. To ensure that a one-rein stop can be accomplished when needed, the rider must make sure the horse will flex its neck laterally by a direct pull on one rein before he or she mounts. The one-rein stop is performed by getting a shorter grasp on a rein on one side at about the middle of the horse's neck. While giving more slack in the rein on the opposite side, the short rein is pulled gradually to the side at about the height of the rider's knee while pushing its hip on that side away with the rider's heel. One rein should not be suddenly pulled in a sharp back or up direction. Either could make the horse fall on its side.

A properly executed one-rein stop will make the horse turn in a circle that gradually spirals into tighter circles. When the horse nears a standstill, the pull rein and heel pressure are gradually released to reward the horse for paying attention to the rider. The horse is allowed to move forward, until it disobeys again. The one-rein stop may be needed several times before the horse decides to maintain its attention on a rider's cues for speed and direction.

A similar technique to the one-rein stop is the *pulley rein (cavalry) stop*. One-rein stops require room to circle, which may not be available when riding on some trails. The pulley rein stop is performed by holding one rein in a fixed position, usually a fist that is pressed into the horses neck just in front of the saddle with direct contact with the mouth (no slack in the rein). The other rein is also held short but gradually pulled back with the rider's upper body while the arm holding the rein remains rigid. The pulley rein stop can stop a horse without the room needed for circling in a one-rein stop while reducing the risk of the horse rearing, and is the only safe stop method if riding in woods or on slopes.

English-style riders are frequently taught an emergency dismount from unruly horses. This requires continuing to hold the reins with both hands while placing the heels of the hands on the horse's withers and kicking both feet free of the stirrups. Using the rhythm of the horse's movement and keeping the rider's legs stretched out, both legs are swung backward and upward in a vault toward either side (usually the left) while pushing the upper body way from the horse's withers and releasing the reins. The rider should bend at the waist while in the air, attempt to land on his feet, and prepare to roll. Some trainers encourage holding onto the mane or reins, but this may increase the risk of being stepped on by the horse or entangled by the reins and dragged.

Dismounting

A routine dismount is similar to mounting a horse, but in reverse. The reins and the horse's neck should be grasped with the rider's left hand while the right hand grasps the horn. The rider's right foot is freed from the stirrup and then the right leg is swung over the horse's rump. It is potentially dangerous for the horse to move during a dismount.

Western-style riders usually continue their right leg swing to the ground and slide their left foot from the stirrup. The swing should also twist slightly so that as the rider touches the ground with his right foot his body will then be facing the horse's right hip. This puts the rider back into the safest position, which is standing next to the horse.

Horses used for English-style riding are generally taller than horses used for western-style riding. A short rider or a tall horse can put a dismounting rider in a dangerously awkward position if she tries to swing her right leg to the ground while the left foot is still in the stirrup. The left leg may still be in the stirrup while the rider cannot reach the ground with her right foot. Therefore, English-style riders are taught to kick free of the stirrups before dismounting.

To dismount from an English saddle the rider swings the right leg over to the left side, then stands in the left stirrup with both legs together, leans slightly over the saddle, braces his or her body up with both hands while freeing the left foot from the stirrup. After freeing the left foot, the rider pushes away from the horse and lands with both feet on the ground while continuing to hold the reins. The English-style dismount is also safer for children and other riders of short stature.

English-style saddles have floppy stirrup leathers and heavy metal, dangling stirrup irons. After dismounting from an English saddle, the irons should be run up the leathers and fixed near the saddle for safety reasons.

Trail riding etiquette and safety

When trail riding, a rider should not ride alone. A cell phone should be carried on the rider's body, not on the saddle or in a saddlebag. If the rider is thrown or the horse runs away, the rider will need a readily retrievable cell phone. An ID bracelet or tag on should be carried by the rider and another one should be attached to the saddle that also contains emergency contact information. If a rider has an accident, first responders may not be allowed to check a wallet or cellphone for an ID. Materials that should be carried in a saddlebag for trail riding include owner information if the horse runs off and is found, hoof pick, knife, self-adhesive bandage material, whistle, rain poncho or slicker, trail map, rope halter and a 15 ft (4.6 m) rope, and duck tape.

> A trail rider on horseback needs to be a calm, confident leader and not a nervous passenger. Safe riding requires being proactive, anticipating possible problems, and knowing how to guide the horse through them.

Riders should not leave the group or let the group leave them. The group should not move until everyone is mounted, and riders should ride as a group at a pace comfortable for the least experienced rider. Approaching or leaving another rider on horseback should be done quietly and slowly.

A trail rider should ride at least a horse's length behind another horse. Traditionally, a horse that is known to kick on trail rides will have a red ribbon tied to its tail. A red ribbon on a forelock signals the horse bites. A green ribbon means an inexperienced trail horse. A yellow ribbon marks a stallion. However, all horses may bite or kick if their personal space is invaded by another horse, so all horses should be treated as if they would bite or kick if someone rides too close. If a rider wishes to stop, he or she should first raise a hand to signal riders behind to prevent a pileup and the risk of being kicked. Caution is also needed if riding next to someone else because some horses will quickly turn and kick the other horse, usually in the area of the other rider's leg. The horse should be turned toward scary objects, such as cars, dogs, or bicyclists, and allowed

to keep its feet moving by zig-zagging at a trot, if needed. The horse should not be turned so that a horse-scary object is directly behind it in its blind spot.

Tie-downs, martingales, or other tack that prevents a horse from freely raising its head should not be used on trail rides, since they could cause a ridden or runaway horse attempting to cross water to drown or a horse fallen on its side from being able to regain its feet without struggling.

When encountering people on bicycles or other equipment the horse is not used to, the rider should try to get the other person to talk to him so the horse realizes the scary object is, in part, human. Riders must be watchful of people with raincoats (or other plastic, crackling sounding apparel), umbrellas, and balloons. Each of these are common horse-scary objects.

If roads must be crossed while on a trail ride, traffic guard riders should be posted along the road in both directions to stop oncoming vehicles. Other riders should cross single file between the traffic guards without large gaps in the line and travel no faster than a slow trot. Paved roads, particularly asphalt, can be slick for horses hooves or shoes if the shoes are not specially made or adapted for pavement. If there is any possibility of a need to ride at night, reflective tape should be attached to the rider and the horse's legs above the fetlocks.

Trail riders need to know the dates for hunting seasons and avoid riding in hunting areas. Even if not planning to go into woods or another area that might be for hunting, when riding horses during hunting seasons, rides should be restricted to midday, and a bright orange hat or vest on the riders, or a rump sheet on the horse, should be worn. Trails should stay along roads or in open fields. Bells can be put on stirrups, and the riders can carry a whistle if hunters need to be alerted. However, horses must be desensitized to whistles beforehand and whistling begun softly to warn the horses before making a loud shrill noise.

When riding in dense bush or woods, looped reins, loose back cinches, and loose breast collars can get caught on branches of vegetation. The rider must be able to bend at the waist and lean over the horse to occasionally duck under tree limbs, and the horse must be tolerant of this. English, Australian, and endurance saddles do not have horns, which allows riders to bend over closer to the horse's neck when riding through areas with trees having low branches.

All horses should be trained to tolerate dismounting on either side. Riders should also practice mounting from either side. When riding in hills or mountains, riders should always dismount on the uphill side. Mounting or dismounting on the downhill side is difficult and dangerous, since the horse may fall toward its rider.

During lightning storms riders need to seek low ground, but remain watchful for flash flooding. Taking cover under trees that are next to rock outcroppings or in water must be avoided. Metal on riding tack and on riders should be removed, if possible. Riders should stand on something that insulates, such as a rubber rain slicker, and crouch with feet together and arms in near the body.

When crossing a stream or river, there should be nothing that could impede a horse's movements, such as tie-downs, lead ropes or mecates, lariats, or martingales. The rider's movements also need to be free; that is, no chaps or spurs. The rider should find the most shallow spot as possible and head the horse diagonal to the current. Slower currents indicate deeper water and should be avoided. Deer or elk tracks at a crossing will indicate a safer area crossing site. When riding in the water, riders should watch the far bank, not the water. Watching the water may cause a rider to lose balance. When a horse is crossing water, it should not be permitted to stand and paw at the water, since this is a fairly reliable sign it intends to lie down in the water.

Swimming a horse in deep water is dangerous and should be avoided. If deep water crossing is unavoidable, remaining in the saddle impedes the horse's ability to swim and the rider's ability to get free in an emergency. Split reins should be tied together and hooked over the saddle horn to reduce the chance of the horse stepping on the reins in swallow water. The rider should kick his feet free of the stirrups and hold the saddle horn while he stretches his legs back and floats on his belly over the horse's rump. If a rider is alongside the horse, the horse attempting to paddle

through the water could kick the rider under the water, seriously injuring him. Alternatively, the rider can slide back over the horse's rump, hold the tail, and float behind the horse. Water can be splashed toward the horse's head to keep it moving forward, if necessary. If caught in deep mud, the rider should get off and lead the horse from either the left or right side.

After any ride, horses should always be made to walk back to the barn. They should not be immediately fed or turned out to pasture after returning. Immediate rewards after returning will encourage horses to rush to return to the barn, which is known as being "barn sour." After returning it is best to ride the horse near the barn for a while before finishing or tie it and let it stand for 10 minutes, or more, before being fed or released to pasture.

Arena riding etiquette and safety

Riding in an arena with other riders can be dangerous if proper etiquette is not followed. Riders going at a faster gait have the right-of-way. They are expected to stay to the outside near the rail. Slower riders ride closer to the center of the arena. When stopping, mounting, or dismounting, a rider is expected to go to the center of the arena. When approaching another rider going the opposite direction, riders should stay to their right. Another horse should not be followed at closer than one horse length. Horses should not be longed in a warm-up arena with riders present.

Key zoonoses

(*Note:* Apparently ill animals should be handled by veterinary professionals or under their supervision. Precautionary measures against zoonoses from ill animals are more involved than those required when handling apparently healthy animals, and these measures vary widely. The discussion here is directed primarily at handling apparently healthy animals.)

Apparently healthy horses pose little risk of transmitting disease to healthy adult handlers who practice conventional personal hygiene. The risks of physical injury are greater than the risks of acquiring an infectious disease (*Table 11.1*).

Table 11.1 **Diseases transmitted from healthy appearing horses to healthy adult humans**

DISEASE	AGENT	MEANS OF TRANSMISSION	SIGNS AND SYMPTOMS IN HUMANS	FREQUENCY IN ANIMALS	RISK GROUP*
Bites, kicks and crushing	–	Direct injury	Bite wounds to face, arms, and legs	All horses are capable of inflicting bites, kicks, and crushing injuries	3
Tetanus	*Clostridium tetani*	Indirect, puncture wounds that inoculate tetanus spores	Rigid muscle spasms that eventually paralyze respiratory muscles	Tetanus bacteria are very common in horse feces	3
Cryptosporidiosis	*Cryptosporidium* spp.	Direct, fecal-oral; indirect via contaminated water	Diarrhea	Uncommon	2
Leptospirosis	*Leptospira* spp.	Direct from urine; indirect from urine-contaminated fomites	Flu-like illness and inflammation of the kidneys	Uncommon	3

* Risk Groups (National Institutes of Health and World Health Organization criteria. Centers for Disease Control and Prevention, *Biosafety in Microbiological and Biomedical Laboratories*, 5th edition, 2009):
  1 Agent not associated with disease in healthy adult humans.
  2 Agent rarely causes serious disease and prevention or therapy possible.
  3 Agent can cause serious or lethal disease and prevention or therapy possible.
  4 Agent can cause serious or lethal disease and prevention or therapy are not usually available.

Direct transmission

Systemic disease

Many zoonoses from horses can cause systemic illness. None are common in adult handlers of healthy appearing horses. Tetanus is the most important zoonotic threat. The horse colon is the ideal habitat for *Clostridium tetani*, the bacterium that causes tetanus. Horse manure or objects contaminated with its dust are a prime source of tetanus infection, which can occur when the bacterial spores gain entrance to a puncture wound. The spores can remain infective for more than 40 years. Untreated, tetanus kills by paralyzing the respiratory muscles of the chest.

Anthrax, caused by the spore-forming bacterium *Bacillus anthracis*, can manifest as a blackened skin infection in horses and cause death in humans. Horses with anthrax can transmit the disease to humans by body secretions or contaminating soil with anthrax spores, which can remain infective for at least 70 years. The disease in humans is variable, depending on the route of infection. Anthrax is very dangerous, but rare in the U.S. Transmission does not occur from normal appearing horses to humans.

Rhodococcus equi is a bacterial infection of foals that can be transmitted to humans, but the risk is not increased by being around adult horses.

Brucellosis (*Brucella* spp.), the cause of abscesses on the withers ("fistulous withers") or poll ("poll evil") in horses, can cause systemic infection in humans. Transmission could occur while treating the disease in horses, but does not occur from a horse without signs of disease.

Vesicular stomatitis virus causes blisters in the mouth and nostrils and on the feet and teats of horses. Handlers of horses with vesicular stomatitis blisters in their mouth can become infected from contact with the blister fluid and develop a rash.

Leptospirosis, a bacterial disease in horses, causes eye inflammation and, less commonly, abortions. The eye inflammation, equine recurrent uveitis, or "moon blindness," occurs after the bacterial disease has subsided. Leptospirosis in humans causes flu-like symptoms and signs and inflammation of the kidneys. Zoonotic leptospirosis in humans is usually acquired from contaminated water by ingestion or by the water infecting mucous membranes or breaks in the skin.

Rabies is a fatal disease in horses and humans. Transmission from the carrier occurs after signs of disease appear. The incidence of rabies in horses has been increasing. As a result, anti-rabies vaccine is now considered a portion of the core vaccines recommended for all horses.

Digestive tract disease

Salmonellosis is a problem that often develops in horses confined to stalls and under stress. Humans can possibly acquire salmonellosis from horses without clinical signs that have *Salmonella* infections and from carriers shedding the bacteria in their feces, but based on the general lack of reported human cases from horses in the U.S., the risks are extremely low.

Cryptosporidiosis (*Cryptosporidium* spp.) is a microscopic parasite that can cause diarrhea and abdominal discomfort in horses and humans. Normal appearing horses without diarrhea can carry and transmit the parasite in their feces.

Skin disease

Some mange mites, such as the straw and hay itch mites, can be transiently transmitted from infested horses to humans. Transmission of the mites is from horses with manifestations of the mite skin disease.

Ringworm (*Trichophyton* and *Microsporum* spp.) is a fungal infection of the skin of horses that can be transmitted to humans when treating the disease in horses. The risk is greatest from horses stabled together for long periods in winter.

Dermatophilosis (*Dermatophilus congolensis*), a bacterial disease of the skin called "rain rot," is transmitted by contact or by stable flies. There is no risk of transmission to humans from normal appearing horses, but transmission may occur when handling exuding or crusting skin sores in horses.

Vector borne

Equine encephalomyelitis viruses (eastern, western, St. Louis, and West Nile) can affect humans, causing brain damage and death, but the viruses are not acquired directly from horses. The viruses are spread over wide distances by passerine birds (blackbirds, sparrows, and jays) and transmitted by mosquitoes.

Anaplasma phagocytophilum (formerly *Ehrlichia equi* and *E. phagocytophilum*) is a form of ehrlichiosis affecting horses and humans that is transmitted by black-legged ticks. Anaplasmosis in humans causes influenza-like symptoms.

Sanitary practices

Persons handling horses should wear appropriate dress to protect against skin contamination with hair and skin scales or saliva, nasal, or other body secretions. Basic sanitary practices should be adhered to, such as keeping hands away from eyes, nose, and mouth when handling horses and washing hands after handling them. Horse handlers should be vaccinated against tetanus every 10 years and horses should be vaccinated annually against rabies and encephalitis viruses, including West Nile virus.

Mosquito, tick, and fly control measures should be implemented. Purposeless standing water should be eliminated. Water in stock tanks, pet bowls, and bird baths should be changed at least once per week. Handlers should wear mosquito repellent during mosquito seasons. Cutting or grazing pastures short aids in controlling ticks. Manure should be composted at least 150 ft (45.7 m) from barns. Fly traps and sprays should be considered.

Means of controlling rodents and birds should include sealing any holes more than ½ in (1.3 cm) diameter with steel wool in rooms with grain. Grain rooms should be constructed of gnaw- and peck-resistant materials. Any gaps between doors and thresholds should be less than ½ in (1.3 cm), and grain should be stored in sealed, rodent-proof bins. Grates on floor drains should have less than ½ in (1.3 cm) gaps. Hay and equipment should be stored on pallets so that rodent presence can be monitored. Lightly sprinkling flour on the floors can aid in tracking rodent activity. One-inch gravel, 6 in (15 cm) deep, and 3 ft (1 m) out from buildings can be an effective rodent barrier. Sufficient water should be maintained in water troughs such that birds cannot stand on the bottom and bathe in the drinking water. Bird netting should be considered for use in rafters.

Rodent baits can be dangerous to children, dogs, cats, and birds. The rodenticide remaining in dead rodents can be poisonous to dogs or cats that consume them. Gentle, rabies-vaccinated barn cats are good barn guardians against rodents, snakes, and undesirable birds. Rabies-vaccinated yard dogs are a deterrent to raccoons, skunks, foxes, and opossums.

Grooming tools, halters, hay nets, waterers, and feeders should be thoroughly cleaned and disinfected when used for a new horse on the premises. Stall bedding should be discarded and stall walls, ceiling, and floor cleaned and disinfected for new horses. An effective disinfectant is 1 cup of household bleach in 5 gal (19 L) of water.

When handling more than one horse from different origins, proper sanitation is required to prevent the spread of disease from horses that have little to no signs of disease. Horses from different origins should preferably not be confined in the same barn or adjacent pens or pastures for 3 weeks. Special precautions are needed if sick horses are handled, and sick horses should be isolated from apparently healthy horses.

APPROACHING, CATCHING, AND RELEASING

Approaches to horses have to be adjusted for the tameness and training level of the horse. Wild horses are captured differently to tame, domestic, or trained horses. Before attempting to capture a strange horse among other horses, the social structure in the herd should be observed and dominant horses removed first.

General considerations

Problems with capturing horses can be minimized by handling exercises. Feeding in stalls for 15–30 minutes at least once per day will permit easier capture, grooming, and a health inspection. Walking up to a horse while it is in a pen or pasture solely to stroke it briefly as a reward for standing still and then walking away will, after being repeated many times, desensitize horses to any work or medical treatment after each approach. Failure to do this results in most tame and trained horses having a flight distance of about 10–30 ft (3–9.1 m).

Calming techniques include using a calm voice when around the horse. A handler who assumes a glancing gaze toward the horse's body and legs, with a lowered chin, drooped shoulders, and arms down and hands near the body will be more successful in catching a horse, yet the most important factor is the handler's speed of approach. Approaching too fast or too slow will negate other body language. The proper speed of approach has to be adapted to the individual horse and is based on experience. If the handler tenses his muscles, uses an unnatural tone of voice, or holds his breath, the horse will become ill at ease.

Familiar unstressed voices aid in putting horses at ease. Grooming or massaging the horse with a curry comb before performing other tasks reduces resistance to other handling procedures. Being in close visual proximity to preferred herdmate horses can be a calming influence, but in some cases this can be an undesirable distraction if the others do not behave. Blocking visual distractions by handling a horse in a stall or small pen with solid walls aids in adapting horses to focusing their attention on the handler and being handled.

Importance of head control and haltering

Control of the horse's head is paramount to controlling a horse and protecting both it and the handler. No horse should be handled or restrained without being able to control its head with the use of a halter or a rope around the upper part of its neck.

Horses are claustrophobic. Some, especially quarter horses, may initially tolerate head restraint and then with explosive force attempt to escape, including flinging the head, which can deliver a lethal blow to anyone nearby. To reduce the risk, a handler should never put his head near the horse's head. If it is necessary to be near the head and keep the horse still, the handler should hold the cheek piece of the halter with the elbow of the same arm against the horse's neck. Proper fitting of a halter permits two fingers under the crownpiece and the nose band.

Control of the head permits control of the hindquarters, which is the primary source of a horse's strength. Handlers should never work with a horse that does not have a halter on with a lead attached. The best method of putting a halter on a horse is the right hand brings the crownpiece over the neck just behind the ears and the halter is then buckled, or tied if a rope halter.

There is an underneath method of putting a halter on that involves having a lead rope in hand and looped around the horse's neck. The handler stands on the left side with his right shoulder under the upper part of the horse's neck. The nose band is placed over the nose. The crownpiece strap is held in the right hand and the buckle in the left hand and both arms are raised, one on each side of the horse's neck. The crownpiece strap is flipped over the neck with the right hand and grasped with the left. The handler then steps to the left side and fastens the buckle. This method puts the handler at undue risk of being struck, run over, or hit by the horse's jaw. It also puts the horse at risk of having an ear slapped by a halter's crownpiece strap being flipped over its head. The underneath method of haltering is not recommended.

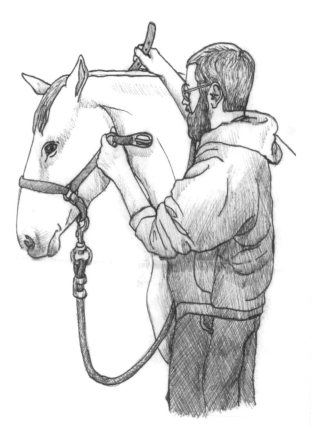

Fig. 11.2 Proper "bear hug" haltering of a horse.

Halters should not be left on a horse in a pen or pasture because they can catch on objects, resulting in possibly fatal injuries to the horse.

"bear hug" technique (**Figure 11.2**). The lead rope should be attached to the halter tie ring or tie loop first.

The handler should approach the horse's left shoulder (also called the *near side*; the right side is the *far side*) at a 45-degree angle to the horse's neck and then rub and scratch the shoulder. The lead rope is then put around the horse's neck just in front of the withers and the handler reaches under its neck to capture the horse by the loop of lead rope around its neck. The loop should be moved to about the mid-neck area. If necessary, the horse is repositioned in the stall or pen. The handler faces forward relative to the horse, releases the lead rope, and holds the halter buckle and strap in the left hand. The handler's right arm reaches over the horse's neck. The unbuckled crownpiece strap is transferred to the handler's right hand, which then allows him to restrict movement of the horse by a loop of his arms and the halter around its neck. The nose band of the halter is placed over the horse's nose with a scooping movement. The

A lead rope should always be used on a halter. A horse should never be led by holding onto its halter. A lead rope should never be looped around a hand or arm or allowed to get caught around a handler's leg. If a halter is an absolute necessity on a pastured horse, a breakaway halter should be used. If head control is needed on a horse that has not been trained to be captured, the use of horse neck straps are another option that is safer than halters on pastured horses. Leather or webbed halters will also lead to skin problems if left on for days in warm weather. Foals, weanlings, and yearlings like to scratch their heads with a hind foot and may catch their foot in a halter, or they will box with each other and catch a foot in another's halter.

The need to catch a horse is sometimes unanticipated. *Temporary halters* can be created with 15 ft (4.6 m) of rope put around the horse's upper neck and tied with a bowline knot. A bight can then be put between the lower part of the neck loop and the horse's throat and then over the horse's nose. A quick release or *slip halter* is similar. A small loop (about 2 in [5 cm] in diameter) is created near the end of a 15 ft (4.6 m) rope and tied with a bowline knot. The rope with the small loop is placed around the horse's neck and then a bight is run through the small loop and then over the horse's nose. When the bight is released from the horse's nose, the loop around the horse's neck also releases, quickly freeing the horse.

Walking behind horses

Horses kick when they are startled, mistreated, or have had no previous handling. Horses that have been handled and not mistreated will kick only if startled or because of other irritations (flies, obnoxious dogs). Kicking is primarily a defensive behavior. An aggressive horse is more likely to bite or strike. Kicking at a nuisance is usually preceded by a lifted cocked leg (a kick threat).

It is easy to startle a horse if approaching it directly from behind. Handlers should always talk to a horse or make other quiet noises, such as whistling, humming, or singing, before approaching its hindquarters. A hand should be kept on the rump as the handler moves around its rump. The handler should stay close enough to be brushing the rump with the side of his body as he goes around. If biting flies are present, it is wise for the handler to be prepared to block the tail with his other arm to prevent possible injury to his eye from the horse's swishing tail.

Key elements of capture

If the horse is alone in an enclosure and avoids being caught, the handler should walk briskly toward it, staring it in the eye with an upright posture and shoulders back. His arms should be kept down near his body. The moment the horse turns its head toward the handler, he should stop, look down, soften his posture, and turn at least 90 degrees away. Intermittent pauses and turning away are used to reward the horse for looking at the handler and not moving. If it stands still, the handler can continue on slowly, not looking directly at the horse, and approaching it at a 45-degree angle to its shoulder. If the horse moves away, the handler should calmly persist. The horse should not be allowed to stand still to eat. The handler should continue with a soft posture, eyes down, and an indirect approach if the horse's head is down. If it raises its

head and moves away, the handler should go back to a brisk, direct, eyes forward, straight posture approach. Again, the handler should pause and turn away briefly if the horse stops and maintains attention toward him. This same approach and pause are continued until the horse can be touched.

After first touching the horse, the handler should walk a short distance away and give the horse a brief break to think about being touched. Then, the handler should approach the horse's left shoulder coming at 45 degrees from the front. The handler should lower his chin and look at the horse's shoulder, not its eye. The handler should keep his shoulders relaxed and slightly drooped. His arms should be at his sides. He should move at a normal pace with confidence. After briefly stroking its shoulder, the handler should stroke its shoulder again with his hand and the end of the lead rope, and then finally put the lead rope around its lower neck. After the lead rope is looped completely around the horse's neck, it is moved toward the mid-upper neck to be able to pull the head around and move the hindquarters away, if needed.

Some handlers recommend training a hard-to-catch horse by keeping it in a small pen and using a breakaway halter with a short lead rope, or for a very difficult horse using a breakaway halter with an extra long lead rope that it has to drag but can be reached by the handler at a distance. However, this method risks the halter becoming caught on a structure. Trying to quickly snatch a short or drag lead on a difficult-to-catch horse is extremely hazardous.

Dangers of using food

Hand-feeding horses or using food in a pen or pasture to capture a horse will teach the horse to invade the handler's personal space and become a nuisance. It can be particularly dangerous if other horses are in the same pasture or pen. Furthermore, treats are not always available when a handler needs to capture a horse. The reward should be standing near the handler and being rubbed only.

> Feeding horses food treats directly from a hand teaches horses to invade the handler's personal space, creating a nuisance and potential danger.

Inside stalls

The horse's attitude should first be assessed. If the horse has its rump directed toward the stall door, the handler should not enter until he or she can get the horse to turn around. A handler can cluck or tap on the walls, escalating this to loud banging, until the horse faces the handler. The stimulus used for getting the horse to face the handler should then instantly stop. This may need to be repeated several times to reposition the horse in the stall.

Most horse stalls only have one exit, the stall door. Therefore, the stall door must always be unlatched when the handler is inside a stall, and a horse should never be allowed to get between the handler and the stall door. A lead should be attached to the halter. The handler's presence should be announced in a soothing voice.

Once the horse is facing the handler, the handler diagonally approaches the left shoulder, puts the lead rope around the horse's neck, and places the halter using the bear hug technique. All handlers should use good manners in a stable by avoiding loud noises or sudden quiet appearances that could startle a horse in another stall with another person.

Doors should be sliding or, alternatively, open toward the outside of the stall. When leading a horse into or out of stalls, the stall door should be fully open. Sliding latches or other protruding hardware should be fully retracted to prevent poking or scraping the handler or the horse.

Pastures, pens, and corrals

Horses should be taught to respond to a whistle or call to come to a stall or pen for grain. The same whistle or call should be used every time grain will be provided to them. A small catch pen adjacent to pastures where horses can be fed, caught, and individually released can improve safe handling of young or otherwise poorly trained groups of horses.

If a horse that needs to be caught has not been taught to come for feeding and is difficult to capture, it should be gathered with herdmates in a pen. The most willing horse to be caught should be captured first and tied outside the pen in a nearby location. The next most willing horse is then caught, taken out and tied, and so on until all the other horses are tied up outside or until the one desired is willing to be caught.

If the last one that is not captured and tied is the one that is desired to be caught, the handler should walk at normal speed with quiet determination directly toward the horse's shoulder. There should not be any efforts to hide the halter. As the horse moves away, the handler needs to apply pressure by continuing to walk toward it. Eventually the horse will stop and look toward the handler. At that moment the handler must stop and turn away. After a 10-second rest, if the horse continues to stand still, the handler can walk a little slower in a zig-zag pattern toward the horse without looking directly at it. The handler should continue until he or she is close enough to rub the horse's forehead and approach its neck to put a lead rope around it. If the horse walks away at any point in the process, pressure should be applied by walking toward it and repeating the release of pressure at appropriate times until it permits capture.

After capturing and haltering, the horse should remain where it was caught and haltered while being briefly groomed, scratched on its withers, and rubbed on its forehead and throat. The handler should then put the lead rope back around the horse's neck to control its movements, take the halter off, and then take the rope off its neck, and walk away before the horse moves. Capture should not be associated only with work or medical treatment, or the horse will develop an aversion to being caught. Catch and release should be repeated daily for as as long as necessary to establish a persistent desired behavior.

Handlers should not work with a horse when other free horses can mill around the handler and the captured horse. If catching or returning a horse in a pasture or pen with other horses is unavoidable, the other horses may try to play with or harass the caught horse, or the horse to be released may attempt to escape and join the herd too soon. A second handler can provide interference, but if the handler is alone handling a horse grouped with other free horses, he or she should have a short whip or stick with a flag to control potential troublemakers.

Trapping horses

Capturing horses by driving them into traps can be time efficient. However, the process of trapping untamed horses forces them to stay still while handlers invade their flight zone. This is counterproductive to the basic training of horses. To learn to be calm around handlers, horses need to be able to move their feet and have some initial control of how far the handler is allowed to invade their flight zone until they learn the handler is a benevolent leader. That is the reason for round pen training.

Feral horses have been trapped or moved by groups of trained handlers using steel tubular horse panels manufactured for small modular pens. The panels are 10–12 ft (3–3.7 m) long, 5 ft (1.5 m) tall, and weigh 50–80 lb. Pressing untamed horses into close confinement with steel tubular panels can be hazardous to the legs of horses, which may kick, strike, or step through the panels, and to untrained handlers who attempt to hold or move the panels against an untamed horse. Some trapping methods involve tying one end of a panel to another fence. If a gap of more than 3 in (8 cm) is left between the panel and the fence, a horse can rear and trap a foot in the gap.

Trapping or moving horses with tubular steel panels should be restricted to catching wild horses, performed by groups of trained handlers, and be overseen by regulatory agencies for humane procedures.

Releasing horses

How a captured horse is released affects how successful the next capture of it will be. Release should be done only after the horse is calm and relaxed. The lead rope should be placed around the horse's neck for control during and after removing the halter. Control of the horse is maintained only with the lead rope around the neck while briefly petting it for standing still and talking to it in a soothing voice. The lead rope should be removed smoothly, and the handler must walk away before the horse can walk away from the handler.

> After releasing a horse, the handler should always move away from the horse; the horse should not move away first or be sent away from the handler.

When releasing a horse into a paddock or pasture, it can get very playful just after release and may try to pull the handler or may kick up as it leaves the handler. A horse should be released when the handler has an immediate exit and in a such a way that the horse has to change direction in order to join its herd-mates. If a catch pen is next to the pasture, the horse should be released in the pen and then given access to the pasture.

If releasing into pasture, the horse should be led through the gate and then turned back toward the gate. The handler needs to be positioned so that he may exit the gate as soon as he releases the horse and moves away. A handler should never attempt to release a horse by reaching over or through a gate or fence.

New horses should be introduced to established herd members in different pastures separated by an alleyway. At other times, they should also be stalled next to each other with a barred grill between stalls. After the excitement of the new horse and the herd seeing, hearing, and smelling each other wears off, the new horse can be pastured or penned with the most submissive herd members. After acceptance by a portion of the herd, all horses can be kept together. However, dominant herd members may still bully the new horse. Introducing them all to fresh pasture at the same time as introducing a new horse will ease the acceptance of the new member.

Special captures
Capture of foals

Capturing a foal requires two handlers. It is imperative to catch and control a nursing mare before attempting to capture its foal. After catching the mare, it should be backed into a flat paneled corner that is strongly built. The handler of the mare should position the mare so that the foal can go between the mare and the wall to hide its face but not escape behind the mare.

The foal handler should not try to stroke the foal before getting it restrained. After the mare is restrained and quiet, the foal handler should move at normal walking speed toward the foal and confine the foal with an arm in front of its chest and the other arm behind its rump (**Figure 11.3**).

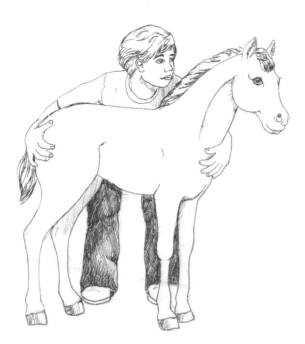

Fig. 11.3 Restraint of foals is blocking of movement, not squeezing them.

Whenever walking behind a foal, the handler should keep his side toward it to protect his abdomen and kneecaps from a kick. The tail should not be held if possible, since some foals will sit down when their tail is held. A foal should never be held just around its neck, as it will rapidly back up and either escape or cause injury. The handler should hold the foal as lightly as possible, and guide it so that the foal is next to the mare in a nursing position. The handler should never be between the foal and the mare. The handler's arms should be used as barrier to excessive movement. The foal should not be persistently hugged or it will resent and resist the restraint. When holding a foal, the handler should turn his head toward its rump to protect his face if the foal struggles and rears suddenly. A gate that does not have a solid panel on the lower half should not be used as a squeeze panel for restraint of foals or small horses.

Large foals may need to be held by two people. The front handler holds under the neck with a knee behind its elbow, and the back handler stands on the same side as the front handler and holds the base of the tail with a knee in its flank. The foal should not be lifted off its feet, as this will add to fear and struggling.

If needed, a small foal can be laid down on its side by a handler standing by its side, bending its head away from the handler and toward the withers. The outside flank should be grasped and the foal gently slid down the handler's legs. Lateral restraint can be maintained by a handler squatting with knee pressure on the foal's neck and reaching between the hind legs and pulling the tail through the hind legs and holding it. Placing a towel over the foal's head and humming to it will increase its relaxation while down. Large foals or weanlings should be chemically restrained for lateral restraint.

Capture of stallions

The capture and restraint of stallions should not be attempted by novices. Only after a high degree of proficiency is reached by the handler in handling mares and geldings should the handling of stallions be attempted. No one, regardless of experience, should handle a stallion without another person within voice range.

The value of a stallion is in passing on genes that are expected to improve the quality of future horses. This supersedes the priority of any other use. Therefore, only stallions of exceptional quality that will be bred to high quality mares should remain sexually intact. Determination of exceptional quality should be based on the unbiased opinions of others, not just the owner. After all, the foals produced will have to be appreciated by others to find future homes and proper care.

Because of their potential value, stallions are often kept in separate enclosures and away from other horses. Their strength, unflappable interest in mares in season, and desire to dominate other stallions make handling stallions more hazardous than handling mares and geldings. Regardless of a stallion's prior handling and training, a handler in an enclosure with a stallion or restraining a stallion on a lead should always be conscious of the stallion's position and demeanor by keeping it in the handler's peripheral vision. No handler should ever ignore a stallion or allow it out of his peripheral vision. A handler should never turn his back on a stallion when leaving its pen or stall.

Wild stallions control mares and challengers to their authority mostly by biting and striking.

If agitated, they are much more likely to bite or strike handlers than mares and geldings. When entering a stallion pen, a handler should back the stallion away if it walks into the handler's personal space. When handling a stallion, the handler should stay at its shoulder or slightly behind it when possible for safety. After the halter is on, it is helpful to back the stallion to signal the handler's authority. Its attention should always be on the handler until just prior to breeding.

Handling of stallions is easier if breeding occurs in a dedicated shed or barn, training occurs in a separate arena, and turnout is a paddock not near the breeding or training sites. Different halters and leads should be used for breeding and for training or exercise. Stallions will recognize the difference and become less excited when the non-breeding halter is used. An extra-long lead rope should be used to handle stallions when breeding because they have to rear up to breed.

HANDLING FOR COMMON CARE AND MANAGEMENT

When handling horses, dangerous objects and situations (junk, dogs, children) should not be in the handling area, and an assistant who does not pay constant attention to the horse should not be used.

Basic equipment and facilities

Handling equipment for horses that attach to the horse's body is called *tack*. Most tack is made of leather, but some is made of nylon or other synthetic materials. Stitching in tack can break and materials can wear out, particularly where leather bends sharply around metal rings and buckles.

Halters and lead ropes

Halters (*head collars* to the British) and lead ropes are the most basic equipment needed to handle and restrain horses. Halters are usually made of leather, rope, nylon, or polyester. Parts of a halter are the noseband, which includes the nosepiece and chinpiece, connecting strap, throatlatch piece, cheekpiece, crownpiece, buckle or tie strings and loop, and tie ring or loop (**Figure 11.4**). Leather and synthetic strap halters have metal nose and cheek connectors.

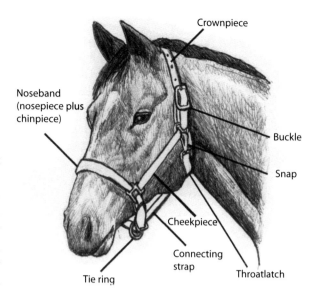

Fig. 11.4 Parts of a halter.

Leather halters will break under pressure and cause little discomfort when pulled against. These characteristics promote disrespect for restraint, and will trap moisture underneath the halter that can cause skin problems. Nylon or polyester will not break, although their metal connectors can. They cause little discomfort when resisted, and trap less moisture and dirt than leather. If near a fire, a nylon halter can melt and glue itself to the horse's skin. Rope halters will not break, causing discomfort if pulled on, and therefore are less resistant to restraint. Rope halters do not trap moisture or dirt.

Leather or nylon strap halters have rings (connectors) that the nosepiece, chinstrap, cheekpieces, throatlatches, and crownpiece attach to. There are noseband, cheekpiece, and throatlatch rings and a single leading or tying ring on the lower aspect of the noseband. The metal rings and the sharply bent leather attachments to the rings are susceptible to breaking under moderate stress.

Lead straps with a chain shank and clip are sometimes used on difficult to handle horses, primarily racehorses and breeding stallions. The chain shank is clipped to a halter and then run through some of the halter rings to exert leverage and pressure on the nose, chin, or gums. Halters with round rings should be employed if a chain shank is being used to reduce the likelihood of the chain binding in the ring.

Although common in Europe and with racing thoroughbreds in the U.S., horses should not be turned out in a pasture or pen with a halter on. If a pasture halter is considered absolutely necessary, it should be a *breakaway halter* with velcro attachments or a leather "fuse" (adjoining leather straps thinner than normal halter straps) joined by a Chicago screw. There is an important disadvantage to breakaway halters in that they may break at a time when restraint is needed. They could also teach a horse that pulling back with a halter on is an effective escape route, which would eliminate an important psychological advantage that handlers usually have with properly trained horses, which is that pulling back does not lead to escape.

Twisted cotton lead ropes are the most comfortable for handlers. They are strong, provide good traction for gripping with the hand, and hold hitches well. Metal halter clips can be attached, but are not necessary for attachment to the halter since a double sheet bend hitch can be used. Braided nylon is available in a variety of colors and is a popular choice, but is slick and does not hold hitches as well. Metal halter clips are clamped on the end of nylon lead ropes. The metal clips or their clamp on the rope is the weakest part of a nylon lead. Lead ropes for only leading and tying horses are usually 9–12 ft (2.7–3.7 m) in length. Longer, heavier lead ropes of 15–20 ft (4.6–6.1 m) are used for longeing or leading other horses, such as pack horses from horseback.

Riding tack

In addition to halters and leads, tack includes saddles, headgear, reins, harness, breast collars, cruppers, and martingales. Many horse handlers, especially veterinarians and veterinary technicians, might not use riding tack, but it is important to know how others use tack on their horses for proper communication and detection of improper use that could cause safety problems to horses or people or produce physical injury to the horse.

Saddles

The major saddle styles in the U.S. include *Western* (with a horn to dally a rope for cattle restraint) and *English* (relatively flat in front without swells) (**Figures 11.5** and **11.6**). *Australian* saddles (with swells in front but no horn) have increased in popularity in the last 20 years. Less common saddle types are racing, endurance riding, and side saddles. The strap that holds the Western saddle on is called the *cinch*. The English riding term for this is *girth*.

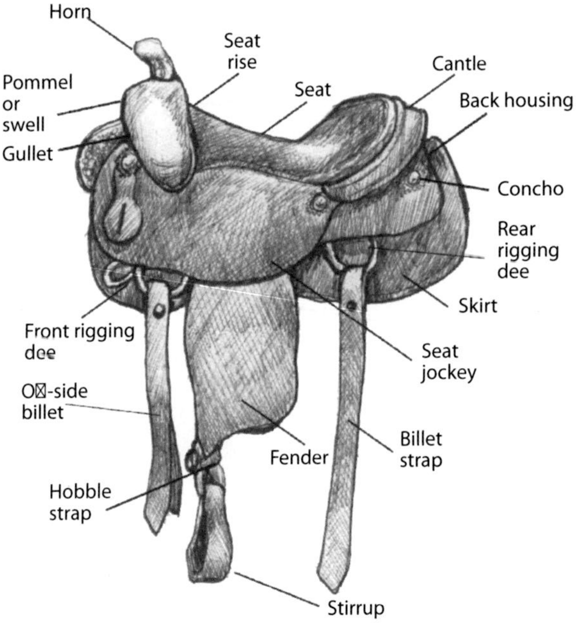

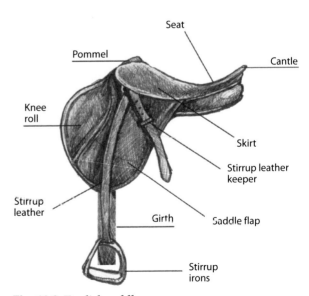

Fig. 11.5 Western saddle.

Fig. 11.6 English saddle.

Western saddles may have one cinch if used to demonstrate leg communication with the horse. Saddles intended for working cattle or trail riding have a back cinch that keeps the saddle from shifting up the back when a rope on a horn pulls the saddle forward or when riding down sloping ground. Western girths may be canvas, neoprene, cotton, nylon, or mohair. String mohair cinches allow better air circulation and are cooler, are cleaned easily, and stretch enough to conform to the shape of the horse.

Two cinches on a saddle is called *double rigging*. Double rigging is preferred for roping, ranch work, and trail riding on sloping ground. The double rigging is termed *full* if the front cinch is below the swell of the saddle and there is a back cinch. A 7/8 *full rigging* has a front cinch that is seven eighths of the distance from the cantle to the swells. The attachment to the saddle is a Y-shape. A *3/4 rigging* is a front cinch located three quarters of the cantle to swell distance and can be either single-rigged (1 cinch) or double-rigged. *Center fire rigging* is one cinch attached at the middle distance from the cantle to the swells. Attachments of cinches to a Western saddle can be D-ring attached to the saddle tree, in-skirt, or flat plate. In-skirt and flat plate attachments reduce leather bulk between the horse's sides and the rider's legs.

There are three main forms of English saddles: *dressage and saddle seat*, *close contact*, and *all-purpose*. Dressage and saddle seat saddles have straight flaps. The cantle on dressage saddles is high, and on saddle seat saddles it is low. Close contact saddles are used for events that include jumping. They have a curved flap and less padding. All-purpose saddles are a combination of both.

English style girths are often leather. Only one girth is used on English saddle. The position of attachment to the saddle is analogous to ¾ attachment on a Western saddle. English girths have double buckles on each end of a single girth. An English overgirth has one buckle on each end of the girth and a strap that wraps around the horse's chest and over the saddle seat. Overgirths are used to stabilize polo saddles.

Saddle blankets or pads help prevent horses getting friction and pressure *saddle sores* on their back. If poorly designed or misfitted, saddles can easily cause back sores on horses. For example, Arabian horses have a narrower ribcage and shorter backs than quarter horses. A quarter horse saddle will cause back skin sores on an Arabian horse.

Western stirrups are generally 5¼ in (13.3 cm) wide *bell-bottomed stirrups* that are used by ropers to stand and be balanced. Bell-bottomed stirrups use a leather wrap on the bottom to reduce friction with the sole of a boot and avoid getting hung up. *Roper* and *Visalia stirrups* are flat bottomed and similar to bell stirrups. *Oxbow stirrups* (also called Rodeo stirrups) are circular and for riding on the arch of the foot, thus reducing the risk of blowing a stirrup, i.e. the foot slipping out. Oxbow stirrups are used by cutting horse riders, barrel racers, and to start young colts under saddle. If hung up and dragged, the rider can free himself easier than with bell-bottomed stirrups by just rolling over on his stomach toward the horse. Oxbow stirrups are less likely to be crushed around the rider's foot if rolled on by a horse that falls. Other options to prevent hangups are breakaway stirrups or stirrups with *tapaderos* (front covers to prevent the foot from going through the stirrup). Tapaderos also keep brush or branches from being caught in a stirrup and help keep feet warmer in cold weather.

English stirrups, which are called *irons*, are metal, open ended, and attached to the *stirrup leathers*, which, in turn, attach to the saddle at the stirrup bar. The stirrup bar latch should be kept in open position. In the open position, the stirrup leathers attachment to the saddle can detach from the saddle if pulled backward, such as when a rider falls off with a foot caught in the irons. English-style riders can safely wear tighter boots than western riders and lace-up boots because of the release bars on the irons on English-style saddles. Stirrup length varies with the type of English riding. Dressage and saddle seat riders need to use longer stirrup lengths, while events involving jumping require shorter stirrup lengths.

Other equipment that may be attached to a saddle include a *crupper*, which is a strap from the back of the saddle that goes under the horse's tail. Its purpose is to prevent the saddle from slipping forward. A *breast collar* (also called *breastplate* or *breast girth*) is a strap that goes across the front of the horse's chest and attaches to both sides of the saddle. Breast collars may be 3-piece, tripping, or pulling. Three-piece collars are Y-shaped, and the lower strap attaches to the middle of the cinch. A tripping collar is a broader strap that attaches only at each side of the saddle. A pulling collar is broad and Y-shaped, and attaches at the middle of the cinch and higher on the saddle, near or to the saddle horn. All breast collars should not press on the chest high enough to press on the trachea. A breast collar keeps the saddle from slipping backwards, and if the cinch fails, the breast collar prevents the saddle from sliding underneath the horse.

Martingales are varied ("standing," "running," "German," "Irish"), but all are straps attached to the cinch or breast collar that runs to the reins or a noseband to prevent a horse from raising its head too high. Most run to rings on their ends that the reins slide through. Standing martingales run to a noseband. Western *tie-downs* are standing martingales. If using martingales, a rider must avoid prolonged, extreme head flexion, which can cause pain and interfere with a horse's respiration. In English riding this is called *rollkur* and is banned by the International Federation for Equestrian Sports.

Bridles

Bridles consist of *headstalls* (leather straps that hold the bit), a *bit*, and *reins* (**Figures 11.7** and **11.8**) English bridles have a *noseband* or *cavesson* and reins

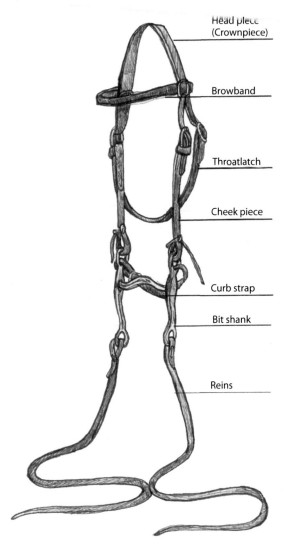

Head piece
(Crownpiece)

Browband

Throatlatch

Cheek piece

Curb strap

Bit shank

Reins

Fig. 11.7 Western bridle.

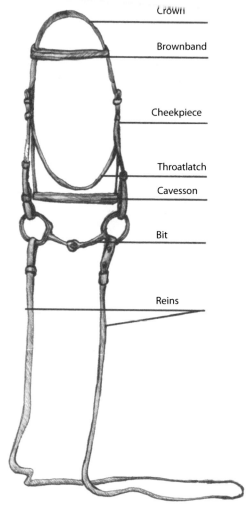

Crown

Brownband

Cheekpiece

Throatlatch

Cavesson

Bit

Reins

Fig. 11.8 English bridle.

the buckle together. Cavessons, when applied, limit the ability of the mouth to open and escape bit pressure. Western bridles do not have nosebands, although separate nosebands may be worn in conjunction with the bridle. Advanced dressage may use a *double bridle*, which has two bits (a curb and a snaffle) in the mouth at the same time and has two sets of reins. A cavesson is always used with a double bridle.

Double bridles include a small diameter snaffle bit (*bradoon*) and a curb bit. The bradoon sits above and behind the curb bit, the Weymouth. Double bridles are used for more sophisticated signaling to the horse. The bradoon is primarily used to raise the head and signal turns, while the Weymouth is used to lower the jaw and collect the horse (push more weight carriage toward its hindquarters).

California (Spanish)-style western riding uses a form of double bridling in traditional training. A young horse is started in a *hackamore* (from the word *jaquima* meaning "halter" in Spanish), which is bitless and puts pressure on the nose and jaw. The hackamore comprises a *bosal* (bo-SELL) that encircles its jaw and nose and a *mecate* (rope made of hair used as reins). A bridle and spade curb bit is added later, with less use of the bosal and gradual reliance on the spade bit until the bosal is no longer needed.

Hackamores

Horses used in Western riding are commonly trained under saddle at 2–3 years of age. Young horses with "wolf teeth," vestigial first premolars that should be removed as a yearling, or erupting adult teeth may not tolerate bits well at this age. For this reason, hackamores are often used on young horses in Western training. Hackamores consist of a bosal similar to a cavesson, a headstall consisting of only a strap that goes behind the poll, and mecate reins. In some cases, a fiador is added to balance the bosal and keep it from rubbing on the nose. A *fiador* is a cord that loops over the poll, is attached to a headstall with a browband, runs underneath the horse's jaw, and connects to the heel knot of the bosal. Pulling on the reins of a hackamore causes the bosal to press on the top and sides of the nose and on the bottom of the lower jaw.

A *side pull* is another bitless bridle that does not cause as much pressure on the nose or jaw as does

the bosal. It is used for training young horses with tender mouths or inexperienced riders with rough hands. It also may be used in place of a bridle in freezing weather to prevent frostbite in the horse's mouth from the bit.

Reins

The reins on Western style bridles are usually separate, called *split reins*. But there are also *loop reins* used for training or for roping, barrel racing, or other sports; mecate (a kind of loop rein with extra length, a third rein, that is used for leading and tying the horse); and romal reins, which are attached with an extension that may be used like a quirt (a short, soft whip). *Romal* (ro-MEL) *reins* have a series of knots called buttons that aid in signaling the location of the reins to the horse.

Split reins are used on working horses because if dropped from the bit they do not form a loop the horse could step through or catch on objects and so unexpectedly trap the horse. If lifted behind the horn of the saddle, split reins will not trap the fingers if the horse lowers its head, and split reins do not catch branches and brush when trail riding. The advantage of loop reins is when dropped from a riding position they fall on the horse's neck. If a split rein is dropped while riding, it falls on the ground and some control of the horse is lost. Reins are usually attached to the bit by leather straps. In some cases, snaps are used. Rubber bands should be used to secure the snaps to reduce the problem of them opening during use.

English bridles have loop reins. Reins in a double bridle need to be distinct by size and texture. The bradoon rein is thicker and textured. The curb rein is smaller and smooth.

With the exception of a mecate, reins should never be used to tie a horse because of the risk of injuring its mouth. Mecate reins can be arranged around the horse's upper neck so that the long extension of the mecate can be a tie, and any pressure from a pullback is put on the horse's neck, not on its bit.

Bits

Bits are metal bars that are placed in the toothless gap of the mouth called the bars, or diastema. Bits are only one aspect of the control of horses. Riders who do not realize this and rely heavily on rein pressure instead of proper use of the seat and legs can injure the mouth of horses and endanger their own safety.

Metals used in making mouthpieces vary. Those that stimulate salivation are preferable. Salivation makes the bit more comfortable and allows the horse to be more relaxed. Cold-rolled steel (sweet iron), copper alloys, and German sliver (nickel silver) encourage salivation; stainless steel does not. Aluminum tends to dry the mouth.

> There are basically two types of bits, snaffle and leverage, with many variations of each.

Snaffle bits are usually the first bit used in training and the most common bit overall. Snaffle bits are usually jointed in the middle. Reins are attached to the snaffle rings, not to shanks (levers), and therefore no leverage is produced by pulling on snaffle reins. Pressure from the reins is directly applied to the mouth. Snaffle bits cause pressure primarily on the individual corners of the mouth. If the horse's head is lowered, there can be some pressure on the tongue and roof of the mouth. Reins should be attached to a snaffle bit above and behind the chin strap (bit hobble). Otherwise, pulling on the reins will tighten the chin strap down on the lower jaw.

Snaffles are direct force bits, meaning they are mild compared with the force possible with leverage bits. The rings that the reins attach to can be round ("O" ring), D-shaped, or oval ("egg butt"). They can be solid, single-jointed, or double-jointed mouthpieces. More severe mouthpieces are twisted wire. There are no shanks or curb straps. Western riding uses a bit hobble that looks similar to a curb strap, which prevents the bit from being pulled sideways through the mouth. Snaffles are fitted to create one or two wrinkles at the corners of the mouth. Snaffles are intended for young horses in training, for inexperienced riders who may pull with force on the reins, and for English riding, which maintains constant contact with the horse's mouth.

Leverage (curb) bits are used primarily in western riding. They are metal bar mouthpieces combined with lever arms called *shanks*. The shortest shanks are 2 in (5 cm), called Tom Thumb shanks. Leverage is a factor of the length of the shank in relation to the

shank that extends above the mouthpiece, called the *purchase*. Short-shanked bits are better for younger horses getting used to the pressures of a curb bit. Longer shanked bits can exert more pressure but also signal the horse earlier than short-shanked bits. Straight shanks apply pressure more abruptly than curved shanks. Ultimately, the severity of any bit is dependent on the rider and the force exerted with the hands. The purchase determines leverage on poll pressure; the shank determines pressure on the curb strap, tongue, and corners of the mouth. These bits magnify the pull on the reins and create a squeezing effect on the poll, lower jaw, tongue, and, in some types of curb bits, the roof of the mouth. Curb mouthpieces are fitted lower in the mouth than snaffles. Curb bits should touch or only create one wrinkle at the corners of the mouth. Most curb bits exert a 1:4 ratio of pressure, meaning one ounce of pull on the reins will result in four ounces of pressure on the mouth of the horse.

A Western curb bit mouthpiece is a solid metal bar that often has a bend in the middle, called a *port*. High port bits (more than 2 in [5 cm] high) or those with a high welded or jointed midpiece such as western-style "correction" bits or "spade" bits may also put pressure on the roof of the mouth. Bits that have a hinge where the bit connects to the shanks are called *loose-jawed* and provide an early signal to the horse. Those that do not have the hinge are called *fixed shank*. A grazing bit is a curb with shorter shanks that curve turn back to allow grazing, although it is generally inadvisable to allow horses to develop the bad habit of trying to graze with a bit in their mouth. The width of a bit should not be more than ½ in (1.3 cm) wider than the mouth. The distance can be measured by putting a wooden dowel in the horse's mouth and marking the width across.

The *Kimberwich bit* and *Pelham bit* are English-style curb bits, since they apply leverage with shanks, although the bit may be solid or jointed. Pelham bits have a second set of ring attachments next to the bit to alternatively exert direct rein pressure. The Kimberwich has large rings next to the bit that look similar to snaffle bit rings, but the Kimberwich rings are offset and will create leverage. The *Weymouth bit* is a straight shanked bit used in a double bridle for advanced dressage.

Gag bits are double-reined bits that have rings on each side with a straight or broken bit attached with small metal tubes that allow the bit to slide up the cheeks to tighten the distance between the bit and the poll. The rings also have shanks attached for leverage. One set (smooth) of reins attaches to the rings for snaffle action and the other (textured) to the shanks for leverage on the mouth and poll. A curb strap is not used with gag bits. Gag bits can be very severe. They are used primarily for warm-ups or retraining periods.

A *Liverpool bit* is a curb bit with several rein attachments for fine-tuning the pressure exerted. This bit permits individualized pressure delivered to horses in team harness, allowing the reins of different horses to be joined together, thus simplifying the signaling to the team by the driver.

Rider aids

Spurs

Spurs are metal riding accessories worn on the rider's heels to reinforce subtler cues to horses to move to the side and gain its attention for instruction. They can encourage collection for precise moves, but the use of spurs shortens a horse's stride and will reduce their forward speed. English spurs have either rounded (*Waterford style*) necks for dressage riding or blunted (*Prince of Wales style*) necks for hunter and jumper riding. English spur necks are shorter than western spurs and designed for close leg positioning when riding. Western spurs have longer necks with rotating rowels. Eight or more points on a rowel or blunted points are mild when used correctly. *Roweled spurs* allow rolling the rowel on the horse's side for further attention, if the horse ignores leg pressure and then rowel pressure. It is important for the rowel pin to permit easy rotation of the rowel. Proper and safe use of spurs requires finesse and should never be injurious to the horse. Short-legged riders should use short-shanked spurs and long-legged riders should use long-shanked spurs to reach and touch the horse only when intended and necessary. If riders cannot push, roll, or bump spur rowels or blunted necks on their facial cheeks in the same manner they plan to use them on a horse's side, such riders should not wear spurs.

Spurs should never be worn when riding bareback. If the rider begins to slide off, the rider may accidentally spur the horse on the opposite side and cause the horse to jump into or onto the rider.

Riding whips

Riding *whips*, *crops*, *bats*, and *quirts* are rider aids carried in the hand. Riding whips, crops, and bats are used primarily by English-style riders. A riding whip is about 3 ft (1 m) long with a lash at the end. A crop or bat is a stiff, 2 ft (0.6 m) long stick with a popper at the end. A quirt is a short riding whip that has been used in Western riding and is similar to a crop, but has two falls (leather straps) at the end. Romal reins are looped reins that a quirt is attached to at the reins' midpoint.

Used correctly, riding whips are not whips but extensions of the rider's arm and used to tap areas of the body to move. Dressage whips are permitted for show riding in dressage events.

Harnesses

Harnesses are worn by horses used to pull wagons, carts, sleighs, plows, or other loads (**Figure 11.9**). Applying a harness to a horse is called *hitching up* (British call it "putting to"). A harness can be a breast strap (breast collar) worn across the chest for pulling light loads. Heavier loads with a breast strap can impair breathing, so they are pulled with a collar and hames harness.

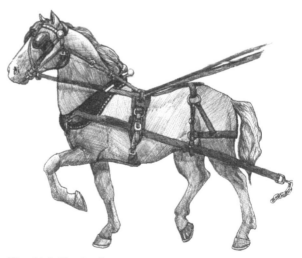

Fig. 11.9 Equine harness.

A *hames* is two curved metal or wooden frames that are padded by the collar. *Collars* are always put on the horse before the remainder of the collar and hames harness. Poor-fitting breast collars or full collars can injure the horse's skin or damage nerves to the shoulder, causing the muscles of the shoulder to become weak and shrink, a condition called "sweeney."

Neck collars should only be used with vehicles that have whiffle trees, which move with the movement of the horse's shoulders. The collar should fit loose enough to allow the flat of the hand to slide under the collar and the horse's trachea. There are two types of neck collars: the *Kay*, or *closed collar*, used for light harnesses, and the *open collar*, which is open at the top and closed with a strap.

Other parts of the harness include *breeching*, which is a strap that goes behind horses closest to the load to aid in slowing or stopping the load being pulled. A Breeching strap should ride halfway between the hocks and point of the hip. It should be loose enough to allow the width of a hand under it. *Traces* are straps that connect the collar to the crossbar of the load (the *single tree*, the British term is "swingle tree"). The saddle or pad is a strap that goes around the chest of the horse and is attached by the girth. The saddle and girth of a light harness is collectively called a *surcingle*. Saddles have tugs and terrets. *Tugs* are loops to hold up the shafts of a wagon. *Terrets* are metal loops to channel the reins. The belly band, loosely attached to the saddle, keeps the shafts of a cart from rising up. The saddle is attached to the breeching's loin strap and the crupper by a backstrap. The crupper is a padded loop that goes under the tail to keep the saddle from slipping forward. The backstrap to the crupper should be loose enough to allow the width of a hand underneath it. Tail hairs are pulled to be short to keep draft horses' tails from getting entrapped by the harness tack. The order of tacking up a harness horse is critical for proper application (*Table 11.2*).

Bridles for harness horses are similar to those for riding horses. Some bridles have *blinders* (also called "blinkers" or "winkers") to block the peripheral vision and encourage the horse to concentrate on just what is in front of him. An *overcheck* attached to a bridle and the pedestal on the saddle prevents the

Table 11.2 **Order of harnessing a horse**
1 Place collar around the neck
2 Fasten hames in the collar
3 Place the harness saddle, back band, bellyband, girth, crupper, loin strap, and breeching on as one unit
4 Put the tail through the crupper
5 Tighten and buckle the girth of the harness saddle
6 Run the false martingale from the bottom of the collar between the front legs and attach to the girth
7 Run the reins through the saddle terrets and then the hame terrets
8 Put the bridle on and attach the reins
9 Attach the overcheck strap from the bridle to the saddle ring
10 Attach the vehicle to the harness

horse from grazing when hitched up and the horse's head from going under a shaft of a wagon if the horse stumbles. Two common bits are the snaffle bit and the Liverpool bit.

Horses closest to the wagon, called *wheel horses*, must be the largest and strongest to stop the wagon on command. In an 8-horse hitch, the next pair are the *body team*, then the *swing horses*, and finally the *lead horses*. The lead horses must be the calmest and ignore distractions to lead the other pairs forward.

Pens and arenas

The facilities needed for routine handling of horses are simple. Pens are usually small outdoor enclosures with loosened soil for better footing that may be used for longeing or training young horses. Arenas may be outdoors or under a roof and may be lined with fencing. Arenas typically also have loosened and dampened ground for safe footing when performing athletic maneuvers or in speed events.

Tying
Lead tying
The risk that a horse may try to pull itself free from being tied must always be anticipated. Horses should only be tied to solid objects that can hold a typical 1,200 lb (544.3 kg) horse pulling with all its strength and that does not rattle, clang, or make any other noise when pulled on. This excludes gates, fence rails, stall doors, and unhitched trailers as safe objects a horse can be tied to.

Unbreakable halters and leads should be used. Slippery nylon leads that do not hold a hitch well should not be used. If a horse pulls back and breaks the halter, lead, lead clip, or object it is tied to, it is much more likely to attempt pull-backs again in the future. Horses should not be routinely tied in a manner that incorporates a string to service as a breakaway, since permitting them to break away with ease at their discretion encourages future pull-backs. A horse should be trained in a safe manner to learn that it will gain untied freedom only when it is quiet and released by the handler.

To create a safer environment for horses that may pull back when tied, leads should be tied with a safety hitch to more easily free a horse in trouble, and a handler should always have a knife ready to cut the horse free, if needed, to prevent injury. When a horse pulls back, it is more likely to become injured if tied too low or with too much lead between it and the hitch. A lead hitch should be tied at or just above withers height, about one arm's length from the hitch (**Figure 11.10**). Tying longer away can allow the horse's neck to get wrapped in the lead rope or the horse to step over the rope. Tying closer can cause many horses to feel claustrophobic and then panic. Tied horses should never be left alone or tied closer than 10 ft (3 m) apart. If tying to a rail, a horse should not be tied so close to the end of the rail that it can move to the other side of the rail. A horse should never be tied to any kind of stall door.

The problem of pulling back usually begins by the horse becoming scared, pulling back, and escaping because of being tied to an insecure object or a halter or lead clip that breaks. Therefore, a horse should not be tied and then introduced to something potentially scary to horses. In potentially horse-scary situations, a handler or handler's assistant must hold the lead rope. Handlers should never duck under a tied lead rope. Horse cannot see under their jaw. This can startle even a quiet horse and cause a pull-back or catch the handler in a very dangerous position. Similarly, handlers should always remain in such a position that they can move away from a horse quickly. They should never sit or kneel on the ground next to a tied horse. If a horse panics and a quick release is needed, the handler should hold onto the lead after the hitch releases so that the horse does not run backwards, fall, and go over on its back, injuring its neck or head.

To discourage pull-backs, some trainers use rubber inner tubes from automobiles around a stout post, to which they tie a horse wearing a non-breakable halter and lead rope. These can injure a young horse's neck from recoil, or the inner tube can break. Holding the end of a long lead rope that slips through a tie ring when a horse pulls back can prevent injury while teaching that escaping by pulling back does not happen. A Blocker tie ring is a metal ring with a curved metal bar in the middle that allows horses to pull back with varying degrees of resistance so that they gradually learn there is no escape by pulling back, but without getting hurt while trying (**Figure 11.11**). Another, older method of preventing pull-backs is to put a loop around the horse's chest with the honda underneath and the standing end of the rope run between the front legs and then the halter. The horse is tied with a regular lead rope an arm's length way from the hitching ring. The chest rope is tied a little closer to the hitching ring than the lead rope. If the horse attempts to pull back, pressure on the chest will inhibit most horses from pulling back, whereas feeling the pull on a halter that seems to trap their head can make them panic.

Horses must never be tied to a hitch ring or rail by their bridle reins. This can easily break the reins or cause the bit to do great harm to the horse's mouth and the incisor teeth. Horses should only be tied with a regular lead rope and halter or a neck loop with a non-slip knot (bowline). Horses should never

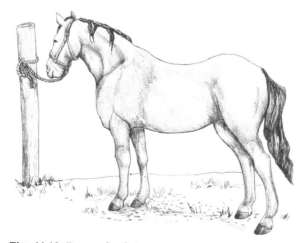

Fig. 11.10 Proper lead tie.

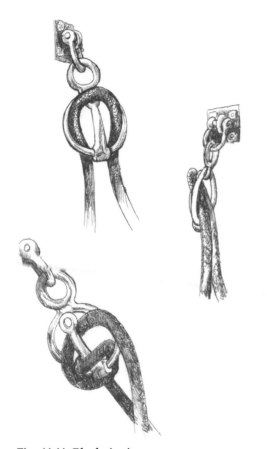

Fig. 11.11 Block tie ring.

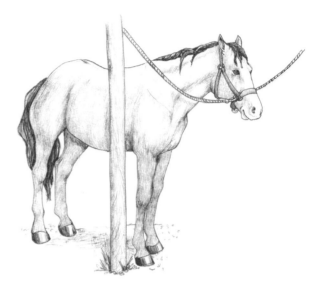

Fig 11.12 Cross-tying.

be tied with a chain shank lead. In addition to injuring the horse, the chain could break and become a lashing weapon. All head restraint riding accessories (tiedowns, martingales) should be disconnected prior to leading or tying horses.

Horses are inquisitive and nimble with their lips. Many will teach themselves how to untie hitches. The end of the lead rope should be dropped through a bight in the hitch to prevent a pull on the end of the lead untying the hitch. A more secure tie is to use a bowline hitch.

Cross-tying

Cross-tying allows a groom to move 360 degrees around the horse easily (**Figure 11.12**). This is advantageous for grooming horses, but cross-ties have several potential disadvantages. Horses have to be trained to tolerate cross-ties, because cross-tying allows little head freedom and horses can feel claustrophobic. If they panic, they are more likely to break free and learn to pull back for freedom, or injure their neck or back, than if tied more securely by a single lead rope. Furthermore, cross-ties are often not available in a safe location.

Accustoming horses to cross-ties should be done gradually. A horse new to cross-ties should be allowed 1–2 ft (0.3–0.6 m) of slack on each side and then closely supervised. Gradually the slack is decreased on subsequent tying occasions until the slack is only 6–8 in (15–20 cm) on each side.

Cross-ties are usually 10 ft (3 m) apart. They should not be more than 11 ft (3.4 m) apart, to prevent a horse from turning and becoming twisted in the tie ropes. Cross-tying should be done where there is a wall close behind the horse so that the horse cannot back up too far. The wall attachments should be 1–2 ft (0.3–0.6 m) higher than the horse's head. The length of the ties should permit the horse to lower its head about 1 ft (0.3 m). Horses that need to lower their head more to clear their airway should not be tied by cross-ties. Cross-tying is often done in barn aisles, but a separate area not used for pass through should be used. If a horse is cross-tied, another horse should never be led underneath a cross-tie in order to move through an aisle. The tied horse must be disconnected from one side and moved over in the aisle and the other horse is led by with its handler on the side that positions him or her between the two horses.

Agitated horses restrained by cross-ties could run forward and flip themselves over on their back, or lose their footing and fall with their head hanging from one or both cross-tie leads. If a horse rears, it can get a leg over a cross-tie line and cause a fall on its side. Because of this, many handlers who use cross-ties use string connections tied to the halter so that they will break easily if the horse tries to escape and will not leave a length of rope attached to the halter of a fleeing horse. Other options are using quick-release snaps and commercial connectors at the wall end of the tie leads that break easily. This option can result in having broken metal connectors on the ends of cross-tie leads on a loose horse, which are dangerous to the horse and handler. Because of its greater versatility and safety, single lead tying is preferable to cross-tying.

Restraint by distraction

Distraction techniques work very well in most horses, but they must be applied with constant rhythmic stimulation. Patting the horse once and then holding the hand still instantly loses its effect. Persistent and rhythmic pats of varying intensity will distract a horse for long periods depending on what procedure requires the distraction technique.

Love pats or pinches

These are rhythmic flat-hand pats or soft pinches. These work well if used intermittently and with varying locations, rhythms, and intensity. Light rhythmic taps on a horse's forehead or behind an eye is often enough distraction to have a horse stand still for exams.

Eye covers and blindfolds

Short duration distraction can be achieved by rubbing the horse on the neck and then sliding the hand back and forth over the head, eventually cupping the hand over an eye. The eye should not be reached for directly, because this will scare most horses. Blindfolding with a small towel can calm many horses. Application also requires an approach-and-retreat sliding method with the blindfold cloth over the horse's neck and head. It can be held in place by tucking the cloth ends under the cheekpieces of the halter.

Front leg lift or hobble

Holding a horse's front leg up using an assistant or a one-leg hobble will cause most horses to stand still. If an examination or treatment is being performed, the front leg on the same side as the procedure should be lifted. If a second assistant holds the leg, he or she should pick the foot up with his or her head toward the horse's rear. After raising the leg, the handler should rotate his or her body so that he or she faces forward with both hands holding the leg up. The hind legs are never lifted up as a means of restraining a horse's movements.

Lifting a left front leg with the left hand while facing the horse's side can permit palpation of the inguinal area with the right hand, reducing the risk of a kick.

Lifting feet
Front foot

To lift a front foot, the horse should first be standing square: front and hind legs on each side equidistant, front legs parallel to each other, and hind legs parallel to each other. The handler then stands alongside the horse facing the horse's rump. Placement of the handler's foot should be at least 10 in (25 cm) to the side of the horse's hoof. Placing the handler's foot too close to the horse or in front of the foot to be picked up increases the risk of being stepped on by the horse. The handler should slide the hand nearest to the horse down the back of the front leg to be picked up (**Figure 11.13**). Many horses accustomed to having their feet picked up will pick their foot up voluntarily at this point. If the foot is not offered by the horse at this stage, then the long hairs on the back of the fetlock are tugged, or the suspensory ligament or the chestnut is squeezed until the foot comes up.

A handler should resist the temptation to push the horse's weight off the leg with the handler's shoulder. This will teach the horse to lean on a handler when holding the foot up or trying to get the foot up. The foot should be held up primarily with a hand on the hoof wall since some horses are uncomfortable with being held at the pastern or coronary band. For the horse to be comfortable and not resist, the leg being held is lifted straight up and not pulled to the outside.

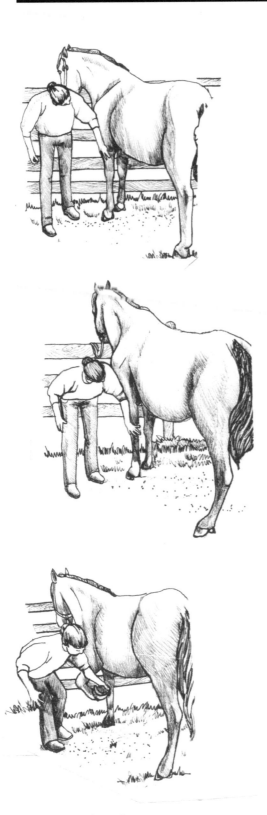

Fig. 11.13 Lifting a front foot.

Holding the horse's foot up for examination or cleaning can be done with one hand. Only if both hands must be free to use hoof nippers or a rasp does the foot need to be straddled and held by the handler's knees.

If the horse struggles with its foot being held, the handler should maintain his hold of the foot until done and it can be gently placed down. The horse should not think it escaped having its foot held by struggling. If the horse leans on the leg being held up, the handler should drop it suddenly and then pick it back up again. This teaches the horse to stay balanced on three legs when the foot is being held up.

Hind foot

To begin picking up a hind foot, a handler should be positioned toward the horse with both hands on the horse. A hind foot should not be attempted to be picked up with one hand with the handler facing backward. The latter method puts the handler at risk of being kicked without prior warning.

The handler starts by standing next to horse's flank with her body touching the horse and out of its kick zone. To pick up a left hind leg, the handler should face the right side of the rump and place his left arm on top of the rump with his hand directed toward the horse's tail. The handler then places her right hand on the horse's rump with her thumb up and slides it down the back of the rump, the upper leg, hock, and finally lower leg. The handler's left hand remains on the horses's rump for the handler's balance and to monitor any resistance by the horse. If the horse moves toward the handler, it can be pushed away when the handler is in this position. Once the right hand reaches the lower aspect of the hind leg, if the foot is not offered by the horse, the hock can be pinched until the foot comes up or the leg can be pulled up toward the horse's abdomen into a flexed position. While holding the cannon bone up and with the leg in a flexed position, the handler moves backward and underneath the hock, resting the horse's left leg over his or her left leg and inside the thigh. At the same time, the left hand on top of the rump is slid down the rump and inside the leg with the handler's left elbow becoming positioned on the inside surface of the hock (**Figure 11.14**). A horse's hind leg should never be straddled in the manner of restraint used for the front leg.

If the horse struggles when holding a hind leg, it is important to hold onto the leg for the safety of the handler and to prevent the horse from learning to escape by struggling. Releasing the leg should be performed when the horse is quiet by reversing the procedure used in picking it up. To release the left hind leg, the handler's left hand is slid up toward the horse's rump while the right hand grasps the cannon bone and flexes the leg, and then the handler takes a step or two backward toward the horse's belly. The leg is lowered toward the ground with the right hand while the left hand is positioned on the horse's rump.

Moving horses

Leading

Leading horses is good mild exercise for horses, especially if done to cool off after strenuous exercise. Leading manners can be ingrained during this exercise. Mechanical walkers are boring and do not provide the opportunity to ingrain proper manners when being led.

Horses are traditionally led on the handler's right side, but there are exceptions. When leading horses around people or horse-scary objects, the handler should stand or walk on the side that puts the handler between the horse and the people or object.

Leading a horse with a long lead and the horse behind the handler can allow a spooked horse to step or jump onto the handler. If the horse invades the handler's personal space, it should be calmly pushed over with the handler's right elbow. Yelling, staring at, or otherwise appearing annoyed with the horse will make the handler appear as an aggressive threat, as opposed to appropriately making the horse uncomfortable with a timely, assertive elbow.

The lead rope should be held about 1–2 ft (0.3– 0.6 m) from the halter with the right hand when leading on the near (left) side of the horse. The remainder of the lead should be folded back and forth like an accordion in the left hand. It should never be looped around the hand or arm (**Figure 11.15**). The halter should not be held without a lead line.

A halter-broke horse should move forward, turn, and stop when the handler does. If it does not, the

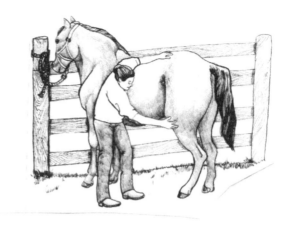

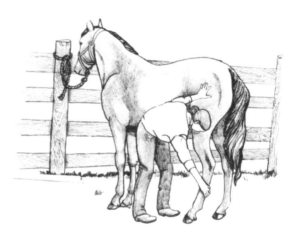

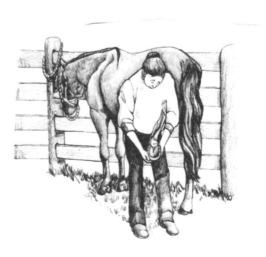

Fig. 11.14 Picking up a hind leg.

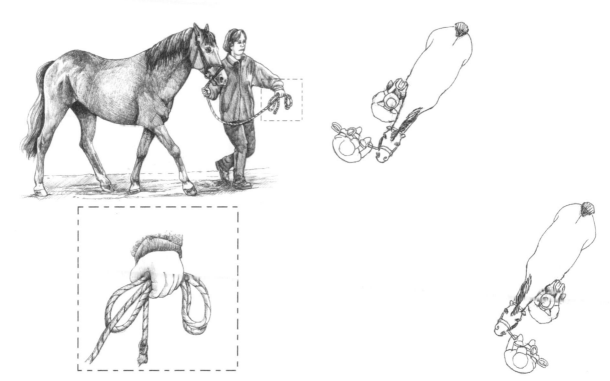

Fig. 11.15 Proper leading of a horse and lead rope management.

Fig. 11.16 The handler controlling a lead rope must stay on the same side as the person performing a procedure on a horse.

handler should not face it and attempt to pull it forward. Without facing the horse, the handler should pull it to the side or in a circle around the handler to get the horse's feet moving, then guide it to walk forward. A handler can also stand near a fence or wall and use a whip in the left hand to wave toward the horses rump when it balks. Alternatively, an assistant can raise his or her arms or a broom when needed while staying out of kick danger range.

Backing a horse with a lead rope can be difficult. On their own, horses do very little backing up. Handlers should never stand directly in front of a horse and attempt to get it to back up, due to the risk of being struck with a front hoof or getting run over.

If leading a horse on a steep slope, the handler should always stay on the uphill side. Otherwise, if the horse spooks or resists, it could knock the handler down the slope or fall onto the handler.

Tying a lead rope to a rope halter with a double sheet bend is safer than using a snap. A metal snap is the weakest part of a lead rope and it can bump the horse's jaw.

Horses trained for western riding should be able to be led by bridle reins regardless of the type of bit used. Horses routinely ridden with an English bridle with two sets of reins and bits should be lead only by the snaffle bit reins. The curb bit reins should be left on the neck and tucked under a run up stirrup strap.

A handler should never lead more than one horse when going through a door or gate. The door or gate must be completely open and fixed in a way that it will not swing while the handler or the horse passes through. The handler should go through before the horse and not permit crowding by the horse. The horse should be backed up, if needed, to protect the handler's personal space. The handler must look forward and proceed with confidence so that the horse will follow. If the handler turns toward the horse or looks directly at the horse, it will not follow.

A horse should be held by a halter and lead rope, not tied, whenever potentially painful or horse-scary procedures are to be done. The person holding a lead rope should nearly always remain on the same side as the person (veterinarian, farrier, etc.) working with the horse, so that if the horse jumps or shies, it moves to the side away from both handlers (**Figure 11.16**).

The only exception to staying on the same side is when assisting someone who is working on the head or neck and sometimes a front leg, so that the restraining assistant needs to stand on the opposite side of the horse to prevent crowding and obstructing the other handler.

Difficult-to-lead horses should be properly trained or retrained to be respectful when being led. When time does not permit retraining before it must be led, a chain shank may be needed rather than a lead rope to provide additional control. *Chain lead shanks*

should be used only when necessary and sparingly or their effectiveness is lost (**Figure 11.17**). A horse should never be tied with a chain shank under its jaw, over its nose, or in its mouth.

A chain shank can be run through the left noseband ring, over the nose and out the right noseband ring and clipped back to itself. This method causes only mild discomfort since it does not constrict on the nose, as do the other methods. Continuous pressure should not be applied with a chain shank, since this will numb the tissue and the shank will become less effective.

A better means of control is to run the chain through the left noseband ring, then over the nose and through the right noseband ring and clip to the right cheek ring. This method is commonly used in leading stallions and young race horses. Pressure on the chain encourages the horse to drop its nose and flex its neck (**Figure 11.18**).

Additional control is gained by the chain being run through the left noseband ring, under the jaw, through the right noseband ring, and then clipped on the right cheek ring (**Figure 11.19**). Clipping to the right noseband ring should not be done, as this will

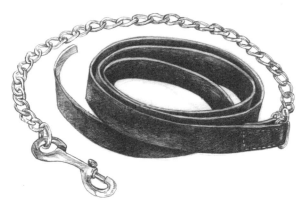

Fig. 11.17 Chain lead shank.

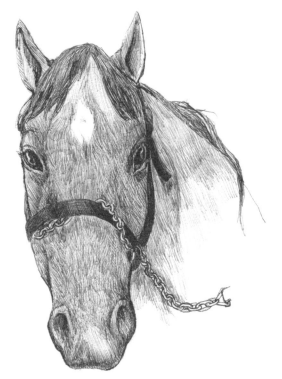

Fig. 11.18 Chain shank over the nose.

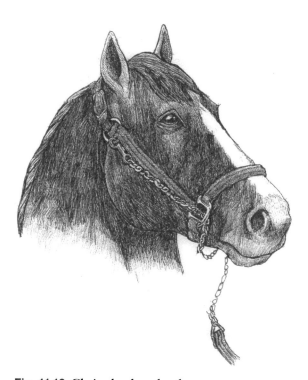

Fig. 11.19 Chain shank under the nose.

twist the halter to the left when the lead is pulled on. Placement of the chain under the jaw may encourage desired forward movement in sluggish horses, and can help raise the head for halter classes. However, this method makes the horse throw its head up, and it is not recommended for saddle horses because it can create a dangerous reaction when the horse is bridled with a chin strap or curb chain. When the strap or chain puts pressure on the lower jaw, the horse may rear or throw its head, injuring the rider.

The most severe use of a chain shank is placing the chain in the horse's mouth, under the upper lip, and on the gums above the upper incisor teeth (**Figure 11.20**). This method, called a gum chain, is often used in the horse racing industry on stallions, but this should be a last resort when handling horses as it violates the rule of using the least pressure possible to get the desired result. There is no gradation of correction possible when using a gum chain on a misbehaving horse. This method does permit a handler to control a horse while having another hand free to complete an examination or treatment procedure. Gum chains require constant pressure to stay in place.

A chain shank should never be run through the halter tie ring and then snapped back to itself. A loop could be formed that the horse can catch on posts or other objects. If the horse lowers its head, it could step through the loop and trap its head, causing a violent effort to get free.

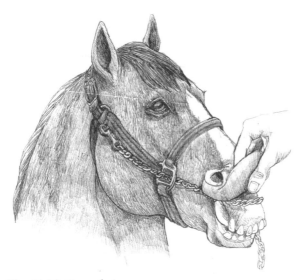

Fig. 11.20 Gum chain.

A loop of rope around the poll and through the mouth above the upper lip works like a lip chain. This is one form of crude head control referred to as a "war bridle." There are other rope restraints of the head or mouth in horses also called war bridles.

A *Chifney bit* (invented by a jockey, Samuel Chifney), also called a round bit or anti-rearing bit, is a restraint device for difficult-to-control horses. It typically has a straight portion that goes in the horse's mouth as a bit. The circular part goes over the horse's lower jaw and has three rings. The side rings are attached to the halter or a headstall with clips. The middle ring is an attachment for the lead rope clip. A pull down with the lead rope will put pressure on the roof of the mouth as well as the tongue.

Leather halters designed for use on stallions during breeding or on undisciplined horses are made of thicker leather and have round rings for use with a chain shank. The increased weight of the halter is a signal to the stallion to prepare for breeding. Lead ropes should be longer for handling stallions in case they try to rear and the handler needs to move further away. Stallions should not be led closer than 20 ft (6.1 m) from other horses.

A foal that has not been trained to be led can be moved by letting it follow its mare, who is being led. A halter and lead rope assisted by a rope loop over the foal's rump can be tried if the mare is not available to be led. A handler should never stand in front of a foal and pull on a lead rope, as the foal may balk and then jump forward into the handler.

Longeing

Longeing (from Latin *longa* meaning "to lengthen") is often spelled phonetically and informally as lungeing or lunging. Lunging is the preferred term in the United Kingdom.

Longeing is an exercise that helps a horse stretch out and expend its initial excess energy ("freshness") before riding or working with the horse. Longeing a horse will help when training it to respond to its handler's body language and voice commands. Other reasons for longeing include checking for lameness and giving the horse mild exercise. Longeing should not be used to physically exhaust a horse. Splint boots, brushing boots, or leg wraps should be used on horses when they are longed to protect their legs during sudden turns.

Longeing can be done as free longeing in a round pen or long-line longeing on a 25–30 ft (7.6–9.1 m) lead line (**Figure 11.21**). Short lines of 16 ft (4.9 m) are safer for both handlers and horses that do not have much experience in longeing. Longeing should not be performed for more than 20 minutes, and less if the horse is under 3 years old.

Round pens for free longeing should be 40–50 ft (12.2–15.2 m) in diameter. If used for mounted training, round pens should be at least 60 ft (18.3 m) in diameter. The pen gate should only open to the inside and abut the post gate to prevent it from accidentally opening if the horse bumps it. Solid walls 6–8 ft (1.8–2.5 m) high that slant outward are much safer for the horse than modular steel pipe pens. Solid walls also eliminate visual distractions during training. However, because of all the openings between horizontal rails, modular steel pipe pens facilitate emergency escapes by the handler if attacked by a dominance aggressive horse. Horses should be allowed 20 minutes alone in a round pen to acclimate to the surroundings before free longeing begins.

When line longeing, the handler should use the hand holding the lead line to point out the direction in which the horse should go and reinforce the command by raising a whip in the other hand. To move the horse to the handler's left (clockwise), the lead line is held in the left hand, the left hand is raised to the 10 o'clock position, while a whip is held in the right hand. If the horse is reluctant to move, the handler should raise the whip with her right hand.

If raising the whip is insufficient to get the horse to move, the handler can escalate the pressure to move by slapping the whip on the ground. Pointing the whip toward the horse's near shoulder will psychologically push the horse away from the handler if it gets too close while circling. The lead line and whip must be switched if the direction of movement is changed to the handler's right (clockwise circles).

The handler must be careful to avoid coiling the lead line around his or her hand or arm or letting it get wrapped around one of his or her legs. Talking with observers should not occur while longeing. Only verbal commands should be given to the horse. The horse should be asked to change pace and directions frequently. When free longing, cutting-horse trainers prefer to have the horse turn its head toward the fence and pilot more sharply when turning. Most other trainers prefer the horse to turn toward the handler when turning rather than turning its rump toward a handler.

After the horse has performed well, it should be stopped and allowed to relax. The horse should never be allowed to run out of air from exertion or excitement, as this can result in the horse panicking, becoming uncoordinated, or acting resentful. The horse should turn toward the handler during rest but not approach unless invited. If it makes uninvited movements that could invade the handler's personal space, the horse should be stopped and backed up.

When longeing a horse in a regular halter, a change in the horse's direction just requires a switch

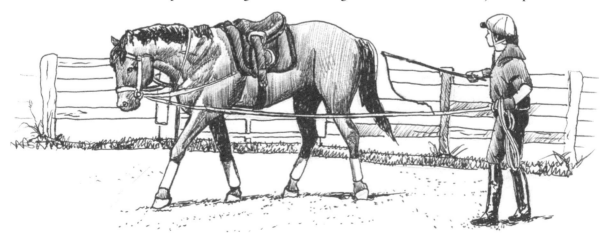

Fig. 11.21 Longeing on a long line.

in the hands in holding the lead line and whip while simultaneously stepping ahead to the horse's shoulder and slightly backward. When the horse changes directions in a fluid movement without heightened excitement, its attitude indicates a safer mental state to be ridden and that continuing to longe is unnecessary.

Long lines

Long lines (British, "long reins") are two lines more than 8 ft (2.5 m) long that run from a bridle through rings in a surcingle around the horse's chest or through stirrups on a western saddle. They are first used with a horse in a round pen. The handler walks a safe distance behind the horse and directs its movements with the long lines. Long lines are used in preparing horses to go under saddle, i.e. be ridden, with proper responses to rein pressure. They are also used in the training of horses to pull carts or wagons and to perform tricks. The Spanish Riding School in Vienna, Austria, uses long lines managed by a handler while assisted by a second handler with a whip to train their famous Lipizzan stallions.

Mechanical hot walkers

A hot walker is a device that mechanically leads (lead or tie walkers) or pushes (panel walkers) horses in a circular path to cool them down after exercise or to provide primary exercise. Horses in a mechanical hot walker should be supervised at all times. Horses are usually walked in pairs and should be placed on opposite sides of the hot walkers. If used for exercise or rehabilitation, the duration should be 20 minutes or less. Horses should never be ridden in a hot walker.

Moving groups of free horses by horseback

Moving groups of free horses while on horseback can be dangerous. A group of saddle horses is called a *remuda* or *cavvy*. The western term for herding horses is "wrangling" from the Spanish word *caverango*, meaning herder of saddle horses. "Jingling" is another term for herding horses, used for when one or two dominant mares have a shiny bell tied around their neck to enable handlers to locate them audibly or visually in environmental conditions with poor visibility.

Two riders, wranglers, are typically used to move horses. The wranglers' horses need to be accustomed to being in groups of horses and not be herd bound (bothered by other horses moving away from them). Experienced herds will follow a lead wrangler's horse, while the second wrangler follows behind to move stragglers a little faster. Horses unaccustomed to being wrangled have to be moved by both wranglers behind the herd, who move them quietly by invading the flight zone of the herd, primarily that of the dominant mares in the center.

A horse has to be trained to be a wrangler's horse, and not every saddle horse can become one. If the herd begins to run, the natural tendency is for a horse to run with the herd. A wrangling horse has to move at the desired speed of the rider in all circumstances and move away from the herd at the rider's will. Older, more dominant horses are usually used for wrangling and they are warmed up under saddle long enough each time to focus on the rider before approaching a horse herd to be moved.

Environmental protection

Fly masks

Fly masks are used to protect the horse's eyes from irritation by flies. They are also used to protect the eyes from flying debris when traveling in stock trailers.

See-through, insect-barrier face masks for horses should be clean with soft points of contact with the skin. There should be darts or rounded inserts to prevent the mask from touching the eyes and eyelashes. Proper fitting allows a finger to fit under the mask at all contact points. Attachments are usually hook and loop (Velcro). The horse must be desensitized to the ripping sound of detaching hook and loop attachments before it can be expected to wear a fly mask.

Before each use the mask should be checked for dirt in the mesh and for damage from prior use. Fly masks should not be left on overnight. A second mask should be worn while the first one is drying after being cleaned. Wet masks should not be worn.

Blanketing

Horse blankets (not to be confused with saddle blankets) are often used to prevent show horses from growing a winter coat. They can be used to keep horses warm in cold weather, but if healthy horses are allowed to acclimate to colder weather, blankets are unnecessary. Once blankets are used for a couple of weeks, they will reduce a horse's ability to adapt to cold weather, which will then necessitate continued blanketing.

Blankets have the disadvantages of possibly causing rub injuries and inducing infection, restricting movement, entrapping legs, and causing overheating and chilling. On the other hand, blankets may be needed for sick or elderly horses, on horses riding in stock trailers in cold weather, or on horses that have been clipped. Clipping may be necessary in horses that do hard work in winter and sweat. Clipping aids in drying them, and blankets are needed to keep them warm when not working. Blankets should be considered for any horse if temperatures go below 0°F (–17.7°C). Lightweight blankets with tight mesh may be used for controlling fly bites.

A halter and lead rope should be on the horse before taking blankets on or off or during adjustments. Blankets have two cinches: a front and back cinch. The front cinch should always be fastened first going on and unfastened last coming off. Caution is needed with horses with long hair coats when synthetic fiber blankets are being adjusted or taken off because of static electricity. When reaching underneath the horse from the left side to grasp the cinches, the handler should face forward to reduce the risk of getting kicked in the head.

Horse blankets can be *standard cut* for stock horses or *European cut* for horses with narrow shoulders. They may have an "open front," which is closed by buckles or snaps or "closed front," which has to be lifted over the horse's head. Closed-front blankets can be put on more quickly and are stronger but are not as adjustable, and some horses may not become accustomed to having the front placed over their head. Insulating fiber strength is measured in Denier. Higher Denier numbers reflect coarser fibers and greater strength.

HANDLING FOR ROUTINE MEDICAL PROCEDURES

Most handling and restraint of horses can be and should be done WITHOUT tranquilization, sedation, hypnosis, or anesthesia. However, certain handling and restraint procedures should be restricted to veterinary medical professionals because of the potential danger to the animal or handler. These require special skills, equipment, or facilities, and possibly adjunct chemical restraint.

Restraint of individual horses or parts of their body
Whole body
Stocks and stall corners
Stocks are standing stalls for examination and treatment of horses (**Figure 11.22**). The dimensions for average horses are 36 in (91.4 cm) wide, 84 in (213.4 cm) high, and 88 in (223.5 cm) long. There is a gate at each end. Horses are led into the stocks from the back gate, and when done they are led forward out the front gate.

Stocks are the safest method of physically restraining horses. Forward, backward, and side to side movement is restricted while in stocks, but the safety of horse stocks should not be overestimated.

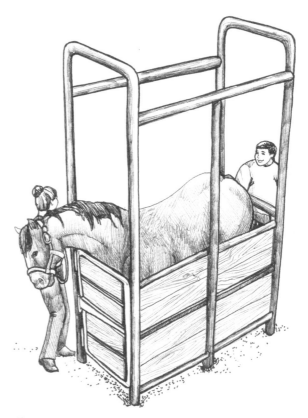

Fig. 11.22 Horse in stocks restrain.

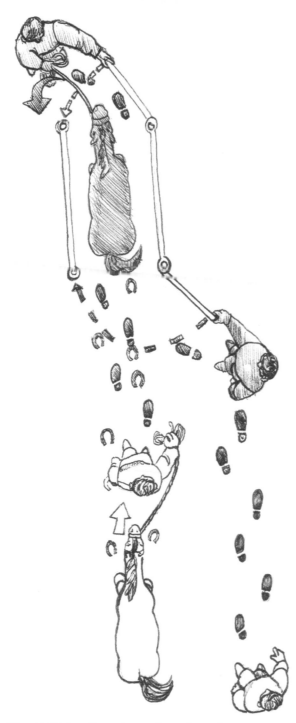

Fig. 11.23 Leading a horse through stocks.

If not further restrained, horses can rear and strike over the front gate and kick over the back gate.

When a mare with a nursing foal must be restrained in stocks, the stock should have a small pen attached to the front of the stocks, so the mare and foal can be face to face until the mare can rejoin the foal.

To move a horse into a stock, it is led into the stock with both gates open, as if going through it. After the handler walks through and passes the front gate, in a calm and quiet manner the front gate is closed first and then an assistant closes the hind gate (**Figure 11.23**). After the hind gate is fastened, the horse's lead rope can be tied. A horse should not be driven into a stock from behind with a front gate closed, or with the handler attempting to lead the horse from the side of the stock.

A halter and lead rope should always be left on the horse. A handler must never approach a horse in a stock while in its blind spot (directly behind it) and startle the horse. A handler or assistant should remain with the horse the whole time it is in stocks.

If stocks are not available, a horse can be backed into a flat-walled, strongly built corner with a ceiling that is high enough that it will not hit its head if it rears. The corners of most box stalls are sufficient. Having the horse's rump in the corner prevents backing and avoidance with right or left movements of its rump. The handler should face the horse at 45 degrees to a shoulder to psychologically inhibit forward movement, and then reinforce this with tone of voice, halter and lead, and some distraction techniques. If a procedure must be done on or near the horse's rump, such as rectal palpation, makeshift stocks can be made in an open area using hay or straw bales for protection of the handler.

Casting

Casting involves laying a large animal down on its sternum or side. Horses are too large and strong to be safely cast without moderate to deep chemical restraint. However, supplementary physical restraint can provide greater control of how horses become recumbent than from chemical restraint alone.

Double side line casting for assisting chemical restraint requires 70 ft (21.3 m) of rope, preferably cotton, and strap and ring pastern hobbles. The rope is folded in the middle and a bowline on the bight is used to create a large collar that goes around the front of the horse's chest with the bowline on the bight knot over its withers. The long lines are run from the withers to the strap and rings placed around the hind pasterns from inside to outside and then back up alongside the shoulders and through the rope collar on both sides.

Casting of horses requires at least three handlers. One handler controls the head with a halter and lead rope. The other two handlers manage the long lines. After the horse is sedated enough to want to lie down, one handler standing in front of the horse pulls a hind leg about 6 in (15 cm) off the ground. The other handler wraps his or her long line around the horse's hip and stands at 90 degrees to the horse on the same side as the front handler. As the horse lies down, both hind legs are pulled up toward the abdomen, wrapped with figure 8's and half hitches with the long lines to keep the legs in flexion, and finally tied to the neck collar. The front legs can be hobbled or tied and a rope connected to the hobble run over the withers and tied to itself. The horse's head should be placed on thick padding and restrained by the lead rope handler sitting on its neck and holding the halter.

Head and mouth restraints

Tongue hold restraint
A fair, not great, examination of the mouth can be performed by grasping the tongue through the bars of the mouth (diastema). One hand is placed on the bridge of the nose while the other, palm down, reaches in the bars of the mouth to grasp the tongue and then pull it to the side.

Full mouth speculums
Examination of the mouth of sedated horses can be aided by a hinged speculum that is placed and cranked open. The McPherson (Hausmann) speculum pries the mouth open by pushing the upper and lower incisors apart and locks in place with ratchets. The PowerFloat speculum is fixated by screw knobs. Full mouth speculums should be used only when a horse is chemically restrained to avoid risk of injury to the horse and handler.

Cradles
Cradles are collars of parallel wooden rods tied with cord that can wrap around the horse's neck to prevent a horse from chewing its front legs and some of the rear parts of its body (**Figure 11.24**). A cradle can also be a deterrent to cribbing and prevents biting and tugging on blankets. Although it permits

grazing, it must be removed for the horse to eat from an elevated feed bunk.

Side sticks
Side sticks are a pole attached to the halter and a surcingle (strap around the chest), which prevent a horse from reaching back to chew any of the back part of its body, but it can still reach the distal aspects of its front legs. Side sticks do not interfere with eating or drinking.

Grazing and cribbing muzzles
Grazing muzzles are used to prevent horses from eating bedding or too much lush grass or from choking on food pellets. Muzzles can allow overweight horses to get pasture exercise and socialization with other horses while being on a restricted diet. A grazing muzzle should be lightweight, provide air circulation, fit well, and have a breakaway safety mechanism for release if it is caught on a fence or other stationary object. They have mesh openings that allow very limited amounts of grass to be grazed.

The fit should allow 1 in (2.5 cm) from the bottom of the muzzle to the lips and 3–4 fingers' width on the side of the muzzle. A grazing muzzle should be removed for an hour twice per day to ensure that the horse drinks and can lick salt. They can drink with it on, but some horses will not.

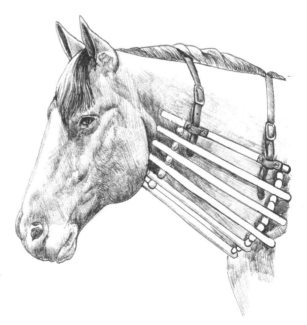

Fig. 11.24 Neck cradle.

The initial cause of cribbing is controversial, but regardless of the inciting cause, it is aggravated by boredom. A horse cribs by grabbing a stationary horizontal object with its incisors, usually immediately after eating grain, flexing its neck, leaning back while grunting, and sucking air into its throat. Grazing muzzles may prevent cribbing. Some stables attempt to eliminate all horizontal objects that horses could crib on. Surgery to prevent cribbing is no longer recommended.

A common problem with the efficacy of grazing and cribbing muzzles is intermittent use. To be effective, they must be used every time the horse has access to grass or to a horizontal object that it can crib on.

Cribbing collar

An alternative to a muzzle for controlling cribbing is a cribbing collar. This is a collar that goes around the ears and throat and causes discomfort when the horse pulls down and back with its mouth. Some collars emit a low voltage electric shock when the horse cribs. There is debate about whether horses should be physically prohibited from cribbing, since this is blocking an emotional and perhaps physiological need to crib, and physical restraint may make the need to crib worse. Since there is risk of a horse in a pasture getting the collar caught on fencing or other objects, at least one attachment should be breakaway. If something startles the horse and it raises it head too high, the strap on some collars can press on the trachea and carotid arteries, causing the horse to stagger or faint.

Horses that crib should be in a pasture with other horses for distraction and confined with electric fencing that they cannot crib on.

Bib

An equine bib is a leather flap that attaches to a halter. Its purpose is to prevent chewing of wounds or blankets. It must be removed to allow the horse to eat. Drinking is possible with the bib in place, but the horse may not attempt it and must be monitored for attempts to drink.

Neck straps

Neck straps are similar to dog collars and are fitted to be worn on the upper neck. The strap's purposes are for identification and minimal restraint. A horse should not be led by holding onto a neck strap. Straps should be breakaway for the safety of the horse at turnout and the safety of the handler who tries to use the strap for more than minimal restraint. Neck straps are less prone to being caught by bolts, limbs and such than are halters on pastured horses. They are primarily used to identify individual broodmares.

Tail restraint

A horse's tail may be tied with a quick release sheet bend and then to its neck with a bowline knot. The tail should never be tied to anything other than the horse's body. To grasp and tie the tail, the right-handed handler stands next to the horse's left hip and slides his or her right hand over the horse's rump and reaches around with the right hand to grasp and pull the tail toward him or her, rather than standing in the kick zone. A sheet bend (tail tie) is begun by laying the rope perpendicular across the tail and folding the tail over the rope.

Placement of rectal thermometers

Rectal temperatures are routinely taken on horses with minimal head restraint. Using a halter and lead rope, an assistant should hold the horse, or if the horse is well tamed it can be tied by the lead rope. In either case, the horse should be positioned near a wall or strong fence. The handler should walk next to the left side of the horse and stand with his body touching the left flank with his left hand on top of the horse's rump. The handler grasps the base of the tail with the left hand and slightly lifts the tail. While holding a lubricated thermometer in the right hand, the handler leans toward the horse's anus. The right hand should be slid over the left hip toward the anus to prevent startling the horse. The thermometer is then inserted into the rectum.

Working with a downed horse
Handler safety

Note: Rescue operations on downed horses should be performed by trained personnel with optimum equipment for safety of the horse and the personnel assisting with the rescue. Ideal methods are available from Technical Large Animal Emergency Rescue, www.TLAER.org However, trained personnel for horse rescues are not plentiful and might not be able to respond quickly enough. A local veterinarian should always be called since the horse will probably require medical care and chemical restraint, and the owner or others with a strong emotional attachment will be unable to make objective decisions during the rescue attempt. The following information is intended to alert routine handlers of the risks if they believe more immediate assistance is required, or if they are asked to help trained personnel.

A recumbent horse rises on its front legs first. Control of front legs is most critical to preventing a horse from rising at an undesired time. A horse lying on its side must lift its head, lie on its sternum, and extend its front legs to rise. Kneeling on the horse's neck or holding the nose up and pulled to the side toward its withers will prevent a horse from regaining its feet. Another person should maintain a strap or rope to the person leaning over the horse to pull the handler away if the horse thrashes before it is restrained. When a horse is lying on its side, it can injure its recumbent-side eye or its facial nerve if its head is not cushioned or flexed upward and held in that position.

> All procedures done on a downed horse should be done with the handler standing behind the horse's back, not on the legs side.

Cast in a stall
Some horses, particularly younger ones, will sometimes attempt to roll in their stall. When they do, there is a risk of being cast in a stall: rolling three-quarters of the way over next to a wall and becoming entrapped from being tipped on their backs with their legs folded against the wall. In this position, they cannot push themselves back or away from the wall, and they will panic, thrashing with their legs and head. Remaining in this position can be fatal for a horse.

To rescue a horse that is cast in a stall, the handler should call for assistance while also calming the horse. The handler should talk to the horse to ensure the horse knows of the handler's presence. As soon as an assistant is present, the handler should position himself near the lower part of the horse's neck while not getting near the horse's legs or trying to step or reach over the horse. The safest method of moving

the horse is to place a rope loop around its neck, work the loop toward the upper part of the horse's neck, and then pull the neck away from the wall and toward the middle of the stall until the horse can get its legs underneath its body. In the absence of a rope, the mane in the mid-neck area can be pulled to move the horse. Pulling by a halter and lead rope to reposition a cast horse could injure its neck. Care must be taken by the handler not to get stepped on or pinned against the wall by the horse as it attempts to stand. An hour after the horse is again standing, it should be observed for signs of colic, which can result from being cast, and swelling in the legs from injuries that may have occurred.

Alternative methods that involve pulling on the horse's legs and rolling the horse toward the handler are not recommended.

Lifting a trapped or injured horse
It is best to lift horses with straps designed for slinging a horse. New, improved hoist slings for horses have been designed in the last 20 years. However, if a sling harness and trained personnel are not available in time to save a horse trapped in a ditch, well, or other life-threatening situation, it may be lifted with a rope sling and a two-block tackle, each with two sheaves, and a ¾ in rope. A halter and lead rope should be applied first. If a halter and lead rope are not available, a temporary one can be made with a rope by a neck loop tied with a bowline knot and then a bight through the neck loop and over the nose. A blindfold should be applied next, preferably with padding over the eyes using a jacket, towels, or a woman's bra.

A rope sling can be made using 50–70 ft (15.2–21.3 m) of ½ in (1.3 cm) or thicker nylon rope by making a collar in the middle of the rope using a bowline on a bight. The collar is placed on the horse's neck with the bowline on a bight on the front of the horse's chest. The rope ends are passed under the front legs, up and under the neck loop collar, crossed over the back, and run under the hind legs (from front to back). It is important not to cross the ropes under the horse. The ropes should be brought up the back of the legs near the base of tail, under the crossed ropes on the middle of the back and under the collar, and then bend the ends back behind the crossed ropes and tie with a quick-release knot. The hook on the traveling block of the block and tackle is attached to the back ropes just behind the withers.

In some situations, a metal rod bent in a C-shape, with the end bent back to bunt the leading edge and with the rope attached to the other end, may be needed to thread the rope under the legs. Blunted hooks on poles should be used to retrieve ropes near the horse's legs or feet. Towels or clothing should be placed under the leg ropes for padding. Lifting should be slow while someone restricts large movements of the head by holding onto the lead rope.

Moving downed horses on glides

Glides (also called "slides" or "skids") are sheets of slick plastic that a downed horse is placed on and moved by sliding the sheet (**Figure 11.25**). The horse is pulled onto the glide after "sawing" or "flossing" restraint straps under its body and around its chest and flank. One person must maintain control of the head with a halter and lead rope while several others pull the horse, back first with the straps around its body, onto the glide. The degree of restraint to maintain the horse on the glide varies, but this often requires chemical restraint, a padded face mask to protect its eyes and facial nerve, hobbles, and straps over the torso. Additional glides may be needed to cover rough surfaces to allow the glide that is carrying the horse to slide more easily.

In emergencies, if a glide is not available, a heavy tubular steel gate at least 8 ft (2.5 m) long can be used as a glide or travois to move a downed horse over rough ground.

Injections and venipuncture
Access to veins

In horses, the jugular vein in the neck is nearly always used to obtain blood samples and give intravenous injections. The cephalic vein in the front leg, transverse facial vein near the eye, saphenous vein, and lateral thoracic vein are dangerous to use in an unsedated adult horse. The medial saphenous vein can be accessed in a foal if the foal is held in lateral recumbency.

Normally, little restraint is needed for jugular venipuncture. A halter with a lead rope is usually sufficient. The handler may use mild distraction techniques when needed. The phlebotomist occludes the vein and collects the blood without further assistance.

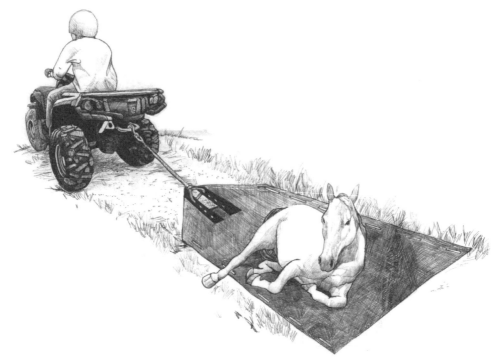

Fig. 11.25 Moving a downed horse on a glide.

Injections

Intramuscular

Most injections in horses are intramuscular (IM) and done in the neck (lateral cervical) area. The preferred lateral cervical location in adult horses is a triangle one hand's width above the jugular vein, one hand's width in front of the shoulder, and one hand's width below the crest of the neck (**Figure 11.26**). Less commonly, injections might be given into the pectoral, triceps, gluteal, or semitendinosus/semimembranosus (thigh) muscles. Injections into the thigh or gluteal muscles should be performed by the handler pressing his or her body against a side of the horse and leaning around or over the horse to make the injections on the opposite side from the one where the handler is standing. To prepare a horse for the injection, the skin around the injection site is gentle pinched a few times immediately before the needle is inserted into the muscle, after which the syringe is attached to the needle.

Intramuscular injections should not be given into the neck muscles of nursing foals. Resulting soreness may prevent it from nursing. The thigh muscles should be used for IM injections in nursing foals.

Subcutaneous

Subcutaneous (SC) injections are poorly absorbed in horses and can result in severe reactions. They are very rarely administered in this species. The lateral cervical area is used when SC injections are indicated.

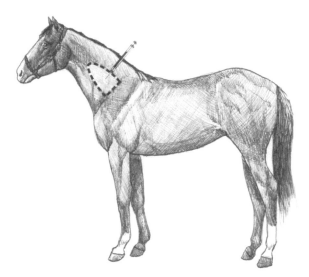

Fig. 11.26 Preferred site for IM injection in horses.

Intravenous

Intravenous injections in unsedated horses are nearly always given into the jugular vein.

Administration of oral and ophthalmic medications

Oral

Although giving oral medications to horses is usually not difficult, it is helpful if the medication or its vehicle tastes pleasant to the horse. Tablets can be crushed with a mortar and pestle, small plastic pill crusher, or a medication-dedicated coffee grinder. Crushed medication may be added to a paste of applesauce, corn syrup, molasses and brown sugar, banana, cherries, shredded carrots, peppermint, pudding, peanut butter, or yogurt to improve palatability. Palatable medications can often be added to the horse's grain or in a treat such as a small amount of alfalfa pellets to successfully administer the medication. If this is not possible or effective, an oral syringe may be used. The paste should not be administered into the cheek pouch. Instead, it should be placed in the interdental space ("bars of the mouth") and injected on top of the tongue. A balling gun to deliver tablets (boluses) should never be used in a horse because of the risk of injury to the horse or handler.

Before giving a paste by oral syringe, there should be no grass or hay in the mouth, which could enable the horse to mix it with the paste and spit it out. To administer the oral medication with a syringe from the horse's left side, the handler should put his or her left fingers on the halter's noseband and their thumb in the corner of its mouth while standing close to the horse's shoulder and bending its nose toward the handler. The syringe is held in the right hand. The back of the right hand is pressed against the horse's cheek and the hand rotated to place the syringe into the left bars of the mouth beneath the thumb of the left hand. After inserting the tip of the oral syringe into the mouth, it is angled toward the throat and the syringe plunger pushed slowly to deliver the medication to the top of the tongue.

Administration of large volumes of oral fluids requires passage of a stomach tube, which is done through a nostril. The horse is restrained with a long-handled nose twitch for the passage of the nasal tube.

Ophthalmic

Horses have the largest eyes of any land animal. The size of their eyes alone puts them at high risk of injuries. Like all animals, horses are protective of painful eyes. Even if they stand still for exam and treatment, they have very strong palpebral muscles that clamp the eye fissure shut. Treatment with dropper bottles or ointment tubes can be attempted by stabilizing the heel of the hand holding the medication on the horse's skull above the affected eye. The handler's other hand pulls the lower lid down to open the palpebral fissure and drop the medication onto the eye or inner surface of the lower lid.

Another method of administering ophthalmic ointment is to wear a sterile glove and place ointment on the gloved index finger. The handler's ungloved hand is used to open the palpebral fissure while the gloved finger scrapes the ointment onto the inside surface of the lower lid.

When ophthalmic medications are administered, the treatment hand should be stabilized against the horses head and move with movements of the head. This should be done with constant pressure rather than the more hazardous method of running a hand under a halter to stabilize the hand.

Reliable administration of ophthalmic medications to horses often requires sedation and placement of a subpalpebral or nasolacrimal tube.

SPECIAL EQUIPMENT

Twitches

Twitches are distraction techniques applied to the neck or nose of horses. Procedures that twitches are used for include passing stomach tubes, standing castrations, treating wounds, and farriery work. Twitches should never be used on a foal.

Twitches provide a temporary diversionary stimulus while a procedure is done that the horse otherwise would not tolerate. Twitches can injure tissue if applied for too long (more than 10–15 minutes), and they should be applied effectively on first attempt. Gently rubbing the skin where the twitch was applied after its removal will improve recirculation of blood in the area and provide a kind release for the horse to remember. Twitches should not be used to try to control a distressed horse that is thrashing, when the area to be twitched has been previously injured, or as a means of discipline and training of horses.

Based on one study, conventional opinion is that twitches work by the release of endorphins. Endorphins are internally produced morphine-like substances in the brain. Human long-distance runners' brains produce endorphins during running, which cause the euphoric sensation and addictive behavior associated with running. Conversely, horses do not become addicted to having a nose twitch applied. In fact, they usually become resentful and anxious about it being used repeatedly.

Endorphins are released to modulate the discomfort and speed the recovery of having a twitch applied. They do not cause the horse to become tractable from an endogenous opiate high. Horses that have had nose twitches used, particularly if used aggressively or for too long, are likely to strike with a forefoot when a handler works near its head. When a nose twitch is used, the horse becomes motionless and submissive to protect its lip from the possibility of being torn, which would risk the horse's survival.

The *long-handled nose twitch*, made from hickory wood, is most commonly used to twitch the nose (upper lip), but it should be used as infrequently as possible and for the shortest possible time. Long-handled twitches are about 30 in (76.2 cm) long with a rope or cord, leather, or chain loop (**Figure 11.27**).

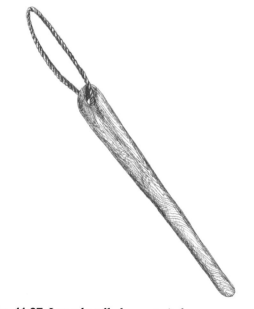

Fig. 11.27 Long-handled nose twitch.

Rope or cord twitches are preferable. The loop applies a clamping effect on the upper lip. The horse should be in stocks or standing with its right side next to a solid wall or fence. The handler holds the stick and halter with the right hand about 1 ft (0.3 m) from the twitch loop, grasps the cheekpiece of the halter, and pulls the head to the left while the handler stands close to the horse's left shoulder. There is risk of the horse striking out with a front leg if the handler stands in front of the horse. The handler places the twitch's loop over the left hand with the little finger outside to prevent the loop from sliding over the wrist (**Figure 11.28**). The horse's upper lip is grasped between the thumb and three fingers of the left hand and the loop is slid over the fingers onto the lip. While keeping the fingers holding the lip out of the way, the handle is twisted clockwise with the right hand, which continues to hold the lead rope (**Figure 11.29**). The left hand assists in keeping the rope from wrapping around the twitch handle. When the twitch is applied, an assistant must continue to hold it as well as the lead rope and should slowly rock or jiggle the twitch handle to continue

the distraction. Within 5 minutes the twitch should be removed by grasping the lip, untwisting the twitch, and removing it in a controlled manner (not pulled off) while desensitizing the horse by rubbing its nose and patting its neck. Neither twisting the loop on nor off should be done rapidly.

A handler should never stand in front of the horse while applying a nose twitch.

A nose twitch can be performed using a bare hand. The upper lip is squeezed between the thumb and the index and middle fingers. This is effective only for a very short period. A leveraged twitch can be improvised with a small loop of rope and a stick. This can be maintained longer than just using a bare hand. Application is the same as with a long-handled twitch.

A *skin twitch* (the "Gypsy Hold") consists of grasping a fold of skin on the neck just in front of a shoulder, which can distract a horse for a short time. The fold of skin should be rolled over the fingers so it can be held in a tight fist and slowly rocked or jiggled.

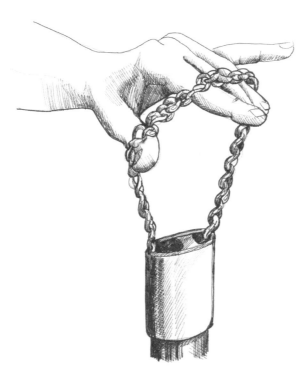

Fig. 11.28 Hand position to apply a long-handled nose twitch.

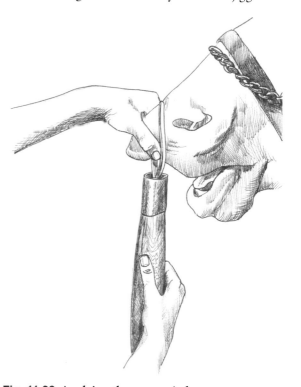

Fig. 11.29 Applying the nose twitch.

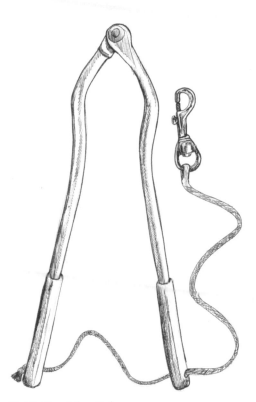

Fig. 11.30 Kendal twitch.

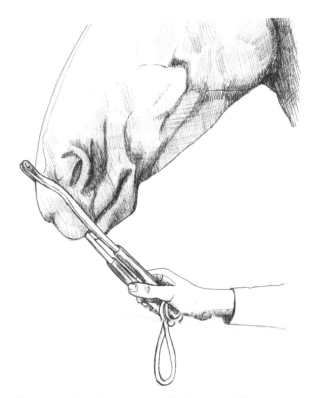

Fig. 11.31 Kendal twitch applied to upper lip.

The *humane* or *Kendal twitch* is a small hinged clamp, curved to prevent excessive pinching, that is placed on the horse's upper lip (**Figures 11.30 and 11.31**) It is no more or less humane than other twitches that are applied correctly. It is intended to be clipped to the halter to free the hands of the handler. However, the twitch can be knocked off by the horse, allowing the twitch to become a swinging menace to the horse and handlers. It is much safer when used by an assistant who continues to keep hold of the twitch as long as it is applied, but this may not be possible if the horse rears or is tall and elevates its head. Like other twitches, a jiggling or rocking motion will prolong the distraction effect. However, the humane twitch is more likely to slip off the nose than a long-handled twitch of rope or cord.

The *Wilform twitch* is a metal square with a screw and a bar that acts as a vice (**Figure 11.32**). It has no bars sticking out to the side. Because of the leverage of the screw, it could be applied too tightly, and if not applied tightly enough, it could be slung off by the horse as a highly dangerous metal missile.

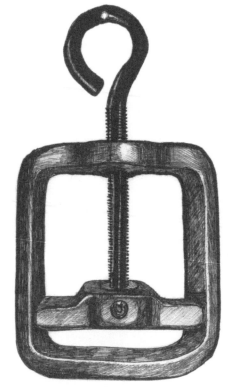

Fig. 11.32 Wilform nose twitch.

The ear should never be held in a manner that might inflict pain.

An *ear twitch* is an ear being roughly pulled on by a hand or a long-handled twitch or even bitten by a handler. Ear twitches should never be used. Good horsemen spend hundreds of hours desensitizing horses to having their ears handled. This could be ruined in one application of an ear twitch. Ear twitching can damage the horse's ear cartilage, blood supply, and nerves. The pain can make the horse head-shy and thus a danger to anyone who tries to halter or bridle the horse afterwards. If the horse becomes disfigured, useless, or unsafe, it may euthanized. In some states in the U.S., ear twitching is illegal.

Hobbles

Hobbles can be useful in restricting a horse's movement. However, hobbles should not be used on horses with a history of neuromuscular problems, those that are sedated, or when a painful procedure is required. A handler who puts any type of hobbles on a horse should remain near enough to immediately provide reassurance and aid to a horse that struggles violently.

Front leg hobbles

Front leg hobbles are also used to teach patience and discipline. They can teach the horse not to panic if its legs become entrapped in wire or with rope. However, some horses can learn to do a modified lope with hobbles on. A horse that is trained to accept front leg hobbles will often be calm to many stimuli that might otherwise bother it. However, using front leg hobbles on a horse for the first time in an emergency could cause it to panic and lead to injury. Hobble training should be done gradually.

Front leg hobbles are also used to prevent horses from traveling extended distances when turned loose (**Figure 11.33**). They may be used for short periods when a rider must be dismounted and cannot tie the horse to a suitable object, and for longer periods to allow grazing. Grazing hobbles should be attached to the cannon bones rather than the pasterns to allow

better clearance of brush and less rubbing of the legs. When multiple horses are hobbled overnight, one horse should be tied, saddled, and fed grain, and so be ready for retrieving escaped horses. The lead horse in the group should also wear a neck strap with a bell to locate a group if they escape. Horses should be allowed to drink before being hobbled. Hobbled horses that try to drink from ponds, lakes, or streams can trip and drown.

It has been suggested that the Tom Fool knot can be used as hobbles for horses. The Tom Fool knot is essentially two bights through a loop in a rope and is similar to the Handcuff knot. However, the Tom Fool knot cannot be applied to a horse's legs without picking each foot up. The knot jams the legs against each other, making it hard for the horse to maintain its balance if it attempts to move. It may have value in restraining the legs of an anesthetized horse.

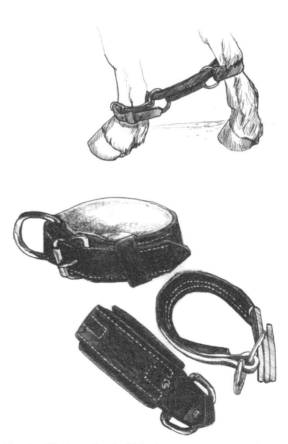

Fig. 11.33 Front leg hobbles limit movement and permit grazing.

One-leg hobble ("Rarey strap")

A one-leg hobble ties a front leg in flexion. It can be used to restraint difficult horses for procedures that require the horse to stand still. If a horse is not trained in advance for a front leg hobble, it should be applied on soft footing and the horse's movements controlled at a distance by the lead rope and halter, since the horse may struggle for a relatively short period before it becomes resolved to the restraint. One-leg hobbles are sometimes used for brief (5 minute) periods to establish leadership over a dangerous horse. Horses with a one-leg hobble applied can still rear and pivot on the hindquarters and can be dangerous to handlers. The one-leg hobble was made popular by an American horseman, John Rarey, who was called to England in the 1800s to assist training a horse for Queen Victoria.

Picket (staking or pegging) hobble

A horse that has been trained for hobbles can be staked with a hobble on one leg. A single-leg leather hobble with an attached metal ring, stake lead rope, and swivel snaps on the stake permit safe grazing within the radius of the stake lead rope. Either a front leg or a hind leg can be hobbled, but hobbling a hind leg is safer for the horse. If staked with a hobble on a front leg, the horse could be tripped and fall should it spook and jump. The stake should be well anchored in the ground but visible above ground and without sharp points.

Side hobbles

Side hobbles are used to discourage kicking or as a transition to training for front leg hobbles. Two straps connected by a line are placed around a front leg and hind leg on the same side of the body. Side hobbles are tolerated better by most horses than front-leg hobbles. They permit more freedom while grazing, while not allowing a horse to lope. Australian hobbles are two side hobbles attached diagonally to the front and hind legs, forming an "X" beneath the horse.

Breeding hobbles

Some breeders use hobbles on the hocks of mares when breeding. Breeding hobbles can be created by using a folded rope with a bowline on the bight knot to form a collar. The long lines are run between the front legs to the strap and ring hobbles over the hocks and then back along the shoulders to the collar. The ends of the long lines are tied to the collar with quick-release hitches.

Breeding hobbles may protect the stallion from being kicked, but the hobbles could also create a new danger of the stallion getting one of his front legs caught in the hobble rope.

Scotch hobbles

Scotch hobbles are used to inhibit kicking. A Scotch hobble is created with an 18 ft (5.5 m) long soft rope. A non-sliding neck loop is made from a bowline knot. A working end of the rope is run from the neck loop to a hobble strap with metal rings on one hind leg pastern and then back through the neck loop. The movement of the pastern can then be restrained or the hind leg lifted slightly (2 in [5 cm]) toward the horse's belly to prevent kicking.

The rope that goes to the pastern should not be run around the pastern because rope burns could result. The end of the rope should be run through the metal rings of a leather or nylon foot strap (hobble) from the inside aspect of the hind leg to outside. A makeshift pastern hobble can be made with 3–4 ft (1–1.2 m) of rope tied by the ends with a sheetbend to form a circular rope. The rope is folded and placed on the back of the pastern and each end pulled forward. The bights on each side provide a channel for the long rope from the neck to slide and not burn the back of the pastern. The handler restrains the horse by a hand on the lead rope and the other hand on the rope to the pastern.

A Scotch hobble can be used to supplement chemical restraint for veterinary procedures by pulling the hind leg up slightly and restraining it from kicking while a horse is being anesthetized. As the horse is anesthetized and the head is controlled with a halter and lead rope, the hobble rope is used to pull the hind leg up and lay the horse down in a more controlled manner. It continues to be used for leg control when the horse is lying on its side for castration or other veterinary procedures on the abdomen or groin.

A Scotch hobble should not be used to lay a horse down that has not been chemically sedated, because struggling can release myoglobin from muscular injury, which can damage the horse's kidneys.

Morral (feedbag)

A feed bag, also called a *morral*, is a canvas bag with grain in it that is strapped over the horse's muzzle (**Figure 11.34**). The morral eliminates wasting of grain and makes horses easier to catch. A horse being fed with a morral should be supervised to reduce the risk of the morral being caught on a fence or other structure, and the horse should not have access to water until the morral is removed. If a horse attempts to drink with a morral on, the bag could fill with water and possibly cause drowning or aspiration pneumonia.

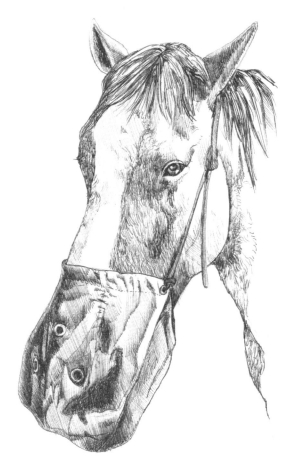

Fig. 11.34 Feed bag for feeding grain.

TRANSPORTING HORSES

Ground transport

Trailers and vans should be road worthy and of sufficient size for the horses to be hauled. Most trailers measure 7 ft (2.1 m) from floor to ceiling, which will accommodate horses up to 16 hands in height. Taller horses require taller trailers. Ventilation is important, even in winter. Closed trailers should have at least one overhead vent per horse. There should be no protrusions or sharp edges inside the trailer or van. Flooring should be non-slip.

Many horses are trailered for the first time when being taken to a veterinary clinic or hospital because of illness or injury. This is too late. Forcing the horse into a trailer (called a "float" in Australia and New Zealand) or a horse van ("horsebox" in Britain) is a setback for training the horse to load properly and is an unsafe situation for handlers. Loading and unloading horses from a trailer is one of the most potentially dangerous activities for a horse handler. Much of the danger can be minimized by early training, routine practice, thorough preparation of the trailer and towing equipment, and careful driving.

Loading

Horses should be trained to be hauled and receive periodic practice as reminders. Before horses can be loaded and unloaded from a trailer, they need to be able to walk on a wooden platform to experience stepping up, hearing the hollow sound made on a plank floor, and backing up and stepping down. Step-up entries are sufficient for small trailers. Large trailers may have a much higher flooring level and require ramps for loading. Ramps should not have a grade of incline of more than a 25 degrees. Distractions, especially dogs, should be removed from the loading area.

Loading and unloading is safer with two people involved. A cotton or leather lead rope is best for trailering. Nylon lead ropes can burn the hands if the horse rushes backwards. Handlers should never be positioned with the horse between themselves and the only exit while loading. There should be direct access to a front exit, and the handler should stand on the other side of a divider, or the horse should be taught to be sent in rather than be led into the trailer. The lead rope should be tied by reaching into the trailer from outside, or there should be direct access to a front exit.

Some handlers run a lead rope around a tie ring or other stationary structure inside the trailer and will then pull the horse toward the trailer, hold it, then pull it closer and hold it, continuing this until the horse loads. However, pulling and holding, and thus forcing the horse to hold its feet still while pulling back, usually intensifies its fear of trailer loading. A better method involves allowing a horse to move its feet by longeing it near the trailer. The handler sends the horse on the longe line toward the trailer. He then lowers his energy, allowing the horse to become more relaxed whenever it investigates the trailer and remains still. This process is repeated until the horse willingly enters and stays still in the trailer This is a training process that should be done in short increments over several days. No reprimands, such as sharp jerks on the lead rope, should ever occur in a trailer. Nothing that might cause fear or pain should ever occur in a trailer. Food rewards are not recommended. Food treats are not always available when horses need to be loaded. In emergencies such as barn fires, food may not be readily available.

With straight load trailers (in countries that drive on the right), for stability the most weight should be distributed on the left side of the trailer by having a single horse on the left side, or if there are two horses, the heaviest on the left side. Having most of the weight on the side closest to the center of the road reduces the risk of the trailer tipping during left turns into a lane that is slanted to the road's shoulder. It also can ease getting a trailer back onto the road if the right wheels drop off the pavement. Slant load trailers eliminate much of the instability of straight load trailers, shorten the length needed, and allow horses to better maintain their balance when the trailer goes around curves. There is more room in the back stall of slant load trailers, so the largest horse should be loaded last.

Horses should be loaded after everything else has been loaded. They should not have to wait after being loaded. The trailer needs to be attached to the tow vehicle and tires chocked so that it is immoveable prior to the horse loading. The trailer's interior should be as bright as possible. Trailer doors should be tied back or otherwise secured so that they cannot be blown open or closed by wind during loading. In warm weather, the driver should check for wasp nests in trailer corners, wheel wells, behind bumpers, in storage compartments, windows, and the trailer tongue. Any old feed that may have been left from a previous trip must be cleaned up in case it has become moldy. Handlers should use their hands to check surfaces for sharp or rough areas, and not just visually inspect the surfaces.

The best method of leading into a trailer requires many training exercises and occasional refresher sessions. Horses should be trained to load without being led in. The handler should never stand in a trailer in front of a horse and attempt to get it to load. If the horse does decide to enter, it could jump into him. Horses not trained for trailer loading can be encouraged by a lasso around their rear, a person waving their arms or a broom behind them, or tapping on the top of the rump with a long whip. However, just making a noise by rhythmically slapping leather chaps or something similar is often more effective. Watching and following a seasoned horse that loads well aids loading horses new to trailers. This should be done during the handling of nursing foals by following their mother into a trailer.

After the horse enters the trailer, the butt bar or chain should be secured before tying the halter lead. The handler who secures the bar or chain should not stand directly behind the horse in case the horse suddenly tries a hasty exit. When past the age of weaning, horses in trailers should be haltered and tied. The lead rope should be tied with a quick release hitch, a Blocker tie ring, or a panic snap to free a horse quickly, if needed. Tying horses should be done through a window from the outside or a forward compartment after they are loaded. Horses should be tied loose enough to brace themselves against the back or side of a trailer and be able to move in order to keep their balance during travel, yet short enough to prevent them from stepping over the lead rope and becoming entangled. Foals or other horses that have not been halter broke should not be tied. The untied horse should be blocked off with a divider or gate and a trained and seasoned horse tied in the back of the trailer.

If trailering a reluctant horse, a stock trailer should be used for more ventilation and visibility, so that it has a less enclosed feeling. Either interior lights should be turned on or the trailer parked so that the sun shines into the trailer. A calm herd-mate should be loaded first. A horse should never be tranquilized before hauling to prevent it from being injured by an inability to keep its balance.

Protective equipment may be used if needed, including leg wraps, bell boots, head bumpers, tail wraps, and blankets. Leg wraps may or may not be helpful. Some horses will not tolerate them, and will persistently stomp their feet and develop bowed tendons. Leg wraps can also get too hot in warm weather. However, if in a turnover accident, horses will fight to regain a standing position but then will quiet down. Injuries often occur to legs in the effort to stand and may be reduced if a horse is wearing leg wraps.

Horses should not be hauled while wearing tack. In addition to the damage that can occur to the saddle, saddle blankets and saddles increase the risk of the horse overheating and having more serious injuries in a vehicular accident.

Use of a rump rope or two handlers grasping each other's wrists behind the horse's rump to force loading can increase the risk of the horse rearing. If using a rope around the horse's rump, about two-thirds of the pressure to move should be applied to the rump rope and one-third to the halter's lead rope. Long ropes can be tied to each side of a trailer, crossed behind the horse and held by two assistants to aid loading a reluctant horse. If these techniques are used, the handler with the lead rope should use an extra long lead rope for safety if the horse rears. Two handlers grasping each other's wrists prevents rope burns to the horse and sideways evasions to loading. Use of a blindfold or backing the horse onto the trailer increases the risk of the horse jumping into or onto the handler.

Nursing foals should always travel with their dam. If other horses are traveling with a mare and foal, the mare and foal should be in a compartment separated from the other horses.

Traveling

Before setting off, a driver hauling horses should plan a route, check the weather, and ensure that the proper paperwork is ready. Travel in the first 2 hours should be especially careful. After 2 hours, the horses should be checked, and rechecked every 4 hours of travel thereafter. Every 4 hours the horses should have at least 30 minutes of trailer rest at a stop. Trailering is particularly tiring on horses since they must stand the entire time. Constant balancing and bracing with the start, stops, and sways of the trailer can be exhausting. At least one night of rest should be provided after each 8 hours of trailering. Signs of discomfort in horses can include restlessness, sweating or trembling, and lying down. Drivers should keep their own rest stops as short as possible while the horses are still trailered.

In preparation for hauling horses, drivers should practice towing and backing the trailer. They must stay alert and avoid driving if tired, injured, or on medications that adversely affect their ability to remain alert or decrease their reaction time.

The lead rope should be tied with enough slack to permit the horse to balance itself while being towed and to reduce the risk of claustrophobia. A break-away halter or tie ring that permits sliding (Blocker tie ring) should be used to inhibit the horse from lowering its head during a normal trip but still permit it to free its head if in a trailer accident. A cotton lead rope should be used for tying in a trailer.

> For trips lasting more than 3 hours, a horse must be able to lower its head. Respiratory secretions are not properly cleared if horses cannot lower their head below the height of their withers within 6 hours. Otherwise, accumulated mucus and other secretions can become media for bacterial growth.

Floor mats increase traction and reduce noise and road heat. For short-distance trips, rubber mats only are sufficient. Bedding on top of the mats only is desirable for longer (more than 2 hours) trips when horses are more likely to urinate in the trailer. Because bedding can reduce the air quality, only low-dust, large-flake pine shavings should be used. Trailer stall dividers should not go to floor, so an adult horse has more room to balance itself. However, if there is a possibility of a foal going under or being thrown underneath a divider, the bottom of the divider should be blocked.

No feed is needed during short trips of less than 3 hours. Feeding should be done 3 or more hours prior to travel and grass hay provided every 2–4 hours to maintain normal gastrointestinal activity. Dust is reduced when horses are fed in a trailer with a manger and with wetted hay cubes.

Stops should occur at least every 4 hours to allow horses to drink and if possible eat grass. Some horses will not drink water that is not from their home. Water should be provided in a familiar bucket. Adding peppermint oil to the horse's water at home and later to water from other sources may induce them to drink water that is not from home. Colic can occur because of reluctance to drink adequately during travel.

Stallions and geldings stretch backwards and spread their hind legs to urinate, and so many will not urinate in a trailer. Stops every 200 miles or 4 hours may be necessary to prevent urine retention. It is important to stop in places away from traffic where the horse can walk around, graze, urinate, and defecate before resuming travel.

Blankets should be avoided in most cases to reduce the risk of overheating. However, in cold weather, the trailer should still be well ventilated, which may necessitate blanketing horses, especially in stock (open) trailers. When hauling in a stock trailer or a horse trailer with windows open for ventilation in warm weather, horses should wear fly masks to protect their eyes from flying insects and debris in the trailer, particularly loose bedding materials.

Proper driving while hauling horses in a trailer takes practice; a horse can be thrown off its feet with fast starts, sudden turns, or quick stops. To test a driver's skills, a bucket of water can be placed in an empty trailer that will be hauled to determine whether a driver can pull a trailer without spilling the water bucket. Drivers must always remember that extra room is needed to stop when hauling a trailer with horses. The normal distance between the towing vehicle and a vehicle ahead of it should be doubled when hauling a horse trailer. Safe driving becomes even more important when hauling horses in adverse weather conditions. Distractions, such as the use of cell phones, should be strictly avoided while towing a horse trailer. Smoking materials should never be thrown from the towing vehicle. Lit cigarettes or matches can be sucked into the horse trailer and cause a fire.

If an emergency stop becomes necessary, horses should not be unloaded next to a highway. An off-road area away from the highway should be sought and unloading done only if necessary. Emergency flashers should be turned on. If pulling off the roadway is not an option, flares or flashing lights should be placed 20, 50, 100, 200, and 300 ft (6.1, 15.2, 30.5, 61, and 91.4 m) behind the trailer. If flares or lights are not available, other people should be enlisted to alert motorists. Two spare tires should be carried owing to the frequent occurrence of two flats at the same time on horse trailers.

A Limited Power of Attorney for Animal Health Care document should be kept in the towing vehicle to direct emergency responders who have legal authority to make decisions on treatment of the horses if the owner is injured in an accident while pulling horses in a trailer. Free forms are available at www.usrider.org. USRider is an equestrian motor plan that provides roadside assistance and towing services for the vehicle and horses.

Unloading

The lead rope should be untied before releasing the butt bar or chain or opening the back door of the trailer. Untying must be done without entering the trailer stall with the horse. Untying horses in stock trailers can be done from outside the trailer. Other trailers may allow the handler to get to the tie ring from a window, a front compartment, or an empty stall adjacent to the horse to be untied. Horses should be trained to wait a couple of minutes after being untied until given permission to come out. After the horse is untied, the handler should open the back door and release the butt bar or chain, go into the trailer and pat the horse briefly for standing still, and then ask it to quietly back up. Before backing a horse out of a trailer, there must be prior assurance that the trailer cannot move and that the doors are secured open and unable to move with a wind gust. If the horse rushes back, a handler could get caught in the trashing. Rushing back is unacceptable and indicates the need for more training for the horse in loading and unloading.

> Unloading can be the most dangerous aspect of hauling horses.

After the horse is unloaded, care should be taken if tying it to the trailer. Ties too close to door latches may catch a lead rope, and wheel wells where a pawing hoof might get caught should be out of range. Horses should never be tied to an unhitched trailer. A scared horse can pull a trailer and cause great damage to itself and anything around it.

Trailer check, maintenance, and towing

Safer trailering requires proper trailer and towing vehicle maintenance. Drivers need to comply with the towing vehicle's manufacturer maintenance schedule. Towing weights should not exceed 85% of the towing vehicle's maximum towing capacity. The vehicle should have a factory-equipped or after-factory-added towing package. Towing packages typically include oversized battery, high-output alternator, wiring harness for the trailer, heavier brakes and suspension, transmission oil cooler, oversized radiator and high-capacity water pump, and an axle ratio that is geared for towing. Oversized extendable side mirrors are also helpful.

Most states do not require yearly safety inspections of horse trailers, but wheel bearings should be repacked every 12 months or 12,000 miles. An annual inspection should include the wiring, brakes, and emergency breakaway cable, pin, and control box. Horse trailers are required to have emergency breakaway systems to activate the trailer brakes if the trailer comes uncoupled from the truck during travel. The trailer battery that activates the trailer brakes in an emergency should be rechecked at least once per year.

Oak planks are best for flooring covered by non-slip rubber mats. Low-dust bedding should be used in areas where the horses may urinate to prevent splashing and encourage elimination. At least once per year, wood floorboards should be checked for rot and aluminum floorboards checked for weakening from oxidation. Floor mats should be removed when washing the interior and left out until the flooring is dry.

Tires should have at least ¼ in (0.6 cm) of tread. Replacing trailer tires should be considered at 6 years, regardless of the extent of wear. Tire failure is a leading cause for serious trailer accidents. Tires for trailers are different from those for trucks. The load rating for most trailers is at least "D," i.e. an 8 ply tire designed ST (stiff sidewalls) to prevent sway and carry heavy loads. Drum brakes should be adjusted every 5,000 miles.

A maintenance checklist should be reviewed prior to each trip (*Table 11.3*).

Table 11.3 Checklist prior to hauling horses

1 Check tire tread, tire pressures, vehicle and trailer lights, brakes, and floor of the trailer
2 Check interior for sharp edges, protruding nuts or bolts, wasp or rodent nests, and spoiled feed
3 Open vents, but do not open drop-down windows if horses could stick their head out during travel
4 Clean and inspect flooring after each haul
5 Inspect all fluid levels in towing vehicle
6 Lubricate the trailer ball and check it for tightness and check coupler on trailer for proper operation and an effective locking mechanism. After hooking up the trailer, make sure the hitch is properly attached and locked in place, the safety chains are crossed underneath the hitch and attached to the towing vehicle properly, and the breakaway emergency stop cable is attached
7 Pull the trailer empty and check the brakes on the towing vehicle and the trailer
8 Load emergency materials for people and horses: first aid kits, A-B-C rated fire extinguisher, blankets, and drinking water
9 Load emergency tools: flashlight and spare batteries, jumper cables, duct tape, extra halters and lead ropes, spare vehicle bulbs and fuses, crowbar, pliers, screwdrivers, wrenches, hammer, traction devices in winter, properly inflated truck and trailer spare tires, vehicle jacks, lug-nut wrenches, three emergency reflective triangles, and four tire chocks
10 Load hygiene tools: broom, shovel, manure fork, bucket, and sponges
11 Secure all tack and supplies to prevent slipping, sliding, or rolling around during travel
12 Carry legal and emergency paperwork: registration papers and titles for the truck and trailer, emergency veterinary contact information, Limited Power of Attorney for Animal Health Care document, veterinary health certificates (Certificate of Veterinary Inspection) if crossing state lines, Coggins test papers, and if needed, a brand inspection certificate

Trailer turnover accidents

If confronted with a trailer turnover accident with entrapped live horses, a handler should approach the trailer slowly to minimize the risk of inciting struggling. A perimeter containment should be set up if a horse becomes free. If the horse cannot stand because its head is tied fast, a knife taped to a pole should be used to cut the lead rope. The handler should not climb or reach into the trailer.

Pickup beds

Most domestic ranch and farm animals can be transported in appropriately prepared pickup beds, including horses. Pickup beds can be floored with mats to improve footing and outfitted with a rack on all four sides that are withers height or higher Seasoned ranch horses can be trained to jump into pickup beds. Transporting them in a pickup bed avoids the expense of a trailer, the time involved in hooking and unhooking a trailer, and the difficulty of backing and parking a trailer.

However, routinely transporting a horse in a pickup is inadvisable because the vehicle being top-heavy increases the possibility of tipping over. The horse is also put at risk of eye injuries, especially if not tied to face backward to the cab or is not wearing a fly mask. In addition, there is no overhead shelter from sun, rain, and hail.

Air travel

Horses have been transported in airplanes for more than 70 years. At least 5 hours should be allowed for a horse to rest before it is loaded onto an air transport plane. Travel containers are similar to a small box stall. The horse is usually cross-tied.

Grain should not be fed immediately before, during, or immediately after flying. A handler needs to stay with the horse during takeoff, turbulence, and landing. Hay should be available and water offered every 1–2 hours. There should be at least one groom for every 3 horses. Chemical restraint is inadvisable since it could affect the horse's ability to balance itself during flight.

The horses should wear only a halter. Leg wraps are avoided since they can come loose during flight and are unsafe to reapply while in flight. Blankets, boots, and head bumpers can cause the horse to overheat. At least one night of rest should be provided after each 2 hours of air travel.

DONKEYS, MULES, AND HINNIES

Donkeys have served as a beast of burden for humans for about 5,000 years. They have been used for riding, pulling wagons and carts, and guarding livestock, especially sheep from canine predators.

At about the same time that horses were becoming domesticated and used in the grassy plains of the Steppes of Asia, other members of the family Equidae, the donkey (ass) from Nubia, in the dry, rocky corner of northwestern Sudan, were being domesticated in Egypt for transportation and the guarding of property.

Six donkeys were introduced to the New World in 1495 at the request of Christopher Columbus on his second visit to the Caribbean islands. Donkeys (*burro* in Spanish; "burro" in English now denotes a feral donkey) were later brought to Mexico and other sites throughout the New World by conquistadors. Donkeys and small mules were further spread in the southwestern U.S. by prospectors and miners. Feral herds of donkeys still exist in the Great Basin area of the West. Mules were preferred for agricultural work in the southern U.S.

Mules are hybrids of the breeding of horses with donkeys. As a beast of burden (packing and pulling wagons and carts), mules have been preferred to horses since ancient times despite the more muscular hindquarters and pulling power of the horse. Mules can thrive on poorer food than horses, eat less per pound of body weight, drink less water (they sweat much less than horses), have thicker skin than horses and are less susceptible to saddle sores, and have much harder hooves, rarely requiring shoes to work. Their durability for work lasts more years than in horses. Donkeys and mules also excel at surefootedness for travel in rocky, mountainous areas.

Mules were used by the Carthaginian military commander Hannibal to cross the Alps to invade Rome in 218 BC and by Napoleon to cross the Alps in 1800 to attack Austrian forces.

Mules were the most desirable draft animals during the western migration in the U.S. Mules were trained to move forward by the command "get up," to turn left by "haw," right by "gee" in the northern U.S. ("yee" in southern states), and stop by "whoa." "Come up" meant start. "Easy" was the signal for slowing down. Large mules from the southeastern U.S. were used to pull wagons across the plain states. Smaller mules from the southwestern U.S. were preferred as pack animals in mountainous passages.

A male donkey is called a *jack* (also called an ass) and a female is a *jenny*. A *mule* is an offspring of a jack and mare. A male mule is a *john* and a female mule is a *molly*. A *hinny* is an offspring of a stallion and a jenny.

Natural behavior of donkeys

Donkeys evolved in rocky, arid, semi-desert conditions, which required the ability to defend themselves from predators since they were unlikely to outrun them. Food was scarce, and large groups could not find enough food in one location. Their social structure became based on family units rather than herds. Hence, their social structure and reaction to danger are very different from those of horses.

The family unit is typically a jenny, foal, and yearling protected by a dominant jack. Less dominant males usually form bachelor groups. Within families and bachelor groups, a donkey will form strong bonds with just one or two other donkeys and become very distressed if separated from its preferred herdmate.

Their ability to flee from danger is less than that of horses, so they are less flighty (less likely to easily startle and run) and more fighty (they are more likely to attack if threatened). They will bray loudly to either communicate with scattered members of the family unit foraging for food or to deter a predator. Mules retain most of these donkey characteristics.

Donkeys have a natural aversion to dogs. Desensitization to dogs usually requires a longer period than for horses.

Donkeys in the wild live in small groups. They tend to bond with a companion and become very distressed if separated. It is best if they bond with another donkey. If they bond with a horse or pony that will be removed from the pasture for training or work, the donkey will become distressed. However, donkeys or mules used as pack animals can become "bell sharp," led by a bell on a buddy horse rather than a lead rope. They are not built for efficient flight, in contrast to horses, so they are less likely to bolt from novelties in their environment and more likely to freeze or fight if believed to be threatened. Donkeys become very territorial and are intolerant of new animals in their environment or smaller animals such as dogs, cats, sheep, and chickens if not desensitized to them. Because of their calm disposition, jennies have been used to teach foals to be led by a halter and lead rope and to develop patience in being handled.

Donkeys vary in size. Minis are under 36 in (91.4 cm), Standards are 36–54 in (91.4–137.2 cm), and Mammoths are taller than 54 in (137.2 cm). Each can carry up to 25% of its weight in combined tack, supplies, and rider.

Mules have longer ears than hinnies. Hinnies have a more horse-looking head and their overall size is slightly smaller than a mule. They do not have a true forelock. The size of the dam affects the size of the offspring. Mules have more donkey-like colors and hinnies have more horse-like colors. Mules are more common than hinnies because mules are larger and have more pulling power. It is also easier to breed a jack to a mare than a stallion to a jenny.

Donkeys

Donkeys are highly gregarious and protective. They are vocal and communicate with a loud noise similar to "hee-haw", called braying.

Approaching and catching

Capturing a donkey that has had frequent handling when it was young is usually easy. Most will approach a handler, and others will stand still when moved to a corner. Separating a donkey from a group is very difficult because they usually have a special buddy and do not like separation. It is best to move the group to the desired location, capture the donkey wanted, and then move the group back. If the buddy has been identified, it should be kept with the desired donkey, if possible. Head collars are convenient means of capture and restraint.

Handling for routine care and management
Routine restraint

As with other animals, as little restraint as possible should be used with donkeys. It is good to talk to

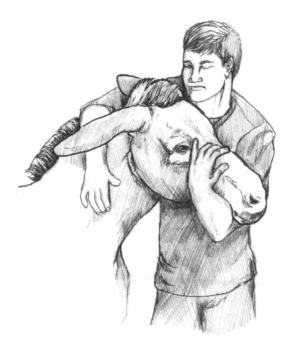

Fig. 11.35 Head hug hold.

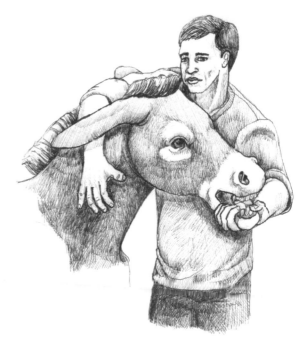

Fig. 11.36 Chin hold.

and pat donkeys, but a handler should avoid stroking their eyes, ears, and flanks, which they resent.

Halters for ponies or horses can be used on donkeys, but many donkeys do not like their ears touched, so their ears should be avoided when haltering. Handlers should unfasten the strap that goes over the poll and refasten. The crownpiece should not be pulled over ears.

Donkeys can often be restrained by a head hug or hug with chin hold (**Figures 11.35** and **11.36**). The chin hold consists of placing a thumb into the bars of the mouth and grasping its chin. A halter or loop of rope around the donkey's neck should also be present and held with the other hand, rather than grasping an ear. If the donkey backs to escape the hold, the handler should go with it and guide it using the chin hold as a rudder to position its rump into a corner of a stall or pen.

Nose twitches are not well tolerated and donkeys will often strike out with a front leg.

Leading and tying
Donkeys that are frequently handled may be led with a halter and lead rope as with a horse. Those that do not lead by a halter and lead rope can be driven by the handler being on the donkey's left side and

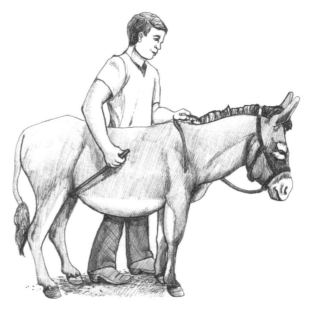

Fig. 11.37 Driving a donkey by tapping with a stick.

reaching over the donkey's flank to tap the donkey's right flank with his hand or a stick (**Figure 11.37**). If three people are available to move the donkey, one can lead while the other two use a tied loop to assist with the rump. Untrained donkeys may be small enough for two handlers to cradle in their arms and carry short distances (**Figure 11.38**).

Depending on the style of training received, saddle donkeys can be guided by taps with a stick on the sides of their neck or by a bridle with a snaffle bit and reins.

On level ground, a donkey can pull up to 300 lb (136.1 kg) when trained with long reins, a proper harness, and a light cart.

Lifting a foot

Donkeys must be taught tolerance in having their feet handled when young, similar to horses. Handlers must not lift the feet as high as is usual in holding horses' feet. Instead, donkey feet should be held lower for their comfort, not above the handler's knee. If they are older and might have arthritis, their feet should be lifted as low as feasible.

Mules and hinnies

Mules are bigger and more independent than horses, but like donkeys they will not entrust as much leadership to humans as horses do. Mules will defer to human dominance, but they are less submissive than horses. They are less herd bound and less inclined to spook and bolt. Mules have exceptional strength and endurance and, from their donkey mother, relatively small hard feet designed for rocks and desert conditions. The manes of mules are roached (cut short) because the mane is stiff and sticks up, getting in the way of a pulling collar. They are less athletic in turning and running than horses. Therefore, mules are superior to horses in some tasks and inferior in others.

Hinnies have a more horse-like appearance than a mule. However, they tend to have more behavioral characteristics of a donkey since they are imprinted by their jenny mother, compared with mules being raised by their mare mother.

Mules and hinnies are handled similarly to horses. Horses do not forget rough handling but may forgive it to a certain extent with gentle handling later. Mules are less prone to forgive. Difficulty in handling mules may be from bad experiences the mule had in earlier life. A mule will remember specific individuals who have been unkind to them and wait for an opportunity at a later time to retaliate.

Adult, conditioned pack mules carry their load on rigid or soft pack (aparejos) saddles made for mules. A saddle pad or blanket is used under a rigid saddle.

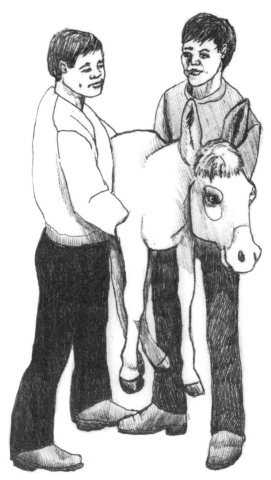

Fig. 11.38 Small, untrained donkeys may be carried by two handlers

Donkeys are tied by their lead rope in the same manner as horses, but tie rings must be placed lower than that for horses. The donkey should be tied at its withers height, or a little above. Donkeys are not as claustrophobic as horses. They can be tied closer than horses to a tie ring.

Riding, guiding, and driving

Adult donkeys can carry people who weigh up to about 100 lb (45.4 kg). They have a much different conformation of their back and thorax than that of horses and ponies. Therefore, saddles must be made specifically for donkeys because pony saddles will not fit properly. Owing to the shape of their chest, the saddle should be fitted with a crupper, a strap that attaches the back of the saddle to the base of the tail to prevent the saddle from sliding forward.

Thick pads are needed for pack saddles. Riding saddle blankets are too thin to be used as a pad for pack riding. Rigid saddles are made of wood (Sawbuck) or aluminum or fiberglass (Decker) and held in place by cinches, breechings, and breast collars. Sawbuck saddles have two cinches; Deckers have one. Rigid saddles are designed to allow the weight to be carried evenly on both sides of the upper chest without pressure on the top of the spine. Heavier loads can be carried more comfortably with the Decker saddle.

Panniers are the detachable bag or box packs that are attached to saddles to carry the load. Manties are canvas tarps that are wrapped around the cargo. Sawbuck saddles are made for panniers, and Deckers will carry either manties or panniers. Sawbuck saddles and panniers are preferred for the southwestern U.S. because packing is easier without the burrs, thorns, and insects that adhere to manties handled on the ground. Decker saddles and manties are more common in the Northwest U.S. because when crossing streams and rivers, panniers would fill with water and so prevent a pack animal from getting up if it slips while crossing. Soft pack saddles also distribute the load weight on both sides of the upper chest. Horses and mules can be used for packing but require a different-shaped pack side bars than do donkeys. The average pack weight for a horse is 175 lb. (80 kg), for a mule 225 lb. (102 kg), and for a donkey 200 lb (91 kg).

When leading a pack animal, the lead rope should not be tied to the lead horse. It should be loosely wrapped around the saddle horn and maintained on the downhill side in case the pack animal falls and the lead rope must be quickly released. When leading multiple pack animals, a breakaway string should be used on each animal's lead rope. The end of the lead ropes should not dangle closer than 18 in (46 cm) from the ground. The most inexperienced pack animal should be the first after the rider's horse. Whenever resting on a slope, pack animals should be trained to face the downhill side. Otherwise if falling rocks startle them, they could jump backward and down the slope or off a ledge.

Mules can also be used for riding. Mules have thicker withers than horses, which cause saddles to slide forward and backward easily, requiring the use of breechings or a crupper and a breast collar.

Army mules had their tail hairs trimmed into the shape of bells around the tail. If the tail was completely shaved, the mule was called a "shavetail". This meant the mule was untrained. One bell meant it was trained only to pack. Two bells indicated it could pack and be driven to pull loads. Three bells, the highest rank, meant it could also be ridden.

SELECTED FURTHER READING

Birke L, Hockenhull J, Creighton E, et al. (2011). Horses' responses to variation in human approach. *Applied Animal Behaviour Science* 134:56–63.

Christensen JW, Ladewig J, Sondergaard E, et al. (2002). Effects of individual versus group stabling on social behavior in domestic stallions. *Applied Animal Behaviour Science* 75:233–248.

Hill C (1997). *Horse Handling and Grooming*. Storey Publishing, North Adams.

Lagerweij E, Neils PC, Wiegant VM, et al. (1984). The twitch in horses: a variant of acupuncture. *Science* 225:1172–1174.

Mackenzie SA (1998). *Equine Safety*. Cengage Delmar Learning, Albany.

McGreevy P (2012). *Equine Behavior: A Guide for Veterinarians and Equine Scientists*. 2nd edition. Saunders.

McLean AN (2005). The positive aspects of correct negative reinforcement. *Anthrozoös* 18:245–54.

McMiken DF (1990). Ancient origins of horsemanship. *Equine Veterinary Journal* 22:73–78.

Miller RM (2010). *Handling Equine Patients: a Handbook for Veterinary Students & Veterinary Technicians*. Robert M. Miller Communications, Truckee.

Moyer E (2008). *Horse Safety*. Bow Tie Press, Laguna Hills.

Payne E, Boot M, Starling M, et al. (2015). Evidence of horsemanship and dogmanship and their application in veterinary contexts. *Veterinary Journal* 204:247–254.

Reeder D, Miller S, Wilfong D, et al. (2009). *AAEVT's Equine Manual for Veterinary Technicians*. Wiley-Blackwell, Ames.

Sarrafchi A, Blokhuis HJ (2013). Equine stereotypic behaviors: causation, occurrence, and prevention. *Journal of Veterinary Behavior* 8:386–394.

Thomas HS (2003). *Storey's Guide to Training Horses*. Storey Publishing, North Adams.

WorkSafe New Zealand (2014). *Best Practice Guide for Riding Horses on Farms*. WorkSafe New Zealand, Wellington.

CHAPTER 12

CATTLE

Cattle have been domesticated and handled by humans for approximately 8,000–10,000 years, beginning in the Middle East and North Africa. They were first raised as a convenient source of meat and for the leather they provided. Later, their value as a beast of burden was realized in northern Europe. Egyptians discovered that cattle could also be a source of milk for humans.

As with the horse and hog, domestic cattle were brought to the Americas 500 years ago by Spanish conquistadors and explorers. Christopher Columbus brought cattle to the West Indies on his second voyage in 1493. Cortez took cattle from Spain to Mexico in 1519. The first domesticated cattle in North America landed in St. Augustine, Florida, in 1528 with the Spanish explorers. The English and Dutch brought other domesticated cattle to New England in the early 1600s.

Oxen were inexpensive and effective draft animals for wagons, and played a large role in the western migration in the U.S. More than one pair, or yoke, were directed by cracking a bullwhip on the opposite side from the direction a turn was desired. The bullwhip was used for its noise, not on the animal to cause pain and injury.

Because of the dry highland plains and the more than 700-year occupation by the Moors from North Africa, the Spanish brought a nomadic herd-based method of handling cattle in a constant search for forage. The British and Dutch brought a territorial method of grazing and handler bonding with individual animals. This included providing shelter from the weather (barns and sheds). Today's herding and handling of cattle in the U.S. is a composite of these two methods. Methods of handling cattle have improved significantly in the last 30 years through the guidance of Temple Grandin. Better methods of herding and moving cattle while minimizing stress have been promoted by Bud Williams, Burt Smith, and Curt Pate.

Most cattle in the U.S. are derived from European breeds, which are of the species *Bos taurus*. The European breeds were selectively bred for either beef or milk production. The Brahman breed of cattle, the species *Bos indicus* from Asia, is bred for beef production. Brahmans and Brahman crosses are more heat and parasite resistant than European breeds. Since Brahmans are raised for these characteristics, and their independence, they are generally not handled as often as European breeds. Some cattlemen consider Brahmans inherently more difficult to handle, but much of this may be more from the difference in handling frequency than difference in the breed's inherited behavior.

The U.S. leads the world in beef production, followed by Brazil and the European Union. It is second in the world to India in milk production and dairy processing.

Sexually intact adult male cattle are *bulls*. Castrated males are *steers*. A steer used for pulling wagons is an *ox*. Adult females are *cows*. Dairy cows are either *dry* (not currently producing milk) or *freshen* (having had a calf and producing milk). Young cattle are *calves*. A young female that has not had a calf is a *heifer*.

NATURAL BEHAVIOR OF CATTLE

Cattle are highly social animals that will form herds whenever possible. Within a herd, three groups tend to develop: female, male, and mixed gender. Female groups contain about 10 cows, possibly with some young males. Male groups are smaller and composed of young males. Older males tend to remain alone when not breeding. Mixed gender groups form during breeding seasons and contain approximately 15 animals. By 7 weeks of age, calves will sleep in groups.

Social hierarchy categories within a herd of cattle include *leaders*, *dominants*, and *submissives* (also called subdominants or timids). When a herd moves, the leaders lead, followed by the dominants, and trailed by the submissives. Roles as leaders, dominants, and submissives can shift among some herd members depending on the activity. In general, the social rank of a cow is well established by 2 years of age and maintained by threat posturing followed by butting when the correct social response does not promptly occur. Young bulls play-fight to develop tactics and test strength. They gradually become more aggressive and territorial.

Higher social rank is based on horn size, age, and weight. The herd bull is the most dominant herd member. The bull does not participate much in herd discipline, except in controlling young bachelor bulls. Other than breeding, its primary objective is to keep the herd separate from other herds. An older, heavier cow with large horns is more likely dominant than smaller, younger cows, or those with shorter or no horns. The most dominant individuals are usually not the most aggressive. Dominant adults tend to break up fights among younger herd members.

Leader cows stay on the periphery of the herd at the edge of their social distance, which is the maximum distance that cows will stray from the bulk of the herd. Leaders are inquisitive and initiate movement of the herd. They are also the most likely to approach a handler first. They are licked by other cattle more often than other herd members. Dominant members maintain a larger personal space than submissives.

Although recognition of herd members is visual, auditory, and olfactory, the sense of smell is more important to cattle than sight or sound for identifying herd members. It is primarily by smell that cows and their calves recognize each other. Most communication among cattle is visual by body posture. In vocalization, the "moo" is used to demand attention from others. A call (also called the hoot or roar) is higher pitched and occurs in a series of short bursts. This is even more demanding and often indicates distress.

Cattle graze by apprehending grass with their tongue for 4–9 hours per day, mostly in the early morning and late evening. During midday, they seek shade to rest and ruminate. Lying down comprises half of the daytime hours. When grazing, cattle spread out more than when moving or resting. When cattle are grazing, dominants move the greatest distance away from possible threats.

Some management practices for cattle do not permit natural behavior. Feedlots are highly concentrated, unnatural environments for fattening cattle for 75–200 or more days. Grazing is eliminated and replaced by multiple feedings of grain and high-energy roughage. Feedlots became popular in the 1950s and 1960s for economic reasons. Feedlot cattle are typically treated with antibiotics to prevent liver abscesses that occur from highly concentrated diets, and hormones to stimulate muscle growth. A beta-agonist may also be fed to reduce the development of fat but that can cause anxiety and loss of hooves during hot weather.

Veal is tender meat from dairy bull calves that are 16–20 weeks of age. Veal calves in the U.S. may be kept in individual tether stalls and unable to turn around so that they remain cleaner until slaughter. Group housing of veal calves is mandated in Europe.

Feedlots and veal calf isolation have some advantages over pasture feeding, such as labor economy, inexperienced animal handler safety, protection from predators, and rapid weight gains. However, weight gain can occur without good handling of livestock, and the risk of cattle being injured, becoming lame, and having bloat and diarrhea is higher in concentrated animal feeding operations.

SAFETY FIRST

Despite their long domestication, cattle are still the most likely farm animals to injure people who handle them. Unlike with horses, flight is not an effective means of defense for cattle. Cattle are more inclined to stop and fight. Most injuries are the result of improper handling or carelessness. Cows determine their rank in a group by shoving, and each is an individual with a particular level of desire to test their rank. Reducing the risk of handler injury requires preventing unnecessary agitation in cattle,

Table 12.1 **Keys to safer handling of cattle**
• Accustom them to handler presence and handling facilities prior to the need to handle them for specific purposes • Respect their ability to injure handlers • Recognize difference in breed, gender, and seasonal aggressiveness • Beware of increased self-defensiveness in isolated herd members • Herd them quietly and slowly using calmly applied pressure and release on their flight zone • Cull overly aggressive individuals

preventing improperly maintained containment and handling facilities, and recognizing signs of the desire of some cattle to exhibit aggression.

Genetic selection of calm cattle is prudent. Overly aggressive individuals should be culled. Walking among calves in their first 3 months of life and gentle handling will pay dividends in being able to work with them later as they age. It is good husbandry to socialize calves to humans within a distance that permits cattle movement without undue stress and allows screening inspections for disease or injury. A flight zone distance no greater than 15 ft (4.6 m) should be the goal. Good handlers move cattle with patience and give them limited options where to go and some time to think about it. If stressful procedures are necessary, they should not be performed by the routine handlers and should be done as gently as practical.

Handler safety

Risks to cattle handlers include being knocked down, trampled, crushed against a wall or fence, stepped on, butted, gored with a horn, kicked, bitten by molar teeth when drenching, and being hit by a tail. It is important to use the minimal amount of pressure and restraint required to move, sort, or treat.

Cattle defenses and offenses

If restrained, cattle will thrash their heads to the side to butt. Adequate head restraint of cattle during handling is critical. Cattle kick one leg at a time with a sweep to the outside and down (*cow kick*). Calves may kick with both hind legs at once. A danger zone from a kick backward is within 8 ft (2.5 m) from the base of the tail. Cattle have no upper incisors, just

a dental pad. A cow's tail is heavy and can inflict pain to any part of the handler's body it hits. A tail can also cause serious injury to eyes. Cattle do not care where they step and will make no attempt to avoid stepping on handlers' feet or running over a downed person. Bulls, cows with nursing calves, injured cattle, or previously mistreated cattle may charge a handler with an attempt to butt and crush. Individual bulls or cows with aggressive behaviors that endanger other cattle or handlers should be culled. One-third of the farm fatalities involving cattle in the Midwestern U.S. are caused by cattle that have exhibited aggressive behavior in the past.

Breed variations

The temperament of cattle is affected by type and breed. *Dairy cattle* are selected primarily for their ability to produce milk. *Beef cattle* are selected for their mothering ability. Beef cows are more prone to maternal aggression and are typically more difficult to handle than dairy cattle because they are not selectively bred for their ability to be handled, and they are not handled very much. When they are handled, it is usually for frightening and uncomfortable or painful procedures.

Among beef cattle, Asian cattle (Brahman) are more excitable, sullen, and aggressive than European cattle breeds. Brahman or Brahman crosses are more likely to lie down in an alley if stressed. They are also more difficult to sort because they more strongly resist being isolated. Large European mainland beef breeds are more excitable than British breeds. Angus cattle are more excitable than Herefords. All these differences are generalizations. They can vary widely among individual cattle and can be markedly altered by good or bad handling.

There are also general differences in dominance aggression between members of breeds. Angus cattle and Brahmans are usually dominant to Herefords and Shorthorns. Ayrshires are dominant to Holsteins, which are dominant to Jerseys.

Gender variations

Bulls are unpredictable and can be exceedingly dangerous. When they are yearlings, they are aggressively playful. As they age beyond 2 years, they can become territorial and more dangerous, particularly during the breeding season or if pastured with other bulls. Territorial aggression is demonstrated by pawing, bellowing, tossing of the head, and standing broadside to the intruder. Handlers should never try to make a pet of a young bull and never handle a bull alone.

Groups of bulls can be maintained without serious fighting if rotation grazing is used, but new members or groups should not be added. Bulls should not be raised alone. They should be moved regularly to reduce the risk of territorial aggression and have a companion, at least one steer or dry cow. Moving bulls should not be done by a handler on foot, and is best done if moved along with a small group of steers or cows. Well-trained dogs can be helpful. A long, strong stick should be at hand, and an emergency escape route should be identified in advance of need. Handlers should be careful of approaching any group of cattle since a bull mingling with them could be overlooked until it becomes aggressive. If moving bulls into a pen, they should be moved at a trot until well inside or they may stop inside the gate and begin fighting because their individual zones have been invaded by competitors. Handlers should not attempt to interfere with bulls that are fighting. Bulls that will be handled often should have a nose ring, and when being led, their heads should be held up by the nose lead.

Cows with calves can be dangerous. When catching a calf with the mother nearby, the calf should be kept between the handler and the cow, and the handler should hold the calf's mouth shut. A long, stout stick should be at hand as an emergency deterrent to the cow. When moving cows with calves, the handler should start the move slowly, allowing time for each cow and calf to find one another. Herding dogs should not be used to move cows with calves.

Handling facility risks to humans

Cattle handling facilities have at least a holding pen, a crowding tub, a narrow alley, and a chute with a headgate. In each area, all surfaces should be free of sharp or rough edges. Nails should be hammered in flat and bolts that are too long should be sawn off. Loose fitting clothes and rolled up long sleeves that can get caught on fences and restraint equipment should be avoided.

Catwalks and walkways more than 2 ft (0.6 m) high should have handrails. Catwalks should be 18 in (46 cm) wide and 36–42 in (91–107 cm) below the top of the fencing, which is slightly higher than waist height when standing on the catwalk. All catwalks should be non-slip.

Cattle should never be handled between the rails of an alleyway due to the risk of injury to the handler's head or fractured hands and arms. Children should not be allowed around livestock yards owing to danger from the animals and their handling facilities.

Exit strategies and fending off attacks

The most common emergency exit for cattle handlers is to scramble over or under a fence. The need for a rapid escape is most likely when handling a bull, a cow with a calf, or an otherwise aggressive cow. Other possible escapes in a pasture can be climbing nearby trees or farm or ranch equipment.

> Cattle handlers must always have a predetermined, feasible emergency exit from a pen or pasture.

Usually cattle display advance signs of pending attack or group panic. When cattle are not grazing but relaxed, they hold their head at shoulder height. A head held higher than their shoulders is a sign of fear. A steady stare can be a sign of aggression. More definite signs of aggression are slinging of the head or a lowered head with a fixed stare. The proper response by a handler to signs of aggression is to stand erect, face toward the cow, spread both arms out, and stare at it. Most will move away. Unlike horses, which will jump to the side without looking, cattle first look in the direction they plan to move.

Cattle can outrun a human. Handlers must not try to escape by outrunning an aggressive cow or bull. When a cow showing signs of aggression does not eventually retreat, handlers should walk slowly backward. They should not look away or run, but should seek a safe location and later cull the cow from the herd.

A bull that paws the ground with a broadside display is body language for impending charge. If challenged by a bull, the handler should turn his side to it and walk away on a diagonal path. There should be no attempt to run in a straight line away from the bull. Alternatively, an evasion action can be to run at a right angle to a charge and force the bull to turn in circles. If in a pen with a bull, a handler is already within their flight zone and a charge may occur without prior indication. If a handler is knocked down by a cow or bull, he should not try to stand. It is safer to crawl or roll to safety. Handlers should not work a bull alone. Another handler should be present to distract the bull if the primary handler is trapped or down.

If the possibility of aggressive cattle is expected, the handler should carry a 5 or 6 ft (1.5 or 1.8 m) stick. Just holding a stick up increases the handler's profile and height, which makes the handler look more dominant. With sufficient practice, stockwhips can be made to make a loud crack, which will encourage cattle to move or discourage a challenge to a handler's personal space. However, proper use of a stockwhip is a learned skill. Without sufficient experience in their use, stockwhips can be dangerous to handlers, especially the risk of eye injuries. Sticks and whips should not be used to strike a cow, unless a handler believes a charge is imminent or has already begun.

Cattle safety

Corporate livestock production, with multi-tiered management, increases the chances that animal handlers may not have sufficient experience and training to handle cattle well or that they have become desensitized to procedures that are abusive. Critical-point criteria to assess the welfare of cattle have been advocated by Temple Grandin. These include how many cattle are limping, the percentage of cattle that vocalize during handling (no more than 3/100 head), running into gates or fences (1/100 or fewer), and percentage that fall down (no more than 1/100 head). Acts of abuse include dragging a live cow with a chain, running cattle on top of each other on purpose, prodding cattle in sensitive parts of their body, slamming gates on cattle on purpose, and beating a cow. Plants that supply McDonalds, Wendy's, and Burger King food chains must be audited for compliance with the critical care criteria. Family-owned cattle and pig farms are not audited, although cattle abuse can also occur in these as well.

Handling facility risks to cattle

Cattle handling facilities can present physical hazards to cattle, or can be a psychological barrier that prevents them from moving in ways that keep them from injuring themselves or each other. Facilities should be reviewed for hazard potentials before working cattle. Handlers should drive in protruding nails, saw off bolts that are too long, replace rotten lumber, lubricate gates, and pad clanging steel parts. Floors should be uncluttered, sloped to provide drainage, and roughened to provide traction. The floor of forcing pens and alleyways should be concrete. Fences and gates must be strong enough to hold crowded, pushing cattle. Chutes and alleyways should be solid-walled and wide enough for cattle to move forward easily without being able to turn around.

Handlers should check out distractions in the work area, such as clutter, water puddles, shadows, dangling chains, people in flight zones, and hissing and loud noises. Blood on the ground or floor can cause cattle to balk. Gates should be padded with rubber stops to reduce noise. The yard design should have cattle moving away from the yard entrance in holding pens but going toward the entrance in forcing pens and alleyways. Cattle look for escape in the direction they enter. Movement should be on the level or uphill. Good drainage is important to reduce pools of water that could distract cattle. The bottom half of steel pens should be paneled to prevent legs from being caught. Yard pens should be long and narrow to aid one person moving cattle. Funnel-shaped entrances into alleyways should be constructed from a crowding pen.

Handling methods adverse to cattle care and safety

Unfavorable handling of cattle results in decreased weight gains and performance, decreased immunity and resistance to disease, and bruising and injuries. Common handling procedures that cause stress include disbudding/dehorning, vaccinations, castration, weaning, pregnancy checks, dipping, and drenching.

Yelling agitates cattle. Handlers should speak at a normal volume with a low tone of voice. Talking to an animal in a calm manner can reduce fear in animals and agitation in the handler. The handler should desensitize cattle to things that may be scary to them. Cattle should be worked in groups whenever possible. Individual animals worked alone are easily stressed and panicked. An escaped animal should never be chased. After herding it into an enclosure, a handler should allow 30 minutes for the animal to calm down before trying to draw it back to a familiar group.

Electric prods are painful and will panic cattle into injuring themselves or other cattle. Plastic paddles, flags, and streamers should be used rather than electric prods to move or turn cattle (**Figure 12.1**).

When moving cows with calves, handlers should begin slowly to allow the grazing cows to gather their calves. Cows will hide young calves and graze away from them, returning about every 4 hours to nurse. Rushing a gathering process will result in cows abandoning their calf.

Situations that cause cattle to refuse to move can cause them to injure themselves as well as create inefficiency in their handling. Common causes for balking are seeing commotion or hearing loud noises at the end of the alleyway, seeing a dead end in an alleyway, people being in the way of cattle movement, anything that flaps, strange smells, shadows and drains, and moving into sunlight. Anything that contrasts with the general appearance of ground or flooring will cause cattle to stop, put their head down, and try to focus on what appears unusual. Ways of preventing balking include having a chute with a headgate that faces a holding pen with resting cattle; using small pens and working small groups at a time; using the same flooring throughout the forcing pen and alleyway; having floor or ground that is level or a rising incline; providing a direction of movement into bright, but not blinding, sunlight; using curved alleyways with solid walls that allow cattle to view two body lengths ahead, padding steel working equipment; and reducing the width of the crowding pen.

Feeding and providing water to cattle in holding pens without working them will help desensitize them to being confined and being around handling facilities. The handler should close the gate after they are in and let them stand for an hour. Then the cattle should be let out without having been handled. Later, they should be released by opening up the crowding pen and alleyway, and letting them go through the squeeze chute and headgate without catching them. Familiarization with working facilities without stress will facilitate efficient movement, lower stress, and improve the safety of handling cattle for needed procedures.

Commercial dairy cattle have been selectively bred for milk production without sufficient concern for some other genetic qualities. Their range of movement during a day has been confined, and they are often confined part of the day on concrete. These, and other factors, contribute to a higher susceptibility for lameness in dairy cattle in large-scale operations than in beef cattle on pasture.

Docking tails is an amputation of up to two-thirds of the tail, performed on some dairy cattle to reduce the chance of a soiled tail contaminating milk, handlers, and equipment. Tails are also docked, though less commonly, in feedlot cattle to prevent them from being stepped on in close confinement. The adverse effects of tail docking in cattle include the inability

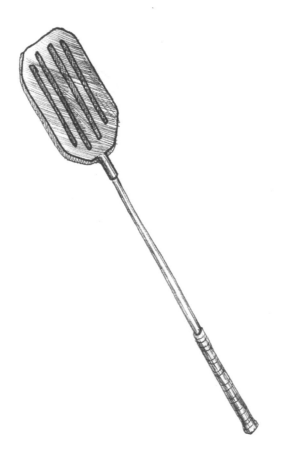

Fig. 12.1 Plastic paddle for moving cattle.

to avoid biting insects, associated abnormal avoidance behaviors, stump infections, and neuromas. Although opposed by the National Milk Producers Federation, the National Mastitis Council, and the American Veterinary Medical Association, tail docking persists in many U.S. states. It is illegal in at least three states and five European countries. McDonald's Corporation has announced that they will not purchase dairy products from groups that practice tail docking. The USDA has proposed a rule that would prohibit tail docking and require lameness monitoring in milk cattle for dairy products to be labeled organic.

Key zoonoses

(*Note:* Apparently ill animals should be handled by veterinary professionals or under their supervision. Precautionary measures against zoonoses from ill animals are more involved than those required when handling apparently healthy animals and vary widely. The discussion here is directed primarily at handling apparently healthy animals.)

Apparently healthy cattle pose little risk of transmitting disease to healthy adult handlers who practice conventional personal hygiene. The risks of physical injury are greater than the risks of acquiring an infectious disease (*Table 12.2*).

Table 12.2 **Diseases transmitted from healthy appearing cattle to healthy adult humans**					
DISEASE	**AGENT**	**MEANS OF TRANSMISSION**	**SIGNS AND SYMPTOMS IN HUMANS**	**FREQUENCY IN ANIMALS**	**RISK GROUP***
Crushing, butting, and kicks	–	Direct injury	Crushing, butting, or kick injuries, which can be permanently disabling or lethal	All cattle can inflict serious injuries. Injuries from adult cattle can be fatal.	3
Cryptosporidiosis	*Cryptosporidium* spp.	Direct, fecal-oral; indirect from contaminated water	Diarrhea	Common, particularly in dairy calves	2
Colibacillosis	*Escherichia coli*, 0157:H7	Direct, fecal-oral	Bloody diarrhea, kidney failure, death	Common	3
Brucellosis	*Brucella abortus*	Direct from secretions, especially placental fluid	Undulant fever, muscle aches, and lethargy	Very low, due to U.S. federal eradication program	3
Q Fever	*Coxiella burnetii*	Direct from body secretions, particularly milk and placental fluids; indirect from inhalation of contaminated dust	Flu-like signs and atypical pneumonia	Moderate in cow-calf operations	2
Leptospirosis	*Leptospira* spp.	Direct from exposure to urine; indirect from urine-contaminated water	Kidney infection	Common in some locations and varies with vaccinations	3
Listeriosis	*Listeria monocytogenes*	Direct from fecal-oral transmission, but most from ingestion of contaminated beef or dairy products	Septicemia, atypical pneumonia, and encephalitis	The incidence in cattle and other farm animals may be as high as 52%	3

* Risk Groups (National Institutes of Health and World Health Organization criteria. Centers for Disease Control and Prevention, *Biosafety in Microbiological and Biomedical Laboratories*, 5th edition, 2009):
  1 Agent not associated with disease in healthy adult humans.
  2 Agent rarely causes serious disease and prevention or therapy possible.
  3 Agent can cause serious or lethal disease and prevention or therapy possible.
  4 Agent can cause serious or lethal disease and prevention or therapy are not usually available.

Direct transmission

Systemic disease

Since 2000, only cats exceed cattle in the number of reported cases of rabies in domestic animals in the United States. Handlers of cattle that appear and act abnormally are at risk because of the lack of awareness of rabies in cattle and the variability of disease signs.

Anthrax, caused by a spore-forming bacterium, can manifest as a blackened skin infection and can be fatal in humans. Cattle sick with anthrax can transmit the disease to humans through their body secretions, by contaminating soil with anthrax spores, and by exposure to an infected animal's hide. There are three forms of the disease: cutaneous (95% of cases – painless ulceration, fever, headache, and possible septicemia), pulmonary (airborne, from infected wool, hide, or hair), and gastrointestinal (from ingesting infected meat).

Listeriosis (*Listeria monocytogenes*) can cause generalized disease in immunosuppressed humans that includes atypical pneumonia. Direct transmission is primarily from cattle with encephalitis, abortion, or mastitis, and abnormal appearing cattle.

Coxiellosis (Q fever) is a bacterial disease that is transmitted by inhalation of dust contaminated by the body secretions of cattle, sheep, or goats (urine, milk, feces, etc.) infected with *Coxiella burnetii*. Infected placental fluids and tissues are especially hazardous. Infected animals can appear healthy. Handlers who work with cattle or swine have the highest incidence of antibodies indicating exposure to *Coxiella*.

Leptospirosis (from *Leptospira pomona* and others) is a bacterial disease of cattle that is transmitted in infected cattle urine or genital fluids. The organism can be transmitted by gaining entrance into a person's mouth, breaks in the skin, or eyes. Viable leptospirosis organisms continue to be eliminated in the urine after cattle have recovered a normal appearance of health.

Cattle are the most common reservoir of enterohemorrhagic strains of *Escherichia coli*, particularly 0157:H7, a bacterium that is in the feces of apparently healthy cattle finished in feedlot operations. If ingested by young or elderly people, it can cause bloody diarrhea and, less commonly, kidney failure.

Most cases in humans are from ingesting undercooked, contaminated ground beef. Cattle handlers may be at risk if their immune system is suppressed, and poor hygiene leads to ingesting the bacteria from cattle feces contamination of their hands or face.

Vesicular stomatitis virus in cattle causes blisters and ulcers in the mouth and nostrils and on the feet and teats. Handlers of cattle with vesicular stomatitis blisters can become infected. Vesicular stomatitis virus causes flu-like symptoms in humans.

Cattle tuberculosis (*Mycobacterium bovis*) is usually transmitted to people by drinking infected raw milk, although it can be transmitted by aerosol over long distances and inhaled. Cattle tuberculosis is now rare in the U.S. due to pasteurization of milk and routine testing of dairy cows.

Brucellosis is a bacterial disease that can cause abortions in cattle and is transmitted to humans by exposure to body secretions (saliva, urine, fetal fluids) or eating meat from infected cattle or drinking unpasteurized milk. The disease in humans is influenza-like and called undulant fever. Its occurrence in the U.S. is very low due to extensive eradication efforts.

Digestive tract disease

Cryptosporidium is a protozoan parasite that causes diarrhea and is transmitted by feces contaminated water. Calves or lambs with diarrhea are the usual source to humans.

Campylobacteriosis (*Campylobacter jejuni* or *C. fetus*) is one of the most common causes of bacterial diarrhea in humans. Contact with infected cattle can be a source if the bacteria gain access to a handler's mouth. Most human cases from cattle are from drinking unpasteurized milk.

Salmonellosis is a bacterial disease of the digestive system that can invade the blood stream and become systemic. Human salmonellosis from handling cattle is rare. Transmission is usually from eating undercooked, contaminated beef. The risk of acquiring salmonellosis is much greater from birds and reptiles.

Taeniasis is caused by *Taenia saginata*, a tapeworm acquired by eating raw or undercooked beef products. It is not transmitted by handling cattle.

Skin disease

Dermatophilosis (*Dermatophilus congolensis*), a bacterial disease of the skin, is transmitted by contact or by stable flies. Ringworm in cattle (*Trichophyton verrucosum*) is a fungal infection that can be transmitted by direct contact. Dermatophilosis and ringworm in humans transmitted from cattle is rare.

Nervous system disease

Bovine spongiform encephalopathy (mad cow disease) is a zoonotic disease acquired from eating infected cattle tissues, not from handling or restraining cattle.

Vector borne

Cattle and humans can develop a malaria-like blood parasite disease called babesiosis (tick fever, Texas fever). Humans with impaired immune systems can develop babesiosis if bitten by *Babesia*-carrying ticks, but cattle *Babesia* organisms have been eliminated from the U.S. except for a quarantine buffer zone along the Mexican border.

Sanitary practices

Persons handling cattle should wear appropriate dress to protect against skin contamination by hair and skin scales or saliva, urine, and other body secretions. Ticks on cattle should be controlled with acaricidal pour-ons, ear tags, or dips. Basic sanitary practices should be adhered to, such as keeping hands away from eyes, nose, and mouth when handling cattle and washing hands in warm soapy water afterwards. No one should eat or drink in an animal handling area.

Handling equipment should be cleaned and disinfected before being used on a new group of cattle, especially those with a different origin, that could be immunologically naive to diseases that a previous group may have carried. Equipment that may be involved includes oral speculums, stomach tubes, dehorning instruments, grooming instruments, balling guns, endoscopes, ultrasound probes, and thermometers. Chutes, alleyways, and concrete flooring should also be cleaned and disinfected.

Special precautions are needed when sick cattle are handled. Sick cattle should be isolated from apparently normal cattle. New herd members should be quarantined for at least 2 weeks to reduce the risk of transmitting a disease that they could be incubating.

Cattle, especially calves, should be kept in a clean, dry enclosure. If handling cattle with diarrhea, handlers should wear gloves and a face shield. Rubber or plastic gloves should be worn when assisting with calving. Cattle should be vaccinated for leptospirosis, and exposure to wildlife, especially rodents, should be controlled.

APPROACHING AND CATCHING

Catching cattle

The degree and frequency of catching and handling cattle varies greatly, as do the reasons. Freshen dairy cattle are handled twice every day for milking, but beef cattle are usually handled just twice a year. Calves are castrated, vaccinated, and ear tagged in the spring. In the fall, the entire herd is vaccinated and calves are given boosters 2–3 weeks later. Disbudding of horned cattle is performed at 2–6 weeks of age. Castration should be performed within the first weeks of birth. Castration may be done on weaned calves, but it should be done using local anesthetic. Dehorning is performed on cattle as soon as possible after 6 weeks of age. Individual cows may have to be restrained and handled at other times to treat illnesses or injuries, check for pregnancy, or artificially inseminate.

Before catching cattle, an inspection of all fences, gates, alleyways, and restraint chutes used for catching should be conducted. Weakened points in the facilities should be repaired, and distractions that might affect the movement of cattle should be removed. The facilities should have been previously cleaned and disinfected, appropriate to their type. The cattle to be caught should be visually inspected prior to catching them. Lameness, labored respiration, lack of appetite, depressed attitude, or other abnormal signs could indicate a need for special handling or rescheduled handling.

The most common approach to catching cattle is to herd them quietly toward or along an enclosure and into an alleyway that goes toward a squeeze chute (British term is "crush") with a headgate (British term is "head bail"). This should be done without a lot of excitement and by using a soothing voice. The herd's collective flight zone should be approached at 45 degrees from behind, moving toward a shoulder of one of the dominant cattle in the center of the herd.

Capture and restraint of calves

Owners should select and train for gentle calves. Weaned calves must be handled gently in order to have gentle adult cattle later. Mother cows can be maternally aggressive and should always be removed from the calves before handling them. Therefore, handlers should always work in pairs when sorting and catching calves.

Capturing a calf

A calf can be caught by hand if herded with its mother into a pen, after which the mother is sorted into another small pen. Small calves may be caught in large pens with a leg crook on a long pole. Branding, castration, and disbudding of calves can be efficiently done by roping calves by handlers skilled in using a lariat. A Nord fork is a head restraint for calves that are caught by a heeler (a person on horseback who ropes the hind legs). The Nord fork when staked restrains the calf's head without risk of choking.

Moving a calf

Small calves can be moved by putting an arm in front of their chest and the other arm around their rump. They are then picked up and carried, or they are walked forward while blocking backward or side movements. Larger calves must be herded in ways similar to adult cattle.

Standing restraint

A calf is backed into a corner by the handler. The handler straddles its neck while facing the calf's nose. A handler can gain access to the jugular vein with both hands by bending over and pushing the calf's head to the side and restraining it with an elbow.

Flanking a calf

Flanking a calf up to 200 lb (90 kg) can be useful in treating the umbilicus (navel), tattooing, branding, ear-tagging, and castration. Small calves can be laid down on their side in the same manner as putting a dog in lateral restraint by reaching over the calf's neck and flank and grasping the front and hind leg closest to the handler's legs (**Figure 12.2**). The calf is lifted up and its legs rotated away from the handler while letting its body slide down the handler's legs. The calf is held on its side by the handler's forearm on its neck and holding onto its lower front and hind legs.

For larger calves, the handler should stand next to the calf's left side with his left arm under its neck. The right hand grasps the calf's right flank skin and the left hand is moved to grasp the right front leg at its knee. The handler's right knee is pushed into the calf's left flank. The calf is lifted in timing with its attempt to jump out of the grasp and its feet rotated away from the handler. The calf continues to be held as it slides down the handler's right leg. To continue holding a calf down, the handler places a knee on its neck and holds the upper front leg in a flexed position.

To tie a downed calf on its left side, a handler straddles the calf's rump in a kneeling position and his right knee is placed behind the calf's hocks. His left hand holds the calf's right front leg and his right hand ties the legs. To tie the legs, the upper front leg is held in backward extension and a constricting loop on a short cord (pigging string) is placed on the leg. Both hind legs are picked up while pulling the front leg back. The pigging string is used to make wraps around all three legs and half-hitches to tie the three legs together. Only one front leg is tied because of the risk of impairing respiration.

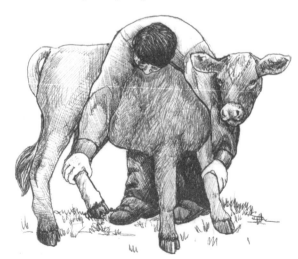

Fig. 12.2 Flanking a small calf.

Another method of tying a downed calf is to use a rope about twice as long as the calf. Both hind legs are tied with an end of the rope using half hitches. The middle part of the rope is crossed beneath the calf, run between the front legs, and placed over the calf's neck. If adjusted correctly, both hind legs are pulled forward to prevent the calf rising to its feet. Castration can be performed with the calf in this position.

Larger calves laid on their side may need to be restrained by two people. One person restrains the head with a knee on the calf's neck while holding the uppermost front leg in a flexed position. The second handler holds and stretches the upper hind leg while sitting behind the calf and bracing a foot against the back of the calf's other thigh. When releasing the calf, the hind legs should be released first.

Packing groups of calves

Calves can be crowded into alleyways for procedures that require minimal restraint, such as vaccinations and pour-on insecticides. Calves can also be drenched (given liquid medications) by moving through the group from front to back. Treated individuals are marked with livestock paint crayons to prevent double treatment or missing a treatment.

HANDLING FOR ROUTINE CARE AND MANAGEMENT

Training cattle to be handled

All cattle should be habituated to being handled by humans, with practice exercises of less than 30 minutes, in order to increase safety of both humans and cattle and to maintain optimum productivity in the production of beef or milk. As with other species, whenever a handler is around cattle, he or she is training them to have good or bad responses in the future, whether the handler realizes this or not. Handling needs to be consistent among all handlers and from one handling to the next.

When handled often, cattle can be moved by hand motions, body language, and verbal directions. Walking among cattle when they are weanling calves with no purpose other than to have them adjust to a handler's presence makes a great difference in how they can be handled later. If dogs or horses are to be used to handle cattle, they should be led as a handler walks among the cattle. Cattle are more likely to remain calm in the future if exposed to what has become routine sights, sounds, and smells. When mingling with them, the handler should wear the same hat, call them with the same call, talk or sing to them in the same way, and otherwise act in the same manner. Direct stares, which could be perceived by cattle as a predator stare, should be avoided. Mingling among the cattle will assist in assessing individual cow behavior. A handler should stand sideways toward the cattle with arms at his side to minimize his appearance until the cattle become more adjusted to his presence. When standing in one spot, the handler should make natural movements with his arms and shoulders. Staying completely still and staring is an image of stalking to a prey animal.

Training is accomplished by putting a small group of calves or untrained cows in a holding pen. After allowing them to settle for 20 minutes, the handler slowly moves them around the inside of the pen's perimeter by briefly invading their flight zone at about 45–60 degrees behind their collective point of balance. Only the edge of the flight zone is worked. Invading the flight zone will cause cattle to run, scatter, or fight. The handler should occasionally stop the cattle in a corner and allow them to rest for a couple of minutes. After a brief rest, they are moved again and stopped in another corner. This exercise is done for up to 30 minutes. Movement should be practiced in both directions and should be repeated daily for at least 3 days. Refresher moving exercises should be done monthly for at least 3 consecutive days. A primary goal of these exercises is to keep the cattle moving at no faster than a walking pace. More than two handlers in a pen is confusing to the cattle. One handler moves the cattle and the other works the gates.

If cattle are to be moved by horseback handlers, cattle moving exercises on horseback similar to walking handler exercises should be practiced. When horseback handlers are moving cattle, there should be no walking handlers in the pen due to the likelihood of being trampled.

Dairy cows have calves to become freshen, but since the milk production is for human consumption, heifer calves are moved in the first day of birth to hutches with small pens. Replacement heifers remain in individual pens for the first 8 weeks of life and are fed a commercial milk replacer. Surplus or market calves are sold at 2 weeks of age. Some bull calves may be kept for veal production, remaining in individual pens or stalls until sent to slaughter by 20 weeks of age. Replacement heifers, being reared in hutches, are not given the opportunity to learn how to follow a herd. They learn to approach handlers for food and mental enrichment and may become aggressive, which can be problematic when they become older and need to be herded. Therefore, young heifers need to be grouped by 9 weeks old with other calves and taught to be herded.

Introduction of heifers to a milking parlor should be quiet and gentle. Food should be provided. If there is an objection to the first handling of the udder (which should be brief and gentle), a tail jack, chest twitch, or flank rope or clamp can be used until the heifer tolerates the handling. The release from restraint should be delayed until after the heifer quietly accepts the food, the parlor, and the gentle handling. Release from restraint should be gradual and associated with the heifer exhibiting calmer behavior. Palpation for insemination or pregnancy diagnosis should not be done in milking parlors. Nothing should occur in a milking parlor that might cause a heifer to avoid going into the parlor in the future.

Basic handling and restraint equipment and facilities

Primary facilities

A handling and restraining site should be along a central fence line to aid in moving cattle toward working facilities at a well-drained point. Fences near and in the working facilities need to be higher and stronger than pasture fencing. Well-designed alleyways and chutes are curved, solid-sided, and constructed of the same material (including color and texture) throughout. The facility should be designed and maintained in a condition that eliminates gouges and cuts (bolt ends cut off, nails pounded in, sharp or jagged metal edges repaired) and is functional and relatively quiet (fence gates, drop down gates, and squeeze chutes lubricated and padded).

Lighting should be bright but diffuse, so that it does not glare into the cattle's eyes. Translucent plastic panels permit diffuse light that eliminates shadows. Dull, subdued colors should be used on painted areas. Lighting should become brighter toward the restraint stanchion or headgate. However, cattle should not be expected to move into direct sunlight, which would impair their vision and raise suspicions of the unknown.

Balking in alleyways and chutes can be more carefully investigated by making a video at cattle height while walking through the cattle passages. The movie can be evaluated for noises, changes in flooring, visibility of handlers, glare of light, and other reasons for discouraging the movement of cattle.

Basic handling facilities for cattle include collecting pens, crowding pens, working alleyways, squeeze chute and headgate, and loading/unloading chutes (**Figure 12.3**). Alleyways, crowding pens, squeeze chutes, and loading ramps should have solid sides to block the cattle's peripheral vision. Industrial rubber belting can be used on alleyway sides and squeeze chutes rather than solid fixed sides to allow direct access to cattle by lifting the belt, as needed, while still blocking the cattle's vision of the outside.

Pens

Types of pens can include holding pens, collecting pens, funneling pens, hospital pens, and quarantine pens. Pens should be numerous, small, and with good gates. Pen fences should be 5–6 ft (1.5–1.8 m) high. For pens in which handlers may be in with cattle, there should be a 16 in (40.6 cm) clearance at the bottom of gates that can provide room for a handler to roll under in an emergency.

Funneling (redirection) pens: crowding pens and bud boxes

Funneling of small groups of cattle into single cattle-wide alleyways can be done with *crowding pens* (tubs) or with small pens with precisely located gates called *Bud boxes*. In crowding pens the handlers are on catwalks outside the pen to work the cattle, and thus are safer for inexperienced handlers or when working with aggressive cattle. Bud boxes require handlers with experience to be in the pen with cattle that enter the pen as a group through a large gate and are then redirected toward a small gate and into a single file alleyway.

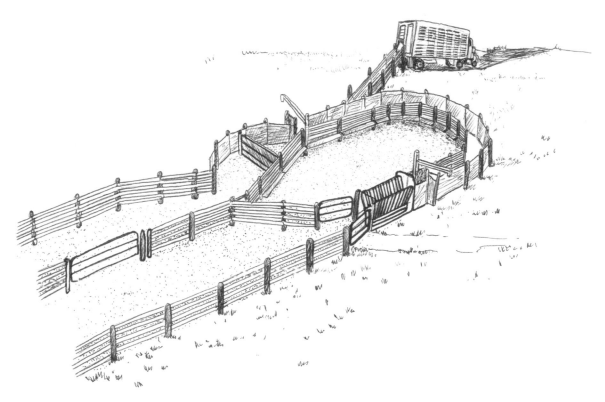

Fig. 12.3 Basic cattle handling facilities.

When using a crowding pen ("forcing" or "sweep" pen), a handler should not fill the pen/tub with too many cattle at a time (**Figure 12.4**). This prevents the movement needed to turn and go the correct direction into an alleyway. Most crowding pens for cattle have a 12 ft (3.7 m) radius designed for 5–10 head, but inexperienced handlers tend to overfill them. When moving them into the alleyway, the large swing gate should follow the cattle and not shove them. Working fewer cattle at a time enables the entire job to take less time. Crowding pens for domestic cattle should be only half to three-quarters filled. Entrances to alleyways from crowding pens must gradually funnel the cattle into the single file alleyway, and there should not be a sharp angle between the crowding pen and the alleyway. Crowding pen walls and gates should be solid to keep cattle from seeing any outside distractions. The alleyway gate should be self-closing or have a self-closing latch.

A Bud box is a pen constructed of pipe rails or thick board planks with a large group gate and a

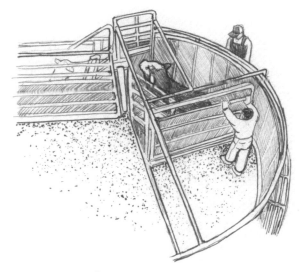

Fig. 12.4 Crowding pen.

small individual cow gate (**Figures 12.5–12.7**). The working principle is to bring cattle into a small pen via a large gate, close the large gate, and herd the cattle around the perimeter of the pen and through a small gate in a corner adjacent to

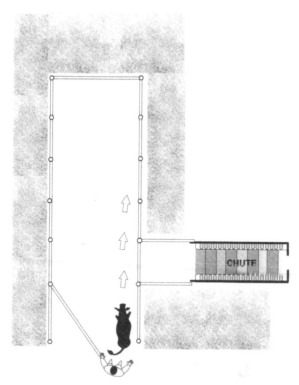

Fig. 12.5 Entering a Bud box.

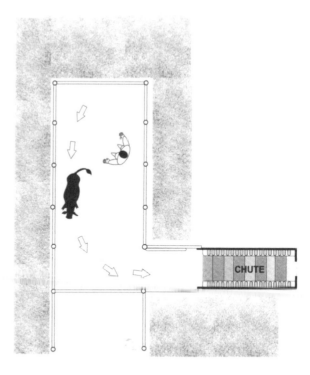

Fig. 12.6 Redirecting in the Bud box.

the large gate. The small gate leads to a single file alleyway. The pen is typically 12 ft (3.7 m) wide and 20 ft (6.1 m) long. If handlers move the cattle on horseback, the width can be 14–16 ft (4.3–4.9 m). The length can be up to 30 ft (9.1 m) if used to fill transport trailers. The portion of the pen opposite the gates can be rounded or have blocked corners to turn cattle more easily. Cattle should be able to see beyond the end of the pen so that they will move into the pen without any hesitation, which a solid end would cause. Four to 20 cattle can be funneled at a time, depending on their size and length of the exit alleyway.

Alleyway (working chute, race)

Many procedures, such as vaccinations, spraying for external parasites, and applying pour-on insecticides, can be performed on cattle without restraining their head in a head catch (stanchion or headgate). They can be pressed together in an alleyway by using blocking gates and butt bars. Working front to back helps keep them tightly together.

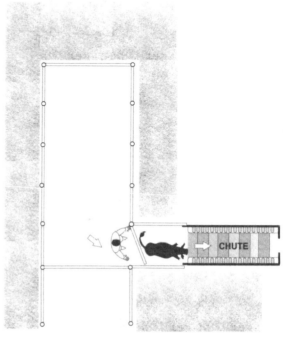

Fig. 12.7 Exiting the Bud box.

A working alleyway should have walls 5 ft (1.5 m) high. If Brahman cattle will be handled, the height should be 66–72 in (167.6–182.9 cm). The center width should be 18 in (45.7 cm) for small calves and up to 28 in (71.1 cm) for adult cows. Large bulls may need up to 32 in (81.3 cm). The bottom should be 15–18 in (38.1–45.7 cm) wide. Flaring the walls outward from the floor keeps the feet of cattle from spreading out and helps prevent attempted turn-arounds and associated balking. Alleyways should be curved with a radius of 12–20 ft (3.7–6.1 m) that permits cattle to see only 2 cattle lengths ahead. The minimum length should be 30 ft (9.1 m), but very long alleyways allow cattle to stand in one place too long, and some will even lie down.

Working alleyways should have solid sides with a catwalk. Handlers should step up on catwalks away from the cattle to prevent startling them with a sudden appearance. Continually speaking in a normal tone also helps cattle be aware of handler presence and avoid startle responses. If solid sides could create ventilation problems, a 1–2 ft (0.3–0.6 m) wide rail at cow eye height may be a useful compromise to a solid-sided alleyway. The solid sides may also be flaps of canvas or rubber, which allow the handler to reach into the alleyway and help move the cattle, if needed. Emergency release panels allow cattle that go down to get out and regain their feet. The gate at the end of the alleyway should be made of bars and not be solid, to allow cattle to see the outside, which will encourage forward movement to the end. Overhead restrainers 5 ft (1.5 m) above the alleyway can stop rearing, turning around, and falling over backwards. Curves in alleyways should be mild enough to permit a view of cattle ahead. No corner in an alleyway should be more than 30 degrees. Drains and grates should be located outside alleyways to avoid being a cause for cattle balking in an alleyway.

Alleyways should have drop-down anti-backup gates rather than metal pipes (butt bars, slip rails), preferably worked with a control rope. If butt bars are used, they should block 6–8 in (15–20 cm) below the average-sized cow's tail head. Concrete in alleyways and crowding pens should be grooved in 8 in (20 cm) squares or diamonds for better footing. Deep groves should not be used in milking parlors or other daily traffic areas due to excessive wear on hooves.

Squeeze chute and headgate

Squeeze chutes are metal boxes with a headgate to entrap individual cattle. Headgates are stanchions (head catches) that close on the cow's neck, preventing it from escaping forward or back but that can also open as a front gate. A squeeze chute can press on the sides of the cow's body, preventing side to side movement. The upper section of the sides have drop-down bars and the lower section has removable panels to provide access to different areas of the cow's body (**Figure 12.8**). Stationary squeeze chutes should be permanently bolted to a floor. Equipment should be padded where steel hits steel. The headgate should move smoothly, quietly, and quickly. Outdoor squeeze chutes should be oriented north-south to prevent cattle from facing the sun when approaching the chute.

Although it is an uncommon procedure in the U.S., cattle should be trained for restraint in squeeze chutes and headgates. After each training step, the cattle should be fed a small amount of grain or choice hay. The first step is to allow the cattle to walk through the chute several times as quietly as possible. The next step is to stop them in the chute without squeezing them and then release. Finally, they are stopped in the chute and the sides squeezed gently and released without any other procedures being done on them. When procedures (ear tagging, vaccinations, castration, etc.)

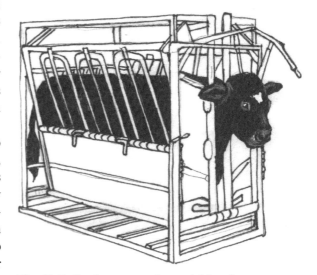

Fig. 12.8 Cattle squeeze chute with headgate.

are performed on them in the future, release from the chute should be timed for when they are not struggling. Release should be into a pen with other cattle and grain or choice hay.

Procedures that are best performed in a squeeze chute and headgate are vaccinations, injectable medications, drenching, bolusing, castration, dehorning, treatment of eye conditions, fertility exams, implanting, ear tagging, branding, bolus administration, stomach tubing, and collection of blood from the jugular vein. All squeeze chutes, including portable ones, should be securely fixed to the ground to prevent tipping or sliding.

Squeeze chutes that are used for dehorning or branding should not be used for artificial insemination. Artificial insemination is best performed in an *AI-dedicated dark box* without a headgate or squeeze. AI dark boxes are 28 in (71.1 cm) wide with solid sides, front, and top. A cloth hangs on the back of the box and drapes over the cow's rump. If wild cattle are handled, the dark box should be the length of two cows, so that a calm cow can be run in first and aid in pacifying the back cow to be inseminated.

The *headgate* in a squeeze chute (British is "cattle crush") entraps the cow's head just behind its ears. Cattle are driven into the chute and caught by vertical bars just as the ears go through and before the shoulders get into the headgate. As soon as the head is caught, a bar is placed behind the cow to prevent it from pulling back on its jaw and ears. Depending on the restraint needed, the sides of the chute may be squeezed against the cow to limit movement. A simple stanchion is a head catch without a chute or headgate.

Headgates can have straight or curved stanchion bars. Curved stanchion bars limit the vertical movement of the head more than straight stanchions, reducing the risk of being butted by an upward head movement, but curved bars can cause choking if the cow goes down. Headgates may have adjunct swinging bars. A head bar is a straight bar that goes over the back of the neck, preventing the head from being thrown upward. A nose bar has a bend in the middle that fits over the bridge of the nose, preventing the head from thrusting forward.

There are four types of headgates: scissors, full opening, positive control, and self-catching. The most common type is scissors. A *scissors stanchion* has halves that pivot from the bottom and squeeze the sides of a cow's neck. It opens from the front, and the bars may be straight or have a curve at the points of contact with the neck. Straight bars allow the head to easily move vertically. Curved bars could put pressure on the carotid arteries and cause the cow to faint. Prolonged procedures, like many veterinary medical procedures, should be performed in straight bar headgates. This headgate may have a head table or nose bar attachments to limit vertical head movement.

The fully opening stanchion has two biparting halves that work like sliding doors. It permits an easier exit for large cows and bulls. The positive control (guillotine) headgates close from above and below, which can cause choking. Positive control headgates were more common when horned cattle were popular. Release is relatively slow, requiring the cow to back after releasing its head, and then opening the front like a gate or releasing from the side of the chute. The self-catching headgate works by a cow's shoulders hitting the stanchion bars and moving them forward to close. This can malfunction or be improperly adjusted for the size of each animal, either way allowing escape.

Butt bars prevent backing up when released through the front. Butt bars also are placed behind the first cow and the last cow in an alleyway. Drop down gates to block backing up are safer than butt bars if counterbalanced to prevent injury to cattle backs. When using a butt bar, the handler should always keep his or her body at the end of the bar in case the other end is suddenly hit by a cow and the handler's end is swung forward or backward. Butt bars in squeeze chutes can break the arm of someone doing a rectal palpation if the cow suddenly goes down.

Single-file alleyways leading to restraint chutes should be curved. *Catwalks* that keep the handler above the sight of cattle help forward movement. Bars or gates that slide across the alleyway or gates that drop down should be used to prevent backups, but a bar or gate should never be placed behind a handler in an alleyway moving cattle. Vertical gaps in an alleyway allow safety escapes or movement from one side of an alleyway to another. When tying a lead rope to a cleat on the side of the headgate, the handler pulls the lead rope with one hand while the other hand wraps the end around the cleat with figure 8s, finishing with a half hitch. The wraps should be done with the heel of the hand to protect fingers from getting trapped if the cow suddenly tugs on the lead rope.

Squeeze chutes and headgates can have either manual or hydraulic action. Manual levers can be ratchet latch or friction latch. Ratchets are noisier. Friction latches can become insecure with wear. Protruding levers on manual chutes are dangerous and can cause operator head and hand injuries and even fatalities. Protruding levers are eliminated with hydraulic chutes. The pressure setting should not squeeze excessively, which would frighten or injure cattle. Most chutes operate at 500 psi and have pressure release valves. Squeezing should be slow and steady to limit movement without unneeded pressure.

Squeeze chutes are V-shaped with the lower portion about half to two-thirds the width of the shoulder space. This encourages cattle to slow down when entering the chute. The lower aspect of the V-shape is about 16 in (40.6 cm) wide and twice as wide at the top. The width of the floor in the squeeze chute should be set to 6 in (15 cm) for 400–600 lb (181–272 kg) calves, 8 in (20 cm) for 600–800 lb (272–363 kg), and 12–16 in (30.5–40.6 cm) for adult cattle. The squeeze should work from both sides to prevent unbalancing the cow. The flooring should be non-slip. Cattle will move into a chute if the flooring is the same color and texture as the alley. If that is dirt, dirt should be thrown onto the chute floor. Application of squeezing the sides should be slow and steady to reduce agitation. Squeeze chutes typically have removable 2 ft (0.6 m) high side panels for access to the lower aspects of the cow with individually removable vertical bars for access to various areas of the cow's upper body. The side should open to enable a cow that is down in the chute to regain her feet.

Handlers should always open and close swinging gates in livestock enclosures, including headgates, with outstretched arms to reduce the risk of being knocked down by a bumped gate. A cow restrained in a headgate will typically put her head down and then jump forward, bumping her shoulders against the gate while raising her head.

> **A handler should never stand near the front of a cow's head in a headgate or lean near its head.**

A collection pen should be located in front of the headgate and the side opening of the squeeze chute. This will enclose cattle that have got too far through the headgate to catch them in front of the shoulders, and so become caught by the hips, at which point they must be released frontwards into the pen. It will also contain cows that go down in the chute and must be rescued by a side-opening gate. Cattle that are normally released from a squeeze chute with a headgate should be penned and provided with water, salt, molasses blocks, or hay to calm down before being released into a pasture. Otherwise, they are likely to run out feeling they have escaped. This leads to harder struggling the next time they are worked in a chute. Unstressed cattle should come out of a squeeze chute and headgate no faster than a walk or slow trot.

Stanchions without squeeze chutes are common in dairies. Self-catching stanchions (headlocks) trap the most dominant cows first at feed bunks, thus allowing others to then find a place to get to food. Stanchions are also incorporated into most veterinary clinic bovine stalls for cattle restraint during exam and treatment.

Loading and unloading chute

A loading chute is a loading platform or ramp used when cattle are moved between a trailer or truck and a working facility. Cattle will best move onto a loading chute directly from a crowding pen or a Bud box. Long single file alleyways to a loading chute should be avoided, and they should face north-south to prevent cattle from facing the sun when loading. Cattle should be loaded single file in a chute that is a minimum of 12 ft (3.7 m) long and 26–30 in (66–76.2 cm) wide. Traction should be provided with cleats every 8 in (20 cm). If concrete ramps are used, the ramp should be stair-stepped 12 in (30.5 cm) deep with 4 in (10 cm) rises. Catwalks alongside the chute are helpful in encouraging smooth loading. Fixed chutes should not exceed 20 degrees of incline. Gaps between loading chutes and transport vehicles should be blocked with self-aligning bumpers and telescoping sides.

Optional restraint facilities

Optional additions include a weighing scale, palpation cage, tilt table, calf tilt table, shed over the working area, concrete flooring, and man-gates and man-passes.

Weighing scales

Cattle scales are inserted at floor level and enclosed as a small pen or stall positioned just before or after the squeeze chute. They should be off the main alleyway and entered only when cattle are to be weighed. Some scales are built into the floor of squeeze chutes, but these can cause balking of the cattle at the chute, and the scales go out of adjustment more often.

Palpation cage

Palpation cages are used for pregnancy exams of cows, artificial insemination, fertility testing of bulls, and castration of calves. Palpation cages have handler gates in the alleyway immediately behind a catch or squeeze chute. The gate swings into the alleyway and away from the chute and can be latched to block other cattle in the alleyway from going forward until their turn in the chute. This allows a handler to inspect or treat a cow from behind by entering behind the caught cow in the chute and to not be injured by other cattle in the alleyway.

Artificial insemination (AI) should be performed in restraint chutes that are not used for painful procedures such as vaccination, ear tagging, and medical treatments. AI dark boxes are preferable. The chute for AI does not need to squeeze or have a head catch.

Tilt tables and rotary chutes

Tilt tables facilitate working on the flank, udder, and feet or legs of cattle. The cow is led or herded next to a vertical table top. The halter rope is tied to restrain the head first. One belly strap goes under the front part of the chest and a second strap goes under the abdomen. Legs are strapped down. The vertical position of the table top is then tilted to the horizontal plane. This type of tilt table can be on a hydraulic pedestal able to go up or down and even be flush with the floor. Smaller tilt tables are transportable for field work.

A *rotary chute* is a squeeze chute on a circular track that turns a cow on either side. After the cow is caught in the squeeze chute, the chute can be rotated 90 degrees until the cow is lying on its side, the side of the chute having become like a horizontal table top. Rotary chutes are safer for both cattle and handlers, but they limit access to the cow's side more than a tilt table.

Cattle should not be held on their sides for more than 30 minutes, as there is a risk of rumen gas accumulation.

Calf tilt table

Calf tilt tables are reduced-size versions of the tilt tables used for adult cattle (**Figure 12.9**). They work best for calves less than 500 lb (227 kg). Use of tilt tables for working calves is slower than the "rope and drag" method. A tilt table also results in greater separation from herd members. However, calf tables are much safer than inexperienced handlers trying

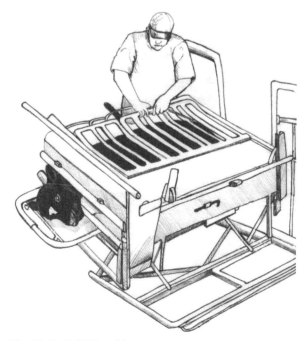

Fig. 12.9 Calf tilt table.

to rope calves. Calf tables also permit handling of calves with fewer people involved.

The "rope and drag" method of working calves is still practiced by some western states ranches. This is not because of tradition, but because some handlers believe that the 30 seconds it takes for 6 efficient calf handlers to vaccinate, ear tag, brand, castrate, and dehorn a calf is less stressful to calves and safer than being sorted, run up alleys, having their neck caught, and being squeezed in a chute. In addition, the procedures being performed on the calves take more time owing to the obstructions to access created by the restraint equipment.

Shed

Sheds are helpful over working alleys and squeeze chutes, especially if equipped with lights, outlets, and water source for cleaning.

Concrete flooring

Concrete floors under the working alleys, squeeze chute, and crowding tub can improve footing and drainage.

Man passes and man gates

Man passes are fence gaps 12–18 in (30.5–46 cm) wide for handler safety escapes. Man gates are 2–4 ft (0.6–1.2 m) wide at convenient locations for handler movement and safety.

Dip tank

Dipping of cattle for ticks has been replaced in most areas by acaricidal sprays, pour-ons, dusts, and ear-tags. Dip tanks should have a funneled entrance that permits only one cow to enter the dip tank at a time. Otherwise, incoming cattle may jump onto a cow that is already in the tank. The in and out ramps should be cleated for traction and not exceed 20 degrees of inclination above water. The slope of the lower aspect of the ramp, which is under water, can be a steeper drop off.

Moving cattle

Other than transporting cattle, there are three methods of moving cattle: leading, driving, and herding. Moving of cattle should be done quietly

and without pain. Moving cattle is preferably done in early morning or evening when it is cool. Cows with calves are best moved in the evening. When the herd is stopped, calves will lie down, and the herd will stay with the calves. Cattle will file memories of places, people, weather, odors, and other environmental stimuli and react on second exposure based on memory, if a reaction is not overridden by logic or reason. Bad handling experiences are remembered by cattle for at least 3 years.

Calling and leading

Leading is the least stressful way of moving cattle. Cattle can be trained to come or follow in anticipation of being fed. If a call or noise is used before and during feeding, cattle will learn to respond to the call. Sweet feed (grain with molasses) or alfalfa hay can be used to train cattle to be led. If cattle are being trained to come to be fed in a pasture, they should be programed to associate food with a call sound, not the sight of a truck, to prevent crowding before distributing the feed.

Having a quiet leader steer or cow can be extremely helpful in moving cattle. In the great Texas cattle drives of the 1800s, nervous leader cattle were killed. Old Blue was a famous longhorn steer who wore a leather collar with a bell and calmly led more than 10,000 head of cattle over 8 years to railheads.

Cattle will follow more easily than they can be herded. Teaching new cattle where to go can be done by leaving small piles of grain or hay in a trail to the destination planned for them. If a cow gets too close, the handler should reaffirm his dominant social status by spreading his arms and waving a herding stick in the air. If that does not result in moving the cow away, he should tap it on the nose with the herding stick.

When walking among cattle to adjust them to his or her presence, the handler can feed them treats from a feeding bucket such as carrots, apples, or sweet feed (molasses and grain). This will teach them to follow when he carries the same bucket. Cows that do not follow can be sorted and kept alone in a pen until the others are moved. The penned cow will seek out the others after she is released. A barrier or platform such as a truck bed should be used when training cattle with food. They respond better when hungry but could become dangerous if the handler is on foot. Cows with nursing calves should not be called. The anticipation of food rewards may train the cow to leave her calf.

Over time, cattle can be taught to follow a quiet, leading handler. Frequent presence among the herd and the appropriate use of rewards, such as access to different food and fresh water, is required. A leader must be consistent. When training cattle to lead or leading trained cattle, a handler cannot switch to herding the herd and then back to leading. If a herd must be herded, other handlers should do it. Once a herd is taught to be led some members should be retained as tutors for new herd members if the remainder of the herd is sold.

Driving

Driving and herding are often used as synonyms, but they are not. Driving cattle is less organized and involves the use of some degree of fear. Moving cattle by cracking whips, yelling, and waving objects is driving cattle.

Driving cattle uses the method that group hunting predators use to move animals for a kill. It is the oldest and most stressful way of moving cattle. At its core, driving involves positioning the cattle between the site to move them to and the handlers. Handlers then invade the flight zone, frightening the cattle to move in the direction desired. Driving cattle effectively toward a desired destination requires multiple handlers. Driven cattle often move at a pace faster than a walk.

Herding: flight zones and balance points
Herding

Herding cattle mimics the means that a dominant herd member would use to move other herd members. It is a less animal-stressful method than driving, but experienced handlers are needed to accomplish herding. A group (herd) of cattle can usually be herded just by a handler's presence within their personal comfort zone. Teaching cattle to follow is preferable, but many circumstances require herding. Herding cattle is accomplished by a rhythmic push on the periphery of

the cattle's flight zone, followed by a slight retreat, slight push, slight retreat, and so on. The pace of herding is at a walk.

Cattle should never be chased. If they are and they are successful in escaping to another side of a pasture or somewhere else they can find rest, they will always attempt to run and escape when their flight zone is approached.

Zones

There are three psychological zones around prey animals: *recognition*, *flight*, and *fight*. Recognition is the largest zone. The flight zone is the most important for herding. If the flight zone is aggressively invaded, the fight zone will be reached. Factors that affect the flight zone include the time of day and season of the year; the weather; previous experiences; presence or absence of herdmates and their proximity; the terrain; the presence of obstacles between the animal and the herder; genetic tendency to be nervous or calm; and the herder's size, angle of approach, speed of approach, and demeanor, as well as the number of herders and dogs.

A typical flight zone for domestic cattle is an oval with a diameter anywhere from 5–300 ft (1.5–91.4 m). Most dairy cattle have a flight zone of 5–10 ft (1.5–3 m). Beef cattle that are around handlers on a regular basis have flight zones of about 15–25 ft (4.6–7.6 m). Beef cattle raised in southern states in the U.S. have a larger flight zone than the same breed raised in northern states because of the regular, close exposures to humans that occur in winter feedings in the north.

Flight zones are dynamic, changing depending on current conditions and past experiences. The easiest method for a handler to reduce a flight zone is to wait, be quiet, and let the animals settle and adjust to his or her appearance and behavior. Squatting or turning sideways reduces a handler's silhouette and pressure on the animals' flight zone.

Balance points
Cattle, like all herd animals, have a side balance point at their shoulder for other animals or handlers to signal movement forward or backward. If the handler is located to the side and forward of the cow's

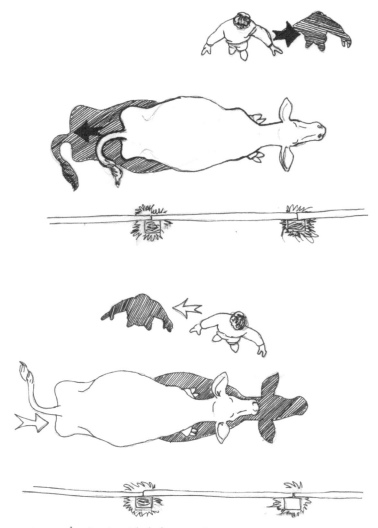

Fig 12.10 Moving a cow forward using its side balance point.

shoulder, she will back up or turn. If the handler is behind and to the side of the cow's shoulder, she will move forward (**Figure 12.10**).

The middle of the nose and middle of the tail are the front and back balance points, respectively. When the handler in front or behind a cow moves to the left, a cow will move to the right. When the handler in front or behind a cow moves to the right, a cow will move to the left (**Figure 12.11**).

Initiating and maintaining movement
Methods by which a handler can cause movement are to stare directly at the animals, face the animals and increase their profile (raise arms, spread legs), and directly approach the animals. Stopping is achieved by removing the pressures to move, such as lowering the handler's arms to the side and standing at a 90-degree angle to the cattle.

It is best to herd in the morning after cattle have eaten. Hunger decreases tolerance to stress. When starting cattle to move after a rest, handlers must concentrate on getting the leaders moving in any direction, and once they are moving to direct their movement.

If cattle are in an alleyway and cannot back up, a handler walking in the opposite direction to the cattle and close to them will encourage the cattle to move forward as the handler passes their side balance points. This can be repeated by the handler making a wide circle away from the cattle to again

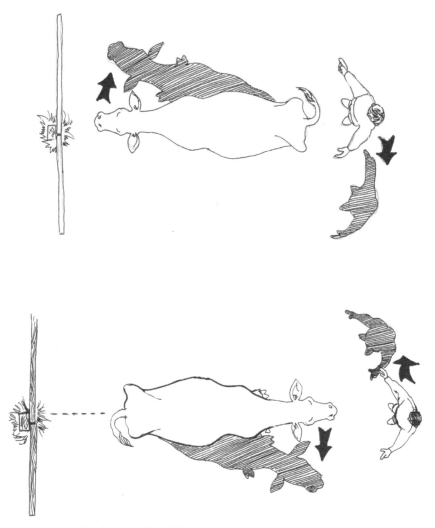

Fig. 12.11 Moving a cow using its front and back balance points.

pass closely to them moving in the direction opposite to the cattle's direction (**Figure 12.12**).

Cattle cannot determine whether a handler has invaded their flight zone if the handler is directly behind them. Herding must be performed from an angle (ideally, 45–60 degrees behind their shoulder) that allows the handler to see an eye of the cow to be moved to ensure the cow can see the handler. The handler should zig-zag while behind the herd in order to be seen alternately with both eyes of the cattle by passing in and out of their blind spot.

Cattle's desire to avoid icy, muddy, or rocky surfaces will adversely affect the direction of movement. Cattle will avoid new objects until they have had time to settle and become curious.

The location of others of their own species and especially their own herd has advantageous drawing power.

Handlers should be mindful of the herd subgroups: leaders, dominants, and submissives. Although one handler can herd a large group of cattle, two handlers are more effective. The forward handler pushes on the herd leaders' flight zone. The rear handler pushes on the flight zone of straggling submissives. Handlers should move in straight lines with confidence and change directions with angles, not curves. Circling movements mimic predator behavior and should thus be avoided. Flight zone pressure on a dominant herd member will make it move toward the center of the

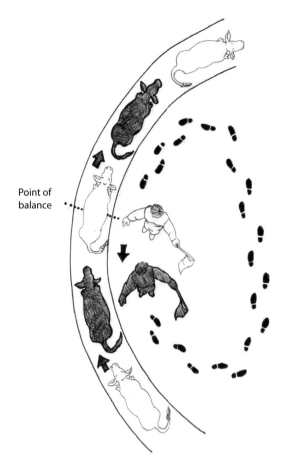

Point of
balance

Fig. 12.12 Passing balance points to move cattle forward in an alleyway.

herd. Handlers who herd cattle must apply pressure from the side, behind the balance point of dominants, not from behind the group. Pressure on a low-ranking herd member may cause it to circle the herd, and if sufficiently frightened, to take off on its own. Submissives, including young calves, follow in the back of the herd. Trying to move a herd from behind will push the submissives into the dominants, an action that is socially intolerable and will leads to the submissives being driven away by the dominants.

Reducing stress on herded cattle includes being moved by a familiar handler, the handler looking away from the animals, pausing in pressing on the flight zone, occasionally taking a well-timed step backward, and reducing his or her profile by presenting a side profile, slouching, kneeling, or turning

away. Fight or flight is decreased by dim light and rhythmic sounds and music, such as a low monotonous tone of singing, humming, or whistling. Fight or flight can also be reduced by leaving agitated cattle alone for 20–30 minutes.

Herding with horses, all terrain vehicles, and dogs

Although cattle are less frightened by a handler on horseback than a handler on foot, they will more readily move when a horse and rider invade their flight zone. Horses increase the size of the herder.

Cattle should not be moved with an all terrain vehicle (ATV). The noise creates a stimulation for driving the cattle, not for herding them. ATVs cannot change directions abruptly and sharply enough to be very effective. In addition, ATVs require too much of a rider's attention for traversing the terrain, and so detract from appropriate attention to herding cattle.

Well-trained herding dogs can be helpful in finding and moving stray cattle on an open range or in large pastures out of brush, but once the cattle enter a collecting pen, few dogs are useful. Herding dogs should generally not be used to move cattle in pens. When being moved a long distance, cattle naturally string out in a single file. They are thus easier to move in a long line than when they are forced to bunch up. This is different to the herding tactics that poorly trained dogs attempt when moving cattle. Their presence around collecting pens can be distracting and disturbing to the cattle, causing danger to handlers by stirring the cattle in close quarters. Dogs should never be used to herd cows with nursing calves. This only results in putting the mother cow in fighting mode.

Moving large herds

Large herds should be herded with eight handlers (four pairs). These are (from front to back) the point, swing, flank, and drag pairs. Prior training of cattle is very helpful. Older cows that herd calmly should be kept as role models for younger ones. To control the rate of movement, handlers go up the sides of moving cattle to slow the herd. To speed the herd up, handlers move down the sides of the herd.

Moving bulls

Moving adult bulls requires taking extra precautions. Trained dogs can be helpful in moving bulls by being a distraction to a bull that gets aggressive toward the handler. Riding a tractor to move bulls is safer than being on foot or horseback. Handlers should work in pairs when handling bulls or beef cows with nursing calves, and neither handler should ever take his eyes off the cattle until they are contained separately from the handlers.

Collecting cattle

Introducing cattle to a collecting facility before handling them there for routine or medical procedures will reduce their stress when the time comes for them to be collected for purposes other than training.

Collecting pens are best located between pastures, so that when changing pastures the cattle have to walk through the collecting pens, with a reward of fresh pasture on the other side. Gates should be located at the top of a rise, not the bottom. Entry to yards should be wide and along a fence line on level ground or uphill.

A collection pen must be strong enough to hold cattle in close confinement and not be constructed of wire fencing. After moving cattle into a collection pen, they should be allowed to settle for 20–30 minutes.

Cattle in small group confinement will bruise or injure each other during sorting, especially if not done quietly and efficiently. Cattle movement in the pen should be directed with flags. Handlers should not yell at or hit the cattle. When most of a group in a crowding pen are facing the alleyway, a handler should slowly swing the crowding gate to have them enter the alleyway one at a time. A drop down gate should be at the entrance of the squeeze chute and is raised to let one cow at a time into the chute. People should not be visible to the front or side of the squeeze chute. Careful use of a *tail twist hold* (released immediately with the slightest forward movement) can be used to train cattle to move forward when touched on the rump (**Figure 12.13**). The use of electric prods should be avoided.

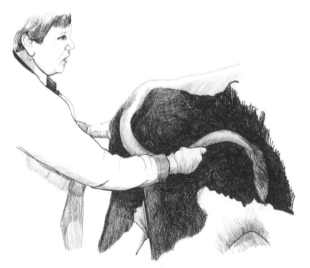

Fig. 12.13 Tail twist to encourage forward movement.

AVMA Policy on Livestock Handling Tools

"The AVMA believes that mechanical aids to direct livestock movement should be used sparingly and not to strike animals. Use of these aids should be secondary to good facility design and an understanding of the specific needs of the species involved. It is important that all people involved in livestock handling be trained in applicable animal behavior and handling techniques and be regularly monitored to ensure that appropriate practices are maintained. Electrical devices (e.g. stock prods) should be used judiciously and only in extreme circumstances when all other techniques have failed. Electrical devices should never be applied to sensitive parts of the animal such as the face, genitalia, or mucous membranes."

Electric prods, also called "hot shots" ("electric goad" in the United Kingdom), should be the last resort to encourage movement (**Figure 12.14**). Their use is frequently inhumane and counterproductive. However, they may be needed in some situations, such as getting downed cows up and into shelter before storms, or making cows move away from a handler knocked down in a pen or chute and in danger of being stomped or crushed. Electric prods deliver 2,200–9,000 volts. Before being used on a cow, they should be discharged

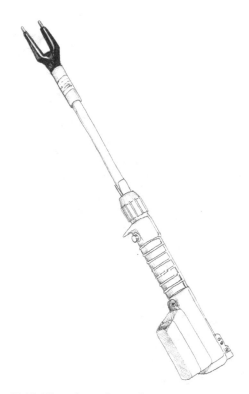

Fig. 12.14 Electric cattle prod.

on something metal near the cow. The sound of the buzz may be enough to cause movement, especially if they have been shocked before. After using it, the end should be touched to a metal surface to ground and discharge any residual electricity.

Sorting cattle

Sorting may be for separating cattle by age, sex, or state of health. Separating cattle from a larger group should be done in pairs, or more, as sorting a cow into a pen by itself can cause it to panic. In addition, a cow that is removed and isolated from a herd for longer than 24 hours will be harassed when it rejoins the herd. Separated cattle should be returned as soon as possible. If the separation has been longer than 24 hours, the cow should be returned when the herd is actively engaged in a diversionary activity, such as grazing in a new pasture or being fed grain. Returned cattle usually assume the same rank in the herd as the rank they left.

One method of sorting is to move them from collecting or holding pens into a sorting pen alleyway 12–14 ft (3.7–4.3 m) wide and then separate them into sorting pens. The handler should plan for the largest cattle to move down the alleyway to the last sorting pen. Sorting can be done more quietly with poles and small flags. It is best to sort out the least excitable first. For example, separate cows from bulls, cows from calves, and older from younger cows. Alleyway sorting requires two handlers.

Sorting can also be done while moving cattle quietly out a pen by stepping in front of a cow's side balance point when wanting to turn it back into the pen. Movements should be slow, deliberate, and measured. The group to be sorted should be calmed for about 20 minutes. The handler should be visible, quiet, and present a small profile (turn to side, squat, sit) during the calming period, but he should never turn his back to animals near an exit.

If an exit from a pen is provided but cattle are reluctant to leave, a shirt or jacket can be tied to a rope and dragged slowly through the pen and out of the gate. Often, the leaders of the group will follow it. If cattle rush through a gate, a handler can stand nearby inside the pen and move slightly toward the gate in front of the leader's side balance point, and then as soon as the cattle slow down, the handler should step back. This back and forth movement may need to be repeated to regulate the speed of additional cattle movement through the gate.

A round pen or a modified Bud box with side pens can facilitate sorting cattle. A handler in the pen can encourage movement of the cattle along the edge of the pen, while a sorting handler opens the appropriate gate at the optimum time. The side pens should have gates that swing either into or out of the sorting pens, regardless of the direction the cattle are moving around the round pen or Bud box. It is best to work small groups of cattle in a sorting pen so they can move more freely.

To facilitate moving cattle through a gate, the gates in holding pens should be placed in a corner that is closest to water or feeding sites rather than the middle of a straight stretch of fence. Slick footing of sorting alleyways should be treated with sand or crushed limestone.

Sorting can also be performed on horseback with trained cutting horses. Sorting with horses requires fewer facilities than sorting using special pens and handlers on foot.

HANDLING FOR COMMON MEDICAL PROCEDURES

Most handling and restraint of cattle can be and should be done WITHOUT tranquilization, sedation, hypnosis, or anesthesia. However, some handling and restraint procedures should be restricted to veterinary medical professionals because of the potential danger to the animal or handler. These require special skills, equipment, or facilities, and possibly adjunct chemical restraint.

Restraint of individual cattle or parts of their body

Restraint of the head of cattle eliminates most of their struggling when restrained. Any other restraint that does not restrain the head well will result in continued struggling. Methods of head restraint include the use of halters, nose leads, nose rings, and stanchions.

Dehorning is done on most horned cattle to reduce hide damage and bruising to other cattle and to increase the safety of handlers and their horses and working dogs. Dehorning also aids working cattle in chutes. Dehorning of cattle should be performed when they are calves.

Head restraint
Rope halters

A halter is the safest method to restrain a cow's head because a cow or bull may go down and be injured if it is tied only by a nose lead, nose ring, or neck rope. However, putting a halter on a cow, especially when it is in a stanchion, can be hazardous for handlers. The most commonly used halter is a rope halter that extends into a lead (**Figure 12.15**).

Rope halters for cattle are made with twisted rope and created with slicing techniques. Care must be taken not to place the nose back portion of the halter lower than the bony part of the nose or the nostrils may become pinched shut, causing the animal to panic.

A cattle rope halter extends into its own lead rope and exits the halter on either the right or left side of the animal's cheek, i.e. it is reversible. When leading a cow, it should be on the cow's left side. If a cow is caught in a stanchion, it should be on the same side of the face as the lead rope, which will be tied to the chute's cleats. To put a cattle halter on properly, remember: "The part that draws goes under the jaws."

Rope halters are used to lead halter-broke cows, calves, and steers. They may be applied while a cow or calf is in a stall, a stanchion, or when restrained by a neck rope and snubbing post. The adjustable portion and lead rope portion should be on the left side of the cow's head. With practice the halter can be held at the crownpiece with the right hand and placed on the cow's head with a backhand movement of the right hand while standing to the left of the cow. The crownpiece goes over the right ear and then the left. The muzzle part should be open enough to fall under the cow's jaw. The halter is then tightened and adjusted into place. This method does not require a handler to be pressed against the cow to place a halter, which would risk injury to his or her hip.

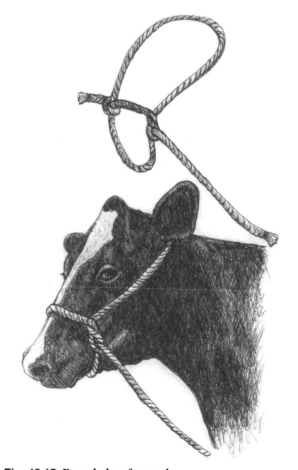

Fig. 12.15 Rope halter for cattle.

Some handlers prefer to use two hands to catch the muzzle first and then place the top part over of the ears. Attempting to place or adjust a halter with both hands requires pushing the handler's hip next to the cow's head. If the handler's hip is not pressed against the cow, a swing of the cow's head may fracture the handler's hip. Furthermore, two-handed haltering can result in bending close enough to a cow's head that a butting injury to the handler's head is possible.

Nose leads

A nose lead is a blunted clamp (also called "tong") that is best placed in the nostrils with a sweeping motion from the side while the cow is in a stanchion and the handler faces it at a safe distance. Functional nose leads should have smooth blunted ends on the tongs, a ⅛ in (0.3 cm) gap between closed tongs, and a smooth rope lead (**Figure 12.16**). Chains on nose leads are undesirable since they can kink, pinch, and pull open. Nose leads should only be used if the neck is restrained in some form of stanchion, including a headgate of a squeeze chute. The use of nose leads to restrain the head is more likely to make the animal more resistant to future handling than will the use of rope halters. Therefore, nose leads should not be used for procedures that have to be frequently repeated.

Halters are generally preferable to nose leads. However, nose leads are less dangerous for handlers to apply, if done correctly. They allow the cow's head to be pulled to either side without being removed and reversed (flipped), as is necessary with a halter. A nose lead also allows the cow's head to be pulled farther to the sides or upward, which can facilitate jugular venipuncture in some cows. Nose leads risk injuring the nasal septum in cattle, but this is very rare if the balls of the lead do not touch when the lead is closed and the lead rope is always kept tight so the cow does not sling its head. A cow restrained by a nose lead should not be tied firmly to a chute cleat in case it goes down and hangs by its nose, which could possibly tear its nasal septum.

When applying a nose lead to a cow, the handler must take care not to lean over the cow's head or be within forward striking distance of the cow's head if it should lunge forward in the headgate. The handler should not approach a cow from a straight-on direction with the nose lead, as this will intensify its efforts to dodge placement of the lead. Nose leads are applied by holding the lead with one hand with the palm up. The handler stands in front of the cow's head while the cow's head is retrained in a head catch or stanchion. The tongs are separated and held open using the ring and little finger. A sweeping movement is used from the handler's right to left if the tongs are held with the right hand. The right tong goes in the cow's left nostril, the left tong immediately follows into the right nostril, and the tongs are quickly closed by a tug on the lead rope. Chain attachments to nose leads do not slide smoothly or reliably without kinking and should not be used with this method.

A less safe method is for the handler to press his or her hip against the cow's head, putting a hand over its head and onto the other side of the jaw, and putting the tongs in while trying to partially immobilize its head. Nose leads should not be applied for more than 20 minutes.

For brief restraint, a handler can grasp a cow's nasal septum with his thumb and middle finger and use his fingers in the same manner as metal nose tongs.

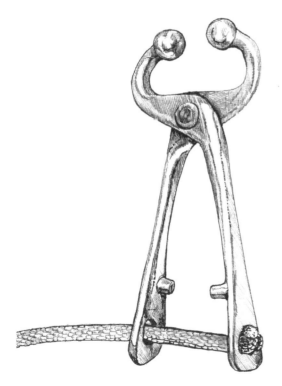

Fig. 12.16 Nose lead with rope attachment.

Nose rings

Nose rings are used in all adult dairy bulls and some beef bulls (**Figure 12.17**). Most have a nose ring placed between 1 and 2 years of age, before they become territorially aggressive. The safest way of moving a bull with a nose ring is with two handlers, one on each side with a bull staff. A bull staff is a pole that has a hook or snap on one end that attaches to the nose ring. A bull staff is usually used in combination with a halter.

Placement of nose rings should be done by a veterinarian since the use of local anesthesia and post-surgical pain relievers are needed. A chute with a headgate and nose bar should be used for nose ring placement.

People should never play with a bull calf, since this can eliminate the natural respect most have for human personal space. A bull calf should be culled if it shows signs of dominance aggression, such as head shaking, staring at people within the bull's enclosure, pawing the ground while facing a person, or deliberately showing his side to a person.

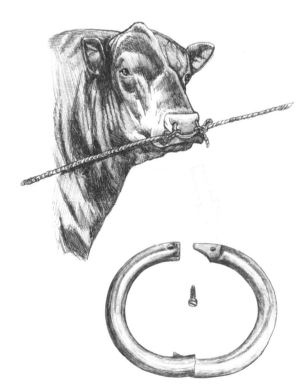

Fig. 12.17 Bull nose ring.

Whole body restraint
Stanchions and tying posts

Stanchions or tying posts can be used to restrain halter-trained or docile cattle. Stanchions or posts should be strong enough to hold adult cattle that might resist the restraint with all their strength. Tie rings on tying posts should be at a cow's natural head height or slightly higher.

Improvised chutes and hay bale barriers

A gate that swings against a wall can be used as an improvised treatment squeeze chute when other facilities are not present. Square bales of hay or straw can be used behind restrained cattle to reduce the risk of the handler being kicked if work is needed round their rump, such as rectal examination.

Rope and snubbing post

If adept with a lariat, a handler can toss a lariat loop around a cow's neck and pull it to a stout stationary post. The restraint should be brief or a halter should placed on the cow's head and the lariat removed. Alternatively, a bight can be run underneath the neck loop at the throat and then placed over the cow's nose to make a temporary halter. This will relieve pressure around the cow's neck. A rope and snubbing post should be used when less stressful means are not available and the need for restraint is more important than the stress that might result.

Chest twitch

A chest twitch is a rope looped around the chest and pulled tight. This may calm a tied, agitated cow.

Casting

Casting methods are ways to lie a cow down and immobilize it when restraint chutes or tilt tables are not available or appropriate for the procedure to be done. Any time a cow is laid on its side there can be risk of displaced abomasum or bloat if handled roughly or forced to remain recumbent for too long. Cows within 2 months of calving should not be cast due to the risk of induced abortion.

An appropriate ground surface should first be selected. The ground selected for casting should be clear, smooth, and loosened dirt or padded. Cattle will lie down if a rope squeezes their chest and their abdomen (half-hitch method) or puts pressure beneath their front legs and over their back (Burley or "Flying W" method). With either method, the lead rope should be held by an assistant or tied low, near the ground, to a sturdy object. Both methods require 40 ft (12.2 m) of rope.

To perform the *half-hitch method* of casting, a loop is placed around the cow's neck and tied with a bowline (**Figure 12.18**). A half hitch is placed around the chest just behind the cow's elbows. The rope is thrown under the cow or a pole with a hook that can be used to retrieve the rope on the other side. Another half hitch is placed around the abdomen, avoiding the udder or prepuce, depending on the gender. The remaining line is pulled back steadily in line with the cow's spine, and the cow is gradually laid down on its side. Cattle should be laid either on their back (ventrodorsal) and propped with hay bales with their front legs stretched forward and their hind legs stretched back with cotton ropes, or on their right side so that the left side can be uppermost and observed for gas accumulation.

If lying on its right side, the front legs are tied with 6 ft (1.8 m) cotton ropes after flexing the leg so that the hoof is near the elbow and restrained with a clove hitch around a pastern, leaving about 8 in (20 cm) extra. The long end is wrapped around the radius and the pastern 3–4 times and then the rope is tied with a slip knot (sheet bend with a bight for quick release) to the 8 in (20 cm) left over from the clove hitch. Similar ties can be used on flexed hind legs with a clove hitch on a fetlock, figure 8 wraps incorporating the fetlocks and tibia just above the hock, and a slip knot tie. Recumbent ruminants rise with their hind legs first. Tying the hind legs securely is of more importance than the front legs.

The *Burley method* of casting cattle was named for Dr. D. R. Burley of Georgia (**Figure 12.19**). It is preferred by dairymen, since the ropes are not placed in front of the udder, and the cow goes down on its sternum and must be rolled over on its side. There is no pressure on the chest or udder and no knot to tie around the horns, neck, or front leg. Therefore, its application and release are quicker. It is also possible to control which side the cow rolls onto. However, it is harder to pull two ropes with enough strength to cast a cow than one rope, as with the half-hitch method.

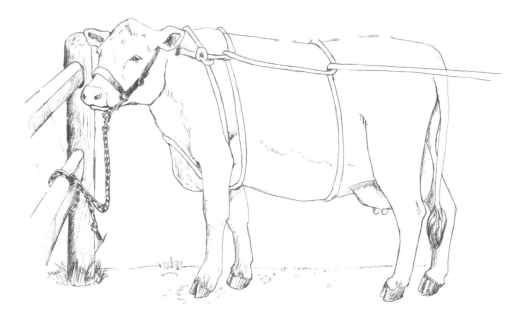

Fig. 12.18 Half-hitch method of casting.

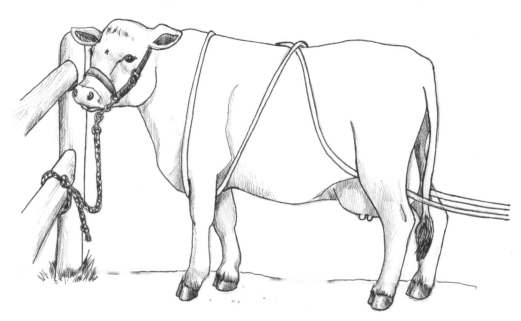

Fig. 12.19 Burley method of casting.

Restraint of the tail

The tail of a cow can inflict serious injury to a handler, since the coccygeal (tail) vertebrae extend almost to the end of the tail. A quick-release sheet bend can be used as a simple and effective hitch. The long hair (switch) of the end of the tail is bent around the tie rope to begin making the hitch. A tied tail should only be secured to the cow's body in case the cow goes down during the restraint. The other end is tied around the cow's neck using a bowline knot to prevent the rope from tightening around the neck (**Figure 12.20**). Alternative ties to further reduce or eliminate the risk of pressure on the windpipe are (1) to put the rope around the neck and behind a front leg on the side opposite to the one that the tail is bent toward, or (2) for horned cattle, having a loop around the horns instead of the neck.

Lifting feet

Lifting a cow's foot should be done for brief periods only (standing on three legs will quickly exhaust a cow and it may go down). A cow's leg should not be lifted by hand, as is done with horses. Dairy cattle can be resentful or sullen and fall on the handler. Beef cattle that are not halter trained will not tolerate an attempt to pick up a front leg.

To lift a front leg on a dairy cow, a rope with a quick-release honda is placed around the pasterns below the dewclaws, and the standing end looped over an adjacent bar or the cow's back and held by an assistant.

Lifting a hind leg is usually done in a chute. A rope with a quick-release honda is placed around the cow's cannon bone and looped over a bar above and behind the leg, and another wrap is made with the standing end around the leg just above the hock. The leg is hoisted and the rope held by an assistant (**Figure 12.21**). If the bar used to lift the leg is not sufficiently behind the cow, the hind leg will not be stretched back and it will have too much freedom to kick back and forth for this to be a safe restraint.

Anti-kicking methods

Calves may kick with both hind legs, but adult cattle usually kick with one. However, they are more flexible in their ability to kick than horses. Cattle can reach forward to their shoulder and sweep outward when they kick.

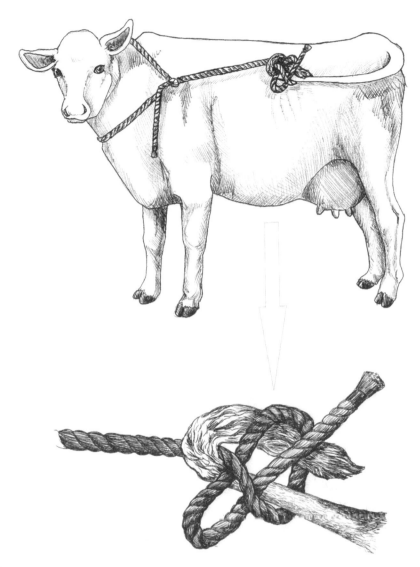

Fig. 12.20 Tail tie.

Tail jacking

Cattle are reluctant to kick if the tail is bent backward toward their spine. The handler stands to the cow's side and grasps the tail about one-third down from the base of the tail. The tail is raised as the handler steps close behind the cow, holding the tail straight up and bent slightly toward the spine (**Figure 12.22**). Only moderate pressure should be used to prevent injury to the tail.

The tail jack restraint hold is used for venipuncture of the ventral vein of the tail; to exam, clean, or treat the mammary glands; and for castration.

Frank pressure

Grasping a flank fold and lifting the skin can inhibit kicking, but the handler's position to apply the hold is dangerous, with a risk of being kicked first or being kicked in spite of the hold.

A rope loop with a honda pulled tight around the flank will inhibit vigorous kicking, but it will not prevent subdued attempts to kick.

Large metal flank clamps that close with a screw mechanism or telescoping rods with springed pin locks exert pressure on the flank to inhibit kicking (**Figure 12.23**).

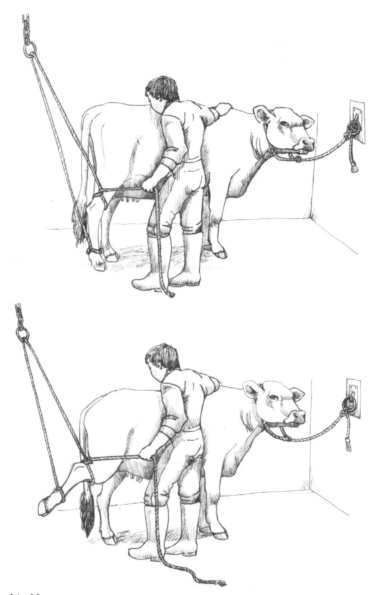

Fig. 12.21 Hoisting a hind leg.

Hock hobbles

Tendon clamps or metal U-shaped hobbles placed above a hock on the Achilles (gastrocnemius) tendon prevent cows from kicking in milking parlors. Hobbles are connected by a chain, which must be long enough to permit the cow to have its hind legs sufficiently apart to keep its balance. Hock hobbles are applied from the cow's side to the opposite side Achilles tendon first and then to the near side tendon.

A 4 ft (1.2 m) cotton rope may also be used to hobble the hind legs. A bight in the middle of the rope is placed above the hock on one leg. The two standing ends are twisted several times to provide sufficient length between the legs for the cow to stand normally. The ends are wrapped around the other leg above the hock and tied with a sheetbend knot.

Working with downed cattle

Downed (downer) cattle are those that have lost their desire or ability to stand and move. Common causes include milk fever, leg injuries, and calving (obturator nerve) paralysis. Downed cattle may recover

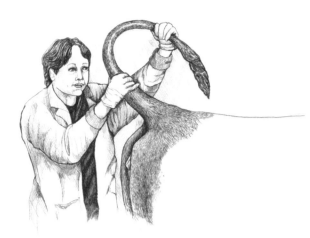

Fig. 12.22 Tail jacking to inhibit kicking.

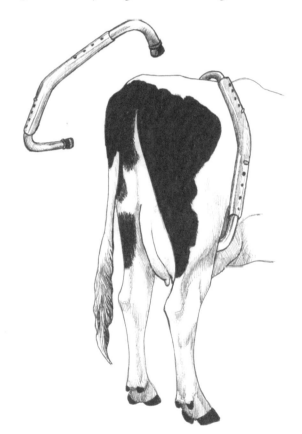

Fig. 12.23 Anti-kick flank clamp.

but need shelter and nursing during the recovery period. Downed cattle cannot be sent for commercial slaughter for human consumption.

Note: Working with downed cattle can be especially dangerous. However, cattle that are down and cannot escape inclement weather may die if not moved to shelter and a more favorable treatment environment. Most of the methods used for rescuing downed horses can be applied to cattle, but, with a few exceptions, financial constraints preclude the extraordinary efforts that are more commonly used on downed horses. A local veterinarian should always be called to provide any needed medical care, sedation, or guidance in a rescue effort.

Getting a downed cow to stand

It is always best to try to have downed cattle stand with their own strength, if possible. First, the handler needs to determine whether the cow is physically able to stand. Second, the handler should make sure that there is sufficient room for the cow to stand and that the surface is non-slip. Third, all of the cow's legs need to be underneath her body. Last, the handler must provide incentive and sufficient time for the cow to stand by clapping or shouting, or slapping on the cow's neck or chest, preferably with a used grain sack or other means of making a noise without bruising. Another method that is often effective is for the handler to rock the cow's body with his knees. In extreme situations, an electric prod should be used sparingly. Twisting or lifting with the tail should not be done due to risk of causing a fracture or paralysis. If the cow stands, she should be permitted several minutes to adapt to standing before encouraging any walking.

Lifting a downed cow

Attempts to lift a downed cow should be done over a non-slip surface to provide traction if efforts are made by the animal to support its own weight. Straps or ropes under the chest and abdomen can be tried on smaller cattle. Placing a large air bag underneath the torso and inflating it can be effective. A *web strap harness sling* may be used underneath the torso and the cow lifted with a pulley system or power lift.

A *hip hoist* is a clamp placed over the pin bones of the hip to lift the rear of a dairy cow (**Figure 12.24**). The pelvic bones of beef cattle are usually not prominent enough to use a hip lift. This avoids any pressure on the abdomen or mammary glands when lifting. The cow must have enough strength in her front legs to support her weight for the hip lift to be effective. The lift does not support the cow's body. It only assists her own efforts to stand.

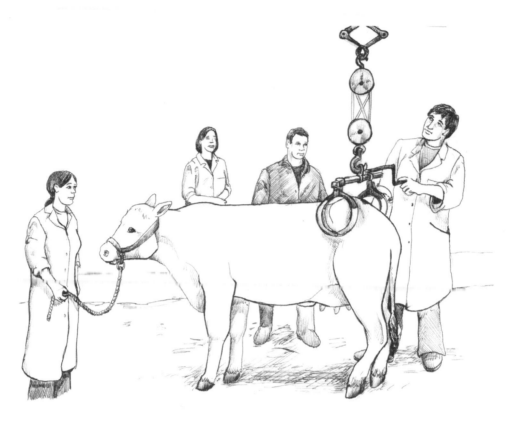

Fig. 12.24 Hip hoist.

Slings and hip clamps are for brief periods of lifting and should not be used for more than 1 hour.

Rehabilitation tubs for aquatic therapy are available for cattle in some veterinary hospitals. These support much of the weight of a cow by the buoyancy of its body. The water should be maintained at 100°F (37.78°C) and the cow's head supported with a halter and lead rope.

Moving a downed cow

Downed animals should never be dragged because of friction injuries to their skin. Downed cattle can be pulled onto a flatbed trailer or a livestock trailer using a glide (heavy canvas may be an adequate substitute), a ramp, and a block and tackle. To move short distances, downed cattle can be pulled or rolled onto a skid, such as a detached farm gate that acts as a travois, and then pulled by a tractor. After removing the cow from the skid, it should be assisted to lie on its sternum, propping it with hay bales if needed. If the cow cannot stand without assistance within a day, it should be assisted with a hip clamp or sling, if available.

Injections and venipuncture
Access to veins

The most common site for collecting blood samples or administering intravenous medications in cattle is the jugular vein. The restraint most commonly used is a squeeze chute with a headgate and a halter. Downed cattle in sternal position can be restrained for jugular venipuncture by using a halter and lead rope, pulling the cow's head to the side of the most accessible hind leg, and tying the lead to the hind leg above its hock.

The coccygeal vein on the lower aspect of the tail can provide access to the bloodstream. The restraint used is the tail jack hold.

The subcutaneous abdominal ("milk") vein is very prominent but should not be used for venipuncture. There is risk to the handler of being kicked and of large hematomas developing on the cow.

Injections

Subcutaneous

Subcutaneous injections in cattle are usually administered on the side of the neck.

Intramuscular

Intramuscular injection sites for cattle are restricted to the anterior neck area only, in accordance with Beef Quality Assurance guidelines. The injections are given about 4 in (10 cm) below the top of the neck and 4 in (10 cm) in front of the shoulder (**Figure 12.25**).

Injections should not be given to cows in alleyways or chutes by reaching through narrow spaces in between bars or planks. Injections should be given in a way that prevents the cow's movements from suddenly pulling away from the needle before the injection can be completed. The back of the hand with the syringe should be laid on the cow's neck and held there until the cow quits moving. The hand and syringe are then rotated and the injection is performed.

Administration of oral medications

Giving tablets (*bolusing*) or liquids (*drenching*) is achieved with the cow in head restraint and using a balling gun or drenching syringe, respectively. Sufficient restraint usually requires a restraint chute for adult cattle. Calves may be crowded into an alleyway and treated individually.

To administer oral medication to a cow restrained in a chute, its halter is removed if it is wearing one. The handler's left hip is placed next to the cow's head while bringing the left thigh underneath the right side of its jaw. The left arm is placed over the cow's head, behind and under its ear, and the hand run down underneath the left mandible (**Figure 12.26**). Care must be taken to keep the handler's head as far from the cow's head as is practical. An oral syringe, a gag, or speculum is put into the right corner of the cow's mouth with the handler's right hand. If necessary, the left hand is used to open the mouth by sticking the hand in the corner of the mouth and pushing up on the palate while avoiding the premolar teeth.

Balling guns are syringes for solid medication called boluses (**Figure 12.27**). Before using a balling gun, the handler should check it for rough or sharp protrusions or edges and file them smooth.

To administer oral medication to a group of calves, the calves are crowded together and the handler wades backward while catching calves and

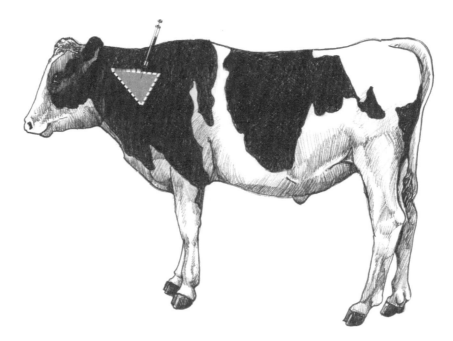

Fig. 12.25 Intramuscular injection site in cattle.

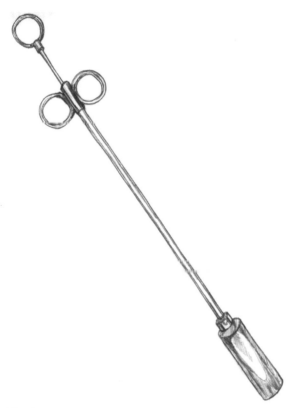

Fig. 12.26 Restraint for oral administration.

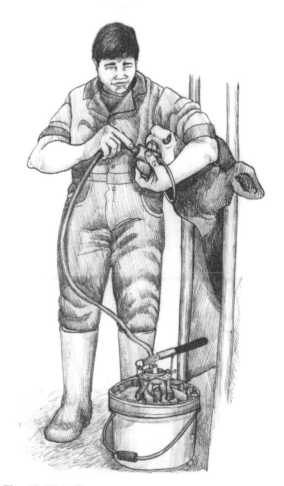

Fig. 12.27 Balling gun.

drenching them. Their packed bodies provide the restraint. Chalk markers are used to identify ones already treated. While standing beside a calf or straddling it, the handler puts his thumb into a corner of the calf's mouth at the interdental space and presses the tongue with the thumb while squeezing the lower jaw to open the calve's mouth. The handler must avoid putting his fingers into the back of the mouth where they could be bitten by the calf's upper and lower premolar teeth. The other hand places the balling gun or oral dose syringe into the mouth and over the hump of the tongue. The plunger on an oral dose syringe must be pushed slowly to prevent the liquid from being sprayed into the trachea.

Mouth speculums (*Frick speculums*) are placed in the mouth in a similar manner to oral syringes. These are cylindrical tubes that are protective conduits for passing soft stomach tubes. As the stomach tube is presented to the back of the cow's mouth, the cow's nose needs to be lower than its poll to reduce the possibility of the stomach tube entering the trachea.

Trimming hoofs and treating feet

Whether, or how often, hoofs need to be trimmed depends on the surfaces the cattle have to walk on. Foot problems and lameness are common in dairy cattle, particularly in their hind feet. Examination, trimming, and treatment are often needed. There are several methods of trimming and means of restraint, including lifting one leg at a time with a rope, casting with ropes, and tilt tables or rotary chutes. Tilt tables and rotary chutes are the most effective and safest for both the cow and the handler.

Mammary examination and treatments

Mammary examination and treatments in dairy cows require restraint in stanchions. Resistant cows must be restrained in squeeze chutes with a headgate. The tail jack hold or hock hobbles may be needed to control kicking.

TRANSPORTING CATTLE

Because of its relative novelty to the cattle, it is more difficult loading well-handled cattle into a truck or trailer than into an alleyway and squeeze chute. As with other aspects of cattle handling, allowing extra time to accomplish the loading with minimum stress is desirable. Stress causes muscle to become dark and tough. If the cattle are going to be marked "dark cutters," they are less valuable. Cattle that are stressed defecate more often, drink less, and lose weight, which also makes them less valuable at their destination. Stress lowers their immune responses to infectious organisms and puts them at risk for infectious diseases.

Cattle trailers should be adaptable to ensure sufficient ventilation, wind protection, and cover from excessive sunlight and inclement weather. Loading ramps should have solid sides, be one cow wide, and not exceed 20 degrees incline. Steps with a 4 in (10 cm) rise are preferred to cleats. If cleats are used, the distance between cleats should be about 8 in (20 cm). No gaps should be left between the transport vehicle and the ramp sides before loading. The loading ramp should be positioned so that cattle do not face sunlight when loading.

Cattle should never be transported if they have not been watered and fed recently. Access to water should be provided up to 2 hours before loading, and to grass hay until the time to load. Legume hay or grain rations should not be given, as they are more likely to cause scours (diarrhea) and, in turn, slick footing.

The transport compartment should be clean and have bedding that reduces the risk of slippage. The cattle should be packed for transport close enough to reduce the chance to fight or fall but not so close as to cause overheating. Partitions should be used to eliminate excess space. To minimize fighting, cattle from different herds or pens should not be mixed during transport. Different sized cattle should be sorted and loaded into trailer compartments by similar weight. Adult bulls should be transported in separate individual compartments. Cattle should not be transported with other species.

Freshen cows (producing milk) must be milked out before being transported. If dairy cattle are in transport for 12 or more hours, they should be unloaded, milked, and fed and watered. Calves that have a dry navel and are able to walk may be transported if they can remain dry and the temperature is not under 60°F (15.6°C). Cows in late pregnancy should not be transported. If transport is unavoidable because of natural disasters or a need for veterinary care, they should be in individual compartments with enough room to lie down. Cattle that are lame at a walk should not be transported. Those with fever should not be transported for anything other than veterinary care.

When transporting cattle in cold weather, they should be checked for signs of cold stress, such as eating bedding material, frozen nasal secretions, and shivering. If signs of cold stress occur, further travel should be delayed if adjustments to the transport vehicle cannot be done to improve protection from inclement weather.

U.S. Code 49, Chapter 805, Section 80502 requires that animals cannot be transported more than 28 hours without stopping for food, water, and rest for at least 5 consecutive hours.

SELECTED FURTHER READING

American Veterinary Medical Association (2014). *Welfare Implications of Tail Docking of Cattle: Literature review.*

Cote, S (2004). *Stockmanship: A Powerful Tool for Grazing Lands Management.* USDA Natural Resources Conservation Service, Boise.

Grandin T (2014). *Livestock Handling and Transport.* 4th edition. CABI Publishing, New York.

Grandin, T, Deesing M (2008). *Humane Livestock Handling.* Storey Publishing, North Adams.

Hansen AL (2006). *Beef Cattle.* Bow Tie Press, Irvine.

Kilgour RJ, Uetake K, Ishiwata T, et al. (2012). The behavior of beef cattle at pasture. *Applied Animal Behaviour Science* 138:12–17.

Stafford KJ (2005). *Cattle Handling Skills.* WorkSafe New Zealand, Wellington.

Thomas HS (2009). *Storey's Guide to Raising Beef Cattle,* 3rd edition. Storey Publishing, North Adams.

Toxel TR, Gadberry, S. *Cattle Working Facilities,* MP239. University of Arkansas, Division of Agriculture.

WorkSafe New Zealand (2014). *Safe Cattle Handling.* WorkSafe New Zealand, Wellington.

Domesticated small ruminants in North America include sheep, goats, and camelids (llamas and alpacas). Sheep (*Ovis aries*) and goats became the first domesticated livestock about 10,000 years ago by nomads in the Middle East. Domestic goats (*Capra aegagrus hircus*) originated in Iran. Llamas (*Lama glama*) and alpacas (*Vicugna pacos*) were domesticated 4,500 years ago in Peru to be used for meat, wool, and transportation. They are now also used as property guardians.

Some sheep and goats have a similar appearance. However, goats carry their tail up unless they are sick or frightened. Sheep carry their tails down, and their tails are often docked to reduce the risk of infections caused by feces smeared on and around the tail. Sheep have a philtrum (groove) in their upper lip; goats do not. Both do not like to get their feet wet and prefer to graze upland areas.

Most goats have horns, and most sheep do not. Sheep horns curl more than goat horns do. There are more than 200 breeds each of domestic sheep and goats.

Llamas and alpacas also appear similar. However, adult llamas are larger, taller, and stronger than alpacas. Llamas have banana-shaped ears while alpaca ears are more like a teddy bear's. Alpacas are about 1–2 ft (0.3–0.6 m) shorter at the shoulder than llamas. Alpacas also have lower set, stubbier tails and a more sloping rump. Two breeds of alpacas exist, while there is only one breed of llama.

NATURAL BEHAVIOR OF SMALL RUMINANTS

Sheep

Sheep have the strongest social ties of any domestic animal. They hate to be alone and act distant or aloof to animals other than sheep. The main defense of sheep is to run as a flock, sacrificing the young, weak, and slow on the periphery of the flock to predators to ensure the survival of the flock in general. In the wild, ewes form flocks of approximately 20 led by the oldest ewe. The oldest ewe with the greatest number of offspring is usually the flock leader. Within a flock, subgroups form, particularly among ewes and their direct descendants. Rams form separate, smaller flocks. Horn size is a significant factor in horned-breed flock hierarchy. The most dominant ewes will position themselves furthest from possible threats. Sheep sleep only 4–5 hours a day, which is much less than cattle.

Sheep spend half of their daylight hours grazing short, young grass and clover. Sunset is a favored grazing time. They like to eat weeds that are up to 8 in (20 cm) long and prefer grazing on higher ground. Sheep apprehend grass with their dental pad and lower incisor teeth and graze closer to the ground than cattle. Cattle cannot graze where sheep have recently grazed. Sheep prefer to graze into the wind to better monitor for the smell of predators.

Sheep communicate through body language, olfactory signals (smell), and vocalizing. Sheep vision is similar to cattle vision, except in those with long wool around their face. These "closed face" breeds have a portion of their range of peripheral vision blocked, a condition referred to as "wool blindness." Sheep have good depth perception, which allows them to move among rocks with sure-footedness. Lowering of the neck and head is a visual submissive posture. Stamping with a front foot is a threat for aggressiveness. Lowering and twisting the head is a horn threat suggesting aggression. Vocal communications include bleating to locate others or relate distress. Ewes "rumble" to lambs, and the "snort" of rams indicates irritation and possible aggressiveness. Odor is important among sheep for identification.

They have three pairs of scent glands: suborbital face glands beneath their eyes, groin glands on each side of the udder, and interdigital glands between the hooves on each foot.

Goats

Goats are herd animals, but unlike sheep, goats can be independent and will scatter when endangered. They are also more inquisitive, quicker, and more agile than sheep. Social status is more evident in goat herds than in sheep flocks. Each herd is led by a dominant female, the *queen*. The head buck is usually the oldest and largest. Wild goats form variably sized groups, but groups of 3–5 does are most common. Bucks group separately, except during breeding seasons. Horns, size, and age determine social dominance among able-bodied goats.

Goats are browsers, eating weeds, leaves, vines, and shrubs while grazing for about half the daylight hours. They are more selective about what they eat than sheep. Goats try to avoid being caught in rain and will seek shelter from inclement weather more often than will sheep.

Goats will nibble to investigate and communicate. They will butt to play or to re-establish their dominance. Bucks will stamp and sneeze when acting aggressive. They will flick their tongue just before rearing to begin a charge to butt an opponent.

Males have scent glands in their skin just behind the horns, just above their hocks on the inside of their legs, and under their tail; these produce strong odors during the rutting (mating) season. In addition, bucks will urinate on their face, beard, chest, and front legs. All these odors are rubbed on territorial markers and possessions, especially during mating seasons. Bucks are much more odoriferous than rams during rutting seasons.

When kids are handled and become frightened, they may shriek with childlike sounds to distract a handler and call for adult goat help.

Camelids

The herd social structure of llamas and alpacas is more similar to sheep than goats. Unlike sheep, males are very protective of their territory, especially male llamas. This instinct prevents overpopulation in areas with sparse vegetation and assures genetic diversity in the wild. Although social animals, individuals act aloof and do not like touching each other. Adult males fight by pushing with their shoulders, battering by swinging their necks, and biting. Kicking may also be used in defense, more so with alpacas than llamas. Camelids, particularly alpacas, produce various vocalizations, but humming is the most common. Llamas may snort or make clicking sounds if agitated, When frightened, camelids may scream.

SAFETY FIRST

The fears of small ruminants are identical to those of cattle. For example, moving into dark areas, loud noises, high-pitched noises, flapping materials, shiny objects, unfamiliar people, and dogs can cause fear in small ruminants. Small ruminants usually move in groups and are distressed when removed from a herd. They will bunch up in 90-degree corners of holding pens. They will not readily intermingle with other breeds and tend to stay near family units within a herd. Their social structures, like cattle, include leaders, dominants, and submissives, and their vision, hearing, smell, taste, and touch senses are similar to cattle.

Handler safety
Sheep

Sheep can be deceptively dangerous. If pressured or startled, adult sheep can bolt en masse and knock handlers down and trample them. Even a single sheep is capable of knocking a handler down often in an attempt to rejoin a flock. Children 5 years old and younger should not be allowed in pens with sheep.

Rams are particularly dangerous. Bending over in a pen with a ram can be perceived as a challenge and can result in being charged. Handlers of sheep should never take their eyes off of a ram.

> Rams are heavier and stronger than the average human and may butt with enough force to kill a handler.

Ram lambs being raised for breeding should be minimally handled. Otherwise, the ram lamb may lose its inherent respect for humans and become dangerous as an adult. It should not be played with by patting it on the head or encouraged to butt. Rams will back up in preparation to charge, with their head tucked low. Stotting, or pronking, is a stiff legged jump that is used by small ruminants to signal alarm to a perceived threat. Moving a ram with one hand under its jaw aids in controlling its attempts to be aggressive. Stepping 90 degrees to the side at the optimum time to prevent a charging ram adjusting its line of attack is an effective defense tactic when needed. Throwing water on a ram during a charge may discourage some from further attempts to butt a handler. A dangerous ram can be hooded with a leather "ram shield" so that it sees only down and to the rear.

Rams that are not familiar with each other will butt one another with risk of serious injury. To allow a few days of acclimation, they should be put together in a small pen to eliminate the ability to get a run at each other. A side hobble (a strap from front to hind leg on the same side) can also be used to discourage butting. Attaching a clog (wood block) to a front leg with a one-leg hobble will also discourage butting (and jumping fences).

Goats

Goats can be very gentle, but they do not tolerate rough treatment and will butt when provoked. Bucks are particularly dangerous after they reach puberty at 5–10 months of age. Signs of puberty include urinating thin streams of urine on their legs, mouth, beard, bellies, and lower aspect of their chest. Scent glands near their horns become active and secrete a strong odor that they will try to smear on animals and people to mark them as their possessions. Intermale rivalry and aggression becomes intense during the rutting season. The rutting season is fall to midwinter for some breeds, particularly dairy goats, but it can be year round for other breeds, primarily meat goats. Aggression can also be directed toward humans, especially by the males. Handlers should never allow a rutting buck to get between them and their route of exit.

A goat handler should never ignore a buck goat during the rutting season. If threatened by a buck, handlers should not stomp their feet or stare at the buck's eyes, because both of these actions are indications of challenge to the buck. Bucks do not back up in preparation

to charge as do rams. Signs of aggression can be staring, ducking the chin to present the horns forward, pressing horns or forehead against an opponent, and rearing with or without a following charge. No one should be allowed to play with or tease a buck. Scratching or pushing on its head must always be avoided.

A handler may get the buck to delay or abort a charge by spreading his or her arms out and standing in an erect position to look as large as possible. If close to the buck, the handler can grasp its beard and hold on to it while walking backwards to an exit. If working with horned goats, a small X-shaped incision can be cut into old tennis balls so that they can be jammed on the end of the horns until the handling procedure is finished. Dangerous buck goats should be culled or a ring placed in their nasal septum as with dairy bulls for safer handling. Children should be forbidden to be around bucks. Adult bucks are especially aggressive to each other during mating season and should be housed individually during that season with aisles separating their pens.

Camelids

Camelids generally have an aloof, non-aggressive attitude and are easy to handle. Males are more likely to bite, strike with their heads and necks, and bump with their shoulders. Alpacas tend to kick in defense. Camelids, especially female alpacas, will spit a fine mist of regurgitated rumen contents when angry. They usually warn a potential spit victim with gurgling sounds. They spit at each other more often than at gentle handlers. A hand towel can be stuffed under the nose piece of a halter to protect against spit when handling a gurgling camelid.

Llamas are highly territorial. As a result, young gelded llamas 18–24 months old that have been socialized with other llamas can be removed and socialized with other species to become guardians for those species, such as sheep. Intact males cannot be housed together and should not be used as guardians.

Camelids, particularly alpacas, may attempt to avoid a handler by holding their head down. The handler must be prepared when near the camelid for the possibility that the head may suddenly be raised up. Otherwise, it could hit an ill-prepared handler in the face.

Camelids are believed to be easier to handle if "imprinted" (handled within the first few hours of life). However, overhandling a young, sexually intact male that is raised in isolation to other camelids can result in a failure to respect human handlers, a condition called "berserk male syndrome." An aggressive male camelid will put its ears back and its face dangerously near the handler's face. It may stick its head forward and horizontal with the ground and charge to bump the handler with its shoulders and try to knock the handler to the ground. If successful in pinning the victim, it will bite at the victim's face, neck, knees, and groin. Excessive handling of young male camelids should be avoided, and orphaned male llamas that have had much human handling should be castrated before weaning.

Many aspects of handling horses can be applied to camelids, such as avoiding feeding treats by hand to discourage crowding and invasion of a handler's personal space, allowing crias to learn by watching well-behaved adult camelids being handled, training them to be led with a halter and lead rope by gentle pressure and well-timed release, and letting them learning patience and respect by being tied with a halter and lead rope for increasing periods of time.

Small ruminant safety
Care of small ruminants
All small ruminants should be handled slowly and quietly. All have relatively fragile bones that can break much more easily than horse and cattle bones. With the exception of some goats, small ruminants have thick wool or long hair that makes them susceptible to overheating and should not be exerted or crowded during warm or humid weather. Newborn lambs may be abandoned by ewes in a flock that is grazing large areas. Penning them together for the first days after birth allows the lambs to become stronger and the ewe to bond better with her lamb. When goats or camelids are used for carrying packs, the packs should be balanced, properly mounted, and not exceed 20% of the animal's body weight.

Predator dangers
Small ruminants are prey to a larger range of carnivores than are horses and cattle. One-third of all sheep and goat losses are from predators. All small ruminants have an innate fear of carnivores, but they can become socialized early in life to the presence of dogs.

All small ruminants need protection from roaming carnivores, such as dog-proof ruminant enclosures or herd guardian dogs or donkeys. The leading predator of small ruminants in western states is the coyote, but in the eastern U.S. it is roaming dogs. Roaming dogs are usually not true predators. They are serial killers that chase sheep for fun rather than food and may maim them without a killing bite. Along with coyotes and dogs, other predators of small ruminants include bears, cougars, bobcats, foxes, feral hogs, and birds of prey (hawks, eagles), and carrion birds (vultures, ravens) also kill weak, injured, or low-ranking sheep. Large flocks of sheep, sheep on open range, and those in areas with abundant predators should have two or more guardian dogs or other guardian animals.

Besides guardian animals, other means for reducing predators include putting bells on some ewes so that there is an auditory alert to a flock being chased. Mesh fencing that discourages predators and gathering sheep in well-lit pens at night near a handler's residence can also be helpful.

Guardian dogs and other guardian animals
Guardian animals are highly recommended for the safety of sheep and goats that are in open pastures. The animal most adapted to guarding sheep is the guardian dog, a member of a breed that has been selectively bred to guard sheep and goats for more than 6,000 years, beginning in the mountains of what is now Turkey, Iraq, and Syria. Most guardian dog breeds for protecting sheep have a similar appearance to sheep, which enables them to visually blend in with flocks.

Guardian animals are intended to protect flocks from predators and serial canine killers. Care must be taken in approaching flocks when a guardian animal is present since a strange handler may be perceived as a predator. Guardian dogs are the most efficient guardians, but more than one are needed. Two should be available to chase away a predator with confidence while a third or more remain to protect the sheep from other predators. Guardian breeds are Akbash, Anatolian shepherd dog, Briards,

Great Pyrenees, Komondor, Kuvasz, Maremma, Shar Planinetz, Spitz, and Tibetan Mastiff.

Single castrated (gelded) male donkeys or llamas can also be acceptable guardians if properly selected, prepared for guarding, and maintained as a member of a sheep or goat herd. Sexually intact male donkeys or llamas are too aggressive to sheep and goats, and sometimes people, and should not be used. More than one castrated male donkey or llama will bond with their own species rather than sheep and goats, if given the chance. Guardians that are not dogs must remain single to be effective. Standard-sized donkeys should be used because miniature donkeys are too small to protect a herd, or themselves, from dogs and coyotes. A female llama can also be an effective guardian if it cannot be used for breeding.

Gelded donkeys or llamas can be effective against coyotes, which do not hunt in packs, and single dogs, but are not effective against packs of dogs or wolves. Donkeys will sound an alarm (braying) and will bite and strike at invaders. Llamas tend to be more selective than donkeys in guarding against real threats to a flock and are not aggressive to innocent dogs, foxes, and other non-threatening pasture invaders.

All guardian animals have to be trained to protect sheep. Guardian dogs are first socialized with sheep at an early age (just after weaning) by being kept in separate, adjoining enclosures with sheep. Socialized guardian dogs can then be allowed in pastures with sheep between 4 and 9 months of age. Guardian dogs should be socialized and routinely handled by owners, but should reside with the flock at all times. A guardian dog's focus should remain on the flock, while herding dogs bond and focus on the handler. Herding dogs should live with the owner; working guardian dogs should not.

Gelded male llamas should be socialized with other llamas until the age of 18 months to 2 years and then socialized for guarding sheep or goats. In that time, a llama will attain the physical size and strength needed and have exposure to the territorial behavior of its elders.

A donkey should be introduced to small ruminants before it is one year of age by being kept in an adjacent pasture or paddock until it bonds with the sheep or goats. Guardian donkeys should be kept away from dogs, including herding dogs.

Llamas and donkeys have different qualities for being a herd guardian. Donkeys are often gregarious and seek human attention; llamas tend to be aloof. Llamas eat the same vegetation and require the same vaccinations as sheep and goats; donkeys have different feed, vaccination, and hoof care requirements. Donkeys tolerate hot weather much better than llamas.

Care must be taken not to overfeed guardian animals or they will become complacent and lethargic.

Key zoonoses

(*Note:* Apparently ill animals should be handled by veterinary professionals or under their supervision. Precautionary measures against zoonoses from ill animals are more involved than those required when handling apparently healthy animals and these measures vary widely. The discussion here is directed primarily at handling apparently healthy animals.)

Apparently healthy domestic small ruminants pose little risk of transmitting disease to healthy adult handlers who practice conventional personal hygiene. The risks of physical injury are greater than the risks of acquiring an infectious disease (*Table 13.1*).

Direct transmission

Systemic disease

Brucellosis is a bacterial disease that can cause abortions in goats and sheep and is transmitted to humans by exposure to body secretions (saliva, urine, fetal fluids) or eating meat from infected goats or sheep or drinking unpasteurized milk from goats. The disease in humans is influenza-like and called undulant fever. It is now rare in the U.S. Most cases are associated with imported goats.

Rabies in small ruminants causes signs of the disease, which are drooling, depression, inappetence, before the transmissible stage. Transmission is not associated with normal appearing sheep, goats, or South American camelids.

Anthrax is a spore-forming bacteria that can cause blackened skin infection and death in humans. Small ruminants with anthrax can transmit the disease to humans by body secretions, soil contaminated with anthrax spores, or exposure to infected animal's wool or hide. Most (95%) cases of anthrax in

Table 13.1 Diseases transmitted from healthy appearing small ruminants to healthy adult humans

DISEASE	AGENT	MEANS OF TRANSMISSION	SIGNS AND SYMPTOMS IN HUMANS	FREQUENCY IN ANIMALS	RISK GROUP*
Butting and trampling (sheep and goats), kicking and biting (llamas)	–	Direct injury	Crushing, butting, or bite injuries, which can be permanently disabling or fatal	All small ruminants can inflict serious injuries. Injuries from adult males can be fatal	3
Cryptosporidiosis	*Cryptosporidium* spp.	Direct, fecal-oral; indirect from contaminated water	Diarrhea	Common, particularly in young small ruminants	2
Brucellosis	*Brucella melitensis*	Direct from secretions, especially placental fluid	Undulant fever, muscle aches, and lethargy	Very low, due to U.S. federal eradication program	3
Orf	Parapoxvirus	Direct, contact with mouth or oral secretions	Blisters and lumps on the hands and face	Common	?
Q Fever	*Coxiella burnetii*	Direct through body secretions, particularly milk and placental fluids; indirect from inhalation of contaminated dust	Flu-like signs and atypical pneumonia	Moderate in cow-calf operations	2
Leptospirosis	*Leptospira* spp.	Direct from exposure to urine; indirect from urine-contaminated water	Kidney infection	Common in some locations and varies with vaccinations	3

* Risk Groups (National Institutes of Health and World Health Organization criteria. Centers for Disease Control and Prevention, *Biosafety in Microbiological and Biomedical Laboratories*, 5th edition, 2009):
  1 Agent not associated with disease in healthy adult humans.
  2 Agent rarely causes serious disease and prevention or therapy possible.
  3 Agent can cause serious or lethal disease and prevention or therapy possible.
  4 Agent can cause serious or lethal disease and prevention or therapy are not usually available.

humans are cutaneous and characterized by painless ulceration, fever, headache, and possible septicemia. Other forms are pulmonary from airborne infected wool, hide, or hair, and gastrointestinal from ingesting infected meat. Another name for pulmonary anthrax in humans is "Woolsorter's disease."

Listeriosis can cause generalized disease in immunosuppressed humans that includes an atypical pneumonia and meningitis. It is transmitted by contaminated meat, milk products, and raw vegetables and fruit. Transmission is not associated with direct exposure to normal appearing small ruminants.

Leptospirosis is a bacterial disease of small ruminants that is transmitted in infected small ruminant urine. The organism from urine or urine-contaminated food or water can be transmitted by gaining entrance into a human's mouth, breaks in the skin, or eyes.

E. coli 0157:H7 is a bacterium that is in the feces of healthy cattle and in that of small ruminants as well. If ingested by young or elderly people, it can cause bloody diarrhea and, less commonly, kidney failure. Most cases in humans are from ingesting undercooked, contaminated ground beef. Small ruminant handlers may be at risk if their immune system is suppressed and poor hygiene leads to ingesting the bacteria from small ruminant feces contamination of their hands or face.

Vesicular stomatitis virus in small ruminants causes blisters in the mouth and nostrils and on the feet and teats. Handlers of animals with vesicular stomatitis blisters can become infected.

Small ruminant tuberculosis (*Mycobacterium bovis*) is usually transmitted to people by drinking raw infected milk, although it can be transmitted by aerosol over long distances and inhaled. *M. bovis* is now rare in the U.S.

Respiratory tract disease

Coxiellosis (Q fever) is a bacterial disease that is transmitted by inhalation of dust contaminated by the body secretions of sheep or goats (urine, milk, feces, etc.) infected with *Coxiella burnettii*. The carrier animals may appear healthy.

Digestive tract disease

Salmonellosis is a bacterial disease of the digestive system that can invade the blood stream and become systemic. Most cases are acquired by eating undercooked eggs, poultry, pork, or beef or handling reptiles or rodents and carrying the bacteria to the mouth. It is a rare zoonosis from small ruminants.

Campylobacteriosis is one of the most common causes of bacterial diarrhea in humans. Contact with infected ruminants, usually lambs or calves, can be a source if the bacteria gain access to a handler's mouth. Most human cases are from unpasteurized milk or undercooked poultry.

Skin disease

Contagious pustular dermatitis (soremouth, orf, scabby mouth) is a poxvirus primarily of sheep and goats, although camelids are susceptible. Humans are also susceptible and can acquire the disease when exposed to secretions of the nose and mouth of infected small ruminants. This is most common on handler's hands after drenching sheep or goats. Dermatophilosis, a bacterial disease of the skin, is transmitted by contact or by stable flies. Ringworm is a fungal infection that can be transmitted by direct contact.

Vector borne

No significant vector-transmitted zoonotic diseases from healthy appearing small ruminants are known.

Sanitary practices

Persons handling small ruminants should wear appropriate dress to protect against skin contamination with hair and skin scales, and saliva, urine, and other body secretions. Gloves should always be worn when handling the mouth or nose of sheep and goats to reduce the risk of *contagious ecthyma* (soremouth, orf). Ticks should be controlled. Basic sanitary practices should be adhered to, such as keeping hands away from eyes, nose, and mouth when handling small ruminants, and washing hands after handling them.

Special precautions are needed when sick small ruminants are handled. They should be isolated from apparently normal small ruminants. New herd members should be quarantined for at least 2 weeks to reduce the risk of transmitting a disease that new animals could be incubating before introducing them to the rest of the herd.

Contact with wildlife should be controlled, especially rodents.

SHEEP

Sheep became domesticated in Mesopotamia about 10,000 years ago. They were originally kept as sources of meat, milk, and skin. Later, they were selectively bred for their ability to grow wool. Sheep were also important symbols in religions. They were part of Greek mythology as the ram with the Golden Fleece, the symbol of kingship. Aries, the ram, was the first sign of the Greek zodiac. Sheep were sacrificed in religious ceremonies by Greeks, Romans, and Hebrews. Several sheep-related terms are used in Christianity, such as flocks, shepherds, pastors, and the Sacrificial Lamb of God.

Domesticated sheep are not native to the Americas. They were brought to the western hemisphere via the Caribbean islands by Christopher Columbus's second voyage in 1493, to Mexico in 1519 by Hernan Cortes, and to the southwest of what is now the U.S. by Francisco Vasquez de Coronado in 1540. The British brought sheep to Virginia in the early 1600s.

Adult sexually intact male sheep are called *rams*. Castrated males are *wethers*. Females are *ewes*. Young sheep are *lambs*.

Approaching and catching

To catch an individual sheep, it is necessary to herd the desired individual with the *flock* into a small catch pen with 10–15 other sheep. Temporary corrals can be created using welded wire at least 40 in (101.6 cm) high and steel T-posts, or similar fencing. Herding flocks into the pen can be facilitated with a properly trained herding-breed dog.

Once the flock is in the pen, the handler should quietly approach the desired sheep straight from behind, staying in its blind spot. The capture is done by placing one arm under the sheep's neck and the other arm behind the rump (**Figure 13.1**). If needed, the sheep may be briefly immobilized by grasping a thigh just above the stifle. This may give time enough to get the other hand beneath the jaws. Handlers should never grab or pull the wool.

If 90-degree corners are present in the pen, the handler can move the desired sheep toward a corner. Cornered sheep will face the handler, who grasps its head and neck with both hands and moves the sheep's front end to the side. As the sheep tries to move forward, the handler grasps the loose skin of both flanks to slow or stop it and then the handler grasps the neck and rump.

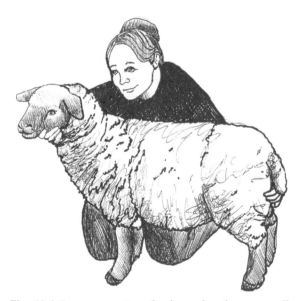

Fig. 13.1 Loose restraint of a sheep that does not pull its wool.

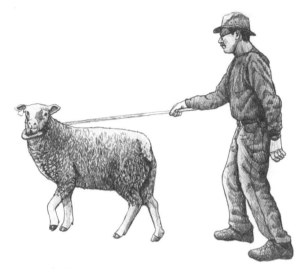

Fig 13.2 Capturing a sheep with a neck crook.

Shepherds crooks are available for either the neck (about 4 fingers wide at the bend) or the hock (less than 2 in [5 cm] wide at the bend) (**Figure 13.2**). Neck crooks are safer for sheep, but leg crooks may be more useful for horned sheep. Leg crooks have the potential to injure legs if used roughly or if the sheep strongly resists.

Handling for routine care and management

Basic equipment and facilities

Sheep-handling equipment, reduced-size versions of the equipment used on cattle, is commercially available. Basic handling equipment for sheep includes a collecting pen, crowding pen, alleyway, and sorting pens. Gates should be drop down. Optional equipment includes a sheep tilt table, squeeze chute with headgate, elevated platform, scales, foot troughs, dipping tanks, and loading ramp (**Figure 13.3**).

The collecting pen should provide 5–6 sq ft (0.5–0.6 m²) per sheep. The crowding pen should have an 8 ft (2.5 m) radius. The alleyway should be up to 28 in (71.1 cm) wide, at least 8 ft (2.5 m) long and 3 ft (1 m) high, with sloping sides that adjust to different sizes of sheep. Higher alleyway sides may be needed for taller breeds. Alleyways are used for individual treatment and sorting. Alleyways should have solid sides but with a 4 in (10 cm) gap at the bottom to allow air circulation

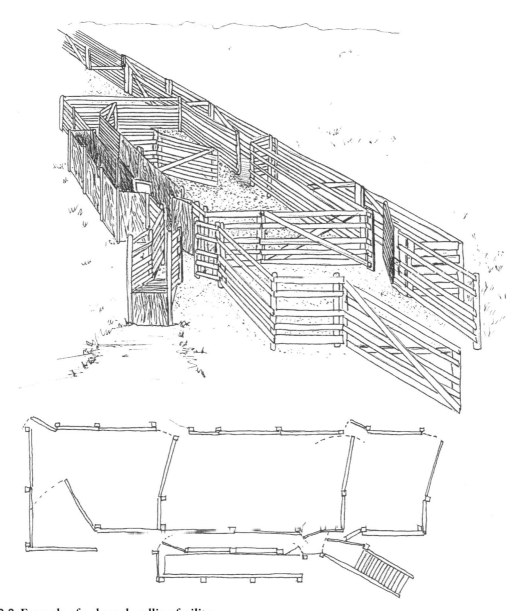

Fig. 13.3 Example of a sheep-handling facility.

from underneath. A squeeze chute tilt table is helpful when trimming hooves, checking fertility of rams, and performing multiple procedures on one sheep.

Because of their thick wool, sheep are better treated for external parasites using dip tanks than with sprays or pour-ons. The alleyway to the dip tank should be curved. Dip tanks should be 12 ft (3.7 m) long on the top and 6 ft (1.8 m) long at the level bottom. The other 6 ft (1.8 m) are cleated slopes. It should be 2 ft (0.6 m) wide at the top and 1 ft (0.3 m) wide at the bottom, and 6 ft (1.8 m) deep. Dipping is best done one week after shearing in the spring. Just two sheep are driven in at a time. Young lambs do not need to be sheared first. Lambs under a month of age should not be dipped.

Packing alleyway

A 3 ft (1 m) alleyway can be used to pack groups of sheep facing the same direction. One handler packs the group with his legs and vaccinates,

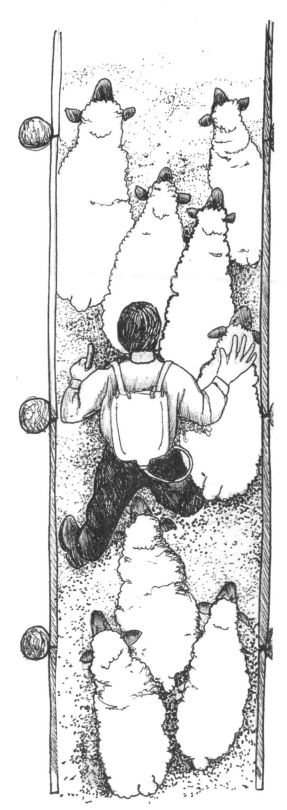

Fig. 13.4 Drenching sheep in a packed alleyway.

drenches, or ear tags one sheep at a time and then pushes finished sheep behind him, gradually working through the whole group (**Figure 13.4**). Adult rams cannot be included since they become aggressive after being turned back behind the handler. The group can be cleared out of a packed alleyway by a herding dog trained to "back" sheep. To back sheep the dog jumps on the sheep's back and moves toward the front of the group, jumps down and turns the sheep, and herds them out of the alleyway.

Moving groups
Leading
Leading sheep can move sheep a short distance by enticing them to follow the handler who provides an opportunity for the sheep to eat a small amount of grain along the way. A ewe with a newborn lamb can be moved by a handler carrying the lamb near the ground (no more than a foot high) so the ewe will follow. Capturing the lead ewe in a flock and moving or leading her will result in the rest of the flock following. A bellwether (leading sheep with a bell on a collar) or a "Judas" goat can be trained to follow a handler and lead sheep.

Herding
Herding sheep is achieved using flight zones and balance points as with herding cattle. Unlike cattle, sheep do not stop and turn or attempt to fight. If a sheep briefly strays from the flock, keeping the flock together will result in the stray sheep returning.

Sheep should be taught to herd in directions dictated by a handler. Teaching sessions in a small pen with at least 6 sheep consist of moving them around the pen at a walk and occasionally stopping them in a corner to rest. Practice sessions should be about 20 minutes for at least 3 consecutive days. Repeat herding exercises should be done once per month.

Herding sheep can be done very effectively by well-trained herding dogs. Herding dogs and guardian dogs can be of great help to shepherds of sheep, but in different ways. A herding dog is not a guardian dog. Herding dogs are usually moderate-sized (30–50 lb [13.6–22.7 kg]) intense, workaholic athletes. Guardian dogs are large breeds often exceeding 100 lb (45.4 kg). Guardians like to rest near flocks and watch sheep during the day, although they are protective and should become aggressive with possible predators. Guardian dogs are effective for goat herds as well, but goats do not flock together in danger like sheep and cannot be herded by dogs as effectively as sheep.

Herding dog breeds differ considerably and can be categorized as gathering, tending, and driving dogs. The gathering breeds are border collies, kelpies, Australian shepherds, collies, and bearded collies. Border collies and kelpies dominate in sheep-gathering competition. A group of 3 sheep will scatter if over-pressured by handlers or herding dogs, but a group of 4 or more will usually not separate when herded. Herding dog trials use 3–6 sheep to better evaluate the dog's technique.

The tending breeds are Belgian Malinois, Belgian sheepdogs, Belgian Tervurens, Bouvier des Flandres, Briards, German shepherd dogs, Beauceron Pyrenean shepherds, and Pulis. These were originally bred with the intent to have them patrol the perimeters of a flock and keep the sheep in a particular grazing area.

The driving breeds are Rottweilers, Welsh corgis, Old English sheepdogs, and Australian cattle dogs. They were originally used on sheep to drive them to market and assist in moving sheep in stockyards.

Sorting panels

Sheep can be moved and sorted by herding into a small pen and using 4 ft (1.2 m) portable sorting panels (hurdles) Groups of 3–4 sheep should be sorted at a time. Sorting individual sheep will cause the sheep to panic.

Restraint of individual sheep or parts of their bodies

Halters

Appropriately sized halters can assist in restraining sheep. Most of the bridge of the nose is cartilage and can be compressed by a poor-fitting halter. The nose strap should go over the bony part of the bridge of the nose and close to their eyes.

Pressing against a wall

Sheep can be restrained against a wall. The handler backs the sheep into a corner with a solid wall. It is pressed against the wall with one of the handler's legs between its neck and shoulder and the other leg against its chest (**Figure 13.5**). Additional restraint can be accomplished with a hand under the sheep's neck near its head.

Straddling

Straddling is restraint for using a bolus gun or drenching syringe on a sheep, taking rectal temperatures, and performing eye or mouth examinations. The handler backs a sheep into a corner, straddles its neck, and holds it still with his knees on both sides of its neck. Straddling the sheep's chest and using one hand under the neck to block forward escape provides more control, but only one hand is free to perform examinations and treatment (**Figure 13.6**).

If the handler is tall enough, straddling can also be used to move a sheep short distances. The handler places a hand under the jaw, straddles the sheep's body facing the sheep's head, and places the other hand on its rump or tail. The handler can then shuffle forward while holding the sheep's jaw and rump. If needed, the sheep can be encouraged to move forward by squeezing its tail head.

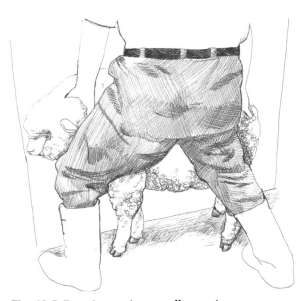

Fig. 13.5 Pressing against a wall restraint.

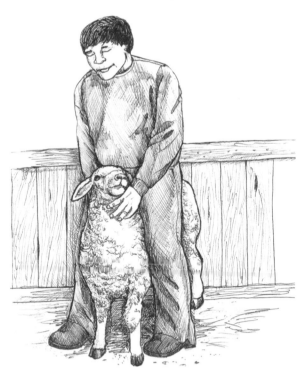

Fig. 13.6 Straddle restraint.

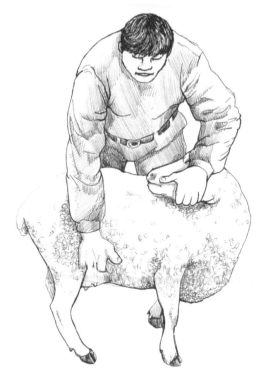

Fig. 13.7 Initiating tipping a sheep.

Tipping

Sheep have a rump padded by wool and fat, and downward positioned tails. This allows them to tolerate being placed on their rump while leaning backward against a handler's legs. However, this will be resented if the tail has not had sufficient time to heal from being docked. The sheep does not have to be lifted in order for it to be tipped ("set up," "rumped"). The handler stands alongside the sheep's body, the sheep's head is turned away from the handler, and its rump is pushed down (**Figure 13.7**). After it sits with the legs away from the handler, its front legs are lifted and body turned slightly so that its back is leaned against the handler's legs (**Figure 13.8**). The sheep is tilted slightly onto one hip, which makes it more comfortable and facilitates the handler freeing both hands to be able to shear. The sheep's head is tucked under an elbow as needed for better visibility and access to the lower chest and neck (**Figure 13.9**). Sheep "chairs" are restraint slings to hold a sheep in a tipped position without the need to lean on the handler's legs (**Figure 13.10**). Sheep are tipped for shearing, crutching (clipping wool from around the rump), and hoof trimming.

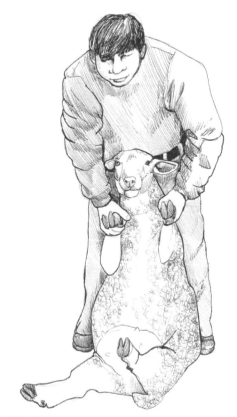

Fig. 13.8 Sheep in tipped position.

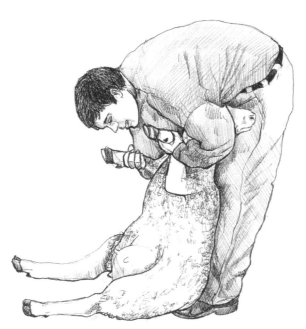

Fig. 13.9 Restraint of head in tipped position.

Backward walk

Moving a sheep a short distance is sometimes easiest by assisting it to walk backwards. The handler straddles the sheep facing forward, picks up the sheep's front legs, and has the sheep stand up on its hind legs. Continuing to hold its front legs, the handler walks backward to his destination while the sheep backpedals (**Figure 13.11**).

Tying up

As with calves, sheep can be restrained by tying their legs with a rope that loops over the back of their necks. Using a fixed loop of rope, a half hitch is placed around each hind leg above the hocks and the rest of the loop between front legs and over the back of the neck. With the sheep on its side, the head is positioned level with the body or pointed up an incline to aid in eructating rumen gas and preventing bloat.

Gambrel

A plastic W-shaped gambrel can be placed on the top of the neck and both front legs placed in the crooks on each side. Sheep cannot lift their legs out of the gambrel while their head is pressed down (**Figure 13.12**). Gambrels are used for restraint during transit or treatment.

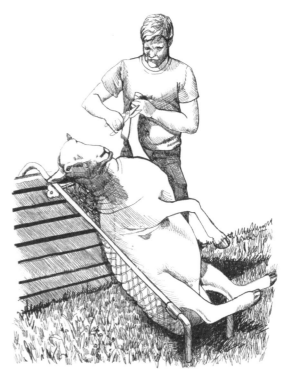

Fig. 13.10 Sheep chair.

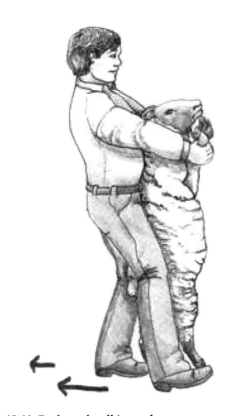

Fig. 13.11 Backward walking a sheep.

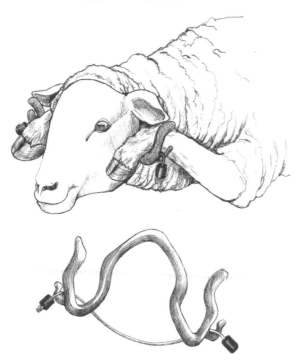

Fig. 13.12 Gambrel for restraining sheep in sternal recumbency.

Trimming hooves

Small ruminant hooves that do not get worn down by rocky surfaces may need to be trimmed as often as every 8 weeks. Every 6 months is about average. Front hooves carry more weight and will wear down faster. To check whether trimming is needed, the rear hooves should be checked. Hoof trimmers for small ruminants look like garden pruners, but true hoof trimmers are sharper and easier to handle than pruners.

To trim hooves, the sheep is restrained to a stationary object and a foot picked up and the leg bent so that the bottom of the hoof is visible without causing discomfort to the animal. Other options are to place the sheep in tipped position against the handler's legs, in a sheep chair, or on a small tilt table. The bottom of the hoof is cleaned with a stiff hoof brush. The edge of the hoof should be trimmed until it is even with the sole. Any softened areas between the hoof wall and the sole need to be scooped out. Any excess growth between the heels should be trimmed. Uneven areas of the sole should be pared, but not enough that pink color appears. A light brush with a rasp can aid in leveling the bottom surface of

the hoof. The dewclaws should be checked and carefully trimmed in small amounts, if needed.

Restraint of lambs

Lambs are captured as if picking up a small dog with a hand under its torso. Small lambs can be carried by one hand with a wrist and forearm under their chest and abdomen and the hand grasping the lamb's front leg nearest the handler's body.

In the first 2 weeks of life, lambs are castrated and their tails are docked to prevent fecal accumulation and flystrike. Both these procedures can be done with the lamb held head up with the its back toward the handler. The handler restrains the lamb's right front and hind legs with the right hand and the left front and hind legs with the left hand. The same hold can be used while the handler sits and holds the lamb on its back (ventrodorsal) on the handler's lap.

Larger lambs can be restrained by straddling the lamb and holding the body by pressing the lamb just behind the shoulders with the handler's calves while the handler blocks forward movement with a hand behind the lamb's jaws.

Another method is to straddle the lamb, grasp each front leg and raise the lamb onto its hind legs and hold its chest between the handler's thighs.

Handling for common medical procedures
Injections and venipuncture
Access to veins
Sheep can be tipped on their rump for jugular or cephalic vein venipuncture. The femoral vein may be accessed with a sheep in lateral recumbency.

Injections
Subcutaneous injections are generally given under the skin behind an elbow, in the inguinal area, or a fold of the flank. Intramuscular injections (IM) should only be administered in the side of the neck, except for nursing lambs (**Figure 13.13**). Nursing lambs should receive IM injections in the semitendinosus and semimembranosus muscles in the back aspect of the thigh.

Administration of oral medications
To drench a sheep, a handler straddles its back, places a hand under its lower jaw, and raises its head

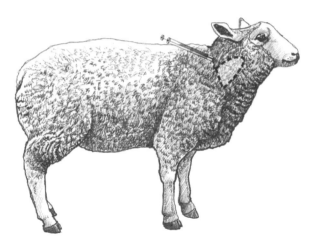

Fig. 13.13 Site for IM injections in sheep.

slightly The nozzle of the drench syringe is inserted between the cheek and the back teeth. The plunger is pushed in slowly, allowing the sheep to swallow the liquid medication. Handlers should wear gloves and not put their bare fingers in the sheep's mouth.

Balling guns are used to administer solid medications. Sheep are caught individually and backed into a wall and straddled. The sheep's head is lifted under the jaw, but its nose should not be lifted higher than the poll. Otherwise, its ability to swallow will be impeded. The balling gun is inserted in the mouth, and the plunger pushes the bolus onto the back upper surface of the tongue. An oral speculum to protect the insertion of a stomach tube is placed in the same way.

GOATS

The domestic goat is a subspecies of a wild goat from eastern Europe and southwest Asia. They were domesticated first in India and then in the mountains of Iran about 10,000 years ago, being kept for their meat, milk, hair, and skin, as they are today. Goatskin bags have been valued for transport of wine and the production of *kafir*, a fermented milk drink. Goats are probably the longest domesticated livestock species thanks to their curiosity and ability to survive in a variety of environments. They were brought to the New World by the conquistadors and became well established on many Caribbean islands.

In some instances, meat-breed goats can be pack or draft animals. Wethers that are at least 34 in

(86.4 cm) high at the withers and weigh 200 lb (90.7 kg) are generally used. Adult goats of that size can pack up to 20–25% of their body weight. Training with small packs can begin at 5–6 months of age. Adult meat-breed wethers of sufficient size and physical conditioning can also be taught to pull small carts.

Methods of handling goats vary and depend on whether they are dairy, meat-producing, or wool-producing goats; brush clearers; or companion pets. Common dairy breeds are the Alpine, La Mancha, Toggenburg, Nubian, Oberhasli, and Saanen. Boer is the most common meat breed. Angora and Cashmere (Kashmir) goats produce fine fibers, mohair and cashmere (Angora wool is from Angora rabbits). Pygmy goats are companion pets.

Adult sexually intact male goats are *bucks* ("billy" is an older term). Castrated males are *wethers*. An adult female goat is a *doe* ("nanny" is an older term). Young goats are *kids*.

Approaching and catching

Approach and capture should be done gently or the goat will become aggressive and try to butt. Signs of aggression in bucks are curled tail over back, raised hair on the back, sneezing and snorting, stamping the forefeet, and rearing up on its hind legs. Goats do not bite or kick.

Domestic goats are curious and will come over to a handler who is doing tasks in their pen. The handler should pat the goat, then gently restrain it by holding it at the base of the skull with both hands or grasp its collar if it has one. A shepherds neck crook can be used if the goat is evasive. Leg crooks should not be used due to the risk of leg injury.

Catch pens

A catch pen is advisable, particularly for meat goats that are not frequently handled. The pen should be used to feed and water in order to desensitize goats to the pen for future captures and handling. To accustom them to a catch pen and handler presence, the handler should feed grain in a small pile for each goat and kneel down near them and talk to them. If a buck is in the group, the handler must be watchful of his actions. Practice captures should be performed at a regular time when the goats are in the catch pen.

Neck chains or collars and halters

Dairy goats often have neck chains or collars for handling and identification. Colored plastic chains or flat web collars can be used to identify groups of goats by age, family, productivity, or other criteria. Dog collars are hazardous because of the metal buckles, which can become caught and cause strangulation. Collars that lace together or plastic chain collars are safer than buckled collars. Other goats will often chew off a herdmate's leather collar. Leather collars also trap moisture and will lead to bacterial or fungal infections. Nylon web or plastic chain collars permit better air circulation to skin and drying than leather.

Plastic chains should break under moderate strain to prevent entrapment on a fence, by another goat's horns, or on other objects. Goats can be led by their collar or a separate leading collar with a leash can be used for leading and tying them for restraint.

Aggressive bucks should wear a neck chain. This allows them to be captured with a bullstaff. A halter with a lead rope can then be placed on their head and control exerted by dual use of the staff and lead rope.

Handling for routine care and management

Basic equipment and facilities

Meat or milk goat handling equipment, reduced-size versions of the equipment used on cattle, is commercially available. Basic handling equipment for meat goats includes a collecting pen, crowding pen, alleyway, and sorting pens. Gates should be drop down. Optional equipment includes a goat tilt table, squeeze chute with headgate, elevated platform, scales, foot troughs, and loading ramp. Since goats are more independent and good jumpers, the sides of alleyways and pens must be higher (up to 6 ft [1.8 m]) than those used for working with sheep.

Moving and separating

Milk and companion goats should be trained to follow rather than attempting to herd them. Goats are more independent thinking than sheep. The Latin word *caprine*, referring to goats, is related to the root for "capricious," meaning doing things on a whim. Rather than herding them, it is more effective to identify the lead goat, usually an alpha doe (the herd queen), and capture and lead her so the others will follow to a smaller pen for sorting or capture. During the breeding season, the alpha male buck will assume leadership and drive them from the rear of the group. By routinely feeding goats, they will follow the handler as they do the herd queen, but if the handler tries to drive them, they are likely to scatter, and if during breeding season, the handler may be challenged by bucks.

Goats do not like to move from light into dark. They like to move to more open spaces, uphill rather than down, into the wind rather than downwind. They do not like to cross water or go through narrow openings, and they hate getting wet.

Goats can be trained to be led by a halter, but most are led by a collar around their neck. Bucks may need a halter and a bull staff clipped to their collar to control their movement, preventing the handler from being butted or stuck by a horn.

Bucks have strong odors that will rub off on handlers. The odors come from scent glands that are especially active during the breeding season and the urine that they spray on their beards and front legs. Handlers should take care not to stand in front of bucks or within urination range of bucks during the breeding season. Because of their odor and aggressiveness at breeding season, bucks are not handled as frequently nor can they be handled as gently as does.

Dogs are generally ineffective in herding goats. Goats will climb, scatter, and fight, all of which are incompatible with effective herding with dogs.

Restraint of individual goats or parts of their bodies

Pressing against a wall

A goat can be restrained by backing it into a corner with a solid wall. The handler then presses the goat against a wall with one leg between its neck and shoulder and the other leg against its chest.

Jaw and neck hold

Small and medium-sized goats can be restrained by a hand under their jaw and the other hand on the upper part of the back of their neck.

Straddling

Some goats can be straddled for restraint. The goat is backed into a corner, and the handler straddles its neck, holding the goat still with his knees on both sides of the goat's neck. Straddling can be hazardous if attempted on horned goats or adult meat goats.

Flanking

A handler can flank a goat by standing next to it and reaching over the neck to grasp the front leg nearest his body. His other hand grasps the flank. While lifting the goat, the handler should slide it down the front of his leg onto its side. The hand on the flank is moved to the bottom hind leg and the handler's elbow presses on the goat's neck while the hand on the front leg continues to restrain that leg.

Platform and stanchion

Milking of goats is typically done with the doe standing on an elevated stand. Some include stanchions similar to cattle chutes with headgates. The goat may voluntarily walk up onto a platform if trained with grain as a reward, or it can be led by its collar to the platform and walked up onto the platform. Stanchions also aid in performing foot trimming and grooming.

Side sticks and neck cradles

Sticks from a halter to a chest strap (surcingle) or neck cradles can be used to prevent chewing on the legs or to restrain a dairy goat who has learned how to nurse itself.

Spanish halter

Spanish halters are similar to a tie-down used for horses. A strap or cord from a halter is run between the front legs and attached to a surcingle. The Spanish halter allows most normal grazing but prohibits the goat from eating from lower tree branches.

Tattooing

Most goat breed registries require an identification tattoo on the ear flap, or in breeds with small ears, the tail web. Restraint for this procedure is by holding the head or having the head in a stanchion.

Trimming hooves

Hooves need to be trimmed about every 8 weeks depending on how abrasive the ground is in their enclosure. Goats are usually trimmed while they stand in the same manner as horses. An assistant handler may be needed to manually restrain the head and is preferred over tying the goat by a halter lead. Elevated platforms or small tilt tables may also be used for hoof trimming restraint.

Restraint for kids

Kid goats are captured as if picking up a small dog. Small kids can be carried with an arm under their chest and abdomen while the hand of the same arm grasps the kid's front leg nearest the handler's body. Kids should never be restrained by an ear, horn, the neck or a leg.

Kids up to 20 lb (9.1 kg) can be held with their heads up and back to the handler and the handler restraining the kid's right front and hind legs with the right hand and the left front and hind legs with the left hand. The same hold can be used while the handler sits and holds the kid on its back on his or her lap. This positions male kids for castration.

Larger kids can be restrained by straddling the kid and holding the body by pressing the kid just behind the shoulders with the handler's legs while the handler blocks forward movement with a hand behind the kid's jaws.

Another method is to straddle the kid, grasp each front leg, raise the kid onto its hind feet, and hold its chest between the handler's thighs.

Kids should be disbudded within 4 days of birth. Horns present a hazard to other goats and to handlers. In addition, the goat may entrap its head in fences or other containment structures more easily with horns than without. Properly performed disbudding will also remove the adjacent skin containing the scent glands. Dehorning older goats should be avoided because of the stress involved and the risk of complications. Restraint for disbudding a small kid is to hold the kid on the handler's lap in sternal recumbency while restraining the head movement with both hands on the neck just behind its ears. Alternatively, a goat-holding box may be used, which is similar to a suitcase but with a hole for the goat's head to stick out.

Handling for common medical procedures

Most handling and restraint methods for goats are similar to those used in sheep, except that goats should not be restrained in the tipped position. Unless they are obese or very muscular, their rump has little padding. Tipping is uncomfortable for goats and they will not tolerate it without a continual struggle. Since goat tails are held in an elevated position rather than against their anus like sheep, tipping goats may also injure their tail.

> Goats should not be restrained in the tipped position.

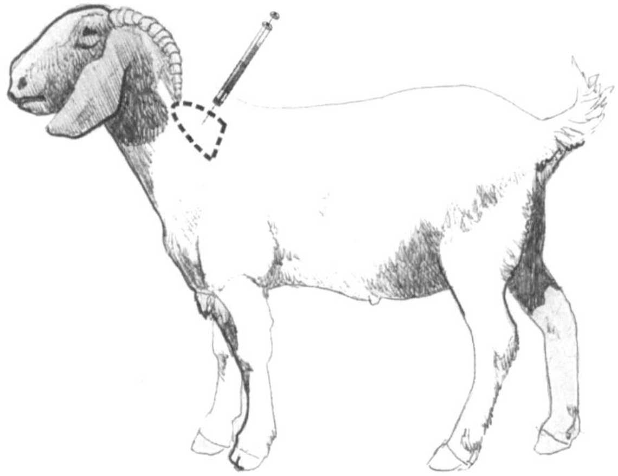

Fig. 13.14　Site for IM injections in goats.

A goat should not be restrained by its horns or by pulling on an ear, which will be resented and cause struggling. Grasping the base of a horn of an adult may be done with little risk of it breaking off, but grasping the end of a horn or anywhere on a young goat's horns may result in the horn breaking off and bleeding profusely.

Some goats become catatonic with fear. The proper handler response is to back off and resume moving or handling in a less intimidating way. The catatonic response is different from fainting in goats, which is a genetic disorder called myotonia. Fainting goats do not really faint. Their muscles will go into involuntary extreme contraction, causing them to stiffen and fall on their side.

Groups in small pens can become aggressive toward small or timid members. Large goats should not be penned with small ones. Horned goats should not be penned with goats without horns, and bucks should not be penned together.

Injections and venipuncture

Access to veins

Goats are haltered and tied or placed in a stanchion for jugular or cephalic vein venipuncture. The femoral vein may be accessed with a goat in lateral recumbency.

Injections

Subcutaneous injections are generally given under the skin behind an elbow or fold of the flank. Intramuscular injections should be administered in the side of the neck only, except for nursing kids (**Figure 13.14**). Nursing kids should receive IM injections in the semitendinosus and semimembranosus in the back aspect of the thigh.

Administration of oral medications

For up to 8–10 US fluid ounces (237–296 ml), drenching is more practical than using a stomach tube. To drench a goat, a handler straddles its back, places a hand under its lower jaw, and raises its head slightly. The nozzle of the drench syringe is inserted between the cheek and the back teeth. The plunger is pushed in slowly, allowing the goat to swallow the liquid medication. Handlers should wear gloves and not put their bare fingers in the goat's mouth. A speculum for insertion of a stomach tube is placed in the same way.

Balling guns are used to administer solid medications. Goats are caught individually and backed into a wall and straddled. The goat's head is lifted under the jaw, but its nose should not be lifted higher than the poll, otherwise its ability to swallow will be impeded. The balling gun is inserted in the mouth and the plunger pushes the bolus onto the back upper surface of the tongue. The balling gun should not be inserted too far, which could impair swallowing and allow the bolus to go into the larynx or trachea.

SOUTH AMERICAN CAMELIDS (LLAMAS AND ALPACAS)

Llamas and alpacas are domesticated camelids indigenous to the Americas and are related to Asian camels. They were domesticated and selectively bred for

4,000–5,000 years by the Incas in the Andean high-lands. The llama is a beast of burden that can carry 25–30% of its weight when conditioned. It is also bred for their meat, hide, and sinew. The smaller alpaca is bred for its fine wool.

Although camelids are ruminants, they have significant differences to sheep and goats. Camelids have long necks that they tend to put through holes in fences, among other places, and get caught or injured. Camelids have a pacing gait like that of Standardbred horses. The front and hind legs on the same side move forward and backward at the same time.

Camelids have poor tolerance to heat and an aversion to dogs. *Kushing* is lying down on their sternum. It can be a means of adjusting to overheating by cooling their abdomen on cool ground, but it also is a passive means of defense. Their overt defense tactics include kicking (they usually do not strike), spitting, and sometimes biting. Spitting is a spraying of rumen contents, which is preceded by a gurgling sound. The spray can be effective at a distance of 6 ft (1.8 m). It is usually a prelude to an attempted escape or an impending attack. Pinning the ears back is another clue to possible aggression. They are adapted to cold but not frigid temperatures (under 10°F [12.21°C]).

There is one breed of llama and two breeds of alpaca, Huacaya and Suri. Suri alpacas are less common. Their longer hair, which curls like dreadlocks and parts on the middle of the back, is distinctive.

Males and some female camelids have vestigial incisors, canine teeth, and large premolars, which become six *fighting teeth* that begin to erupt at 2 years of age and are completely erupted by 4 years of age. There are two pairs on the upper arcade, just behind the dental pad, and one pair below on the mandible. Fighting teeth are sharp and angled backward (**Figure 13.15**). Breeding males should have the fighting teeth sawed off with obstetrical wire for the safety of other camelids and handlers.

South American camelids do not have hooves. They have two toes with large nails and a large soft footpad. Their sternal area is heavily callused for long periods of rest in the sternal position.

Adult breeding males are called *machos*. Castrated males are *geldings*. Adult females are *hembras*, and the young are *crias*.

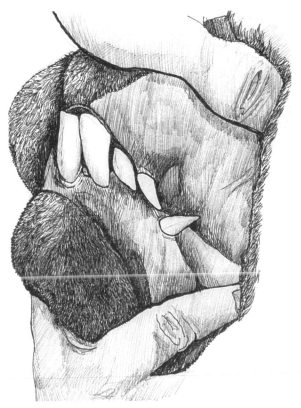

Fig. 13.15 Fighting teeth of a llama.

Approaching and catching

Even docile, well-handled camelids are often resentful of being caught. They can be difficult to impossible to catch in a large pasture. To catch them, they can be herded into a small catch pen or funneled into an alleyway. Herding may be more effective by sweeping, done by two handlers holding a 30 ft (9.1 m) rope about 3 ft (1 m) off the ground and moving the camelids toward a fence. One handler can tie his end to the fence while the other maintains the trapped camelids. The free handler can then catch and halter the desired camelid.

Typically, camelids must be trained to enter small catch pens that are 10 × 30 ft (3 × 9.1 m) or smaller, where they are often fed to desensitize them to the enclosure. They should be approached in a calm, direct manner with an approach and retreat method similar to catching an evasive horse. Rushing an approach can cause camelids to panic and injure themselves. Camelids that are frightened should be caught in a shelter or building with one or more calm companions to decrease the chance of it trying to jump over a fence.

The basic restraint of a camelid is for the handler to wrap an arm around the camelid's neck near its head and pull it close to the handler's body. The handler's other hand pushes down on its shoulders or holds the camelid's shoulder and chest close to his body. An alternative hold is to grasp the base of the tail. However, grasping the tail may cause some to kush. Pinning them against a solid wall may also assist with restraint. The ears should never be used for restraint. Causing pain or fear from handling their ears will make them swing their head and neck dangerously in an effort to escape.

Dogs should not be allowed within sight or sound of camelid catch pens.

Handling for routine care and management

Basic equipment and facilities

Catch pens

Catch pens for camelids are small pens 10 × 30 ft (3 × 9.1 m) or smaller and at least 5 ft (1.5 m) high. Two or more camelids should be herded into a catch pen for ease of sorting and to reduce the anxiety of camelids separated from the main group.

Stocks

A restraint chute similar to a horse stock is advisable for ease of restraint of llamas. Alpacas respond better to loose restraint with a halter and lead rope. Camelid stocks are tall and narrow. If they are not constructed of anchored posts, a stock should be bolted to the floor to prevent it from being tipped over on its side. The size should be 2 ft (0.6 m) wide, 5.5 ft (1.7 m) long, and 45 in (114.3 cm) to the top rail. There should be access to the camelid from all sides. A front and rear cinch attached to side rails is required to keep camelids from kushing in the stocks. Cinches should be 8–10 in (20–25 cm) apart for llamas and closer for alpacas. A third cinch may be needed for some camelids to go over the withers to prevent rearing or jumping. Cross-tie rings should be in forward positions to prevent the tied camelid from moving backward in the stocks. Quick-release ties should be used if lower cinches are not used to prevent kushing.

Moving and separating

Camelids are extremely herd-oriented and are best moved as groups. Separation of individuals from the herd is done best by using a series of catch pens that gradually get smaller until an individual can be caught. Another method of separation involves two handlers holding a 30–40 ft (9.1–12.2 m) rope about 3 ft (1 m) off the ground. Blindfolds should not be used in an attempt to move camelids because they will kush.

Restraint of individual camelids or parts of their bodies

Halters and lead ropes

Camelids can be taught to be haltered and led. This is basic training for llamas that will be used as pack animals. They are principally handled from the left side and led from their left side. Camelid halters should be used to prevent pinching of their nostrils. Placing the halter is done with a bear hug approach as with haltering horses. Pony halters should not be used because the noseband is too low for camelids. The noseband should be at least 1½ in (3.8 cm) above the end of the bony part of the nose. At least two fingers should be able to be placed under the lower aspect of the band and the jaw so that the animal can chew. The cheekpieces should be at least 1 in (2.5 cm) below the eyes. Halters should be removed when not handling the animal because of the risk of it catching on brush, fences, and other objects.

Handling crias

Crias are handled similarly to foals by boxing in their movements with the handler's arms without squeezing them. Small crias can be flanked and laid in lateral recumbency or pressed against a solid wall as with sheep or goats.

If a cria kushes in resistance, a handler can bend down on his knees and straddle its chest and hold the upper area of its neck. Crias can be kept in the kush position by *chukkering*, using a folded loop of rope over the back in front of the pelvis with the ends of the loop around the fetlocks of the flexed hind legs. This prevents them from being able to rise. In this position, another handler can perform jugular venipuncture or administer oral medications.

Crias should be handled for brief periods (less than 20 minutes) on a regular basis to gradually desensitize them to being haltered and led, loosely restrained, and have their legs and feet handled. This will prepare them for necessary toenail trimmings 3–4 times per year if their enclosures are not abrasive enough to wear the nails down.

Llamas as pack animals

Llamas can be excellent pack animals. Alpacas are not large or strong enough to be effective as a pack animal for anything other than the equivalent of a child's backpack.

Llamas should be trained for packing beginning at 1 year of age and led behind experienced older llamas while packing. Blankets or other soft, lightweight objects should be carried during initial training. Less than 30 lb (13.6 kg) should be carried until llamas are at least 3 years old. All pack llamas should be gradually conditioned prior to a long pack trip.

Conditioned adult pack llamas carry their load on specifically made rigid or soft pack saddles. A saddle pad or blanket is used under a rigid saddle. Rigid saddles are made of wood, aluminum, or fiberglass and held in place by two cinches. Rigid saddles are tent-shaped (crossbuck design) to allow the weight to be carried evenly on both sides of the upper chest without pressure on the top of the spine. Panniers are the detachable packs that are attached to saddles to carry the load. Soft pack saddles also distribute the load weight on both sides of the upper chest.

Pack saddles are placed on llamas in a similar manner to how riding saddles are put on horses. The llama should be brushed first. The saddle pad and saddle are placed just behind the shoulder blades; the front cinch is applied first and then the back cinch. Tightening the cinches should be gradual, done at three separate times. After the last tightening, the handler should still be able to get three fingers underneath both cinches.

If packing is intended in areas with steep slopes, a breast collar (strap that goes from each side of the saddle and around the front of the chest) to keep the load from shifting backward and a crupper (strap that goes from the saddle and under the tail) to keep the load from shifting forward will be needed. Neither should be so tight that fingers cannot be slipped underneath the breast collar and crupper.

Each side of the pannier should be weighed to ensure an evenly distributed load. There should not be more than a 2 lb (0.9 kg) difference in weight between the two sides. The heaviest part of the pack should be closest to the llama's body to prevent the load from being top-heavy or shifting.

Handling for common medical procedures

Injections and venipuncture

Access to veins

Venipuncture is generally from the jugular vein or the ventral tail vein. The jugular vein is not externally visible in South American camelids. They have thick skin in the neck and large transverse processes of the cervical vertebrae that obscure the vein. The most accessible points are high in the neck or low in the neck. The high location is preferred because of the proximity of the carotid artery to the lower region of the jugular vein. The cephalic vein may be accessed if the camelid is in a kushed position.

Injections

Intramuscular injections are generally given in the triceps muscle in the front legs or the semitendinosus and semimembranosus muscles of the hind legs. Intramuscular injections should not be given in the neck of camelids regardless of age. Subcutaneous injections are given under the loose skin low on the chest just behind the elbow.

Administration of oral medications

Oral administration of liquids is the same as with sheep and goats, except that straddle restraint is not possible. Restraint is similar to that used for horses and achieved with a halter and lead rope or camelid stocks.

TRANSPORTING SMALL RUMINANTS

Loading chutes

Loading chutes for sheep and goats can be side by side and should be solid walled on the outside to prevent seeing handlers and high enough to prevent attempts to jump out. Partitions between chutes for sheep should be see-through so that they can see other sheep moving forward. There should be narrow divisions in the loading chutes to prevent animals from being able to turn around in the chute. Cleats are needed in the floor to eliminate or reduce slipping.

Sheep and goats

As with transporting all livestock, the driving of the vehicle should be smooth. Accelerating or stopping suddenly should be avoided. Turning corners should be slow enough for the animals to shift their weight and stay on their feet.

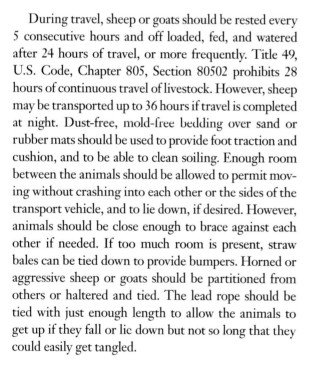

Sheep or goats should not be transported alone. They should be transported with at least a favored herdmate.

During travel, sheep or goats should be rested every 5 consecutive hours and off loaded, fed, and watered after 24 hours of travel, or more frequently. Title 49, U.S. Code, Chapter 805, Section 80502 prohibits 28 hours of continuous travel of livestock. However, sheep may be transported up to 36 hours if travel is completed at night. Dust-free, mold-free bedding over sand or rubber mats should be used to provide foot traction and cushion, and to be able to clean soiling. Enough room between the animals should be allowed to permit moving without crashing into each other or the sides of the transport vehicle, and to lie down, if desired. However, animals should be close enough to brace against each other if needed. If too much room is present, straw bales can be tied down to provide bumpers. Horned or aggressive sheep or goats should be partitioned from others or haltered and tied. The lead rope should be tied with just enough length to allow the animals to get up if they fall or lie down but not so long that they could easily get tangled.

Goats must be transported in completely enclosed containers to prevent escapes. Dog crates can suffice, if they are large enough for the goat to stand up and lie down comfortably. Goat-sized livestock crates are available for the bed of pickup trucks. Crate doors should be doubly latched.

Unshorn sheep, alpacas, and Angora and cashmere goats are especially susceptible to heat stress. They need to be provided extra space and ventilation and travel in early morning or late in the day and at night if transported in warm weather.

South American camelids

South American camelids can be trained to travel in horse trailers or in the back of station wagons, minivans, or pickup trucks with stock sides. They kush during travel, and because of this they occupy relatively small space during travel. If they have enough room to stand, as in a horse trailer, and are tied, they should be tied with enough lead line to be able to kush.

SELECTED FURTHER READING

Birutta, G (1997). *Storey's Guide to Raising Llamas*. Storey Publishing, North Adams.

Hoffman C, Asmus I (2011). *Caring for Llamas and Alpacas: A Health & Management Guide*, 3rd edition. Rocky Mountain Llama and Alpaca Association, Monument.

Mateo JM, Estep DQ, McCann JS (1991). Effects of differential handling on the behaviour of domestic ewes (*Ovis aries*). *Applied Animal Behaviour Science* 32:45–54.

Sayer M (1997). *Storey's Guide to Raising Meat Goats*. Storey Publishing, North Adams.

Simmons P, Ekarius C (2001). *Storey's Guide to Raising Sheep*. Storey Publishing, North Adams, MA.

WorkSafe New Zealand (2014). *Safe Sheep Handling*. WorkSafe New Zealand, Wellington.

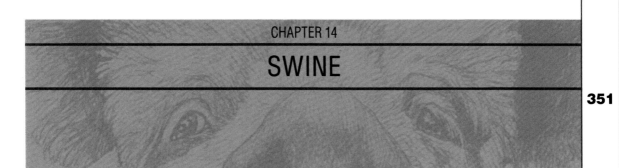

Domesticated swine (*Sus domesticus*) are referred to as hogs or pigs depending on their size. Hogs were domesticated from wild boars about 11,000 years ago in southwestern Asia and China. They were raised for their meat, hides, bones (tools and weapons), and hair (bristles for brushes). Egyptians sowed seed in ground that was loosened by the sharp points of the hogs' hooves. The genome of domesticated hogs is very similar to wild hogs.

The domesticated hogs of Europe came from southwestern Asia. They were later brought to the New World by Spanish explorers. Christopher Columbus brought hogs on his second voyage to the Caribbean islands in 1493. However, it was Hernando de Soto who brought 200 pigs with him in May 1539 to the North American continent. Hogs were a supplement to game meat as de Soto and his men explored Florida and other regions of modern-day U.S. Pigs could travel with the explorers because they follow for being fed better than they can be herded, while they ate additional food that was locally available along the way. The collared peccary, which is native to the southwestern U.S., belongs to a different family (*Tayassuidae*) from domestic swine (*Suidae*).

Young swine that are still nursing are called *piglets*. From weaning to 120 lb (54.4 kg) swine are referred to as *pigs*. An older name for pigs is *shoats*. Starter pigs weigh 10–40 lb (4.5–18.1 kg). Pigs between 40 and 80 lb (18.1 and 36.3 kg) are feeder pigs. After 120 lb (54.4 kg), swine are called *hogs*. Finisher hogs are more than 150 lb (68 kg) and less than 220 lb (99.8 kg). Butcher hogs are 220 lb (99.8 kg) and above. A sexually intact male is a *boar*. Males are typically castrated before puberty and then called *barrows*. Female pigs or hogs that have not had a litter are *gilts*. Once they have a litter they are referred to as *sows*.

NATURAL BEHAVIOR OF SWINE

Swine in the wild live in groups, called "sounders," of 2–6 sows and their pigs. The sows will often pair up for foraging and sleeping. Once young males near puberty, they are driven away by older, more dominant boars. They finish their development in bachelor groups until they are ready to challenge the dominant boars. The dominant boars tend to remain solitary except at breeding seasons.

Hogs defend themselves by pushing and biting. The bullet shape of their body is a passive means of defense that affords considerable protection from predators and adversaries. Their body shape facilitates a quick escape in thick bush and increases the difficulty of being caught, especially if the body is wet and muddy. They move in loose groups as a herd, but if alerted to threats to a herd member by squealing, other hogs will come to the member's defense.

Body size strongly affects social status in hogs and pigs. The superior social rank of heavier pigs is established in early play contests. Success in pushing other pigs away from food or other possessions reinforces social rank. Group interaction is important to hogs. Hogs cannot reach most of their body with their mouth or their hind legs. In groups, they groom each other with their mouths. Deprived of this, they spend much of their time trying to scratch themselves on objects. Grunting vocalizations are auditory social contacts that are nearly constant if moving or nursing piglets.

Hogs are adapted to temperate climates. They are most comfortable at temperatures between 55 and 85°F (12.8° and 29.5°C). During hot weather, their activities in the wild are primarily nocturnal. In the daytime, they wallow in mud and rest. When cold weather occurs, their activities become more crepuscular and diurnal. When resting in cold weather, they huddle together to conserve body heat.

The natural behavior of swine is to forage for food (grubs, worms, roots, nuts) and investigate their surroundings by rooting with their snout for about 7 hours a day. Hogs have a disk-shaped snout cartilage that aids their ability to root. They root to find food and create wallowing areas to cool themselves. They are highly intelligent and require much mental stimulation to prevent self-mutilation or aggression toward other hogs. Deprived of these mental challenges, food possession becomes more important and aggressiveness to other hogs increases. They are capable of living in a wide variety of habitats, but they prefer woodland marshes that provide escape from sunburn and heat, chances to wallow in mud to control flies and other external parasites, and their favorite foods, including acorns and earthworms. They have an extraordinary sense of smell, excellent hearing, but poor vision. Boars "champ" their teeth and produce some frothy saliva containing pheromones. They mark their territory with saliva and urine.

The U.S. has become the largest exporter of pork products in the world. Most hogs in the U.S. are now raised in total indoor confinement on concrete. This prevents their primary natural behaviors of rooting and wallowing. The natural 7 hours of rooting are exchanged for 2 hours of eating from a pan or trough in a pen. Tails are docked to prevent tail biting, which results from the lack of the mental stimulus they would normally get from rooting. The inability for baby pigs to ingest dirt from the sow's teats while nursing and rooting, which they normally begin to do in the first week of being born, will lead to iron deficiency anemia if iron is not administered to baby pigs as a preventive treatment. Providing straw bedding for hogs to root and chew reduces aggression, skin damage, and joint injuries. When they are prevented from rooting, they lie on their sternums more than their sides. This can be stressful since they get greater rest laying on their sides.

Crowding and confined access to food generates most aggression in hogs. Hogs in large commercial operations have been given beta-adrenergic drugs to reduce fat in their muscle. Common side effects of beta-adrenergic drugs are nervousness and aggression. Breed affects social rank in mixed groups. Large Whites are more aggressive than Hampshires, which are more aggressive than Durocs. Large Whites are the most common breed used in pork production in the U.S.

SAFETY FIRST

Handler safety

Restrained swine squeal very loudly. Handlers should not cause pigs to squeal in the presence of sows for procedures such as treating navels, clipping needle teeth, docking tails, notching ears, castration, or administering injections, because the mother sow or other sows may become agitated enough to become aggressive and dangerous.

Handlers should always wear moldable ear plugs when working indoors with swine. Squealing is a significant danger to hearing. For example, feeding time in a swine building can have a squealing intensity that reaches 95–130 decibels. Hearing loss can begin at 85 decibels. If a handler must raise his or her voice in order to be heard by someone who is standing an arm's length away, the decibels are above 80 and ear protection should be worn. Cotton balls and ill-fitting plugs are inadequate protection.

When working in hog total confinement buildings, respiratory problems are a risk. Causes of respiratory difficulty in swine buildings can include dust (particularly particles of feed and fecal matter) and gases (especially ammonia from urine and hydrogen sulfide from feces). Wearing a respirator may be necessary. Disposable dust masks with two straps provide protection against inhaling larger particles, but do not provide protection against small particles of dust or gases.

Other injuries to handlers from hogs can be from biting or colliding with handlers. The most dominant boar should be handled first so that the smell of subordinate boars will not stimulate aggression. Breeding boars or nursing sows weigh more than 500 lb (226.8 kg) and are often aggressive and dangerous, especially if they have been mishandled in the past, including not having been allowed to socialize with other hogs when they were young.

> Handlers should always leave themselves two exits from a hog pen, always remain within reach of stationary objects to hold to prevent being knocked down, and never back a grown hog into a corner.

Sows attempt to knock intruders in their space down and then bite them. Boars will attack intruders while they are still standing. Boars can be extremely aggressive, if provoked. Wild boars were hunted in the Middle Ages with a boar spear, which had lugs (short bars perpendicular to the spear blade) to prevent the boar from running up the spear handle and attacking the hunter after being impaled. Aggressive adult hogs, particularly boars, may try to bite the inner aspect of a handler's thigh and could sever the femoral artery. This can quickly lead to life-threatening hemorrhage. Handlers should always keep a barrier (panel, fence, or other partition) between themselves and the boar being handled. It is also advisable to wear knee boots and steel-toed shoes when in hog or pig pens. If charged by a sow or boar, a slap on its snout with a shovel or cane may be enough distraction for a handler to quickly escape.

Gates in hog pens should only be used for moving hogs in and out. Handlers entering a pen should climb over the pen wall or fence since hogs can escape with speed and force if the gate is unlatched for a handler to enter.

Handlers who work with hogs during breeding should not be involved when breeding sows or boars are handled for painful procedures, such as vaccination or blood collection. Hogs are more likely to remain calm if they do not associate previous pain or restraint with a handler.

Swine safety

Hogs and pigs are very intelligent and individualistic. They do not herd well in groups. Each one that becomes trapped in an enclosure will look for an opening and root to try to escape. Pigs will pile on top of each other seeking escape. They have poor vision and their "fight or flight" response activates quickly. They overheat, tire easily, and can die of heat stroke if not handled with as little stress as possible and quickly.

The primary means of defense and offense of hogs is biting. Hogs are more aggressive when hungry. They will become agitated and sometimes aggressive by "mob action" if a member of the group seems in distress.

Hogs and pigs should be desensitized to humans near their flight zones by handlers entering their pen, getting the pigs up as quietly as possible, having them move quietly around the pen, and then leaving when the animals are relatively calm.

To decrease fighting when mixing sows or pigs, groups should be established according to size, extra food should be provided during initial introduction, and hay, straw, and toys made available for mental stimulation and diversion. A new hog or pig being added to an established group is best introduced in a dark room.

The incisors and canine teeth are often clipped in one-day-old piglets to reduce injuries to the sow's teats and to litter mates.

Key zoonoses

(*Note:* Apparently ill animals should be handled by veterinary professionals or under their supervision. Precautionary measures against zoonoses from ill animals are more involved than those required when handling apparently healthy animals and vary widely. The discussion here is directed primarily at handling apparently healthy animals.)

Seemingly healthy domestic hogs pose little risk of transmitting disease to healthy adult handlers who practice conventional personal hygiene. The risks of physical injury are greater than the risks of acquiring an infectious disease (*Table 14.1*).

Direct transmission

Systemic disease

Leptospirosis (*Leptospira* spp.) is a bacterial disease of hogs that is transmitted in infected hog urine and genital fluids. Common sources for hogs are stagnant water that wildlife have access to, and rats. The organism can be transmitted by gaining entrance into a human's mouth, breaks in the skin, or eyes.

Table 14.1 Diseases transmitted from healthy appearing swine to healthy adult humans

DISEASE	AGENT	MEANS OF TRANSMISSION	SIGNS AND SYMPTOMS IN HUMANS	FREQUENCY IN ANIMALS	RISK GROUP*
Bites	–	Direct injury	Bite wounds to hands and legs, death can occur from torn or severed arteries	All swine are capable of inflicting bites	3
Salmonellosis	*Salmonella* spp.	Direct, fecal-oral	Diarrhea, systemic disease and abscesses	Common	3
Swine Influenza	Influenza A, H1N1, and H3N2	Direct, airborne	Respiratory disease and possible death	Requires a rare mutation of common swine influenza virus	4
Leptospirosis	*Leptospira* spp.	Direct from contact with urine; indirect from urine contamination of water	Kidney infection and flu-like symptoms	Hogs recovering from leptospirosis can appear normal and shed the bacteria in the urine	3
Yersiniosis	*Yersinia enterocolitica*	Direct and indirect, fecal-oral	Diarrhea and occasionally reactive arthritis	Common and can transmit disease while appearing healthy	2

* Risk Groups (National Institutes of Health and World Health Organization criteria. Centers for Disease Control and Prevention, *Biosafety in Microbiological and Biomedical Laboratories*, 5th edition, 2009):
1 Agent not associated with disease in healthy adult humans.
2 Agent rarely causes serious disease and prevention or therapy possible.
3 Agent can cause serious or lethal disease and prevention or therapy possible.
4 Agent can cause serious or lethal disease and prevention or therapy are not usually available.

Brucellosis (*Brucella suis*) is a bacterial disease that can cause abortions in sows and inflammation of the testes in boars. It can be transmitted to humans by exposure to body secretions (saliva, urine, fetal fluids) or eating meat from infected hogs. The disease in humans is influenza-like and called undulant fever. The disease is now rare in hogs in the U.S. because of federal and state surveillance and eradication.

Listeriosis (*Listeria monocytogenes*) is from a bacterium that can cause generalized disease in immunosuppressed humans, including an atypical pneumonia. Transmission is primarily by contaminated food products.

Streptococcosis suis is a bacterium that can cause serious illness in hogs and can be transmitted to handlers. In humans, *S. suis* infection can result in meningitis and sepsis. The incidence is rare.

Respiratory disease

Although rare, bovine or avian tuberculosis can occur in hogs. Infected hogs can transmit the disease to handlers through body secretions. Affected hogs do not appear healthy at the time they are able to transmit the disease.

Bordetella bronchiseptica is a cause for respiratory bacterial infection that can be acquired from hogs. In humans, it usually requires an impaired immune response to cause severe or prolonged infection.

Hogs are susceptible to both avian and human influenza. Concern exists, particularly when hogs are kept in close confinement and under stress, that influenza viruses can mutate through an antigen shift to a more virulent strain that affects humans. Should this happen, an epidemic could result, but this is not a significant risk to handlers from apparently healthy hogs that are not over-crowded and under stress.

Digestive tract diseases

Campylobacter infection is one of the most common causes of bacterial diarrhea in humans. Contact with infected hogs can be a source if the bacteria gain access to a handler's mouth. Most human cases are from unpasteurized milk or undercooked poultry.

Salmonellosis is a bacterial disease of the digestive system that can invade the blood stream and become systemic. Most cases are not from handling hogs but are acquired by eating undercooked eggs, poultry, pork, or beef or by handling reptiles or rodents and carrying the bacteria to the handler's mouth.

Yersiniosis (*Yersinia enterocolitis*) is a bacterial diarrhea that is usually acquired from handling raw pork, especially intestines. However, transmission can occur from both sick and normal appearing hog feces.

Trichinosis, caused by *Trichinella spiralis* and *T. nativa*, is a parasitic disease of muscle. It is not transmitted by handling hogs, but by ingestion of undercooked pork products. *Trichinella* spp. have been eradicated in confinement-raised hogs through the exclusion of rodents as food for hogs.

Taeniasis (*Taenia solium*) is a tapeworm acquired in humans from eating raw or undercooked pork products. It is not transmitted by handling swine.

Skin disease

Vesicular stomatitis virus causes blisters in the mouth and on the snout, feet, and teats of hogs. Handlers of hogs with vesicular stomatitis blisters can become infected and develop blisters on infected skin.

Erysipeloid is caused by a bacterium (*Erysipelothrix rhusiopathiae*) and can be transmitted from infected hogs or pork (erysipelas in swine) to humans through cuts in the skin. In hogs, it causes arthritis and diamond-shaped skin patterns. In humans, it causes skin sores. Transmission is not from healthy appearing hogs.

Vector borne

There are no significant vector transmitted zoonotic diseases from healthy appearing swine.

Sanitary practices

Persons handling hogs should wear appropriate dress to protect against skin contamination with hair and skin scales or saliva, urine, and other body secretions. Basic sanitary practices should be adhered to, such as keeping hands away from eyes, nose, and mouth when handling hogs and washing hands after handling them.

Special precautions are needed if sick hogs are handled, and these should be isolated from apparently normal hogs. New herd members should be quarantined for at least 2 weeks to reduce the risk of transmitting a disease that new animals could be incubating before introducing them to the rest of the herd.

Influenza vaccinations in handlers should be current, and handlers ill with influenza should not handle hogs. Wild birds should not be in contact with hogs. Hogs should be vaccinated for leptospirosis, and wildlife, especially rodents, should be controlled in swine-raising facilities.

APPROACHING AND CATCHING

In total confinement operations, hogs are restricted to crates in which they are already caught and restrained, or to small pens in which catching is relatively easy. Regardless of whether hogs are in crates, small pens, large pens, or on pasture, care must be taken not to startle them, especially sows with piglets, by being either too quiet or excessively noisy. Hogs will become quickly agitated by the presence of a stranger. A startle reaction in hogs is to vocalize with a woof sound, jump to their feet if recumbent, and then freeze in place. Normal level noise should be made at a distance so that hogs moderate their alert response before the handler gets near them.

Special precautions should be taken to prevent being bitten on the legs and knocked down in a hog pen. When entering a pen of hogs, a handler should wear knee-high boots and stay near a fence or something else that is firmly stationary to grab to maintain his or her balance if pushed. Handlers may carry a panel or pole to keep curious hogs from crowding them. Hogs in total confinement are deprived of normal mental stimulation and become excited by the presence of a handler whom they also associate with being fed. Smelling a handler's legs and inquisitive bites of boots is common. However, this can become dangerous if the hogs are large or have not been fed recently, or if blood is present anywhere in the pen. Hogs are omnivores and will become very excited if blood is nearby.

Swine on pasture or in hog lots are usually taught to come for feeding by being called. Traditionally, the commands "suey" and "pig-pig-pig" have been used to call hogs.

Hogs can be taught to appreciate being rubbed and scratched on the back, but this must be done firmly since light touches will be suspicious of danger. Minor procedures, such as vaccinations, can be done without stress on many hogs by restricting their movement, providing food, using a soothing voice, and scratching their shoulders and behind their ears during the procedure. The handler should never put his hands within range of a hog that can turn and bite.

When collecting swine of different sizes, the largest hogs should be sorted out first. Sorting out by largest size to smallest should continue to reduce the risk of smaller pigs being trampled and crushed. Larger hogs or pigs are also more easy to separate from smaller pigs than are smaller pigs from larger pigs or hogs.

Pigs less than 50 lb (22.7 kg) can be caught as they run along a wall of a pen by the handler facing the same direction and sweeping an open hand back and under them to grasp the nearest hind leg, then picking the pig up and grasping the other hind leg. For example, a pig running to the left would be caught by its left hind leg by the handler's right hand. Sorting panels or gates can be used as traps to catch larger pigs.

HANDLING FOR ROUTINE CARE AND MANAGEMENT

Basic equipment and facilities
High volume facilities
High volume swine facilities may have collecting pens, crowding pens, alleyways, drop-down gates, squeeze chutes, and scales. Pigs will jam up and pile on top of each other if funneled from crowding pens into alleyways. The transition from a crowding pen to an alleyway should have an offset entrance to prevent jamming and piling (**Figure 14.1**). Crowding pens for pigs should have a radius of 6 ft (1.8 m). A Bud box can also be used to funnel swine into an alleyway or into sorting pens. Alleyways and ramps should be two pigs width wide with a see-through middle partition.

Restraint crates
Most restraint on confinement hogs is done in their crates or single alleyways. This permits inexperienced handlers to handle and restrain hogs for various reasons relatively safely. Handling and restraint of pigs and hogs raised in hooped pens or on pasture requires more skill.

Hog snares, sorting panels, snubbing ropes, and manual restraint
Specialized restraint facilities are not needed for routine handling and restraint of swine. Most procedures can be done with minor distractions (scratching the shoulders of a hog, gently holding a pig's thigh), hog snares, panels, snubbing ropes, leg holds, and holding small pigs in the same manner of small dogs.

Holding piglets
Within 1 day to 2 weeks of age, piglets have their needle teeth clipped and ears notched, are given iron dextran injections, and the males are castrated. In close confinement operations, the tails may be docked. Vaccinations may also be started before weaning. Nursing pigs (piglets) are less than 20 lb (9.1 kg) and can be easily picked up and handled like a puppy. They should be removed from the sow's sight and hearing for all procedures to be done, but not for more than 1 hour.

Leg holds on pigs
Leg holds are performed on pigs up to about 50 lb (22.7 kg). Handlers should wear ear plugs, coveralls, and high-topped boots.

An inverted standing leg hold ("head stand" hold) is accomplished by grasping each hind leg at the hocks, and the pig is picked up by its hind

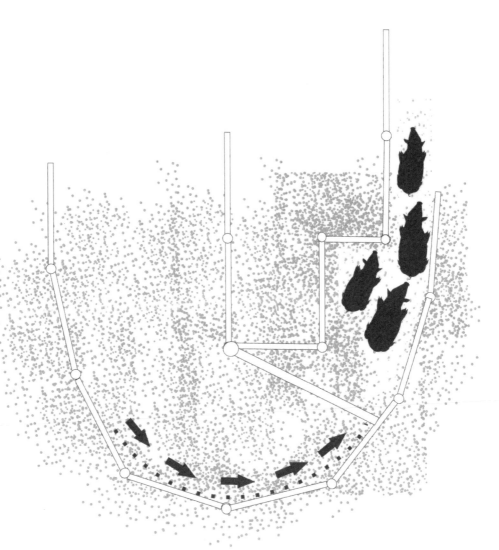

Fig. 14.1 Offset entry into alleyway prevents piling of pigs onto one another.

legs with its back toward the handler. The pig's torso is caught between the handler's legs. The pig's chest and shoulders are held by the handler's legs (**Figure 14.2**). This hold is used for castration and subcutaneous injections. High-topped boots are needed to protect the handler's legs from bites that pigs will attempt when held in this position.

Holding a pig in an upright standing position is less common than holding a pig in an inverted standing position. Oral medications and subcutaneous injections may be administered while pigs are held upright and standing. Holding the front legs allows the pig to bite the handler's hands, so gloves are

recommended. The hold is begun by straddling the pig and grasping the front legs. The handler then squeezes the sides of the pig's neck with his wrists while holding the pig's front leg to avoid being bitten. Small pigs may be caught by a hind leg and then moving the grasp to a hand holding both front legs. The flanks are immobilized with the handler's legs (**Figure 14.3**).

Hog snout snare

Swine more than 50 lb (22.7 kg) are usually captured with a snare (a hollow rigid tube with a wire that goes through the tube and forms a capture loop at the end) (**Figure 14.4**). Large hogs should

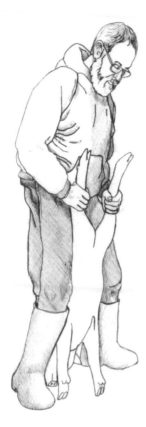

Fig. 14.2 Inverted standing leg hold.

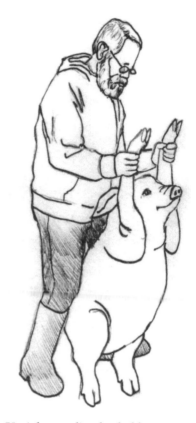

Fig. 14.3 Upright standing leg hold.

be positioned so that their attempt to back up while being snared is blocked, since they may be too strong to hold still after the snare is applied. The loop is placed inside the hog's mouth, and the loop is closed tightly around the upper jaw of the snout (the maxilla) (**Figure 14.5**). Care should be taken to get the snare loop far enough back in the mouth so that when it is tightened it does not squeeze the soft tissue of the end of the nose, where it would cause pain, shut the nostrils, and probably slip off.

After tightening the snare, the handler moves in front of the hog, as the hog will lean back and try to pull out of the loop (**Figure 14.6**). Snares will lose their effectiveness with time. Their use should be for less than 10 minutes. The use of snares with hogs that have tusks can be dangerous when trying to remove the snare, in part because the snare must be placed behind the tusks and can be hard to remove. Swine should never be pulled forward with a hog snare.

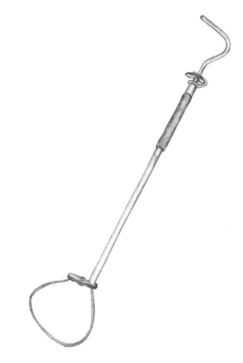

Fig. 14.4 Hog snout snare.

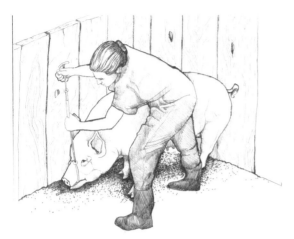

Fig. 14.5 Inserting a hog snare.

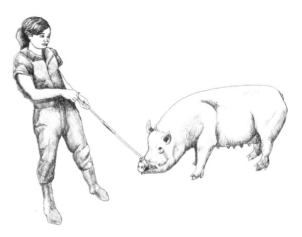

Fig. 14.6 Restraining a hog with a snare.

Snubbing rope

For large hogs that are too strong for a handler to restrain with a snare pole, restraint may be achieved with a lariat and quick-release honda if an assistant handler is available. Long-handled (3 ft [1 m]) bull nose tongs can be used by the assistant to squeeze the neck behind the ears, which will briefly restrain the hog and make it open its mouth (**Figure 14.7**). The handler

stands to the side behind the hog's head and places the bottom of the lariat's loop in its mouth around the upper jaw and then pulls the loop down tight on its upper jaw (**Figure 14.8**). The tongs can then be removed and the rope is run around a tie ring or similar tie point higher than the hogs head, and the hog is pulled near to the snubbing post. When tying the snubbing rope, the tie should be close (within a foot [33 cm]) of the snubbing post to reduce the risk of the hog loosening the snare and spitting it out. If an assistant plans to continue holding the other end rather than tie it, it is helpful to tie the end to a short rod or pole to maintain a sturdy grip as the pig pulls backward.

The use of a snubbing rope with a quick-release honda permits easier and safer removal than does a snare in a large hog with tusks, but it does not allow any pushing away option if the hog becomes

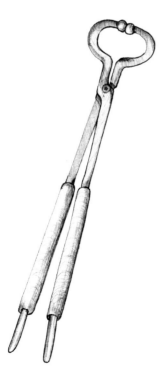

Fig. 14.7 Long-handled bull nose tongs used to put pressure on a hog's neck.

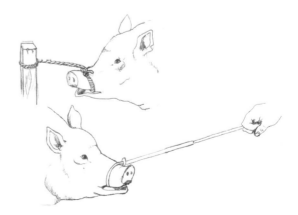

Fig. 14.8 Snubbing rope restraint.

aggressive and moves forward rather than pulling back. Two snubbing ropes that are cross-tied will reduce the risk of the handler being chased. Quick-release hondas should have a leather tether that will allow safer and quicker release of the latch.

A hog should never be pulled forward with a snubbing rope. However, the hog may be allowed to move backward with a handler holding the rope while a second handler guides it by grasping its tail.

Snout rings

Hogs confined in dirt lots or pastures will root the ground with their snouts. If rooting is excessive, pigs about 40 lb (18.1 kg) can be caught with a snout snare and then metal snout rings are clamped into the edge of the cartilage of the nose. Pigs less than 50 lb (22.7 kg) can be caught by an assistant and held in an upright position by their front legs. Leather gloves should be worn and the pig's front legs should be pulled back along the edge of the pig's face to block its ability to bite. Boars are not ringed since they use their nose to push on the female during breeding. If excessive rings are used or poorly positioned, they could interfere with the pig opening lids of self-feeders.

So-called "humane" snout rings are clamped into the nasal septum, leaving the rim of the snout free to open feeder lids without restriction.

Moving pigs and hogs

Training pigs for moving

Swine are not as whimsical as goats but much more independent, and they are more willing to try an individual escape than are sheep or cattle. In warm weather, swine should be moved outdoors in early morning or late afternoon only, to reduce the risk of overheating. Hogs move best if moved in small groups. Groups of 3–6 are recommended. Large groups tend to scatter or, if cornered, they may pile on top of each other. Alleyways for moving hogs should be 18–20 in (46–50.8 cm) wide. Trained adult hogs should be able to be moved by the handler walking next to the hog, just behind its shoulder, and guiding it with a cane by taps on the shoulders and neck.

In total indoor confinement operations, piglets are not allowed to learn to follow their mother. At weaning, they are separated from older swine.

Handlers of indoor confined pigs should begin to train them for being herded just after weaning. Training should involve being rubbed and scratched for short periods after being fed. Small reward treats should be offered. Later training periods should include being gently pushed in different directions and being briefly picked up and gently put down. Eventually, moving them in groups of 5 or 6 in a small pen (10 × 10 ft [3 × 3 m]) and up ramps without generating any excitement should be practiced.

Distractions to eliminate

Like cattle, swine are reluctant to walk on strange flooring, move toward darkness, or go past a dangling or wiggly object on fences. They should be moved toward better-lit areas (but not blinding light), over familiar flooring without sharp contrasts in color or texture (cover with bedding if needed), and in alleyways without clutter for herding. Portable solid sorting panels can block distractions and aid in directing the movement of swine. Side-by-side alleyways with a see-through septation panel in the middle facilitates forward movement, allowing two pigs to move abreast.

Canes, poles, and paddles

Canes and poles can be useful in moving hogs. After brief introductory training, gently tapping the sides of the pig's or hog's face, neck, and shoulders with a cane or pole can redirect a hog without generating excitement. If canes or poles are used abusively, hogs may become frantic or aggressive. Rattle paddles can be more effective for hogs that are not trained to accept canes and poles.

Sorting panels

Sorting panels (also called "hurdles") are flat panels of wood, plastic, or metal that are helpful in sorting, loading, and restraining pigs and hogs. They should be at least as tall as the hog and at least two-thirds as long (**Figure 14.9**). Panels have small holes along the top edge or one side for the handler's hands, but they should not have holes that allow the hog to see through or it will not change direction, and instead will try to push through or under the panel. The smoothest side of the panel should be presented to the hog. The top should be tilted toward the handler and the bottom

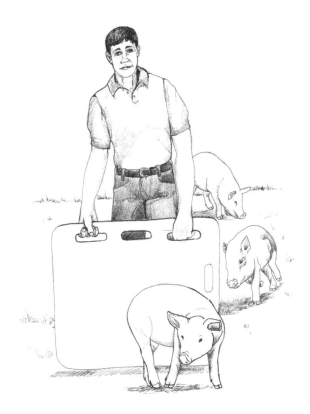

Fig. 14.9 Sorting panel.

pressed on the floor and braced with the handler's foot to prevent the hog from rooting under the bottom.

Backing bucket

If a hog's head is covered with a bucket, it will move backward quickly. The speed and direction of retreat can be guided by a second handler holding its tail to move a hog short distances. If hogs are in an alleyway and cannot turn, a scoop shovel in front of their face may aid in backing them toward a desired destination.

Rope harness

A rope harness for a pig can be created by putting a non-constricting loop tied with a bowline knot over its neck and a half-hitch around its thorax. The harness can be effective for controlling the movement of pigs up to about 100 lb (45.4 kg).

Plastic trash can on wheels

Weanling pigs and small pigs can be moved short distances with less stress to the pigs in a plastic trash can on wheels or a wheelbarrow with high sides.

Carrying or lifting pigs

Small pigs (less than 10 lb [4.5 kg]) can be scooped up with a hand under the body or caught by a hind leg and then grasped under their torso for their comfort and a feeling of security. They should never be grabbed by their ears.

Larger pigs (10–50 lb [4.5–22.7 kg]) can be caught by a hind leg, held by both legs proximal to their hocks, and swung between the handler's legs for procedures involving the back half of their body. The pig is pinned with the handler's knees behind their shoulders while being held inverted by the hind legs. Hogs will attempt to raise their head and push away from the handler with their front legs. High-topped boots are advisable because some hogs will bite the handler's legs during this technique.

For procedures involving the front half of their body, pigs are caught by a front leg and restrained by holding both front legs with their body pinned between the handler's legs. This method is best performed with thick leather gloves to protect the hands from the possibility of being bitten during the restraint.

Hogs more than 50 lb (22.7 kg) should be lifted into an inverted position by two people, each holding one hind leg.

HANDLING FOR COMMON MEDICAL PROCEDURES

Most handling and restraint of hogs can be and should be done WITHOUT tranquilization, sedation, hypnosis, or anesthesia. However, some handling and restraint procedures are restricted to veterinary medical professionals because of the potential danger to the animal or handler. These require special skills, equipment, or facilities, and possibly adjunct chemical restraint.

Restraint of individual hogs and pigs or parts of their bodies

Whole body restraint

V-troughs

V-shaped troughs can be used to restrain pigs under 50 lb (22.7 kg) on their backs for blood samples from the cranial vena cava. V-troughs can be tilted head down or head up depending on the needs of the procedure being performed.

Canvas slings

Canvas slings with holes for each leg and an access hole for the neck can be used for collecting blood from the cranial vena cava in hogs under 50 lb (22.7 kg). This is less stressful and more comfortable for the hog, and it provides better restraint than V-troughs, but it is not as flexible in holding a variety of sizes of pigs as the V-trough.

Lateral restraint and casting methods

Placing a small pig under 50 lb (22.7 kg) in lateral recumbency can be done by reaching over its torso and grasping the front and hind leg on the side nearest the handler's body, picking it up and gently sliding it down the handler's body and onto its side.

For larger pigs up to 80 lb (36.3 kg) the same technique can be used by first snubbing the pig by its snout and tying it low to a post. A short rope with loops on each end is used. The loops are placed below the dewclaws on a front and hind leg on the same side. The handler stands on the side with the tied legs, and the mid part of the rope is pulled under the hog and upward, causing the hog to lie on its side. The handler continues to hold the rope and places a knee just behind the hog's shoulder to maintain the restraint. Laying pigs in lateral restraint should be smooth and allow the animal to slide down the handler's body or legs into lateral recumbency.

For hogs more than 100 lb (45.4 kg), a hock hobble can be used to lay a hog in lateral recumbency. A hock hobble is a snubbing rope applied around the upper jaw with the standing end then run to a hind leg, where a loop is applied above the hock. The snout is then pulled toward the hind leg, forcing the hog to lie on its side.

Large hogs, those over 300 lb (136.1 kg), can be laid on their side using half-hitches around the trunk of their body in the same manner as using half-hitches to cast cattle. The hog is caught with a snout snare, and, using a rope at least 15 ft (4.6 m) long, a loop is placed around the neck and tied with a bowline knot. The standing end of the rope is then placed around the chest and flank with a couple of half-hitches. Steady pulling on the end of the rope will cause the hog to lie down on its side.

Restraint of the head

Restraint of the head using halters or stanchions is not possible with swine. Hog snares or snubbing ropes restrain the head as much as is possible without chemical restraint.

Asian pot-bellied pigs

Asian (miniature) pot-bellied pigs, from Vietnam, have fat rolls over their eyes and a pot-belly, and are swayback. Pot-bellied pigs became a fad pet in the U.S. during the 1980s. Although less popular now, they are still occasionally kept as pets and not treated like livestock. Handling and restraint are more like the techniques used for dogs than for swine raised for meat production. Support slings can be useful in physical restraint of pet pigs.

Dogs and pot-bellied pigs in the same household can cause problems because of competition for food and toys. Pot-bellied pigs are uneasy about being picked up. They will struggle and can easily be dropped and injured.

In moderate climates, they may be housed outdoors or indoors. However, they are very sensitive to heat and cold weather. The preferred temperature range is 65–75°F (18.3–24°C). Outdoor housing should provide at least 50 sq ft (1.9 m²) for each pig. Hay or straw should be provided for rooting and chewing. A shelter (3-sided shed or large dog house) from severe weather and sunlight should be provided. The pen and enclosure should be movable and relocated as soon as the pen's dirt has been rooted throughout the pen. If the pig is housed on concrete, the pen should be cleaned daily and fresh hay or straw added 3 or 4 times per week.

Pot-bellied pigs need to have regular hoof trims about every 6 months if confined in pens with dirt and no abrasive surfaces (rocks, concrete, etc.). Males should be castrated at 2–3 months of age. If they are not, boars more than 2 years of age can grow to more than 100 lb (45.4 kg) and become aggressive and dangerous. Permanent canine teeth (tusks) should be trimmed at 1 year of age and annually thereafter. This requires chemical restraint.

Injections and venipuncture
Access to veins

The blood vessel used for venipuncture in hogs is usually the right jugular or cranial vena cava (but not in miniature pigs). The left jugular is less desirable because it lies close to the phrenic nerve, which could be inadvertently injured and cause paralysis of the diaphragm. The lateral saphenous or central or lateral ear veins are used less commonly. Restraint depends on the size of the pig or hog and usually involves a snare, single-file alleyway, or crate.

The coccygeal vein of the tail may be accessible in large hogs that have not been docked, and in adult miniature pigs.

The jugular vein is used for venipuncture of pigs less than 30 lb (13.6 kg). They are laid in ventrodorsal recumbency on a handler's lap or in a V-trough. The pig's head is tilted down and the front legs pulled back by an assistant. The phlebotomist holds the head extended with his non-dominant hand while performing venipuncture. Alternatively, canvas slings can be used for restraint to perform venipuncture on a jugular vein.

Injections

Intramuscular

Intramuscular (IM) injections are given to hogs in the side of the neck, 2–3 in (5–8 cm) behind and below the ear (**Figure 14.10**). Physical restraint is often not necessary. Due to the lack of muscle elsewhere, small piglets are given IM injections in the semitendinosus and semimembranosus muscles of the hind leg.

Subcutaneous

Pigs are given subcutaneous injections under the loose skin of the axilla behind a front leg or the flank fold while restrained by the inverted standing leg hold (**Figure 14.11**). Hogs are injected at the base of the ear, often without restraint.

Administration of oral medications

Oral administration of medications to swine is done by adding the medication to their feed or water. Although oral examinations can be performed with a hand paddle oral speculum, this is not practical for repeated administration of oral medications. Piglets or small pet pigs may be medicated by being held vertical, head up, while an assistant administers liquid medication with an oral syringe.

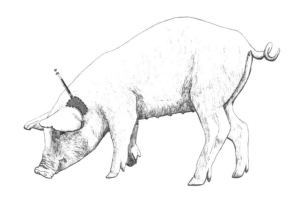

Fig. 14.10 Intramuscular injection site in hogs.

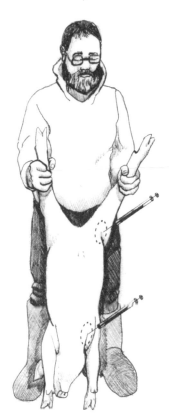

Fig. 14.11 Subcutaneous injection site in pigs.

TRANSPORTING SWINE

When possible, swine should be loaded into transport vehicles from a level surface (a loading platform) rather than up a ramp into a transport vehicle. If a loading ramp is necessary, it should be less than 20 degrees with cleats. Cleats on ramps for adult pigs should be 8 in (20 cm) apart and closer for smaller pigs. Swine will move up solid ramps better than slatted ramps with gaps. The ramp should be covered with bedding used in transport vehicle.

Loading chutes for hogs should have solid outside walls to prevent them from seeing handlers, have 22–30 in (55.9–76.2 cm) wide divisions to prevent them from turning around in the chute, and allow a handler to walk behind them. Center partitions in the chute should be see-through so hogs can see other hogs moving forward. Small groups (3–6 pigs) should be loaded at a time.

Transport vehicle partitions should be used to pen up to 20–25 hogs together. Mature hogs from different groups should not be mixed together, as there would be fighting. Mature boars should be penned individually. In hot weather, transported swine should be in a covered vehicle, bedded with moist sand, have openings in the trailer sides for ventilation, and be hauled in the coolest part of day. Extra space for each hog should be allowed and the vents

adjusted to promote ventilation during travel. In cold weather, the top and most side openings should be closed, and straw or wood shavings bedding provided. The transport vehicle should be cleaned and disinfected after each use.

SELECTED FURTHER READING

Kilbride AL, Mendl M, Statham P, et al. (2012). A cohort study of preweaning piglet mortality and farrowing accommodation on 112 commercial pig farms in England. *Preventive Veterinary Medicine* 104:281–291.

Klober K (2009). *Storey's Guide to Raising Pigs*, 3rd edition. Storey Publishing, North Adams.

Parsons TD, Deen J (2015). How complexity of animal welfare issues can foster differences within the veterinary profession. *Journal of the American Veterinary Medical Association* 247:240–241.

Stephens DB, Perry GC (1990). The effects of restraint, handling, simulated and real transport in the pig (with reference to man and other species). *Applied Animal Behaviour Science* 28:41–55.

Poultry are birds raised for food or fiber. They include chickens, turkeys, ducks, geese, guineafowl, and ratites (ostriches, emus, and rheas).

Chickens (*Gallus gallus domesticus*) were domesticated from *Gallus gallus*, the red jungle fowl, in India and southeast Asia about 8,000 years ago as a source of meat, eggs, feathers, and leather. Turkeys are indigenous to North America and the Yucatan peninsula of Mexico. They were domesticated from the wild turkey (*Meleagris gallopavo*) about 2,000 years ago by Mesoamericans as a source of meat and feathers and introduced to Spanish conquistadores by the Aztecs. Turkeys were brought to Europe around 1519 by the Spanish and then spread throughout Europe. The name "turkey" came from a misidentification with guineafowl, from the country of Turkey. They were originally called turkey fowl and later just turkeys.

Ducks may have first been domesticated from the mallard, *Anas platyrhynchos*, in China and southeast Asia 6,000 years ago. They are raised for their meat, eggs, and down feathers. Ducks can also aid in controlling slugs and snails. Mallards are dabbling ducks, meaning that they tip their heads into the water and filter water through their beaks for food without completely submerging their body.

Geese were domesticated from the greylag goose, *Anser anser*, by the Egyptians about 5,000 years ago and also kept for their meat, eggs, and down. They were later valued by the Romans and by people during the Middle Ages throughout Europe. Geese can also eat overgrown grass and weeds without compacting the soil, fertilize lawns with their manure, guard property as a trespasser and predator sentinel, and control snakes. They will also eat small frogs, mice, and baby rats.

Guineafowl (primarily *Numida meleagris*) were domesticated 4,500 years ago in Africa for meat, eggs, and pest control. They were brought to Europe in the 15th century by Portuguese explorers and to North America by early settlers. They are sometimes kept as predator sentinels for other poultry.

Ostriches, emus, and rheas are open-grassland birds that do not fly. Ostriches (*Struthio camelus*) are from Africa. They were raised first for their feathers in the late 1800s to be used in hats and fans and later in the 1900s for their meat, eggs, leather, and oil. In the 1980s, ostrich raising became popular in the U.S., in part because of a ban on trading with South Africa. Interest in raising emus and rheas followed. Emus (*Dromaius novaehollandiae*) are from Australia and have been raised for meat, eggs, feathers, leather, and oil. Rheas include greater rheas (*Rhea americana*) and lesser rheas (*Rhea pennata*), which are both native to South America. They have been raised primarily for their feathers and to a lesser extent for meat, eggs, leather, and oil. Ostriches are the largest birds in the world (6–9 ft [1.8–2.7 m] tall and up to 350 lb [158.8 kg]). Emus are the largest bird in Australia (5 ft [1.5 m] tall, weighing about 150 lb [68 kg]), and rheas are the largest birds in the Americas (4–5 ft [1.2–1.5 m], weighing about 80 lb [36.3 kg]). Ostriches can run at 40 mph, which is faster than any other two-legged animal in the world. Wild males have harems of 2–7 females. Ostriches do not stick their heads in the sand, but they will lie flat on the ground as a passive defense.

All adult female poultry are *hens*, although a female goose may be called a *goose*. A female chicken under 1 year old is a *pullet*. Male adult poultry are *cocks*; more specifically, a male chicken is a *rooster*, a male turkey is a *tom*, a male duck is a *drake*, a male goose is a *gander*. A castrated male chicken is a *capon*. A young male chicken under 1 year old is a *cockerel*, a cockerel at 8–12 weeks of age is a *broiler*, and a pullet or cockerel that is 3–5 months old is a *roaster*. A young turkey of either sex is a *poult*, and a young male turkey is a *jake*. Young geese are *goslings*, and young ducks are *ducklings*. *Ratites* are large, flightless birds without a keel bone.

NATURAL BEHAVIOR OF POULTRY

All poultry are highly social and disturbed by isolation. In their natural environments, they spend nearly all their waking time foraging for food by pecking seeds, worms, larvae, and insects to eat, picking up sand and gravel for their gizzards, and investigating their surroundings. Dust-bathing occurs in the middle of the day several times per week. Areas with trees are preferred by small poultry to be used for roosting at night.

Strange birds of the same species added suddenly to an established group will be attacked and injured or killed. Owing to the danger from predators, females prefer to hide to lay eggs, and young birds are closely bound to wherever their mother goes.

Young poultry with prominent keel bones and large pectoral muscles, such as some domestic chickens, turkeys, and ducks, are capable of flying short distances and will perch or climb onto elevated resting spots. Turkeys will also spontaneously run short distances in a playful manner. Ratites have small pectoral muscles, no keel, and cannot fly.

Normal behavior of unstressed adult turkeys with sufficient room for exercise includes wing-flapping, feather ruffling, leg stretching, and dust-bathing. In the wild, they feed on leaves, seeds, berries, and insects by foraging and pecking off the ground and lower plants. Turkeys can fly short distances and they roost in trees at night.

Most chickens and turkeys are raised commercially in high-density confinement. Aggressiveness is enhanced by overcrowding. Head pecking of submissive or injured birds can be brutal and eventually kill the new member of the flock. Feather pecking is also common in poultry confined on metal or concrete surfaces. In these environments, birds do not have the opportunity to forage or receive the mental stimulation it provides.

Guineafowl stay in close groups and are ravenous foragers, eating flying and crawling insects, ticks, worms, grubs, and snails. They will surround and attack small rodents, marauding birds, and snakes. They sleep in trees at night.

Ducks and geese get natural exercise by paddling through water. It is important for them to have sufficient water to immerse their bill and eyes in order to clean their face.

Ratite refers to a type of bird with a flat raft-like sternum and small pectoral muscles that cannot fly. All ratites have muscular legs and elongated nails and are capable of swift running and lethal kicks. Ostriches are the most aggressive and powerful. Ratites are not domesticated and can only become marginally tame.

SAFETY FIRST

Handler safety

Most poultry protect themselves with escape by running or short flights. When escape is not possible, they will peck, scratch, and bat their wings. Chickens and turkeys may attack a handler perceived to be weak, particularly small children. Injuries can occur from poultry wings during panic flying within an enclosure or from being improperly held. Aggressive chickens will peck and scratch, and roosters with spurs will use them to poke and scratch. Turkeys can inflict severe blows with their wings, but geese are more likely to use battery with their wings as a defense or offense. Geese will also peck with their beak and rake with their toes. Ducks are less prone to resisting handling with defensive pecking and scratching.

Indoor confinement of poultry can expose handlers to excessive noise, and ear protection must be considered. Respiratory problems are also common in poultry handlers when the poultry are confined indoors. The primary causes of respiratory problems are organic dust composed of feathers, bacteria, and fungi, and ammonia from excrement containing urea. Appropriately rated respiratory masks should be worn and poultry houses frequently cleaned and well ventilated.

Ratites, especially ostriches, are unpredictable and potentially dangerous. The natural predator of ostriches is the African lion, which they can usually outrun and, when necessary, fight with a forward kick that can be fatal. Adult males during the breeding season are especially dangerous. They have a powerful forward and downward strike with a leg and sharp claws on two toes that can that can rip a handler's abdomen open or tear a femoral artery. Emus and rheas also strike forward with their feet. They both have three toes with a sharp claw on each.

> A handler should never stand directly in front of a ratite.

Male ratites are very territorial and aggressive during breeding seasons, especially ostriches. An agitated male will stand tall and bump its chest against objects, hiss, gape its mouth, and flap its wings. A handler should never go into an ostrich pen without an assistant nearby. Humans cannot out-run an ostrich. If a handler is charged in the open by a male ostrich, it is recommended to lie flat on the ground to avoid a forward kick. Ostriches cannot kick low at an object on or near the ground.

Ratites will peck at any shiny object. Handlers should not wear sunglasses or jewelry when around ratites.

Poultry safety

Chicken pullets and turkey poults have their beaks trimmed because of territorial aggression and risk of feather picking and cannibalism (**Figure 15.1**). Hatcheries trim chick beaks using a beak-trimming machine at 6–8 days of age, but this can be performed up to 16 weeks of age. Turkey poults are trimmed at 2–5 weeks of age. This is done by cutting approximately one-half of the upper beak and blunting the lower beak. Beak-trimming machines cauterize the cut as it is made, which prevents regrowth. If manual nippers are used, the beak will regrow.

The causes for feather picking and cannibalism can be varied, but overcrowding and boredom are factors. Providing at least 4 sq ft (0.4 m²) of space for each chicken in a coop and 10 sq ft (0.9 m²) in runs with an opportunity to forage, i.e. investigate and search for food, often prevents or eliminates feather picking in chickens.

Chickens will also peck at rooster combs, and roosters can cause injuries with their claws that lead to cannibalism of the injured bird. These problems are important in raising chickens in concentrated confinement. Preventive procedures used in commercial breeding of chickens are dubbing of the comb, removal of the comb of young roosters, and toe dubbing, the removal of toes of breeding roosters.

The snood of turkeys is particularly vulnerable to being pecked by other turkeys. The snood may be excised up to 3 weeks of age in situations where fighting or pecking has been a problem. Clipping of the two inside toes to remove the nails may be done at hatcheries to prevent scratches and skin tears to other turkeys when the turkeys are older and kept in close confinement.

Proposed rules to the USDA to permit organic production of poultry labeling would prohibit beak trimming, desnooding, dewattling, and removal of combs. Poultry would have to be allowed sufficient room for freedom of movement and the ability to engage in natural behaviors. The incidence of lameness would also have to be monitored.

Although providing poultry spaces to forage outdoors can eliminate common aggression injuries, poultry with access to the outdoors are endangered by a wide variety of predators, such as hawks, owls, foxes, coyotes, and roaming dogs. Rodent control is important indoors and outdoors. In addition to eating grain and spreading disease, rats will kill chicks and poults. Ducks are able to escape from predators in the wild more effectively than other poultry. Although most species of duck sleep on the ground and are more vulnerable to predators, they can sleep literally with one eye open and escape by water or air.

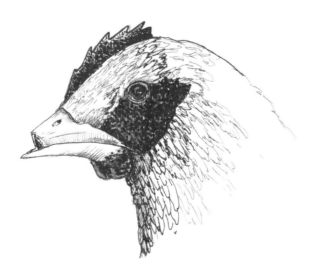

Fig. 15.1 Debeaked chicken.

Handlers signaling their presence near poultry by speaking in a normal tone and moving smoothly, rather than erratically, reduces the risk of small poultry piling up from being startled and smothering.

Key zoonoses

(*Note.* Apparently ill animals should be handled by veterinary professionals or under their supervision. Precautionary measures against zoonoses from ill animals are more involved than those required when handling apparently healthy animals and vary widely. The discussion here is directed primarily at handling apparently healthy animals.)

Apparently healthy poultry pose little risk of transmitting disease to healthy adult handlers who practice conventional personal hygiene. The risks of physical injury are greater than the risks of acquiring an infectious disease. However, most poultry are not routinely handled, and feathers can hide signs of many illnesses (*Table 15.1*).

Direct transmission
Systemic disease

Avian influenza (fowl plague) is caused by an influenza A virus that is able to mutate to a form that can affect humans as a potentially fatal systemic disease with predominately respiratory signs. The disease in

Table 15.1 Diseases transmitted from healthy appearing poultry to healthy adult humans

DISEASE	AGENT	MEANS OF TRANSMISSION	SIGNS AND SYMPTOMS IN HUMANS	FREQUENCY IN ANIMALS	RISK GROUP*
Bites and clawing	–	Direct injury	Bite wounds to face, arms, and legs	All poultry are capable of inflicting bite or claw wounds, or both	2
Salmonellosis	*Salmonella enteritidis* and other spp.	Direct from handling poultry; indirect from fomites (cages, bowls)	Diarrhea, systemic disease and abscesses	Common	3
Campylobacteriosis	*Campylobacter jejuni, C. coli*	Direct, fecal-oral	Diarrhea	Common, but transmission primarily by eating undercooked poultry	2
Avian influenza	Influenza A, H5N1 virus	Direct from poultry respiratory secretions	Influenza signs and symptoms (respiratory)	Possible if exposed to wild birds; outbreaks devastating to poultry flocks	3
Ornithosis	*Chlamydophila psittaci*	Direct from respiratory secretions or fecal matter	Pneumonia	Rare	3
Newcastle disease	Avian paramyxovirus	Direct	Conjunctivitis	Rare in U.S. due to vaccine	2
Poultry mites	*Dermanyssus gallinae*	Direct and indirect from fomites	Itchy skin with red bumps	Common	2

* Risk Groups (National Institutes of Health and World Health Organization criteria. Centers for Disease Control and Prevention, *Biosafety in Microbiological and Biomedical Laboratories*, 5th edition, 2009):
  1 Agent not associated with disease in healthy adult humans.
  2 Agent rarely causes serious disease and prevention or therapy possible.
  3 Agent can cause serious or lethal disease and prevention or therapy possible.
  4 Agent can cause serious or lethal disease and prevention or therapy are not usually available.

birds is highly contagious, affecting fowl, turkeys, pheasants, ducks and many wild species, but rarely waterbirds and pigeons. Clinically, there is a short course and very heavy mortality. Infected birds that survive have a nasal discharge, white spots on the comb and wattles, and swelling of the head and neck. Some strains, notably H5N1 and H7N9, have emerged as the cause of rare, but fatal, human infections. Precautions include keeping poultry away from wild birds and promptly reporting any possible cases of avian influenza to state agriculture and public health authorities. The risk of avian influenza in handlers of poultry that are apparently healthy and not overcrowded or stressed is extremely low, particularly if the poultry are protected from contact with wild birds.

Listeriosis (*Listeria monocytogenes*) is a common bacterial disease in poultry. Affected birds usually appear healthy. Transmission to humans is by ingestion of poorly processed poultry products, raw poultry, or undercooked poultry.

Tuberculosis (*Mycobacterium avium*) is a rare disease of poultry. Free range poultry may acquire it from wild birds and transmit it to handlers, but poultry usually do not live long enough to acquire and transmit the disease.

The systemic dimorphic fungal diseases histoplasmosis and blastomycosis can occur in birds and be transmitted in their feces. However, the infectious form develops in excreted fecal matter. These diseases are not transmitted directly from handling birds but possibly from their contaminated containments, such as roosts and cages.

Respiratory disease

Ornithosis (*Chlamydophila psittaci*) is a bacterial respiratory disease of poultry caused by the same organism that causes psittacosis in caged companion birds. The bacteria can be transmitted to humans by exposure to infected bird nasal secretions or feces. Humans can develop pneumonia if infected with ornithosis.

Newcastle disease, caused by Newcastle disease virus, affects domestic poultry, causing severe nervous and respiratory signs usually resulting in death of the bird. However, Amazon parrots may be able to carry the virus without signs. It can infect humans causing mild conjunctivitis and influenza-like illness.

Digestive tract disease

Salmonellosis can cause severe diarrhea and sometimes enter the bloodstream from the digestive tract to infect organs throughout the body. Overcrowding and other stresses cause increased transmission and susceptibility to salmonellosis. Basic sanitary handling eliminates most risk to handlers. Salmonella from poultry is primarily acquired from undercooked poultry or eggs.

Nearly all poultry should be considered carriers of campylobacteriosis, even if they have no signs of disease. It is one of the most common causes of bacterial diarrhea in humans. Contact with poultry can be a source if the bacteria gain access to a handler's mouth. Most human cases are from drinking unpasteurized milk or eating undercooked poultry.

Skin disease

The avian red mite (*Dermanyssus gallinae*) can be directly or indirectly transmitted to humans. The bite of the mite can cause intense itching and pinpoint red bites in the skin.

Erysipeloid is caused by a bacterium (*Erysipelothrix rhusiopathiae*) that can be transmitted from infected turkeys to humans through cuts and abrasions in human skin. Erysipeloid dermatitis in humans is a swollen, itchy, skin rash.

Vector borne

There are no vector transmitted zoonotic diseases from healthy appearing poultry.

Sanitary practices

Persons handling poultry should wear appropriate dress to protect against skin contamination through feathers, skin scales, urine, and other body secretions. Basic sanitary practices should be adhered to, such as keeping hands away from eyes, nose, and mouth when handling poultry and washing hands after handling them. Eating and drinking in poultry-containment or handling areas should be prohibited. Cleaning of food and water bowls and handling equipment should be done outside of human living quarters.

Special precautions are needed when sick poultry are handled, and these should be isolated from apparently normal poultry. New flock members should be quarantined for at least 2 weeks to reduce the risk of transmitting a disease that new birds could be incubating before introducing to the rest of the flock.

APPROACHING, CATCHING, AND ROUTINE HANDLING

Chickens

Chickens that are handled early in life and frequently as adults will offer no resistance nor appear distressed when gently handled. Those in large groups and having little to no experience of being handled in the past will pile on top of each other in a corner, resulting in injuries and fatalities. If caught, such a chicken will flap its wings and scratch trying to free itself.

Chickens that are handled on a regular basis will eat grain from a handler's hand. They can be easily picked up by grasping them on both sides of the body and restraining the wings next to their body. The wings should not be held tightly enough to impair the chicken's respirations.

Untrained chickens may be captured by hand while in a small enclosure or after a small group is herded to a corner of their enclosure using a folding mesh wire panel. Each panel unit should be 2 ft (0.6 m) wide and 3–4 ft (1–1.2 m) high for adult chickens. The handler should pin the group close enough together that they have just enough room to stand. If they pile on top of each other, more room should be provided. If a small enclosure is not available or the bird is on free range, a capture net can be used. Nets can be used on other poultry too, but the net should be the appropriate size for the bird, have a useful handle length, and possess a padded rim.

If the time of day is not important for the capture, all poultry can be caught more easily in an environment of subdued or blue light. Waiting until evening when they are roosting may be the least stressful time to capture chickens. Placing a cloth over a restrained chicken's head can simulate nighttime and calm the bird.

When capturing a chicken, the wings and body are grasped with both hands at the same time to immobilize the wings (**Figure 15.2**). The grip should be firm

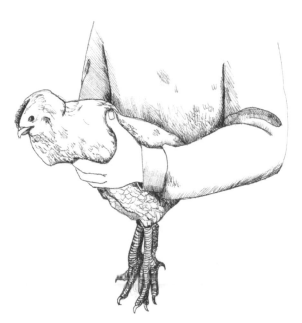

Fig. 15.2 Restraint of a chicken.

enough to provide restraint, but care must be taken not to impede the respiratory movements of the chest. Capture should be as quiet and smooth as possible to avoid upsetting the rest of the flock. The chicken must be held firmly since, if untrained, there will be repeated attempts to escape after periods of rest. The body should always be supported during restraint, and chickens should not be carried only by the legs to avoid injuring the bird. During a release, the handler should return the bird to the ground or floor gently. The bird should not be dropped to the floor.

Restraint of a bird can be done with one hand over its back, making a ring around its neck with thumb and forefinger while supporting the body by loosely wrapping the other three fingers around its body and trapping the legs between the ring and small fingers.

Birds older than 13 weeks should be carried by both wings and both legs. Poultry should never be held by the head, one wing, or one leg. The result will be injury to the bird and possible injury to the handler from the bird struggling in panic. The panic will also spread through the rest of the flock. Grabbing chickens by the leg and holding them upside down increases the risk of injury. Being returned to a flock with an injury could result in a chicken being attacked by other members of the flock. Chickens from battery cages are more likely to have demineralized bone from lack of exercise, and fractures may result from being restrained by the legs.

To remove a chicken from a cage, the handler should reach in and pin the body down and then turn its head toward the cage door. While keeping the hand on top of the bird, the handler should then slide the other hand underneath the bird to grasp the legs, with the index finger between the legs and the thumb just above the hock on one side, and the other fingers above the hock on the other side. The leg tendons are squeezed to extend the legs backward. With the handler using both hands, the bird is removed from the cage head first. The chicken can be carried in the same position with its head between the handler's arm and body. To return the bird to a cage, it is rotated in the handler's hands and placed in the cage head first and placed on its feet.

Guineafowl

Guineafowl are approached, captured, and handled in the same manner as chickens.

Turkeys

The handler should herd 10 or fewer turkeys into a catch pen with a sorting panel in the same manner as chickens. The turkey to be captured is approached from behind. The handler kneels and grasps a wing where it joins the body and the legs between the hocks and the feet, holding the hocks straight, and then places the turkey's breast on a platform, such as a bale of straw. If no platform is present, the breast can be rested on the handler's knee. A mature bird,

which may weigh more than 50 lb (22.7 kg), should be lifted from a kneeling position by the handler's leg strength while his or her back remains straight in order to prevent back injury. Turkeys can be carried by a handler with one arm, holding the legs with the hand and wrapping the arm around the bird's body with the head directed behind the handler.

Domestic turkey hens are generally docile, but toms can be aggressive and should be watched more closely when a handler is in a pen with one. Male turkeys normally have a pale or blue-colored head. Aggressiveness may be signaled by the fleshy parts of the head becoming engorged with blood and red colored.

Waterfowl

The trachea of birds has complete cartilaginous rings and can withstand more compression than the trachea of mammals. Geese and ducks, with their long necks, can be safely captured for restraint by grasping their necks and then their wings and feet (**Figure 15.3**). Compression on their chest must be mild to avoid inhibiting their breathing.

Ducks

The handler grasps the duck's neck from behind without firmly pressing on the trachea and esophagus in front. While pulling the duck upward, the wings are grasped near their attachment with the body with the other hand. The hand on the neck is then moved beneath the body to support the duck's body weight (**Figure 15.4**). The chest, abdomen,

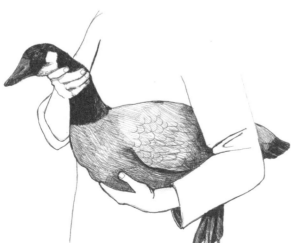

Fig. 15.3 Restraint of a goose.

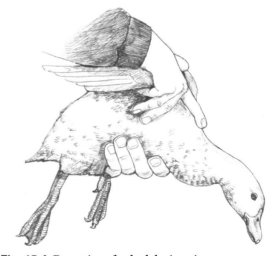

Fig. 15.4 Restraint of a duck by its wings.

and legs should not be restrained. A second method is to grasp the neck and then tuck the body under the other arm and against the handler's side, with the duck's head pointing behind the handler.

The release from being held should be with a sliding movement near the ground as if the duck is landing on water so the feet will extend and support the body.

Ducks are nocturnal feeders and have excellent night vision. Dimming lights in a handling room is not effective in reducing their reactivity.

Geese

Geese can usually be captured after herding into a small enclosure. They walk slowly and should not be hurried or they will become panicked and stressed. Catch pens should not be overcrowded. Too many geese in the enclosure at one time can cause piling, and suffocation might result. If a catch pen is not available, a neck crook or an appropriately sized and constructed net may be used. A handler should remain mindful that geese can cause painful blows with their wings and deep scratches with their feet.

To capture a goose, a handler grasps its neck and then the base of the wings. Both wings can be held with one hand. After the goose is picked up, the handler must maintain his or her grasp on the neck, just below the goose's head, or the goose may peck at the handler's face.

Ratites

Ratites should be herded into a small collection pen for capture. An approach to an adult ratite should always be from behind. Ratites can strike forward with their toes.

If a chick weighs less than 12 lb (5.4 kg), the handler should support the whole body. If it weighs 12–30 lb (5.4–13.6 kg), the handler should put a hand around the bird's body, pick it up, and allow the legs to dangle.

Juveniles are 4–12 months old. They should be moved to a small collection pen with solid walls or caught with portable panels that have been covered with plastic or plywood. A T-shaped or V-shaped long-handled push pole is helpful in directing and sorting ratites. High-topped leather boots and leather chaps can provide some protection against a forward kick. Juveniles may be moved by being held loosely in front of their chest with one arm and the other arm behind its rump while walking beside it.

Plywood or plastic shields can be used in a manner similar to hog-sorting panels to move ratites, but an adult ostrich can still knock a handler with a shield down with a kick. Movable squeeze chutes can be constructed that are designed like a large notebook binder.

Putting a hood over a ratite's head will make it more manageable. Commercial ratite hoods can be used, or a lightweight sleeve or sock with the toe cut out will suffice. Non-aggressive ostriches can be lured by grain in a bucket and hooded by grasping their beak with a hood everted over the hand. The hood is rolled off the hand and over the ostrich's head. Hoods should cover the eyes and about one-third down the neck, but not cover the nostrils. If the ostrich tolerates the hood, it may be possible to lead it without incident. Large ostriches should be led by three handlers, one on each wing and one to gently push the bird forward and guide it.

Eight-foot-long neck crooks can be used on ostriches just below the head to get their head down below the level of their back, thus preventing them from striking forward. The ostrich will pull back when its head is restrained. Thus an assistant is needed to keep the bird from backing up while its head is being held down. The first handler, while keeping the crook on the bird's neck, must move forward to place a hood.

An emu's or rhea's head or neck should not be grasped or hooded, because they do not tolerate handling of the head as well as ostriches. Emus have thin, fragile skin. Their head and neck have little muscle or soft tissue protection from injury, and their trachea can be easily collapsed. Emus and rheas are approached from behind and grasped around their wings, lifted up, and tipped back slightly, or they can be slowly pushed toward the ground and straddled while holding their neck.

Level loading bays to transport vehicles are recommended because ratites are reluctant to walk up inclines. Transport vehicles should provide enough room for the bird's head when it is standing.

HANDLING FOR COMMON MEDICAL PROCEDURES

Injections and venipuncture
Access to veins
Small poultry
Small poultry are held on their side on a table for venipuncture. The handler uses one hand to hold the legs with one finger between the bird's legs, while the other hand elevates the uppermost wing over the bird's back. The phlebotomist accesses the wing (brachial) vein (**Figure 15.5**).

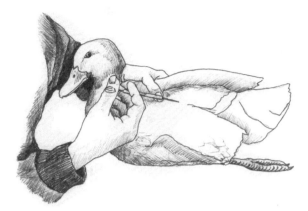

Fig. 15.5 Venipuncture of a brachial vein in the wing of a goose.

Ratites
A brachial vein is used for venipuncture in adult ostriches. The neck cannot be adequately restrained to safely access the jugular vein in ostriches. The ostrich is hooded and restrained with its head below the level of its back with an assistant to keep it from backing up while the wing vein is accessed. Rheas or emus are grasped around the wings from behind and picked up slightly and back. Venipuncture is done from a jugular vein or medial metatarsal leg vein.

Injections
Intramuscular
To administer an intramuscular (IM) injection, a handler holds small poultry by both legs with one hand with an index finger between the legs, and the other hand holds both wings at their base. The injection is given by another person into the pectoral muscle of the chest (**Figure 15.6**). Ratites are held in the same manner as for venipuncture to administer an IM injection into the pectoral muscles or thigh muscles.

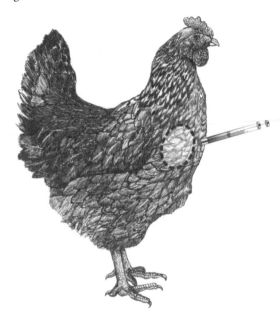

Fig. 15.6 Intramuscular injection site in poultry.

Subcutaneous
Subcutaneous injections are given to poultry in the wing web at the base of the wings. The same restraint as needed for IM injections is used.

Administration of oral medications
Most vaccines and medications for flocks are administered in the drinking water or by aerosol and do not involve handling or restraint.

SELECTED FURTHER READING

Damerow, G (2010). *Storey's Guide to Raising Poultry*, 3rd edition. Storey Publishing, North Adams.

Drowns, G (2012). *Storey's Guide to Raising Poultry*, 4th edition: Chickens, Turkey, Ducks, Geese, Guineas, Game Birds. Storey Publishing, North Adams.

Gauthier J, Ludlow R (2013). *Chicken Health for Dummies*. John Wiley & Sons, Somerset.

Greenacre CB, Morishita TY (2014). *Backyard Poultry Medicine and Surgery: A Guide for Veterinary Practitioners*. Wiley-Blackwell, Ames.

Ackerman N, Aspinall V (2016). *Aspinall's Complete Textbook of Veterinary Nursing*, 3rd edition. Elsevier, St. Louis.

Anderson RS, Edney ATB (1991). *Practical Animal Handling*. Pergamon Press, Oxford.

Angulo FJ, Glaser CA, Juranek DD, et al. (1994) Caring for pets of immunocompromised persons. *Journal of the American Veterinary Medical Association* 205: 1711–1718.

Ballard B, Rockett J (2009). *Restraint and Handling for Veterinary Technicians and Assistants*. Delmar Cengage Learning, Clifton Park.

Ballard B, Cheek R (2017). *Exotic Animal Medicine for the Veterinary Technician*, 3rd edition. Wiley-Blackwell, Ames.

Baker WS, Gray GC (2009). A review of published reports regarding zoonotic pathogen infection in veterinarians. *Journal of the American Veterinary Medical Association* 234:1271–1278.

Bassett JM, Thomas J (2013). *McCurnin's Clinical Textbook for Veterinary Technicians*, 8th edition. Elsevier, St. Louis.

Battaglia RA (2006). *Handbook of Livestock Management*, 4th edition. Prentice Hall, Upper Saddle River.

Beaver BV, Hoglund DL (2016). *Efficient Livestock Handling. The Practical Application of Animal Welfare and Behavioral Science*. Academic Press, Waltham.

Broom DM, Fraser AF (2007) Handling, transport and humane control of domestic animals. In: *Domestic Animal Behaviour and Welfare*, 4th edition. Oxford University Press, Oxford, pp. 199–215.

Campbell KL, Campbell JR (2009). *Companion Animals*, 2nd edition. Pearson Education, Upper Saddle River.

Centers for Disease Control and Prevention: *Injury Prevention & Control*. www.cdc.gov/injury

Colville JL, Berryhill DL (2007). *Handbook of Zoonoses: Identification and Prevention*. Mosby, St. Louis.

Crow SE, Walshaw SO, Boyle JE (2009). *Manual of Clinical Procedures in Dogs, Cats, Rabbits, & Rodents*, 3rd edition. Wiley-Blackwell, Ames.

Dary D (1989). *Cowboy Culture: A Saga of Five Centuries*. University Press of Kansas, Lawrence.

Fowler ME (2008). *Restraint and Handling of Wild and Domestic Animals*, 3rd edition. Wiley-Blackwell, Ames.

French D, Tully T (2005). Restraint and handling of animals. In: *Textbook for Veterinary Technicians*, 6th edition. (eds. DM McCurnin, JM Bassert) WB Saunders, Philadelphia.

Gimenez R, Gimenez T, May KA (2008). *Technical Large Animal Emergency Rescue*. Wiley-Blackwell, Hoboken.

Grandin T (2010). *Improving Animal Welfare: A Practical Approach*. CAB International, Cambridge.

Grandin T (2014). *Livestock Handling and Transport*, 4th edition. CAB International, Cambridge.

Grandin T, Deesing M (2008). *Humane Livestock Handling*. Storey Publishing, North Adams.

Grandin T, Johnson C (2005). *Animals in Translation: Using the Mysteries of Autism to Decode Animal Behavior*. Scribner, New York.

Grandin, T, Johnson C (2010). *Animals Make Us Human: Creating the Best Life for Animals*. First Mariner Books, New York.

Herron ME, Shreyer T (2014). The pet-friendly veterinary practice: a guide for practitioners. *Veterinary Clinics North America Small Animal Practice* 44:451–481.

Holtgrew-Bohling K (2016). *Large Animal Clinical Procedures for Veterinary Technicians*, 3rd edition. Elsevier, St. Louis.

Leahy JR, Barrow P (1953). *Restraint of Animals*, 2nd edition. Cornell Campus Book Store, Ithaca.

National Association of State Public Health Veterinarians Animal Contact Compendium Committee (2013). Compendium of Measures to Prevent Disease Associated with Animals in Public Settings. *Journal of the American Veterinary Medical Association* 243:1270–1288.

National Association of State Public Health Veterinarians. *Compendium of Standard Precautions for Zoonotic Disease Prevention in Veterinary Personnel*. http://www.nasphv. org/Documents/VeterinaryStandardPrecautions.pdf, 2015.

National Center for Infectious Diseases. *Healthy Pets Healthy People*. Retrieved from http://www.cdc.gov/healthypets/child.htm, October, 20016.

Pickering LK, Marano N, Bocchini JA, et al. (2008). Exposure to nontraditional pets at home and to animals in public settings: Risks to children. *Pediatrics* 122:876–886.

Romich JA (2008). *Understanding Zoonotic Diseases*. Thompson Delmar Learning, Clifton Park.

Sheldon CC, Sonsthagen T, Topel JA (2006). *Animal Restraint for Veterinary Professionals*. Mosby, St. Louis.

Smith B (1998). *Moving 'Em: A Guide to Low Stress Animal Handling*. The Graziers Hui, Kamuela.

Vanhorn B, Clark RW (2010). *Veterinary Assisting: Fundamentals & Applications*. Delmar Cengage Learning. Clifton Park.

Warren DM (2015). *Small Animal Care & Management*, 4th edition. Delmar Cengage Learning, Clifton Park.

Note: Page numbers in **bold** refer to figures; those in *italic* refer to tables or boxes.